Infection Control in Small Animal Clinical Practice

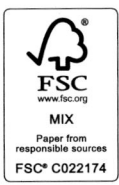

FSC
www.fsc.org
MIX
Paper from
responsible sources
FSC® C022174

Infection Control in Small Animal Clinical Practice

Edited by

Fergus Allerton and Kelly L. Bowlt Blacklock

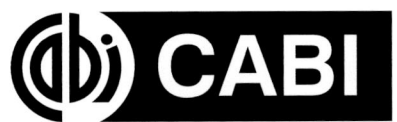

CABI is a trading name of CAB International

CABI
Nosworthy Way
Wallingford
Oxfordshire OX10 8DE
UK

CABI
200 Portland Street
Boston
MA 02114
USA

Tel: +44 (0)1491 832111
Fax: +44 (0)1491 833508
E-mail: info@cabi.org
Website: www.cabi.org

T: +1 (617)682-9015
E-mail: cabi-nao@cabi.org

The views expressed in this publication are those of the author(s) and do not necessarily represent those of, and should not be attributed to, CAB International (CABI). Any images, figures and tables not otherwise attributed are the author(s)' own. References to internet websites (URLs) were accurate at the time of writing. CAB International and, where different, the copyright owner shall not be liable for technical or other errors or omissions contained herein. The information is supplied without obligation and on the understanding that any person who acts upon it, or otherwise changes their position in reliance thereon, does so entirely at their own risk. Information supplied is neither intended nor implied to be a substitute for professional advice. The reader/user accepts all risks and responsibility for losses, damages, costs and other consequences resulting directly or indirectly from using this information.

CABI's Terms and Conditions, including its full disclaimer, may be found at https://www.cabi.org/terms-and-conditions/.

A catalogue record for this book is available from the British Library, London, UK.

ISBN-13: 9781789244953 (paperback)
        9781789244960 (ePDF)
        9781789244977 (ePub)

DOI: 10.1079/9781789244977.0000

Commissioning Editor: Alexandra Lainsbury
Editorial Assistant: Lauren Davies
Production Editor: James Bishop

Typeset by Exeter Premedia Services Pvt Ltd, Chennai, India
Printed and bound in the UK by Severn, Gloucester

Contents

Contributors

Fergus Allerton, BSc, BVSc, CertSAM, DipECVIM-CA, MRCVS; Willows Veterinary Centre & Referral Service, Highlands Road, Shirley, Solihull, B90 4NH, UK. E-mail: fergus.allerton@willows.uk.net

Lindsey Ashburner, VN, VTS; Royal (Dick) School of Veterinary Studies, University of Edinburgh, Roslin, UK. E-mail: Lindsey.Ashburner@ed.ac.uk

Jocelyn Bisson, MA, VETMB, DIPECVIM-CA(ONC); Royal (Dick) School of Veterinary Studies, University of Edinburgh, Roslin, UK. E-mail: Jocelyn.bisson@ed.ac.uk

Kelly L. Bowlt Blacklock, BVM&S, DipECVS, PGCert, PhD, SFHEA, FRCVS; Royal (Dick) School of Veterinary Studies, University of Edinburgh, Roslin, UK. E-mail: Kelly.blacklock@ed.ac.uk

Craig R. Breheny, BVM&S, DipECVIM-CA, SFHEA, MRCVS; Royal (Dick) School of Veterinary Studies, University of Edinburgh, Roslin, UK. E-mail: cbreheny@ed.ac.uk

Brandy A. Burgess, DVM, MSc, PhD, DACVIM (LA), DACVPM; Associate Professor, College of Veterinary Medicine, University of Georgia, 501 D. W. Brooks Drive, Athens, Georgia 30602, USA. E-mail: Brandy.Burgess@uga.edu

Rungtip Chuanchuen, PhD; Head, Research Unit in Microbial Food Safety and Antimicrobial Resistance, Faculty of Veterinary Science, Chulalongkorn University, Pathum Wan, Bangkok 10330, Thailand. E-mail: chuanchuen.r@gmail.com

Caitlin Forbes, RVN; Vets Now, 123–145 North Street, Glasgow, UK. E-mail: caitlin.forbes@vets-now.com

Sian-Marie Frosini, BVetMed, PhD, MRCVS; Royal Veterinary College, University of London, London, UK. E-mail: sfrosini@rvc.ac.uk

Andrew Gardiner, BVM&S, Cert SAS, MSc, PhD, MRCVS; Royal (Dick) School of Veterinary Studies, University of Edinburgh, Roslin, UK. E-mail: Andrew.Gardiner@ed.ac.uk

Owen Glenn, Royal (Dick) School of Veterinary Studies, University of Edinburgh, Roslin, UK. E-mail: Owen.Glenn@ed.ac.uk

Martyna Godniak, RVN; Royal (Dick) School of Veterinary Studies, University of Edinburgh, Roslin, UK.

Emily Gorman, RVN, VTS; Royal (Dick) School of Veterinary Studies, University of Edinburgh, Roslin, UK.

Eleanor Haskey, BSc, RVN, VTS(ECC), PGCERT, FHEA, VPAC A1; Emergency and Critical Care Nurse, The Royal Veterinary College, Hawkshead Lane, Brookmans Park, Hatfield, AL9 7TA, UK. E-mail: ehaskey@rvc.ac.uk

Rosanne Jepson, BVSc, MVetMed, PhD, DipACVIM, DipECVIM, FHEA, MRCVS; Royal Veterinary College, University of London, London, UK. E-mail: rjepson@rvc.ac.uk

Thawanrut Kiatyingangsulee, BSc, PhD; Senior Professional Veterinarian, National Institute of Animal Health, 50/2 Phahonyothin Rd, Lat Yao, Chatuchak, Bangkok 10900, Thailand. E-mail: tawanrut@hotmail.com

Steven Murphy, Dip AVN (Small Animal), Dip HE CVN, RVN; Southern Counties Veterinary Specialists, Unit 6, Forest Corner Farm, Hangersley, Ringwood, UK. E-mail: ste.murphy1988@gmail.com

Tim Nuttall, BSc, BVSc, CertVD, PhD, CBiol, MSB, MRCVS; Royal (Dick) School of Veterinary Studies, University of Edinburgh, Roslin, Edinburgh, UK. E-mail: Tim.Nuttall@ed.ac.uk

Lucas Pantaleon, DVM, MS, DACVIM, MBA; Veterinary Advisor at DVM One Health, Versailles, Kentucky, USA. E-mail: lucaspantaleon@gmail.com

Kathryn Pratschke, MVB, MVM, MScClinOnc, CertSAS, DiplECVS, FRCVS; Royal (Dick) School of Veterinary Studies, University of Edinburgh, Roslin, UK. E-mail: Kathryn.Pratschke@ed.ac.uk

Alan D. Radford, BSc, BVSc, PhD, MRCVS; University of Liverpool, Liverpool, L69 3BX, UK. E-mail: A.D.Radford@liverpool.ac.uk

Tom Reilly, RVN, DipAVN(SA), DipHE, CertVNECC; Head of Clinical Support Services, Willows Veterinary Centre and Referral Service, Highlands Road, Shirley, Solihull, B90 4NH, UK. E-mail: tom.reilly@willows.uk.net

Mellora Sharman, BVSc, MVM, PGradCert, PhD, FANZCVS, DECVIM-CA, FHEA, MRCVS; VetCT, Broers Building, 21 JJ Thomson Avenue, Cambridge, CB3 0FA, UK. E-mail: mellora.sharman@vet-ct.com

Helen Silver-MacMahon, MSc, PSCHF, CERT VNECC, DIPAVN (SURG), CERT SAN, RVN; Research and Development Director, VetLed, Sunnybank Cottage, Bullocks Farm Lane, Wheeler End, High Wycombe, HP14 3NQ, UK. E-mail: helen@vetled.co.uk

Shabbir Simjee, BSc, MSc, PhD; Chief Medical Officer, Elanco Animal Health, Form 2, Bartley Way, Bartley Wood Business Park, Hook, RG27 9XA, UK. E-mail: SHABBIR.SIMJEE@elancoah.com

David A. Singleton, BVSc, MSc, PhD, MRCVS; University of Liverpool, Liverpool, L69 3BX, UK. E-mail: D.A.Singleton@liverpool.ac.uk

Katie Smyth, RVN; Vets Now, 123–145 North Street, Glasgow, UK. E-mail: katie.smyth@vets-now.com

Faye Swinbourne, BVM&S, MVETMED, DIPECVS, MRCVS; Lumbry Park Veterinary Specialists, Selborne Road, Alton, GU34 3HL, Hampshire, UK. E-mail: faye.swinbourne@cvsvets.com

Denis Verwilghen, DVM, MSc, PhD, DES, Dipl ECVS, Dipl EVDC(eq); University of Sydney, Camperdown, NSW 2006, Australia. E-mail: denis.verwilghen@sydney.edu.au

Martin L. Whitehead, BSc, PhD, BVSc, CertSAM, MRCVS; Chipping Norton Veterinary Hospital, Banbury Road, Chipping Norton, Oxon, OX7 5SY, UK. E-mail: martincnvets@gmail.com.

Nicola J. Williams, BSc, PhD; University of Liverpool, Liverpool, L69 3BX, UK. E-mail: Njwillms@liverpool.ac.uk

Alison Young, Royal Veterinary College, Hawkshead Lane, North Mymms, Hertfordshire, AL9 7TA, UK. E-mail: ayoung@RVC.AC.UK

Acknowledgements

A very sincere thanks to all our friends and colleagues who have worked with us on this book over 2 long years. Our journey together has been impacted by the personal and professional challenges associated with the COVID-19 pandemic, which has brought the need for improved infection control into sharp focus. However, we have been buoyed by the arrival of new family members and the constant opportunities to learn from each other.

With regard to infection control, the call to action has never been stronger: we hope this book will highlight the importance of this call and provide some useful ideas for readers to easily implement in every veterinary workplace. The future and well-being of our families tomorrow will be enormously impacted on how well we answer this call today.

Fergus Allerton and Kelly L. Bowlt Blacklock

Dedication

To Beatrix, Ernest, Clémentine, Eléonore, Constance and Eugénie

Section 1: Introduction to Infection Prevention and Control

The word 'infection' evokes images of 19th-century surgeons, operating bare-handed in unwashed frock coats. Up to 60–90% of their more unfortunate patients would develop hospital gangrene following procedures such as limb amputation, writhing in agony for days until death mercifully intervened. With the advent of safe anaesthesia, new antibiotics and aseptic techniques, the future looked bright for medicine and we became complacent, assuming we would be safe from the horrors of the past. However, reality paints a different picture. Infection prevention and control in healthcare is more vital today than it has ever been to protect not only the patient but also the caregiver. For example, in 2016/2017, there were an estimated 834,000 healthcare-associated infections in National Health Service (NHS) hospitals in England alone, accounting for 28,500 patient deaths, costing the NHS £2.7 billion, and resulting in 79,700 days of absenteeism among front-line healthcare workers (Guest *et al.*, 2020).

The philosopher, George Santayana said, 'Those who cannot remember the past are condemned to repeat it.' Therefore, the following chapters aim to illustrate the history and epidemiology of infection control. In the age of increasing antimicrobial resistance, the lessons from the past about practices and attitudes have never been more important for a safe future.

Reference

Guest, J.F., Keating, T., Gould, D. and Wigglesworth, N. (2020) Modelling the annual NHS costs and outcomes attributable to healthcare-associated infections in England. *BMJ Open* 10: e033367.

1 Historical Perspective

ANDREW GARDINER*

Royal (Dick) School of Veterinary Studies, University of Edinburgh, Roslin, UK

1.1 Introduction

In the last quarter of the 19th century, the veterinary control of infection was central to the development of germ theories of disease. In *Spreading Germs: Disease Theories and Medical Practice in Britain 1865–1900*, a comprehensive history that makes frequent reference to veterinary medicine, Michael Worboys writes:

> In most historical accounts of the germ theory of disease, the 'Golden Age of Bacteriology' dawned in Germany in 1876 when Koch showed that a specific bacillus was the necessary cause of anthrax, also known as splenic fever. Immunology, Jenner apart, is said to have begun four years later in France, when Pasteur produced a protective vaccine by attenuating the bacillus of chicken cholera. Research on contagious animal diseases was, therefore, the source of key moments in the history of germ ideas and practices. This pattern continued in virology when in 1898 the first pathogenic animal virus identified was that of foot-and-mouth disease.
>
> (Worboys, 2000, p. 43)

According to McGrew (1985, p. 35), germ theory was 'probably the most important single concept in the history of modern medicine'. Today, Wikipedia describes it somewhat elliptically as 'the currently accepted scientific theory for many diseases' (Wikipedia, 2022). Worboys argued that there was no single germ theory. Instead, there were a number, sometimes overlapping and merging, sometimes competing, often contingent, and all informing contemporary attitudes to infection and its spread within countries, cities, farms, hospitals, and bodies. In light of the recent COVID-19 viral pandemic, this conclusion seems especially apt.

Germ theories dictate germ control practices in the clinic and elsewhere, a major concern of this book. Subsequent chapters focus on companion animals, but in order to consider infection control in historical perspective, we must look beyond dogs and cats. It is true that some small animal vets were advocating advanced measures of infection control well before what is usually considered the main rise of small animal practice in the mid-20th century, and that a famous textbook of small animal surgery, first published in 1900, promoted methods akin to those in human surgical practice (Hobday, 1900). Nevertheless, our story begins earlier, and with infection not in the bodies of individual dogs and cats, but in the collective body of the livestock herd in relation to a major veterinary disease that John Simon, Medical Officer of the Privy Council in 1874, stated was 'the start of everything' in relation to germs, communicable diseases and laboratory research in medicine (Worboys, 2000).

1.2 Germ Theory Meets Veterinary Practice

In 1865, cattle plague became rampant in Britain as part of a rapidly worsening European epizootic. The following January, a National Prayer Day was held in the hopes of eliciting divine intervention. Cattle plague had come and gone throughout history, always leaving economic ruin in its wake. Arguments concerning the cause of these periodic outbreaks, and especially this latest colossal one, went to the heart of 19th-century debate on the cause and control of infection. Some believed that disease always arose through proximity to sick individuals. Large outbreaks might occur when healthy individuals were simultaneously infected or when spread was especially rapid. Others believed that diseases like cattle plague and human cholera emerged spontaneously, perhaps as a result of local

*Andrew.Gardiner@ed.ac.uk

© CAB International 2023. *Infection Control in Small Animal Clinical Practice* (eds F. Allerton and K.L. Bowlt Blacklock)
DOI: 10.1079/9781789244977.0001

atmospheric conditions, poor drainage or unsanitary surroundings. General conditions, such as sudden changes in weather, might explain multiple outbreaks at the same time in different locations, a phenomenon that seemed to run counter to ideas of contiguous spread. This theory of 'spontaneous generation' – the idea that new life forms emerged *de novo* given the right conditions – also offered an answer to a question that had challenged medical science: if a spreading disease never arose spontaneously, where had the first case come from? By 1866, combination theories held wider currency: a disease might arise spontaneously and then propagate contagiously, for example. Different theories and emphases split the medical and veterinary communities, and in 1862 contributed to the formation of Glasgow Veterinary School when James McCall (a contagionist) fell into dispute with his Edinburgh employer William Dick (who favoured generation). At any rate, as the latest devastating outbreak of cattle plague took hold, veterinarians found themselves at the centre of an argument about infection in animal bodies and how best to deal with it. It was an argument that had economic and political dimensions as well as medical and scientific ones, and one that would link theory to practice in some aspects of veterinary infection control but not others.

Cattle plague was eventually brought under control by a policy of quarantines and slaughter. It was a controversial policy, condemned as barbaric, inhumane and unscientific by critics, but it was supported by several Royal Commissions. Farmers and those in the meat trade, initially opposed to mass slaughter, were won over by the promise of compensation. More broadly, the success of 'stamping out' proved that epidemic disease (whether animal or human) was contagious. The theory of spontaneous generation, at least the 'pure' variant of something arising *de novo*, had been dealt a serious blow by a large-scale epidemiological experiment worked out in real time.

There was success, too, for the emerging veterinary profession, who policed and implemented the draconian new controls, thereby establishing a precedent for livestock epizootics that persists to this day, albeit with ongoing controversy – witness the response to the 2001 foot-and-mouth cull (10 million animals killed, most of them healthy) and to the recent playing out of infection-control policy at an individual level in the case of Geronimo the alpaca, culled by the State because of a positive result in a disputed tuberculin test. At post-mortem, Geronimo proved negative for TB (Ambrose, 2021; Humphries, 2021).

Why is cattle plague relevant to infection control in small animals? The key issue is about infections in bodies, whether that is the collective body of the livestock herd/flock or the body of an individual animal. A theory of germs, and the germ practices deriving from this, must account for both.

1.2.1 Lister and 'something in the air'

Around the time of the great cattle plague, in the mid-1860s, Louis Pasteur conducted a series of laboratory experiments to show that the decomposition of purified fluids could be prevented if they were protected from air. Pasteur's theory assumed *panspermism* – the presence in the air of minute living organisms – and was designed to disprove spontaneous generation. Pasteur's opponents, especially the scientist Félix-Archimède Pouchet, argued that such living organisms were not the cause but the result of decomposition and that the same decomposition could take place in the absence of any contamination. Pasteur used pure fluids, meticulously clean and sealed flasks, and careful observation, but the argument dragged on. For an interesting review of the Pasteur–Pouchet controversy that links the episode to the state of experimental science at this time, see Roll-Hansen (2018). Pasteur's ideas informed British surgeon Joseph Lister, who applied them to the context of surgery and wounds (Fig. 1.1). Lister delivered his famous paper 'On the Antiseptic Principle in the Practice of Surgery' to the British Medical Association in 1867. The paper contributed to debate on the cause of wound infections and sepsis (sepsis at this time meaning not systemic bacteraemia but local wound infection or putrefaction). Many practising surgeons believed that sepsis was caused by chemical (not biological) means: septic poisons arose from tissue degradation and could spread locally, deepening the wound infection. If living organisms were involved, it was because they were generated within the putrefying wound; they were not the cause of it. Lister's ideas ran counter to this, claiming infection originated outwith the body. One consequence, which aligned with Pasteur's sealed flask experiment, was that the healthy 'sealed' body, or the carefully protected wound, was germ free. If infection took hold after surgery, it was the surgeon's (or hospital's) fault.

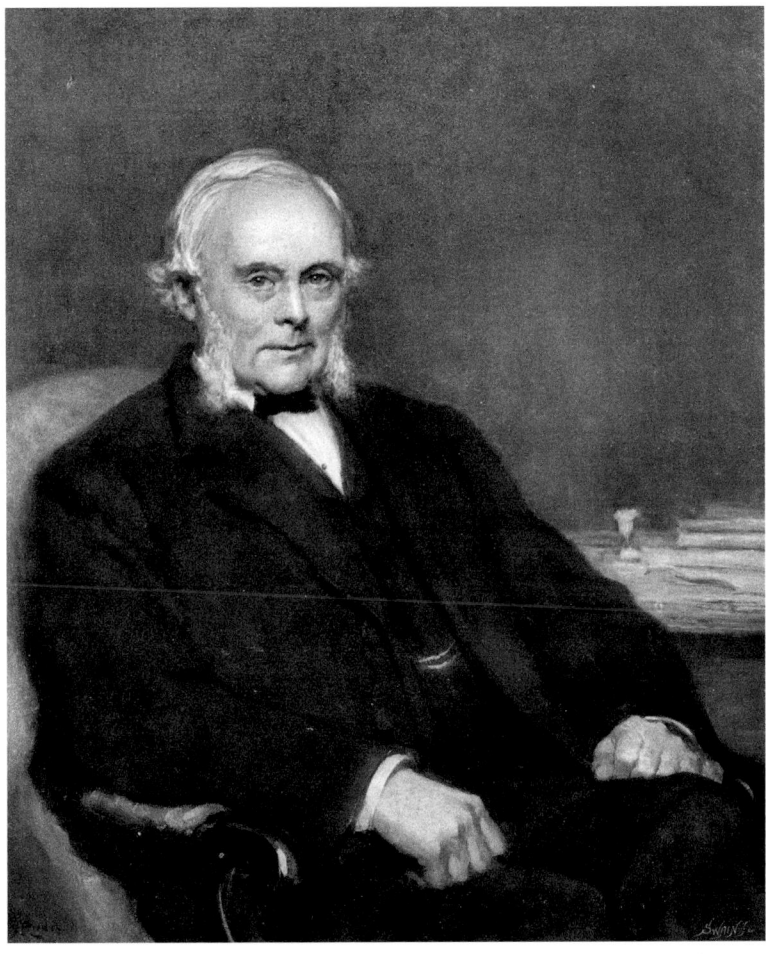

Fig. 1.1. Joseph Lister (1827–1912). Credit: Wellcome Collection. Attribution 4.0 International (CC BY 4.0).

The most iconic aspect of Listerism, often seen in historical images, was the carbolic spray designed to create an antiseptic environment in the vicinity of the surgical wound.

Surgeons of this period favoured empirical methods that worked in their operating theatres and wards, and Lister was often challenged when he linked his ideas to controversial germ theories and panspermism. Nevertheless, it would be wrong to portray Lister's antiseptic surgery as revolutionary; rather, it was part of a gradual process of change as theory and practice interacted with pre-existing ideas on the origin and propagation of infection. Some of Lister's ideas – the use of carbolic acid, for example – were not new. His experiments, like Pasteur's, often involved flasks and fermentation rather than the animal experiments favoured by microbiologists of the period (and vigorously criticized by anti-vivisectionists). This may have led to his work being viewed as abstract and theoretical, more like chemistry than biology. Lister himself came to emphasize techniques and theatre practices over theoretical justifications, which helped give his methods wider currency among pragmatic surgeons, who sometimes used what might be termed 'Lister-lite', i.e. they picked certain elements of Lister's techniques and worked them into their own protocols. There is intriguing evidence that Lister may have taught veterinary students in Edinburgh. A revision to an accounts ledger of the Dick Veterinary College, dated 21 January 1874, shows that a fee due from Lister for a visit

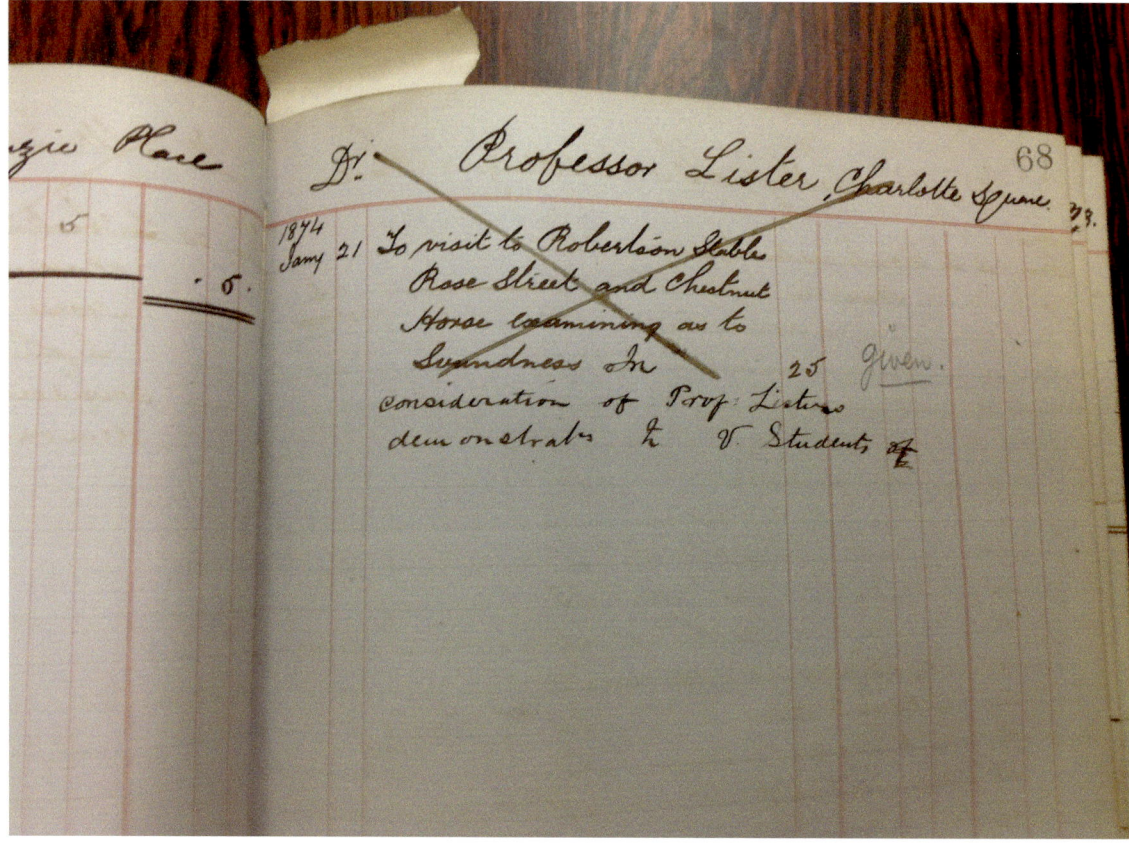

Fig. 1.2. Veterinary ledger entry from 1847 waiving the fee for a soundness examination on Lister's horse in recognition of a demonstration given to veterinary students. Credit: Used with permission from the Centre for Research Collections, University of Edinburgh, Edinburgh, UK.

to Robertson Stables, Rose Street, 'and examining Chestnut Horse as to soundness' was cancelled 'In consideration of Prof Lister's demonstration to V. Students' (Fig. 1.2). Exactly what was Lister demonstrating? He was not publishing widely at this time, but the following year wrote a series of articles for *The Lancet* on improvements in his antiseptic techniques. Perhaps the veterinary students got a preview of this material? If so, it is interesting in the light of Worboys' account of antiseptic surgery in veterinary medicine ten years later:

> The most famous of all germ practices – antiseptic surgery – found no significant place in veterinary surgery. Wounds on large animals only very rarely became septic, despite being dirty and uncovered, while in surgery itself, as late as 1884, the main problems were said to be: tethering, not losing instruments, and finding a soft place for the animal to lie, such as 'a dung-heap covered in straw'.
>
> (Worboys, 1992)

Worboys is referring to George Fleming's *Textbook of Operative Veterinary Surgery* (1884), a standard reference at the time. It is worthwhile noting that the curricula of veterinary colleges varied widely in the 19th century. Edinburgh retained connections with medical education, and Dick, who died in 1866, had been mentored and supported by the comparative anatomist and surgeon John Barclay (Gardiner, 2007). It is possible that his college may have offered its students some teaching by another famous Edinburgh professor, even if only a one-off demonstration of some new-fangled techniques in infection control.

Andrew Gardiner

1.2.2 'The operation, at first sight, appears to be a terrible business'

The contemporary reader of Captain W. Wallace Kerr's article in the *Veterinary Record* of 10 January 1925, might argue that the operation remained 'a terrible business' at second and subsequent sights, too. In a report titled 'Castration of male and female pigs', Kerr gives an insight into operative veterinary surgery in the first quarter of the 20th century, as well as an indication that the profession was beginning to register the decline of horse transport, a change that would eventually lead to the growth in small animal practice. Kerr begins by noting that the castration of pigs (a term that included the spaying of females) was carried out by lay castrators and viewed as 'dirty work' by the veterinary profession. Castrators toured farm districts performing operations on pigs, calves and colts. Their skills, passed down through generations in the manner of a guild, were in high demand, as up to 1000 pedigree pigs could be kept on farms 'run on the most modern and intensive lines'. Even at sixpence a pig (Kerr's own fee, which exceeded that of the castrators), the operation was economically viable 'as, when one becomes expert, as many as fifty pigs can be operated on in an hour' (Kerr, 1925). For vets, there might also have been the chance, once on large premises, of finding further, more lucrative work.

After outlining the benefits of the procedure in terms of practice economics, Kerr describes the operation in considerable detail, illustrated with photographs. It is this, he warns the reader, that appears 'a terrible business'. The castration of young male pigs without anaesthetic is still routinely performed in Europe (not the UK) using a technique very like Kerr's. What is most alarming to the modern reader is the idea of abdominal surgery (i.e. flank laparotomy) being performed without anaesthesia on female pigs. These considerations apart, and with no wish to prosecute a historical veterinarian in the court of the present, it is Kerr's description of infection control that is relevant to our present concerns. During the procedure, the author recommends that the needle and suture thread is held between the teeth 'or inserted in the left breast of [the surgeon's] operating coat ready for use'. Under 'Observations', Kerr reflects on his operating technique and notes that 'antiseptics and disinfectants have been conspicuous by their absence [...] these have not been used or even suggested'. Referring the reader to specific pages in the most recent edition of Fleming's *Veterinary Surgery*, Kerr considers the precautions 'absolutely impracticable and superfluous'. He goes on:

> Disinfection of styes, yards, etc. have not been done, the operating knife, needle, suturing thread have not been sterilised, the operator's hands have not been antiseptically treated, no antiseptic precautions have been advocated whatsoever. The seat of operation has not been treated before, during or after the operation, with respect. [...] The writer would be more than interested to have the views of the 'antiseptic advocate' on the question, viz.: 'How is the female pig immune in such a high degree to extraneous bacterial infection and contamination in the abdominal cavity and what is the secret of her resistance?'

Is this a historical manifestation of the classic tension between theory and practice, or between elite practice (veterinary schools) and 'real-world' vetting? Kerr is clinically interested in this absence of serious wound infections and even wonders if the peritoneal fluid of the pig is prophylactic against sepsis and could be used to this effect in other species. Of course, there could have been more problems than Kerr was aware of, but if significant numbers of pigs had died from peritonitis, farmers would have neither requested nor paid for such surgeries, whether carried out by veterinarians or lay castrators. We have to consider that wound infection may indeed not have been a significant problem in surgery of this type. Kerr, who also practised with small animals, considered that the same operation carried out in dogs and cats would be met with 'harassing sequelae and fatal results'. He does not seem an inattentive clinician. For spay operations in small animals, he employed general anaesthesia and antiseptic measures, yet still did not achieve the success rates he saw with his pigs. Even assuming that one dead dog might weigh heavier on a veterinary surgeon's mind than several dead pigs, Kerr's report, originally a paper read to the Yorkshire Division of the National Veterinary Medical Association, illustrates that infection control was highly contextual. The author himself remarked, 'The pig generally is treated like one, and in most instances lives in filthy surroundings. Before and after being spayed it can be covered in the said filth, yet survive and not even show the clinical effects of septic poisoning.'

A recent report examined the impact of individual sterile surgical kits on the recovery of neutered street dogs in India (Reece, 2021). In a study benefitting from both high patient numbers and impressive standardization of surgical technique, a switch from using shared to individual surgical packs had no impact on recovery time or complications in operated street dogs. The author quotes the surgeon William Halstead, who believed gentle tissue handling to be as important as asepsis in avoiding post-operative infection, and possibly more so (Imber, 2011), a sentiment echoed by the progressive small animal surgeon William Weipers in the 1930s (see Box 1.3). Reflecting on his results, Reece nevertheless advocates best surgical practice when possible because to do otherwise 'flies in the face of accepted wisdom and professional common sense'. Reece describes a contemporary situation in which evidence from clinical practice seems to trump theory and harks back to the informed empiricism that characterized 19th-century surgeons wrestling with germ theories and their implications. It is interesting currently because of the enthusiastic adoption of evidence-based medicine within veterinary medicine, at least as an aspirational idea, and because evidence-based medicine has been labelled a 'tyranny' by some critics (Bonisteel, 2009; Roitberg, 2012). Historians of medicine might ask: what was medicine based on before if germ theory, the 'most important single concept in the history of modern medicine', was established almost 130 years before the Cochrane organisation (see www.cochrane.org)?

1.3 Infection Control and the Small Animal Clinic

Veterinarians have probably always treated small animals. The first curriculum of William Dick's veterinary school in Edinburgh mentions dogs, and they also featured in the course at London, but in both places dogs were completely eclipsed by the attention given to the horse. Within the wider profession, there was a belief that to specialize in small animals, or even take them seriously, was unmanly. A problem for veterinary historians is the silence not just of dogs and cats but of all animals in the historical record, which has tended to focus on great men and notable institutions rather than ordinary practitioners and their patients. There is an assumption that small animal practice began in earnest around the middle of the 20th century. While this is generally true, it ignores some interesting and

significant activity before this. Recent scholarship provides a more nuanced history of the development of small animal veterinary medicine (Gardiner, 2014; Hipperson, 2017; Skipper, 2020) and reveals considerable diversity in terms of who was treating dogs and cats and how they were going about this. Clearly, more histories of practice are needed, but this is no easy task. Late 19th and early 20th-century veterinarians, like family doctors, had no need to keep extensive clinical notes because most worked single-handedly and remembered their patients personally. It can therefore be difficult to discover what practitioners were actually doing in terms of infection control, which is not anyway the kind of information that would be recorded in patient notes. Contextual reading of day and accounting books, when these survive, might help to an extent; for example, were vets treating lots of post-operative wound infections? Such materials may be found in regional archive collections relating to local businesses. Institutional archives often have more extensive records and can sometimes be useful in discovering what was being taught in veterinary schools. Student notes, a rare commodity, are rich sources. Information can also be garnered from published literature of the period (textbooks, journals, magazines, government reports, memoirs) and, perhaps most precious of all for more recent history, from oral testimony. In its linking of science and sentiment in ways akin to human medicine, small animal practice provides a particularly interesting context for the study of infection control. With large animals, economic value is always a limiting factor in terms of the range of procedures and extent of treatment of complications. Busy horse hospitals existed in larger cities, but nothing specific has yet been written on infection control. Army records for horse treatment in World War I may well be a rich source, but small animals will probably not feature here.

In her paper on Edwardian dog doctors, Alison Skipper describes elite canine veterinary care in early 20th-century London, focusing on a small cadre of canine veterinarians mostly working in the West End (Skipper, 2020). The paper's emphasis is on how this group of early canine practitioners interacted with their wealthy clients, the 'dog fancy' and the wider profession, and the work fills an important gap in the history of small animal veterinary medicine. One of the key actors, Frederick Hobday, can be regarded as an historical pivot figure, linking the profession's

Andrew Gardiner

longstanding focus on equine practice (soon to decline) with its future orientation towards companion animals. Hobday is best remembered for the operation to treat laryngeal paralysis that is named after him. He did not invent the treatment; rather, he refined it from a technique pioneered at Cornell University. However, Hobday was a major figure in surgery generally, and authored an influential small animal textbook that gives us insights not just into elite care (for wealthy dog owners) but also at an urban grassroots level, as Hobday was involved in the 'poor clinic' at the Royal Veterinary College where students treated a great many animals under supervision. This teaching hospital running on charitable lines allowed Hobday access to a large caseload that he used to generate information on best practice.

Hobday's Surgical Diseases of the Dog (the words *'and Cat'* were added later) was first printed in June 1900 and underwent many reprints well into the 1940s, changing editorship after Hobday, knighted for services to surgery and veterinary education, died in 1939. This book, which would have been found on the shelves of practices up and down the country, gives us some interesting insights into infection control in the surgical context across this key period in veterinary history (Fig. 1.3). The non-surgical context in the early 20th century centred around distemper, and Skipper notes that the 'vetting in' process at major dog shows arose from a need to detect and exclude cases of distemper. Biosecurity measures (disinfection of tables, veterinarians washing hands) centred on the threat of this devastating disease. The discussion that follows will focus on surgery and veterinary premises, before moving on to antimicrobial drugs, but an excellent account of distemper and its control is given by Bresalier and Worboys (2014).

1.3.1 'The greatest enemy of the surgeon are micro-organisms'

Invoking both Pasteur and Lister, Hobday discussed antisepsis and asepsis in the first chapter of his book, but acknowledged that asepsis may not be attainable in every circumstance. This was likely to be a significant understatement for most veterinary premises at this time. Drawing on 'careful records taken upon more than a thousand wounds in veterinary patients', probably from the poor clinic in Camden but also including his fashionable private practice in central London, Hobday made the following five-stage recommendation for preparation of the surgical site, which he stated would achieve primary union in more than 90% of surgical cases:

1. The hair is shaved with a razor.
2. The skin is then scrubbed for 2 min with soap, hot water and disinfectant.
3. The skin is scrubbed with ether spirit or soap to remove grease and debris.
4. An antiseptic is then applied. (Hobday lists a number of these but turpentine, used in human surgery, is to be avoided, with iodine tincture or iodized chloroform suitable 'for the majority of operations'.)
5. If possible, the wound site is bandaged over with a pad containing antiseptic for an hour prior to surgery.

Suitable antiseptics listed were carbolic acid, Izal, Lysol, Dettol, corrosive sublimate, boracic acid (useful for corneal wounds), perchloride of mercury and flavine. The physical removal of debris using soap and water is emphasized over disinfectants and antiseptics, reliance on which, Hobday cautioned, could lull practitioners into a false sense of security. He also presented a case history of fatal carbolic acid toxicity in a cat (Box 1.1).

The following year, writing in the *Veterinary Record*, London practitioner E. Lionel Stroud extolled the value of the antiseptic approach outlined by Hobday but cautioned, 'The use of carbolic acid in dogs, and especially toy dogs, cannot be too strongly condemned, toxic symptoms, and sometimes death, frequently ensuing when this antiseptic is applied' (Stroud, 1905).

There were therefore some problems with Listerism in the veterinary clinic, caused by large surface area to volume ratios in small patients. 'It is well to bear in mind that most disinfectants are of small value in the strengths which can be safely employed,' Hobday concluded, emphasizing physical cleaning with soap and water. Even so, pre-surgical immersion of animals in antiseptic or antiparasitic baths was mentioned in some textbooks well into the second half of the 20th century, albeit using safer products. Other pre-operative preparations, aside from Hobday's charming injunction to ensure the patient is 'in reasonable health and spirits and feeling well', included admitting the patient to hospital several days before the operation to allow them to acclimatize, and

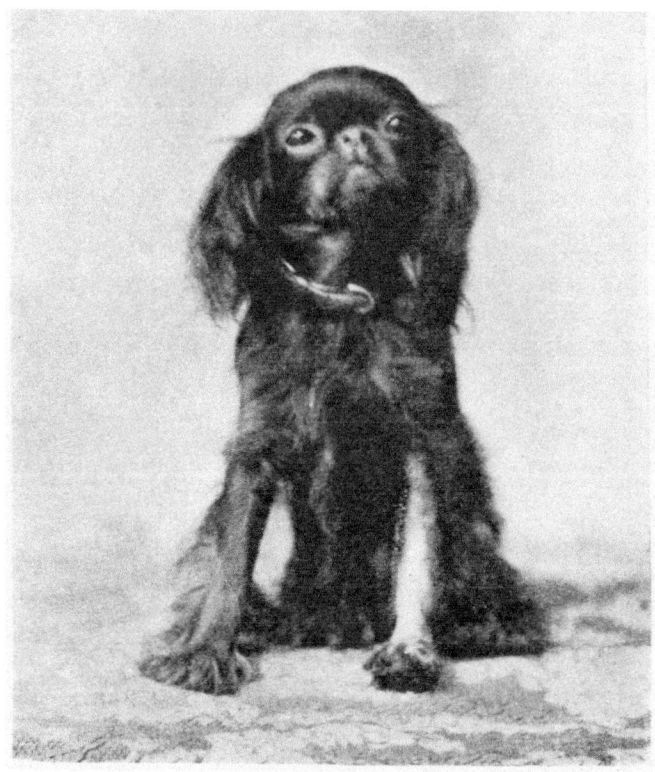

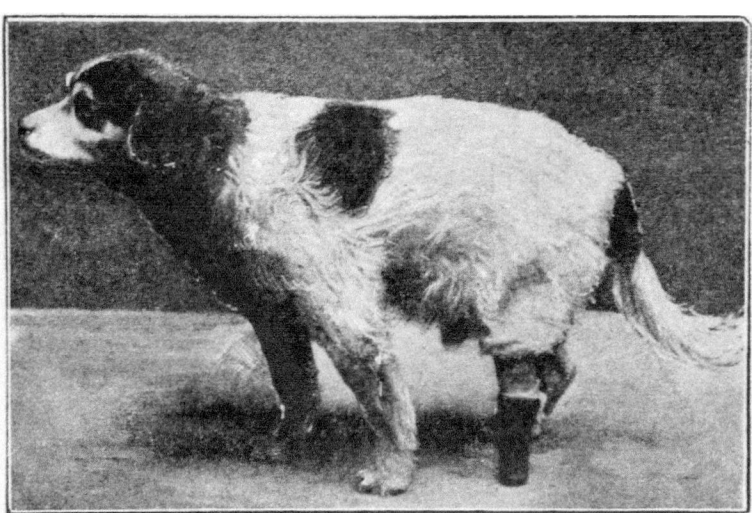

Fig. 1.3. Page from Hobday's *Surgical Diseases of the Dog* showing that limb protheses are not a new idea. The fashion for artificial dog limbs fell away (as the prostheses themselves often did) when it was discovered that dogs coped well with three and sometimes even two legs. False teeth for dogs were another Hobday innovation. He collaborated with a London dentist. Reprinted from Hobday, F. (1900) *Surgical Diseases of the Dog*, with permission from Elsevier.

Andrew Gardiner

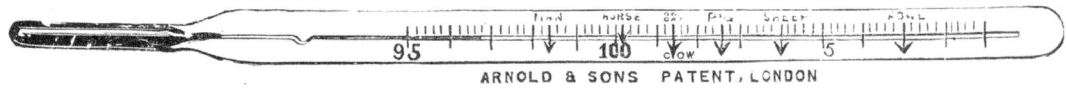

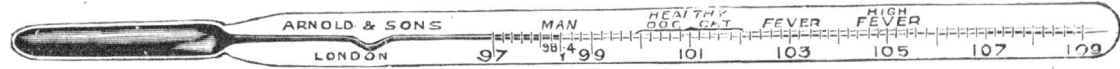

Fig. 1.4. Hobday's thermometers, manufactured by Arnold & Sons. One provides comparative temperatures of different species, including humans, and the other indicates fever ranges in the dog and cat. Reprinted from Hobday, F. (1900) *Surgical Diseases of the Dog*, with permission from Elsevier.

the administration of enemas - procedures lifted straight from human medicine.

Post-operatively, monitoring of the temperature was undertaken to give warning of septic infection, early signs of which included 'general dullness of the patient, loss of appetite, haggard facial expression [pre-empting facial pain scales], a thready or imperceptible pulse, and a rise of temperature'. In an indication that temperature recording was perhaps not undertaken as often then as now, Hobday provided evidence of his own investigations into the normal reference range for dogs and cats. He designed a thermometer, patented by Arnold & Sons, which facilitated easy quantification of fever (Fig. 1.4). He recorded the temperature of over 200 dogs and found the average to be 101.5°F (38.6°C). The average for 41 cats was 101.7°F (38.7°C). Benign variations could be caused by age, condition, temperament and whether the temperature was measured after food, prolonged rest or exercise. There was also some natural diurnal variation. This led Hobday to give the normal reference range

for the dog and cat as 100–102°F (37.8–38.9°C), with fever coming in at 103°F (39.4°C) and high fever at 105°F (40.6°C), although it was noted that some racing greyhounds recorded a temperature of 105–106°F (40.6–41.1°C) straight off the track.

The operating theatre depicted in Hobday's book represented the ideal, i.e. a dedicated, minimally furnished space with tiled walls for easy cleaning (Fig. 1.5). However, only progressive practices would have had such a facility; most operations would take place in less formal surroundings. Attention to detail with instruments and equipment was essential. 'Merely to plunge instruments into an antiseptic solution, as is so frequently done, about a minute before operating is of no value at all,' Hobday warns. Fifteen minutes of immersion in a clean pie dish or an enamelled bowl of antiseptic or at least 3 minutes of boiling in an ordinary saucepan or fish kettle was required, although he adds that Arnolds marketed an instrument sterilizer of convenient size and shape. To do otherwise 'is apt to bring discredit on principles which, when carried

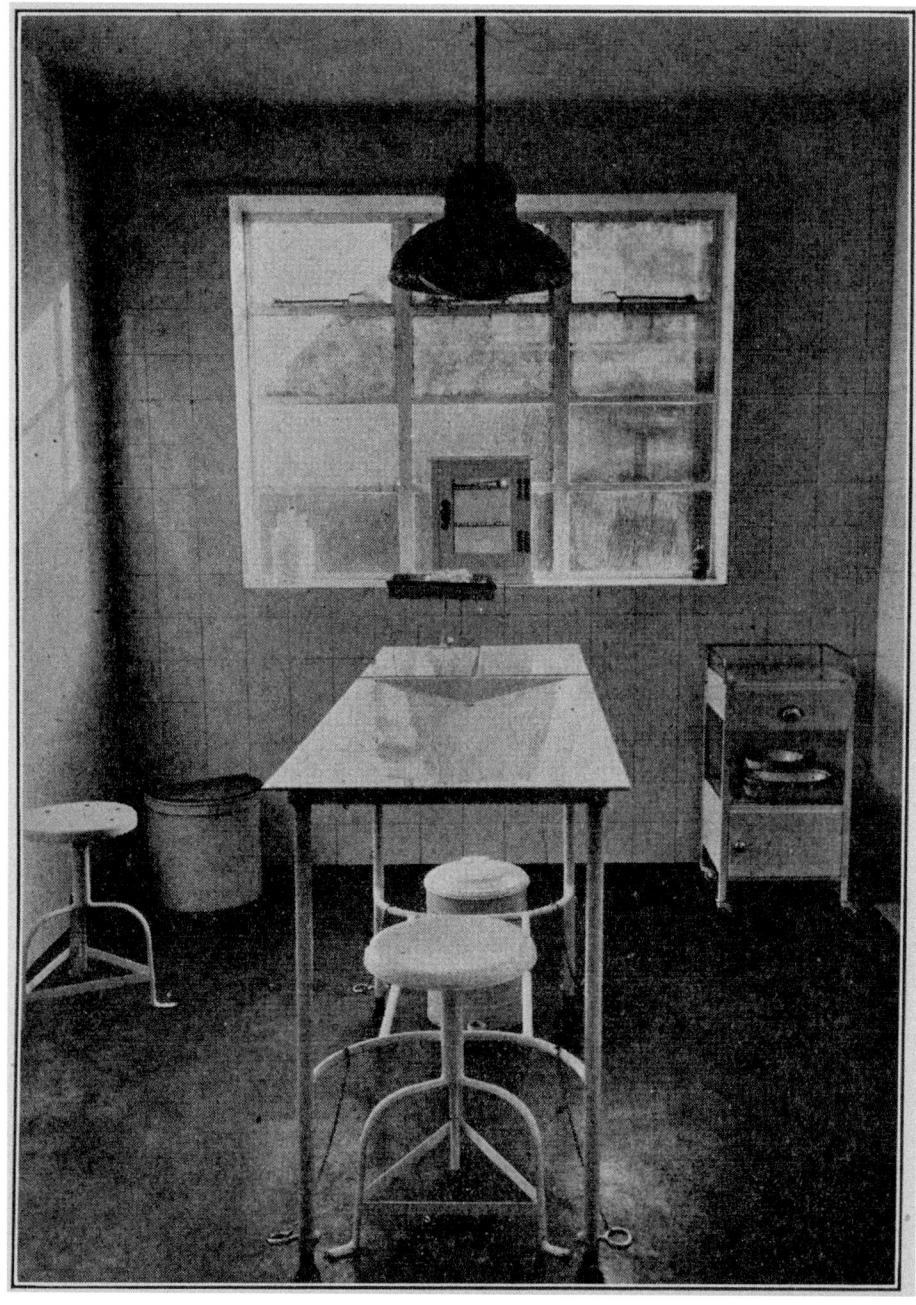

Fig. 1.5. Hobday's operating theatre, as illustrated in *Surgical Diseases of the Dog*. In the first half of the 20th century, most general veterinary practices utilized less formal surroundings. Reprinted from Hobday, F. (1900) *Surgical Diseases of the Dog*, with permission from Elsevier.

Andrew Gardiner

out properly, have been the means of saving many thousands of valuable lives.' For preparation of the surgeon, Hobday said, 'in these days of aseptic and antiseptic surgery, it seems hardly necessary to say that the operator should pay particular attention to the condition of his hands, nails, etc.' Strict adherence to a scrub routine was essential:

1. Scrub hands for 5 min with soap and hot water containing some antiseptic; pay particular attention to the nails using a clean nail brush.
2. Repeat with ether, spirit or ether soap.
3. Hold the hands for some minutes in clean antiseptic solution.

If the surgeon touched anything that was not rendered aseptic, the hands should be disinfected again before proceeding. Any break in the chain of sterilization could ruin an otherwise successful operation. Rubber gloves were deemed essential for abdominal and orthopaedic procedures and, according to Hobday, formed 'a useful adjunct' to the outfit of the operating surgeon. Some of the antiseptics, especially carbolic acid, Lysol and creolin, had adverse effects on the surgeon's skin, and in those situations it was permissible to perform the scrub routine while wearing rubber gloves. There is no mention of gowns, masks or hats, although it is likely that some kind of gown or smock would be used. His position with gloves is especially interesting given that this was by no means universal, even

by the late 1990s. The author first encountered full surgical attire (sterile gown, gloves, mask and hat) in 1997 when working for an animal welfare charity, The Blue Cross. The organization was in possession of a hospital-grade autoclave, which could take large bulky packs. Previous posts in private practice in Scotland and northern England had never featured the full protocol and the author's perception is that surgical gloves, outside veterinary schools, some charities and large hospital-style practices, were the exception rather than the norm.

The transcribed extracts from veterinary oral testimony recorded by Sue Bradley provide a fascinating insight into how asepsis was taught and applied in the 1930s and 1940s (Boxes 1.2 and 1.3). Mary Brancker, the first interviewee here, was taught by both Hobday and another influential surgeon and educator of the time, J.G. Wright. The second, Alistair Clarke, was taught by the small animal specialist William Weipers, who was the Dean of Glasgow Veterinary School from 1969 to 1974.

Clarke's testimony is interesting in relation to Kerr's article on pigs and suggests that significant changes had taken place regarding asepsis on the farm over a 20-year period. In 1925, Kerr seemed committed to the antiseptic approach in dogs and cats while fascinated by the apparent resilience of his pigs to a total lack of asepsis. The apparent rift in technique across species lines (small animal versus farm) was probably narrowed somewhat

---

Box 1.2. Extracts from Mary Brancker interviewed by Sue Bradley, An Oral History of Veterinary Practice, British Library catalogue reference C1519/01/35-36.

Mary Brancker, CBE, FRCVS (and first woman president of the British Veterinary Association) qualified in 1937 from the Royal Veterinary College, where she was taught by J.G. Wright.

SB: You've mentioned Professor Wright. Please can you tell me how you remember him?

MB: [...] He was highly intelligent. He was a very good surgeon. And he was very keen on asepsis, which was a comparatively new idea, so we were all brought up on the fact that you washed your hands and you sterilized your instruments, and you were quick so that you kept the animal under the anaesthetic for as short a time as possible – all these modern things, John George Wright.

[...]

SB: Could you talk a little bit about what he brought to the profession?

MB: What he brought to it? Asepsis. Before that... well, you washed things, but you didn't fuss too much. But with him, you had to boil everything and sterilize it, and if you put it down in the wrong place, you didn't use it again, you took another sterilized instrument. You were very, very careful. Whereas Professor Wooldridge, who ran another clinic at the same college, would lean over an operation he was doing with a cigarette in his mouth. People say the ash is sterilized – whether it is or not, I don't know. But with his fingers that had taken the cigarette in and out of his mouth, he would prod the various bits of the operation and so forth. So there was a difference between the two.

Box 1.3. Extracts from Alistair Clarke Interviewed by Sue Bradley, An Oral History of Veterinary Practice, British Library catalogue reference C1519/02/17.

As a veterinary student in Glasgow from the late 1930s, Clarke saw practice with William Weipers, a leading small animal surgeon and teacher who had a local practice in Queen's Crescent, Glasgow.

SB: Do you remember what you learned when you were with [Weipers]?

AC: I learned surgery. To be gentle. You were dealing with an animal; you weren't dealing with a thing.

[...]

SB: Did he ever wear gloves when he was working with…

AC: No. He never wore gloves. No. You kept your nails short, though. You could if you wanted, but he preferred you not to wear gloves, because you felt the tissue then – you knew what you were doing. Whereas with gloves you didn't feel the tissue you were dealing with. He was a super vet.

[...]

SB: So when you were watching him using his hands, as you've described, can you describe the scene?

AC: You covered the whole body, except for a little bit, with sterile cloths that had been sterilized in … I forget what they call it again, now, the thing they sterilized the cloths [in]. And you put a cloth that way and a cloth that way and a cloth that way, and left just a wee bit hole in the middle. And that's where you did your operation through; you didn't touch any other part of the body unless you had to in the course of the operation. And you learnt to be gentle. He said, 'If you're not gentle, you're bruising tissue, which is leading to sepsis. You've got to be careful.' He was very good, Bill Weipers.

[…]

SB: In his surgery, how would you have made [your hands] sterile?

AC: Well, you could scrub your hands. We had a professor of pathology, and he said the best thing to get your hands sterile is a very high concentration of soap and water, and you do it for a long while, and you scrub, scrub, scrub, scrub, scrub, scrub. And then your hands are as near sterile as you can get them. But if you touch anything else, that's it, finished. You would have to go and start… And you can't afford to waste time when you're doing an operation. Oh, we were taught well.

Clarke qualified in 1947 after his studies had been interrupted by wartime service, and became assistant to Frank Christopher in Newcastle upon Tyne, where his work included farm practice.

AC: They had what they called a 'tea strainer'. You had a big [metal] dish with handles at the end and a lid. You could lift it out - it had holes in the bottom - and strain it off. You could get your sterile instruments [from] there – and you daren't ask for another one [instrument] from one of the men that were helping you, because he had been mucking the byre or something, and his hands weren't by any means clean [laughter], so it was very handy when you had a student with you – he could hand you the things you wanted. But you were dealing with animals in a byre or stable, where you didn't get a lot of contamination with human beings like you would in a hospital, so you can get away with things. […] But you had to be as sterile in your work as you could. But it was very hard to keep your sterility going.

by a spectrum of approaches existing within small animal practice itself. We get a sense of this in Hobday's 'as is so frequently done' comment about inadequate immersion of instruments. 'Kitchen table' small animal surgery will no doubt have been performed by vets in informal or makeshift theatres, with instruments improperly sterilized, especially in those practices where small animals remained marginal. All of this must be seen against a changing context for small animal practice generally, especially in the 1930s: how it was performed, by whom, where, and how the specialty began to be reinvented as a new branch of veterinary

medicine linking science to sentiment and offering opportunities for a profession facing the decline of horse transport. The People's Dispensary for the Sick Animals of the Poor, an organization in almost constant conflict with the veterinary profession during this period was, it can be argued, central to this early development of British small animal practice over 20 years before the formation of the British Small Animal Veterinary Association (Gardiner, 2014). Their premises, especially the Ilford Sanatorium and a large hospital in Paris (the organization was international at this time), provided a kind of 'hospital medicine' for animals. The medical side was run not by a veterinary surgeon but by a doctor, such was the founder's antipathy towards the veterinary profession, which she saw as obstructive to her welfarist aims. This was before the review of the Veterinary Surgeons' Act restricted animal treatment to members of the Royal College of Veterinary Surgeons, so the People's Dispensary could train its own staff at its busy sanatorium, where there were different wards, operating theatres, X-ray departments and even an ambulance service; the only restriction was that those treating animals were not designated 'veterinary surgeons', instead they were 'technical officers'. The charity developed a network of clinics throughout Britain and was expansive, confrontational and immensely successful in terms of fundraising. The practice of asepsis probably varied between flagship hospitals and provincial clinics, but the general feeling within the veterinary profession was that veterinarians had to improve their small animal offering in order to be able to compete with what was, in effect, an alternative veterinary profession. The Christmas 1933 edition of the Veterinary Record editorialized at length on the facilities required for small animal work, even suggesting that providing 'imposing' surroundings was a moral duty for the profession (Anon, 1933). Infection control would indeed be recast as a moral issue, but not until the second half of the 20th century, when a veterinary patient interest group took up the issue of the facilities, equipment and procedures needed to ensure adequate asepsis in the face of multi-resistant bacterial infections. Before that, it had seemed, as if pharmacology would solve everything through the advent of miraculous new drugs.

1.4 Antimicrobials

There have been two recent reviews of the history of antimicrobial use in veterinary medicine (Prescott, 2017; Lees *et al.*, 2021). Space limitation restricts us to a brief synopsis here, and the reader is referred to these comprehensive source papers for more detail. There is relatively little focus on small animals in either paper. An abbreviated timeline, adapted from Prescott (2017), is presented in Table 1.1, and runs from the pre-antibiotic 'antiseptic' era to the current 'stewardship' era.

Sulphanilamide was first used in veterinary medicine in 1937 when it was given to treat bovine mastitis (Allott, 1937). The compound had been discovered around 30 years before by the Austrian chemist Paul Josef Jakob Gelmo. Marketed as Prontosil by Bayer, it found early adoption in veterinary medicine because it was not patented and was therefore cheap. Some infections previously thought incurable could now be treated effectively. After World War II came the 'wonder drug' era, with most new compounds being derived from fungi. At one point in the history of microbiology, it was thought there would eventually be 'a microbe for every disease'. The 1940s and 1950s generated similar optimism around antimicrobials, with many new compounds appearing. In his *Veterinary Therapeutics*, Boddie (1952) mentions the large number of sulfonamides then available but notes that 'clinical experience has led to the discarding of many of these and the number in regular use in veterinary therapeutics is, fortunately, quite small.' On antibiotics, he lists penicillin, streptomycin, chloromycetin, aureomycin and terramycin, although the last three were difficult to obtain.

A feature of antibiotics is that they are all drawn from a small range of compounds. As Table 1.1 shows, resistance to these drugs actually began to emerge relatively quickly (i.e., by the 1960s). The same drugs were used in humans and animals, which brought the two medicines into conflict. There was early adoption of antibiotics as growth promoters in livestock agriculture – an effect discovered accidentally when pigs and poultry fed waste material from antibiotic manufacture showed rapid weight gain. This subtherapeutic use of antibiotics would prove controversial in the years ahead, although a review in 2004 showed that less than 4% of human resistance problems were attributable to farm-animal sources (Bywater, 2004). Prescott (2017) pointed out that, historically, the concept of using antibiotics to promote growth was not restricted to veterinary medicine. Until the 1950s, infants who were not thriving were given low doses of tetracyclines for prolonged periods to promote weight gain. This 'growth-promoting' treatment was phased out only when it was realized that tetracyclines discoloured tooth enamel (as they do in young animals). Controversy over residues and resistance continued and emerged more forcefully in the 1970s and 1980s following the publication of the Swann Report in 1969, the first large-scale enquiry into antibiotic resistance. The report was wide-ranging and made a number of recommendations, including veterinary prescription for certain drugs and restrictions on which drugs could be

Table 1.1. Antimicrobial timeline: a broad overview by decade. Reproduced and modified from Prescott (2017) with permission.

Decade	Phase	Events/drug discovery
Pre-1935	Antiseptic	Discovery (not clinical use) of *sulfanilamide* (1908) and *penicillin* (1928)
1936–1940	Sulfonamide	First sulfa drug use in veterinary medicine (1937)
1940s	'Wonder drug'	Rapid drug development for treating war wounds; most drugs developed from fungi; initial military use only; penicillin and streptomycin available for animals from 1950 *Bacitracin, chloramphenicol, neomycin, polymyxin, streptogramins, tetracyclines, penicillin and streptomycin*
1950s	'Wonder drug'	Tetracyclines and chloramphenicol used widely (and empirically) in animals; intramammary use in dairy cows; antibiotics used as growth promoters begins in USA *Erythromycin, nitrofurans, aminoglycosides, vancomycin, and virginiamycin*
1960s	Early resistance	Plasmid-based resistance elucidated; new drugs begin to be developed to counter resistance; Swann Committee, 1969 following *Salmonella* transmission from calves to humans led to restrictions on veterinary prescribing in UK; MRSA emerges in humans (Jevons, 1961) *Methicillin and other penicillinase-resistant penicillins, spiramycin, gentamicin, cephalothin (first cephalosporin), ampicillin, amikacin, tylosin and flavomycin*
1970s	Resistance	New drugs successful in countering resistance; FDA alert regarding subtherapeutic penicillins in animal feeds (1972) – no action taken; chloramphenicol banned in food animals due to possible idiosyncratic blood dyscrasias (including aplastic anaemia) resulting from consumption of tissue residues; resistant *Salmonella* spreads from calves to humans *Trimethoprim-potentiated sulfonamides, carbenicillin, second-generation cephalosporins and β-lactamase inhibitors added to aminopenicillins*
1980s	Resistance growing	Detailed studies on drug utilization and distribution commence in food animals; bans and moratoria on certain drugs in food animals because of residues *Third-generation cephalosporins, quinolones, fluoroquinolones*
1990s	Resistance crisis	Further restrictions on veterinary uses and enhancement of monitoring activities; banning of certain growth promoters *Azithromycin, tilmicosin, tiamulin, florfenicol*
2000s	Resistance crisis +	Emphasis on rational and prudent drug use and emerging ideas of antibiotic stewardship; WHO global strategy to contain resistance with implications for veterinary use in food animals; MRSA and MRSP emerge in dogs
2010s	Global action	National plans and international cooperations developed to cope with crisis; need to coordinate across human/animal health lines; rising consumer awareness; United Nations statement on coordinated global action required; G7 adds resistance to its agenda; resistance labelled 'a threat to humanity' *Avilamycin developed for animals only (broiler chickens). Had previously been marketed in Europe and other countries in the 1990s.*
2017 onwards	Stewardship	Search to develop animal-only antibiotics, alternatives to antibiotics and other innovations; necessity for implementation of codes of practice as part of response to global resistance crisis; a One Health agenda promoted to avoid unhelpful agriculture versus medicine conflicts around public health

FDA, US Food and Drug Administration; MRSA, methicillin-resistant *Staphylococcus aureus*; MRSP, methicillin-resistant *Staphylococcus pseudintermedius*; WHO, World Health Organization;

Andrew Gardiner

used for growth promotion (i.e. not those used in humans). Uptake of the Swann recommendations was patchy in the USA for political and economic reasons, including lobbying by agricultural and pharmaceutical interests, but the report was influential in UK and Europe.

One of the problems highlighted by both Prescott (2017) and Lees *et al.* (2021) was the surprisingly long lag between antibiotic drug discovery and rational dosing based on pharmacokinetics. Studies on the latter only began in the 1980s and were focused on agricultural use. Antibiotics were therefore widely used for a long time (decades) without proper dosage regimens based on science, and it is only very recently that companion animal prescribing has been surveyed with a view to developing protocols on drug choice, dosing and treatment duration (Murphy *et al.*, 2012; Buckland *et al.*, 2016). Freedom in small animal prescribing probably encouraged the routine prophylactic use of antibiotics in surgical patients. The fifth edition of *Canine Surgery*, edited by Archibald (1965), included a chapter on 'Sterile technic' in which the aseptic protocols seem identical to those in human operating theatres. However, veterinary textbooks represented the institutional (veterinary school) environment and were often quite far removed from what was seen in general practice where veterinarians would often be operating in multi-purpose spaces with minimal assistance, not dedicated operating rooms with support staff and large-scale sterilization facilities. It is therefore likely that antibiotics were used to provide aseptic 'cover' in these situations, somewhat analogous to Lister's carbolic spray. Such a practice might now be deprecated, but we should avoid presentist attitudes when considering a period where there was no antibiotic crisis and rumblings of resistance seemed fixable with new drugs. A 'wake-up call' to a potentially serious resistance problem in companion animal practice was first published only in 2007 (Lloyd, 2007, 2012) following the first published plea for stewardship in the veterinary world in 2005 (Morley *et al.*, 2005).

Three years earlier, a Samoyed dog called Bella developed methicillin-resistant *Staphylococcus aureus* (MRSA) infection following cruciate ligament surgery at a London veterinary practice. MRSA was identified in people in 1961 and quickly became a critical public health issue, but this was the first recorded case in a dog, the infection presumably acquired from a human during or after Bella's surgery. Bella was eventually euthanized due to complications. The traumatic experience of nursing her sick dog led Jill Moss to establish what was, in effect, the first veterinary patient interest group. Patient interest groups or associations are common in human medicine, where they are often centred on poorly understood diseases (e.g. chronic fatigue syndrome/myalgic encephalomyelitis) or diseases associated with social stigma (e.g. HIV/ AIDS). Groups lobby for recognition, funding and action, often in the face of hostility and exclusion from professional bodies, who tend to defend monopolies of knowledge from lay 'outsiders' (for an account of interest groups in human medicine, see Wehling *et al.*, 2015). Successful interest groups or patient associations respond by accumulating significant first-hand knowledge, discovering new information and recruiting (or being approached by) sympathetic 'insiders' desirous of change. Jill Moss revealed that she acquired MRSA when nursing her dog, so from the outset there was an important One Health dimension to the campaign, which received considerable media attention in a climate of high anxiety about 'flesh-eating bugs'. Adopting a science-driven message, The Bella Moss Foundation began to exert leverage and gain influence. This required a move from the particular (Bella's individual case) to the general (humans and animals together). In Jill Moss's own words: 'This was the turning point. I focused less on the veterinary practice neglect for Bella, and more on the bigger picture' (Bella Moss Foundation, 2021). Quite quickly, the organization moved from the periphery to the centre and started working with expert bodies, government, industry, patient advocacy groups and concerned individuals. The focus was on hygiene protocols, responsible antibiotic use and education/communication, as well as support for other companion animal owners who had encountered MRSA or other serious infections in their animals. A strong One Health dimension was retained: the Foundation's Honorary Patron was Claire Rayner, President of the Patients' Association and frequent media spokesperson on human health matters. The Bella Moss Foundation is therefore important not only in the context of infection control in companion animal practice but also in terms of patient advocacy within veterinary medicine.

In the broader history of infection control, a refocus on hygiene brings us back to core principles of asepsis in what might (pessimistically) be called the 'post-antibiotic' era or (optimistically) the era of 'responsible antibiotic use and stewardship'. Writing about the mid-1990s, when the extent of the resistance problem began to be fully appreciated, Prescott notes, 'The very serious nature of the crisis led to a re-examination within the human medicine community of all aspects of antimicrobial use and even to the apparent rediscovery of the importance of basic infection-control procedures such as hand-washing' (Prescott, 2017). The same shift has taken place in veterinary medicine.

In an optimistic account written in the 1950s, antibiotics were said to have 'advanced the practice of medicine farther than any other single factor in any of the previous centuries' (Hussar and Holley, 1954). If this sounds uncannily like the quote on germ theory given near the start of this chapter, perhaps it is an example of a maxim usually attributed to Mark Twain: 'History doesn't repeat itself, but it often rhymes' – with the cautionary postscript that grand scientific claims sometimes need revision.

Acknowledgements

I would like to thank Sue Bradley, Centre for Rural Economy, Newcastle University, Newcastle upon Tyne, UK, for help with the oral history extracts; Fiona Brown, Academic Support Librarian, University of Edinburgh, Edinburgh, UK, for the cancelled vet bill for Lister's horse; Brian Mather, Digital Education Unit, Royal (Dick) School of Veterinary Studies, for help with processing historical images from Hobday's book; and Stephen Page, Advanced Veterinary Therapeutics, Australia, for help with the antimicrobial chronology.

References

Allott, A.J. (1937) The treatment of bovine mastitis with sulfanilamide. *Journal of the American Veterinary Medical Association* 91, 588–596.

Ambrose, T. (2021) The unsuccessful fight to save Geronimo the Alpaca: a timeline. *The Guardian,* 31 August 2021. Available at: www.theguardian.com/world/2021/aug/31/the-unsuccessful-fight-to-save-geronimo-the-alpaca-a-timeline%20 (accessed 5 October 2022).

Anon (1933) Small-animal surgery and surgeries. *Veterinary Record* 51, 1387.

Archibald, J. (ed.) (1965) Sterile technic. In: *Canine Surgery: A Text and Reference Work.* American Veterinary Publications, Santa Barbara, California, pp. 95–109.

Bella Moss Foundation (2021) Bella's story. Available at: www.thebellamossfoundation.com/bellas-story (accessed 5 October 2022).

Boddie, G.F. (1952) *Veterinary Therapeutics.* Oliver & Boyd, Edinburgh, UK, pp. 135–146.

Bonisteel, P. (2009) The tyranny of evidence-based medicine. *Canadian Family Physician* 55(10), 979.

Bresalier, M. and Worboys, M. (2014) "Saving the lives of our dogs": the development of canine distemper vaccine in interwar Britain. *British Journal for the History of Science* 47, 305–334. DOI: 10.1017/s0007087413000344.

Buckland, E.L., O'Neill, D., Summers, J., Mateus, A., Church, D. *et al.* (2016) Characterisation of antimicrobial usage in cats and dogs attending UK primary care companion animal veterinary practices. *Veterinary Record* 179(19), 489. DOI: 10.1136/vr.103830.

Bywater, R.J. (2004) Veterinary use of antimicrobials and emergence of resistance in zoonotic and sentinel bacteria in the EU. *Journal of Veterinary Medicine B: Infectious Diseases and Veterinary Public Health* 51, 361–363. DOI: 10.1111/j.1439-0450.2004.00791.x.

Fleming, G. (1884) *A Textbook of Operative Veterinary Surgery.* Baillière, Tindall & Cox, London, pp. 4–8.

Gardiner, A. (2007) Elephants and exclusivity: an episode from the 'pre-Dick' history of veterinary education in Edinburgh. *Veterinary History* 13, 299–309.

Gardiner, A. (2014) The "dangerous" women of animal welfare: how British veterinary medicine went to the dogs. *Social History of Medicine* 27(3), 466–487. DOI: 10.1093/shm/hkt101.

Hipperson, J. (2017) Professional entrepreneurs: women veterinary surgeons as small business owners in interwar Britain. *Social History of Medicine* 31, 122–139.

Hobday, F. (1900) *Hobday's Surgical Diseases of the Dog and Cat,* 1947 interim edition. Baillière, Tindall and Cox, London, pp. 1–13.

Humphries, W. (2021) Geronimo's owner threatens legal action after tests fail to find evidence alpaca had TB. *The Times,* 10 December 2021. Available at: www.thetimes.co.uk/article/destroyed-alpaca-geronimo-did-not-have-tuberculosis-latest-tests-show-khswprjd9 (accessed 5 October 2022).

Hussar, A.E. and Holley, H.W. (1954) *Antibiotics and Antibiotic Therapy.* MacMillan, New York.

Imber, G. (2011) *Genius on the Edge: The Bizarre Double Life of Dr. William Stewart Halsted.* Kaplan Publishing, London.

Jevons, M.P. (1961) 'Celbenin'-resistant Staphylococci. *British Medical Journal* 1(5219), 124–125.

Kerr, W.W. (1925) Castration of male and female pigs. *Veterinary Record* 2, 19–24.

Lees, P., Pelligand, L., Giraud, E. and Toutain, P.-L. (2021) A history of antimicrobial drugs in animals: evolution and revolution. *Journal of Veterinary Pharmacology and Therapeutics* 44(2), 137–171. DOI: 10.1111/jvp.12895.

Lloyd, D.H. (2007) Reservoirs of antimicrobial resistance in pet animals. *Clinical Infectious Diseases* 45, S148–S152. DOI: 10.1086/519254.

Lloyd, D.H. (2012) Multi-resistant *Staphylococcus pseudintermedius*: a wake-up call in our approach to bacterial infection. *The Journal of Small Animal Practice* 53(3), 145–146. DOI: 10.1111/j.1748-5827.2011.01193.x.

McGrew, R.E. (1985) *Encyclopedia of Medical History*. McGraw-Hill, New York. DOI: 10.1007/978-1-349-05429-9.

Morley, P.S., Apley, M.D., Besser, T.E, *et al.* (2005) Antimicrobial drug use in veterinary medicine. *Journal of Veterinary Internal Medicine* 19(4), 617–629. DOI: 10.1111/j.1939-1676.2005.tb02739.x.

Murphy, C.P., Reid-Smith, R.J., Boerlin, P., Weese, J.S., Prescott, J.F. *et al.* (2012) Out-patient antimicrobial drug use in dogs and cats for new disease events from community companion animal practices in Ontario. *Canadian Veterinary Journal* 53(3), 291–298.

Prescott, J.F. (2017) History and current use of antimicrobial drugs in veterinary medicine. *Microbiology Spectrum* 5(6), ARBA–0002. DOI: 10.1128/microbiolspec.ARBA-0002-2017.

Reece, J. (2021) Surgical asepsis and instruments. *Veterinary Times* 51, 4–5.

Roitberg, B. (2012) Tyranny of a "randomized controlled trials." *Surgical Neurology International* 3, 154. DOI: 10.4103/2152-7806.104748.

Roll-Hansen, N. (2018) Revisiting the Pouchet-Pasteur controversy over spontaneous generation: understanding experimental method. *History and Philosophy of the Life Sciences* 40(4), 68. DOI: 10.1007/s40656-018-0229-7.

Skipper, A. (2020) The "dog doctors" of Edwardian London: Elite Canine Veterinary Care in the early twentieth century. *Social History of Medicine* 33(4), 1233–1258. DOI: 10.1093/shm/hkz049.

Stroud, E.L. (1905) A few operations on the generative organs of the bitch. *Veterinary Record* 29 July, 76–79.

Swann Committee (1969) Report of Joint Committee on the Use of Antibiotics in Animal Husbandry and Veterinary Medicine. London: Her Majesty's Stationery Office.

Wehling, P., Wiehöver, W. and Koenen, S. (eds) (2015) *The Public Shaping of Medical Research: Patient Associations, Health Movements and Biomedicine.* Routledge, London.

Wikipedia (2022) Germ theory of disease. Available at: https://en.wikipedia.org/wiki/Germ_theory_of_disease (accessed 5 October 2022).

Worboys, M. (1992) "Killing and curing": veterinarians, medicine and germs in Britain, 1860-1900. *Veterinary History* 7(2), 53–71.

Worboys, M. (2000) Veterinary medicine, the cattle plague and contagion, 1865–1890. In: *Spreading Germs: Disease Theories and Medical Practice in Britain, 1865–1900.* Cambridge University Press, Cambridge, UK, pp. 43–72.

2 Epidemiology of Nosocomial Infections

TIM NUTTALL*

Royal (Dick) School of Veterinary Studies, University of Edinburgh, Roslin, UK

2.1 Introduction

A nosocomial (derived from the Greek *nosokomeion* meaning 'hospital') infection is one that has been acquired in or is associated with a healthcare setting (Stull and Weese, 2015). This implies that the infection was not present or incubating in the patient at admission. Not all infections that occur in healthcare settings are nosocomial – for example, a patient could have been incubating an infection at admission. In addition, a post-admission infection does not necessarily mean that the causative organism was *acquired* in the healthcare setting, only that the setting was *associated* with factors that led to the infection. For example, a staphylococcal surgical-site infection could be due to nosocomial contamination or endogenous colonization from the skin or mucosal microflora. However, it was the surgery that led to the infection.

In human healthcare, the term nosocomial or healthcare-acquired/associated infection (HAI) is preferred over hospital-acquired/associated infection (confusingly also termed HAI) to emphasize that such infections are not restricted to hospitals and can be associated with other clinical or care settings (e.g. primary care clinics, rehabilitation centres, outpatient clinics, nursing homes, diagnostic laboratories etc.). In a veterinary context, nosocomial infections or HAIs can be considered as anything that occurs outside the normal home, community or animal production setting. This could include primary practices, referral hospitals, diagnostic laboratories, physiotherapy facilities, boarding kennels and catteries, zoological collections, rescue centres, and wildlife rescue and rehabilitation centres (Stull and Weese, 2015).

HAIs are a growing concern and a threat to human and veterinary healthcare (Boerlin *et al.*, 2001). They increase the risk of complications, leading to greater morbidity, mortality and costs associated with veterinary care. The consequent damage to reputation can have financial and professional consequences to the veterinary or care centre and their staff. In addition, many HAIs and associated challenges such as antimicrobial resistance (AMR) are common to medical and veterinary healthcare (Ghosh *et al.*, 2011; Walther *et al.*, 2017). It is therefore important to consider HAIs and AMR as one integrated ecosystem that encompasses humans, animals and the environment (Wieler *et al.*, 2011; Gentilini *et al.*, 2018). This holistic One Health-oriented approach will facilitate improvements in care through shared understanding and best practice.

This book is a guide to preventing and managing HAIs in veterinary practice and other care settings. However, a thorough understanding of the most important HAIs and how they occur is necessary before effective infection control policies can be developed and implemented. This chapter will therefore discuss emerging infectious and/or AMR organisms, the sources of infection and the routes of transmission.

2.2 Sources of Infection

The source of infection is anything that allows an infectious disease to contact a susceptible individual, while the reservoir of infection is the natural habitat of the potentially infectious organism. The source and reservoir are the same if the infection is acquired by direct contact. However, the source may be separate from the reservoir with

*Tim.Nuttall@ed.ac.uk

© CAB International 2023. *Infection Control in Small Animal Clinical Practice* (eds F. Allerton and K.L. Bowlt Blacklock)
DOI: 10.1079/9781789244977.0002

Table 2.1. Potential sources of infection. Data from Stull and Weese (2015).

Source of infection		Examples
Natural habitat or reservoir	Environment	Soil- and water-borne organisms, e.g. *Pseudomonas aeruginosa*
	Human	Human-specific pathogens, e.g. *Staphylococcus aureus* (including MRSA)
	Animal	Animal-specific pathogens, e.g. *Staphylococcus pseudintermedius* (including MRSP), *Microsporum canis* and canine parvovirus
Animate	Carrier	Asymptomatic carriage of potential pathogens; this includes transient carriage and persistent colonization
Inanimate	Fomite	Contamination of surfaces and equipment with viable organisms; many organisms can survive in healthcare and other animal-associated environments

MRSA, methicillin-resistant *Staphylococcus aureus*; MRSP, methicillin-resistant *Staphylococcus pseudintermedius*.

Table 2.2. Potential routes of infection. Data from Stull and Weese (2015).

Route of infection	Definition	Examples
Direct contact	Physical contact with an infected or colonized human or animal source or its products	Skin and mucosal surfaces Airborne droplets and aerosols Splashes and aerosols Vomit and diarrhoea Urine Blood Pus Mucus Other body secretions
Indirect contact	The organism can survive outside the host to contaminate animate or inanimate surfaces	Environmental contamination Fomites Surfaces, hand touch sites and equipment Animate mechanical carriage
Common-source/vehicle infections	The organisms are acquired from a common source but do not spread directly or indirectly between animals	Contaminated products Vector-borne disease

indirect exposure via an animate carrier or inanimate fomite. Contact with a potentially infectious organism does not always result in infection or colonization, which depends on the innate and adaptive defences of the individual (Table 2.1).

The terms carrier, carriage and colonization are often used interchangeably. However, they have more specific meanings that are important in infection control:

- A carrier is an asymptomatic or non-clinical animate reservoir of a potentially infectious organism. In veterinary healthcare, this could be a person or another animal.

- Carriage refers to contamination and mechanical carriage without colonization. This is most common on (but not restricted to) the hands. It is transient and the organisms are usually quickly lost outside the healthcare setting.

- Colonization arises when the contaminating organisms are able to establish and reproduce in the person or animal such that they become part of the resident microflora on the skin, at mucosal surfaces, in the gut or elsewhere. This is often long lasting and persists away from the healthcare setting.

Transmissibility and contagion are also terms that are used interchangeably. However, contagion should be used where there is spread of infection following close contact. It follows that while all contagious diseases by definition are transmissible, transmissible diseases need not be contagious between individuals. For example, canine parvovirus is transmissible and highly contagious between dogs. In contrast, methicillin-resistant staphylococcal infections are transmissible to vulnerable patients through direct and indirect contact but would not be considered contagious (i.e. infection requires specific risk factors).

The transmissibility of an infection is determined by the ability of the causative organism to spread from an infected to a susceptible individual. This can be horizontal (i.e. within an exposed population) or vertical (i.e. between succeeding generations). Vertical transmission can involve genetic (rare in nosocomial diseases) or non-genetic (e.g. egg, placental, parturition, milk) mechanisms. The latter are sometimes considered examples of horizontal transmission, reserving a strict genetic definition for vertical transmission.

Transmissibility can vary from very high (e.g. canine parvovirus and dermatophytosis) to very low (e.g. *Mycobacterium leprae*, the cause of leprosy in humans), although this will vary according to expression of virulence factors by the pathogen and the innate defences and immune status of the exposed individual. Some infectious diseases show little to no transmissibility, for example soil- and water-borne organisms such as *Blastomyces*, *Histoplasma*, *Pseudomonas* and *Clostridium* spp.

2.3 Routes of Infection

The route of infection is the way by which the organism colonizes and spreads within clinical settings to allow contact with a susceptible animal. There are many ways that HAIs can spread within clinical and healthcare settings (Table 2.2).

2.3.1 Direct routes of infection

Direct contact transmission

Direct contact with contaminated skin and/or mucosal surfaces is one of the most common and important routes of infection. This can include touch, wounds, bites and intercourse.

Physical separation of patients, hand washing and gloving are all considered essential baseline measures to prevent the spread of infections (Stull and Weese, 2015). Close physical contact (including cuddling and kissing animals) is important in human–animal bonds. This has great benefits for the animals and their owners, including physical and mental health. However, while close physical contact is necessary and unavoidable in routine and clinical care, precautions must be taken to avoid the transmission and spread of potential pathogens. In particular, direct mucosal-to-mucosal contact should be avoided (Naziri *et al.*, 2016).

Airborne aerosols

Airborne transmission is associated with small droplets or aerosols that can contain viable microorganisms (Greene *et al.*, 2012; Stull and Weese, 2015). Droplets rarely travel for more than 1–2 m, although aerosols with particles less than 100 µm in size can travel further. Droplets and aerosols greater than 5 µm rarely remain airborne for more than 60 s, but smaller particles can remain in air currents for much longer and therefore can travel further. Microbes that can survive some degree of desiccation can survive in droplet nuclei, which can travel on dust particles for considerable periods of time and distances. This allows wide dispersal through air currents and ventilation systems. Droplets and aerosols can also contaminate a variety of surfaces resulting in indirect spread via fomites.

Airborne droplets and aerosols are most commonly associated with respiratory infections (e.g. *Mycobacterium tuberculosis*, *Bordetella bronchiseptica*, influenza viruses) and are generated by coughing and sneezing. However, aerosols can also be generated from air conditioning (e.g. *Legionella* spp.), urine (e.g. *Leptospira* spp.), vomit and diarrhoea (e.g. canine parvovirus), clipping, scrubbing and/or bathing the skin (e.g. *Staphylococcus* spp. and dermatophytosis), clinical procedures (e.g. dental treatment, drills and oscillating saws) and cleaning the environment (especially with high-pressure hoses or dry sweeping and brushing).

Methods of control include separation of patients, isolation, building design, air handling and ventilation, and airway protection for patients and staff (Greene *et al.*, 2012; Stull and

Tim Nuttall

Weese, 2015). Cleaning techniques should be assessed for aerosol risks.

Oro-faecal transmission

Contamination from vomit and/or diarrhoea resulting in oro-faecal contamination is the main route of transmission for gastrointestinal infections (Stull and Weese, 2015). This can result in direct exposure or indirect exposure through contamination of surfaces, water and food where the organism can survive in the environment. Splashing, aerosols and/or mechanical carriage facilitate spread beyond the immediate source.

Methods of control include physical separation, containment, scrupulous disposal, effective cleaning and disinfection, protection of food and water supplies, and rigorous hand hygiene.

Urine, blood and other bodily fluids

The main route of transmission with urine, blood and other bodily fluids is through direct contact. However, urine and (to a lesser extent) other fluids can readily spread or form aerosols, resulting in more widespread dispersal and exposure. Urine is easily spread or aerosolized during urination and cleaning, whereas spread is most commonly associated with interventional procedures for other body fluids.

The most important infection risk to other animals and humans from urine are *Leptospira* spp. However, the risk from other bacteria found in the genitourinary tract should also be appreciated. These can include a wide range of Gram-negative and Gram-positive bacteria that may show AMR (such as extended-spectrum β-lactamase-producing and AmpC-producing *Enterobacteriaceae*, multidrug-resistant *Pseudomonas* spp., methicillin-resistant *Staphylococcus aureus* (MRSA) and methicillin-resistant *Staphylococcus pseudintermedius* (MRSP)) (Wieler *et al.*, 2011; Walther *et al.*, 2017). Urine is a major source of *Encephalitozoon cuniculi* in rabbits (Keeble, 2011). Most of these organisms may be found in both clinically affected animals and non-clinical carriers. Saliva, mucus and/or pus may contain similar bacteria, as well as *Actinomyces*, *Nocardia* and *Clostridium* spp. and other anaerobes, viruses and fungi. In contrast to humans, blood-borne nosocomial infections are uncommon in veterinary healthcare. Feline immunodeficiency virus and feline leukaemia virus would be the most familiar, although other viruses may be significant in particular animal settings. It is also important to screen blood donors for *Bartonella*, *Mycoplasma*, *Anaplasma*, *Rickettsia* and *Ehrlichia* spp. and other endemic infectious diseases where endemic in the local population (Wardrop *et al.*, 2016).

Control measures include separation between animals to eliminate direct contact, splash and aerosol risks, containment using collection devices and/or absorbent pads or barriers, careful handling of fluids, scrupulous disposal, effective cleaning and disinfection, and rigorous hand hygiene. Procedures should be planned and performed carefully with suitable measures to prevent contamination, which should include skin, mucosal and airway protection for patients and staff.

2.3.2   Indirect routes of infection

Indirect transmission of infection involves transferring the infectious organism from its reservoir to a susceptible individual via an intermediate. These can be animate or inanimate fomites (also known as vehicles). The organism must therefore be capable of contamination of the carrier or fomite and then temporary survival under these conditions.

The most important animate fomites are hands – these spread organisms between animals, humans and hand touch sites (Stull and Weese, 2015; Oh *et al.*, 2018). Inanimate fomites include anything

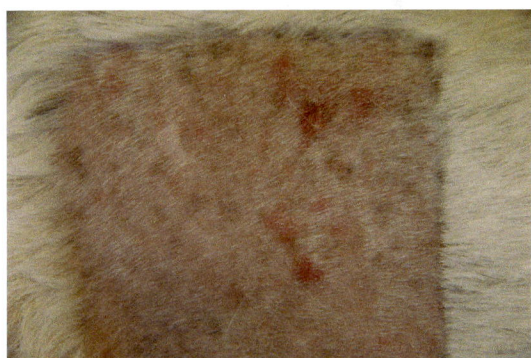

Fig. 2.1. Nosocomial *Pseudomonas aeruginosa* folliculitis and furunculosis in a dog following bathing with a contaminated shampoo. The dog recovered but required treatment with a systemic fluoroquinolone antibiotic.

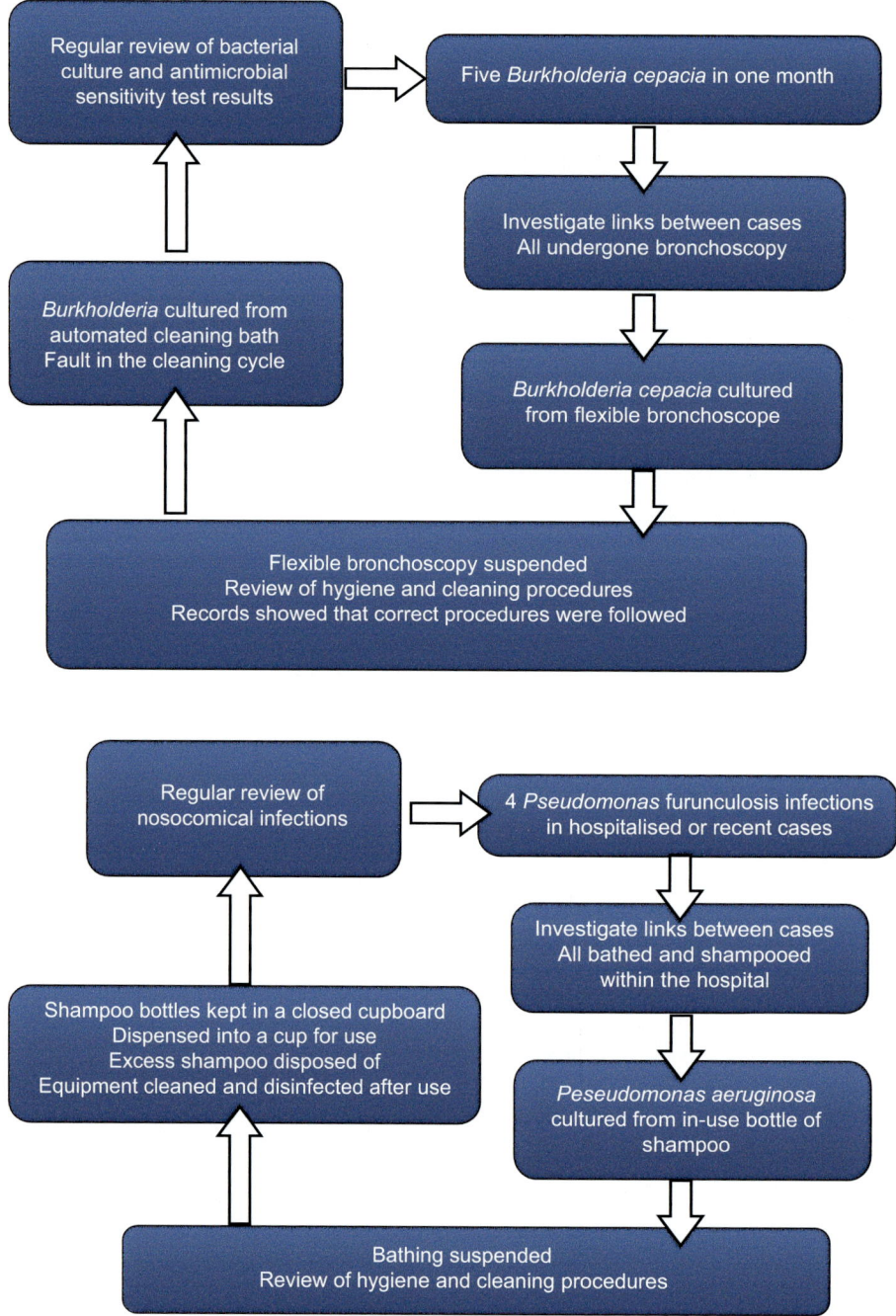

Fig. 2.2. Examples of common-source infections in veterinary practice.

that can become contaminated directly or indirectly by an infectious organism. These include surfaces, equipment, surgical instruments, kennels and cages, food and water bowls, and muzzles, leads and harnesses. Hand touch sites are especially important – these include door, cupboard and drawer handles, phones, keyboards, tablets and other portable devices, stethoscopes, otoscopes and ophthalmoscopes, scissors, forceps and pens. Environmental contamination is particularly important where the source or reservoir of infection is short term (e.g. the organism is only briefly shed or the animal spends only a short time in the clinic) but where the organism can survive for extended periods in the environment, e.g. canine parvovirus, dermatophyte spores, MRSA, MRSP, and *Pseudomonas* and *Acinetobacter* spp.

Control measures are used to prevent fomite contamination and dissemination. Infection control policies should identify risks and interventions appropriate to the site and type of work. Effective hand washing and disinfection is the single most important way to reduce nosocomial infections (Stull and Weese, 2015). However, visual cleanliness is misleading and should not be relied upon. Microbial contamination may not be immediately apparent – bacterial colonization with up to 10^6

organisms ml^{-1} may not change the visual appearance or odour of fluids and surfaces (Sabino and Weese, 2006; Oh *et al.*, 2018). Staff should therefore avoid relying on simple visual assessment of cleanliness and instead adopt a microbiological cleanliness mindset. This involves thinking about the invisible microbiological risks and avoids the trap of assuming a surface, solution or item is clean because it looks clean (Langdon *et al.*, 2020). Adopting regular protocols and procedures will help ensure microbiological cleanliness. These should consider the threat of local and remote contamination from hand touch, aerosols, splash and other risks. Depending on the situation and risk, this could include daily, weekly or monthly cleaning tasks, correct use of personal protective equipment, instructions for clean and sterile tasks, and cleaning and disinfection of surfaces and equipment after use. Standard operating procedures and checklists will help with training, adherence and audit (Stull and Weese, 2015).

2.4 Common-Source Infections

Common-source infections arise from the simultaneous exposure of susceptible individuals to a

Table 2.3. Examples of biofilm-associated contamination and infection.

Route of infection	Examples
Environmental contamination	Stagnant or pooled water (including water tanks)
	Food and water bowls
	Drains, filters and U-bends
	Shower heads, baths and taps
	Water and waste pipes
	Floors and other surfaces
Medical equipment and devices	Endoscopes and otoscopes
	Scissors and forceps
	Intravenous and urinary catheters
	Feeding tubes
	Orthopaedic implants and other prostheses
	Contact lenses
Infections and dysbiosis	Dental plaque
	Inflammatory bowel disease
	Cutaneous bacterial overgrowth syndrome
	Otitis externa and otitis media
	Uroliths, cystitis and other genitourinary tract problems
	Endocarditis
	Intervertebral disc disease
	Upper and lower respiratory tract disease
	Chronic wounds

fomite/vehicle or vector contaminated by an infectious organism. Fomite- or vehicle-borne common-source infections are an important source of infections in veterinary healthcare and other animal care. They can result in serious outbreaks affecting multiple animals. Examples include contamination of soaps, shampoos, diluted antiseptics and cleaning solutions (especially with *Pseudomonas* spp.; Fig. 2.1), drugs, multidose vials (which could include preservative-free propofol and other drugs), water (e.g. with *Pseudomonas* spp., *Leptospira* spp. and *Escherichia coli*), foods (e.g. with *Salmonella* and *Campylobacter* spp.), parenteral feeding solutions, intravenous fluids and blood products (Hohenhaus *et al.*, 1997; Sabino and Weese, 2006; Kessler *et al.*, 2010; Perry *et al.*, 2022). Other examples include improperly cleaned and sterilized equipment used in multiple patients (e.g. otoscopes, laryngoscopes, endoscopes and endotracheal tubes) (Pelligand *et al.*, 2007).

Vector-borne diseases are a subset of common-source infections that are transmitted by another animal. This may involve simple mechanical transmission through external carriage of the infectious agent from one site or individual to another (e.g. flies moving between faecal matter, foods and wounds). Some organisms (e.g. *Salmonella* and *Shigella* spp.) can survive passage through the intestinal tracts, so faecal contamination is possible. In obligate vector-borne infections, the organism must pass through one or more life stages in a vector before infection of the final host is possible. Examples include *Yersinia pestis* and *Bartonella henselae* in fleas, *Leishmania* spp. in sandflies, and *Rickettsia*, *Babesia* and *Borrelia* spp. in ticks. Mosquitos are important vectors of *Trypanosoma* spp. and a number of viral infections.

It is important to be aware of common-source infections and to take appropriate action to prevent contamination and dissemination. Clinical audits can be used to identify clusters of infections suggestive of common-source infections. Good record keeping will then allow tracing to identify likely sources for testing (Fig. 2.2).

Vector-borne disease is less common in healthcare settings but can be significant in other animal care facilities. Pest control measures should address the risks and seek to limit exposure. Important invertebrate vectors include flies, mosquitos, fleas and ticks. Ticks that can complete their life cycle indoors (e.g. *Rhipicephalus sanguineus*, the brown dog tick) can become a serious problem. Vertebrate

vectors include rodents and pigeons (clinically significant *Cryptococcus* spp. can be isolated from pigeon droppings; Siqueira *et al.*, 2022).

2.5 Biofilms

Biofilms are common in natural environments, homes, industrial settings and healthcare facilities, and they will form on virtually any non-shedding surface in wet or humid conditions (Hall-Stoodley *et al.*, 2004). Their presence and importance are often underappreciated. Biofilms are complex and dynamic populations of microorganisms that adhere to each other and to a substrate. The microbes in a biofilm may be one species or comprise a highly complex and interactive mixed population. The cells are embedded within a slimy extracellular matrix composed of extracellular polymeric substances, which are a complex array of polysaccharides, proteins, lipids and DNA produced by the organisms within the biofilm.

Microbes form biofilms in response to a number of different factors, which include binding to specific or non-specific surface attachment sites and environmental influences (e.g. physical or chemical signals, population factors, availability of nutrition, and exposure to subinhibitory concentrations of antimicrobials and disinfectants). These influences regulate gene activity resulting in altered microbial behaviour and physiology – the cells in a biofilm are physiologically distinct from planktonic cells (i.e. living in a liquid medium) of the same organism. Subpopulations within the biofilm may differentiate to specialize in motility, matrix production, nutrient sharing and sporulation. This can make biofilms highly persistent and (from a microbial point of view) a successful strategy.

Biofilms can form on any living or non-living surface (including rock, wood, metal, plastic, skin, teeth, mucosal surfaces, and medical and surgical devices) (Table 2.3). Biofilm formation has five stages (Fig. 2.3):

1. Initial attachment. Planktonic microbes initially adhere to a surface by weak reversible van der Waals forces; hydrophobic bacteria have a greater attraction to the substrate.
2. Irreversible attachment. The attached microbes anchor themselves using cell adhesion structures such as pili.

Tim Nuttall

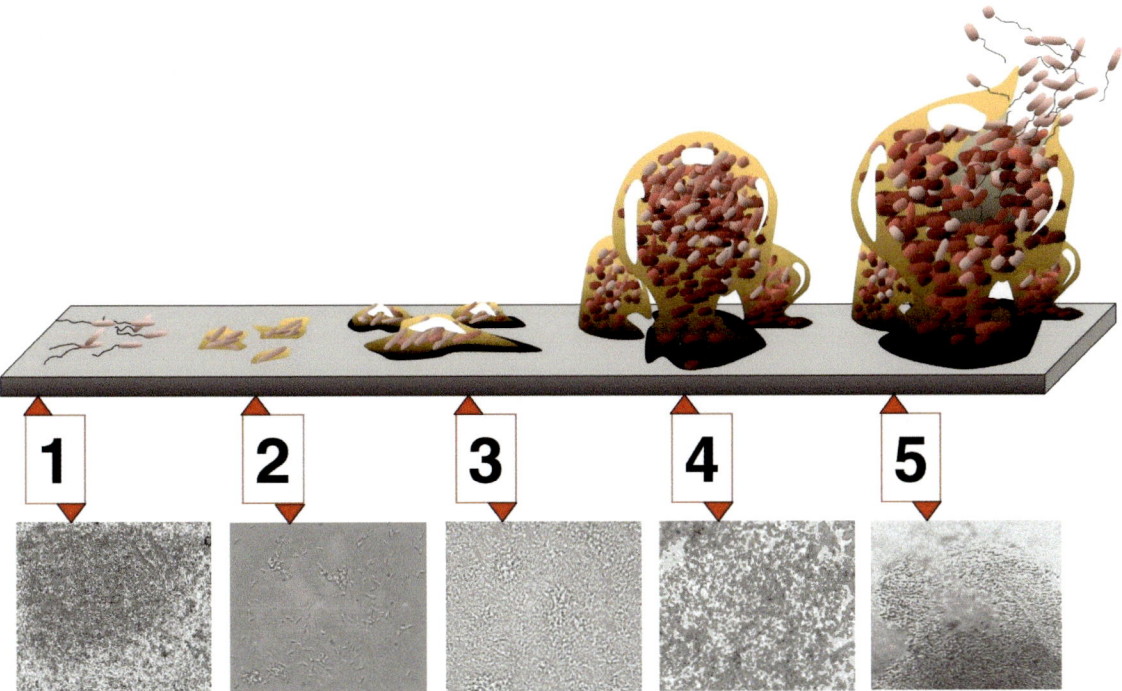

Fig. 2.3. Biofilm development and maturation. (1) Initial attachment. (2) Irreversible attachment. (3) Maturation 1. (4) Maturation 2. (5) Dispersal. Each diagram is paired with a photomicrograph of a *Pseudomonas aeruginosa* biofilm. All photomicrographs are shown to the same scale. From: https://en.wikipedia.org/wiki/Biofilm (accessed 17 October 2022).

3. Maturation 1. The attached cells communicate using quorum-sensing molecules (e.g. *N*-acyl homoserine lactone) and the biofilm grows by cell division, recruitment and matrix production; microbes that are ordinarily less able to attach to surfaces (e.g. less motile or more hydrophilic) can now adhere to the matrix or colonizing organisms.

4. Maturation 2. There is further development and specialization of the biofilm matrix and embedded cells; the mature matrix may also contain material from the surrounding environment, including inorganic and organic debris, minerals, cells, and fibrin and other proteins.

5. Dispersal. This enables biofilms to spread and colonize new surfaces; enzymes and other substances produced by cells in the matrix (e.g. dispersin B, deoxyribonuclease and nitric oxide) contribute to dispersal but may also be useful in helping remove biofilms from inanimate and animate surfaces.

Biofilms have a profound impact on treatment and infection control. Once established, they facilitate adherence to surfaces enabling bacteria to persistently colonize body tissues, medical devices, equipment and environments. The biofilm organisms can then share nutrients and are sheltered from environment factors such as drying, heat, cleaning, disinfection and antimicrobials, as well as innate and adaptive immunity.

Table 2.4. Biofilm prevention measures.

Growth prevention	Attachment prevention
Antibiotics and antimicrobials	Modified polymers
Biocides and biocide coatings/impregnation	Highly smooth surfaces
Metal ion coatings/ impregnation (e.g. silver)	Ozone
Water purification	Positive surface charge
	Hydrophobic surfaces

Table 2.5. Risk factors for nosocomial infections. Data from Ghosh *et al.* (2011), Greene *et al.* (2012) and Stull and Weese (2015).

Route of infection	Examples
Facility-associated factors	Increased animal density and contact
	Mixing of ill and healthy animals
	Stress
	Prolonged hospitalization and intensive care unit stay
	Exposure to infectious and/or AMR organisms through other patients, staff and/or the environment
	Contamination of surfaces, equipment and products
	Selection for AMR organisms by antibiotic and disinfectant use
Compromised physical barriers and defences	Loss of skin and mucosal barrier integrity (including inflammatory conditions such as atopic dermatitis)
	Reduced respiratory mucociliary escalator activity
	Reduced skin and mucosal turnover and repair
	Altered urine specific gravity, pH and flow
Foreign material	Surgical implants
	Other implants (e.g. sutures, drains, intravenous and other catheters, feeding and tracheostomy tubes)
Surgery	Pain and debility
	Surgical risks and prophylaxis
	Contaminated or clean-contaminated procedures
Procedures and interventions	Major dental disease and procedures
	Bronchoscopy, nebulizers and ventilation
	Urinary and gastrointestinal tract endoscopy
	Soiling and/or decubital ulcers in non-ambulatory patients
Underlying conditions	Debility with reduced nutrition and/or fluid intake
	Primary immunosuppression
	Compromised innate and adaptive immunity following treatment

AMR, antimicrobial resistant.

The structure of the biofilm protects the organisms from antimicrobials and disinfectants, reducing their efficacy. Exposure to sublethal antimicrobial concentrations within biofilms selects for antimicrobial and disinfectant resistance, which can then spread within and between populations through transfer of plasmids and other mobile genetic elements (Singer *et al.*, 2016). Some organisms within biofilms may also have altered physiological susceptibility to antimicrobials - i.e. persister cells that show reversible antimicrobial tolerance (Van den Bergh *et al.*, 2017).

Biofilm prevention and management should be addressed in infection control policies. The aims are to prevent surface attachment and microbial growth. However, it is very important to use these measures alongside (and not instead of) basic procedures such as thorough physical cleaning and drying of surfaces, repairing or replacing damaged surfaces and equipment, and high standards of

asepsis, surgical technique, wound care and patient management (Table 2.4).

Biofilms should be suspected in all nosocomial infections, especially those that involve implants or other devices. Standard cultures based on growth of planktonic organisms, however, may result in false-negative cultures and/or underestimate the numbers of microbes in biofilm-associated infections. Antimicrobial susceptibility tests are also based on planktonic growth and therefore will *overestimate* susceptibility and *underestimate* the minimum inhibitory concentrations (MICs) of antimicrobials where there is a biofilm at the site of infection (Singer *et al.*, 2016). This must therefore be considered when interpreting the results and selecting treatment. *N*-acetyl cysteine (NAC) has been shown to damage biofilms, lower the MIC and enhance the efficacy of systemic antibiotics in humans (Manoharan *et al.*, 2021; Aksoy *et al.*, 2022; Guerini *et al.*, 2022). It is therefore

Tim Nuttall

Table 2.6. Precautions that can be taken with raw food-fed animals.

Personal protective equipment for handling
Barrier nursing
Switching to a cooked or commercial balanced diet
    prior to or during hospitalization
Strict separation and safe handling of raw foods
Keeping raw foods refrigerated or frozen until used
Sufficient cooking to eliminate bacterial pathogens

---

possible that NAC and similar anti-biofilm compounds may aid treatment of biofilm-associated infections in animals. A commercially available Tris-EDTA-NAC solution can facilitate removal and treatment of biofilms in ear canals, although an *in vitro* study found most interactions between NAC and enrofloxacin or gentamicin were indifferent to antagonistic (May *et al.*, 2019).

2.6   Patient Risk Factors for Nosocomial Infections

The majority of the organisms implicated in nosocomial infections (especially bacteria) are opportunistic, i.e. they are not primary pathogens and have limited ability to cause disease in healthy individuals. These infections are therefore rarely acquired in the community. However, healthcare and other animal care facilities increase the risk of

infection by concentrating organisms and increasing exposure among vulnerable animals.

General risk factors should be considered when designing facilities and infection control policies. Individual patient risk factors should be considered when planning consultations, procedures and/or inpatient care (Table 2.5) (Eugster *et al.*, 2004). In particular, the impact of procedures and treatment in breaching barriers to infection, facilitating retrograde flow of commensal organisms, promoting biofilm formation and selecting for AMR organisms must be taken into account (Ogeer-Gyles *et al.*, 2006). For example, intravenous and urinary catheters breach normal defences (skin barrier and urine flushing), allow entry of surface commensals (from the skin and prepuce/vulva), are frequently contaminated with bacteria and facilitate biofilm formation (Greene *et al.*, 2012; Aksoy *et al.*, 2022)

Pre-existing conditions that compromise skin and mucosal integrity and/or increase the population of potential pathogens can also increase the risk of nosocomial wound, implant-associated and other infections. For example, atopic dermatitis affects 10–15% of all dogs, with a much higher prevalence in some breeds such as West Highland white terriers. Uncontrolled atopic dermatitis results in chronic skin inflammation and cutaneous dysbiosis skewed towards *Staphylococcus pseudintermedius* and *Malassezia pachydermatis* (Nuttall

Table 2.7. Classification of infection risk. Data from Greene *et al.* (2012).

Class	Characteristics of organisms
Class 1	Organisms cannot readily survive outside the host
	Minimal transmission and low zoonotic potential
	Easily controlled with hygiene measures
Class 2	Organisms cannot readily survive outside the host
	Higher transmission risk following close contact with the carrier, bodily fluids and/or vector
	Low zoonotic potential
	Easily controlled with routine hygiene measures and vector/fomite control
Class 3	Organisms may survive outside the host
	Higher transmission risk following close contact with the carrier, bodily fluids and fomites
	Low zoonotic potential
	Require risk assessment with regard to reducing contact, hygiene and disinfection, and personal protective equipment
Class 4	Organisms may survive outside the host
	May be resistant to cleansing and disinfection
	Highly transmissible following contact with carrier, bodily fluids and fomites
	High zoonotic risk
	Require isolation with high level hygiene, disinfection and personal protective equipment

Table 2.8. Examples of bacteria associated with healthcare-acquired infections (HAIs). Data from Ogeer-Gyles *et al.* (2006), Greene *et al.* (2012), Stull and Weese (2015) and Walther *et al.* (2017).

Organism	Comments	Suggested classification[a]
Gram-positive aerobes		
Coagulase-positive staphylococci (CoPS): Methicillin-susceptible *Staphylococcus pseudintermedius* (MSSP), *S. aureus* (MSSA) and *S. schleiferi* (MSSS) Methicillin-resistant *Staphylococcus pseudintermedius* (MRSP), *S. aureus* (MRSA) and *S. schleiferi* (MRSS)	Common HAI (Walther *et al.*, 2017) Methicillin-susceptible CoPS are usually susceptible to a wide range of antibiotics Methicillin-resistant CoPS show restricted antimicrobial susceptibility; treatment must be based on culture and antimicrobial sensitivity testing	Class 2 Class 3
Coagulase-negative staphylococci (CoNS): *Staphylococcus epidermidis*, *S. haemolyticus*, *S. saprophyticus*, *S. sciuri* and many others (Fig. 2.4)	Methicillin resistance is common (Schmidt *et al.*, 2014) Methicillin-sensitive and -resistant CoNS are carried by most healthy animals and their pathogenicity is low The clinical significance of cultured isolates is uncertain; these should be carefully reviewed alongside the history, clinical signs and cytology before starting treatment	Class 1
Streptococci	Common oro-pharyngeal and respiratory tract commensals Variable pathogenicity; streptococcal fasciitis is rare but peracute and life-threatening (Quilling *et al.*, 2022) Clinically significant antibiotic resistance is uncommon	Class 1
Enterococcus faecalis and *E. faecium* (Dotto *et al.*, 2018)	Common gut commensals Most common in urinary tract and wound infections Multi-drug antibiotic resistance is common Systemic antibiotic treatment selects for AMR carriage	Class 2
Gram-positive anaerobes		
Clostridium spp.	Gut carriage and environmental contamination Uncommon in HAIs but a potential zoonosis *Clostridium difficile* is difficult to eliminate Spores are resistant to disinfectants	Class 3
Bacillus anthracis	Rare in HAIs but a potential zoonosis Spores are resistant to disinfectants	Class 4
Gram-negative aerobes		
Enterobacteriaceae: *Escherichia coli*, *Klebsiella pneumoniae*, *Enterobacter cloacae*, *Citrobacter freundii* and *C. koseri*, and *Proteus* and *Salmonella* spp. (Gibson *et al.*, 2011; Wieler *et al.*, 2011; Timofte *et al.*, 2016)	Frequent cause of HAIs and becoming more common Readily contaminate veterinary facilities and can be difficult to eliminate (Tuerena *et al.*, 2016) Potential zoonoses; some *E. coli* and *Salmonella* isolates may cause severe disease in humans AMR is increasing; ESBL producers are resistant to all β-lactam drugs except amoxicillin-clavulanate, and AmpC-producers are resistant to all β-lactams Systemic antibiotic use selects for AMR carriage Raw food feeding increases the risk of carriage and shedding (Wales *et al.*, 2019)	Most are class 2; ESBL- and AmpC-producers are class 3; *Salmonella* spp. are class 4

Continued

Tim Nuttall

Table 2.8. Continued

Organism	Comments	Suggested classification[a]
Pseudomonas aeruginosa and *Burkholderia* spp.	Uncommon causes of HAIs; associated with invasive and severe infections Readily establish in moist environments Readily form biofilms, making treatment and eradication difficult Significant inherent and acquired antibiotic resistance limits treatment options	Class 3
Campylobacter jejuni	Low pathogenicity in animals Carriage is common and risk is increased with raw food feeding (Wales *et al.*, 2019) Potential HAI through faecal–oral transmission Zoonosis	Class 3
Bordetella bronchiseptica	Common HAI among dogs Highly contagious through aerosols and fomites Potential zoonosis	Class 2
Leptospira spp.	Rare HAI in animals but contagious and zoonotic Direct contact with infected urine Indirect contact via contaminated water	Class 4
Serratia marcescens, *Morganella morganii* and *Acinetobacter baumannii* (Boerlin *et al.*, 2001; Kuzi *et al.*, 2016)	Uncommon HAIs in animals but of growing concern Nosocomial adapted and difficult to eliminate Highly invasive and cause severe infections Widespread drug resistance and limited treatment options	Class 3
Other bacteria		
Mycobacterium tuberculosis complex	HAIs unlikely in animals Zoonotic potential through direct and indirect contact	Class 4
Mycobacterium avium complex	Usually acquired from environment and HAIs unlikely in animals Zoonotic potential through direct and indirect contact	Class 4
Rapidly growing mycobacteria	Usually acquired from environment and HAIs unlikely in animals (although contaminated water may be significant in some situations) Zoonotic potential through direct and indirect contact	Class 4
Mycoplasmas	HAIs unlikely but possible through direct contact May have zoonotic potential	Class 1

AMR, antimicrobial resistance; ESBL, extended-spectrum β-lactamase.
[a]See Table 2.7

et al., 2019). Wherever possible, the inflammation and dysbiosis should be corrected prior to any procedures to reduce the risk of nosocomial infections. If this is not possible, preparation of the patient, the procedure, aftercare and other treatment should take into account and mitigate the risks as far as possible. With atopic dogs, this may include using minimally traumatic skin preparation and/or concurrent management of the inflammation and dysbiosis alongside the primary reason for hospitalization.

Hospitalized patients must be monitored for any signs of nosocomial infections. In most cases, this will be covered in their daily (or more frequent) clinical checks (e.g. temperature, pulse, respiration, demeanour, appetite, vomiting/diarrhoea, coughing, fluid intake and urination). These checks should be thorough and should include organs that may not be relevant to the primary problem (e.g. skin, mucosal surfaces, eyes, lymph nodes), as well as wounds and insertion sites (e.g. inflammation, discharge, venous cording).

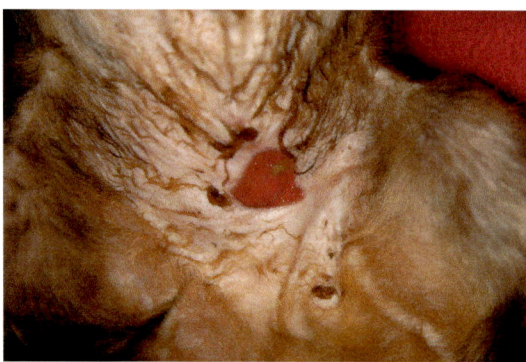

Fig. 2.4. A post-operative wound infection with a methicillin-resistant, coagulase-negative *Staphylococcus* (CoNS) infection; these cultures may be reported as commensal growth only. Cytology is important to determine the significance of this result – in this case the presence of intracellular cocci confirmed that the CoNS isolate was clinically significant.

2.7 Risks Associated with Raw Food Feeding

It is beyond the remit of this chapter to discuss the claimed health benefits or otherwise associated with raw food feeding. However, it is likely that this is associated with microbiological risks to in-contact animals and humans. These include potential pathogens such as *E. coli* 0157 and 0155, *Salmonella* spp., *Campylobacter jejuni*, *Listeria monocytogenes* and mycobacteria, as well as carriage of AMR (Wales *et al.*, 2019). The risk to healthy humans and animals is probably low with routine and simple hygienic precautions. However, the risk within healthcare environments is greater in terms of shedding, contamination and transmission to vulnerable patients. The consequences could be severe. Various human health and veterinary bodies, including the British Small Animal Veterinary Association (BSAVA, 2017), American Veterinary Medical Association (AVMA, 2022), Canadian Veterinary Medical Association (CVMA, 2018), Royal College of Nursing (RCN, 2019), UK Health Security Agency (PHE, 2019) and the US Centres for Disease Control and Prevention (CDC, 2022), have expressed caution about raw food feeding, particularly in terms of exposure of at-risk animals or humans to potential pathogens. It is therefore prudent to exercise caution when handling or hospitalizing raw-fed animals, to avoid raw feeding within healthcare or other environments wherever possible, and to practice strict and effective hygienic precautions when handling raw foods if this is necessary (Table 2.6).

2.8 Infectious Organisms in Veterinary Care

A very wide range of microbial organisms can be associated with HAIs in veterinary settings. These include bacteria, protozoa, fungi and viruses. Nosocomial bacterial infections may be antimicrobial susceptible and relatively straightforward to treat. However, AMR can reduce the therapeutic options making treatment more challenging. Infections with AMR bacteria are rare in the community and are more commonly associated with veterinary care. Antimicrobial stewardship is therefore an essential partner to infection control (Table 2.7).

2.8.1 Bacteria associated with HAIs

Most bacteria associated with HAIs are commensal and opportunistic pathogens (Table 2.8) (Greene *et al.*, 2012). Infections are rare among healthy animals in the community and are associated with specific risk factors (see section 2.6). Many of these organisms will be carried and shed by animals entering veterinary healthcare and other animal facilities. They readily colonize these environments where they can be widely disseminated (see sections 2.2 and 2.3).

Polymicrobial bacterial (or occasionally mixed-organism) infections are seen in a variety of circumstances (Table 2.9). The complex interaction between the organisms in polymicrobial infections, particularly those involving biofilms, can increase morbidity and mortality through increased virulence and AMR. However, it is often difficult to determine the clinical significance of multiple bacteria on cultures – this could represent a clinically significant polymicrobial infection or a single infection with other contaminating bacteria. The latter is particularly true where growth of a potential pathogen is accompanied by bacteria with limited virulence (e.g. a skin wound with *S. pseudintermedius* and a mixed growth of coagulase-negative staphylococci). Cytological review of samples before culture is very helpful in these circumstances – the relative abundance of the different bacteria along with knowledge of

Tim Nuttall

Table 2.9. Examples of polymicrobial infections. Data from Greene *et al.* (2012).

Infection	Organisms/comments
Peritonitis	Gram-negative bacteria Occasionally Gram-positive bacteria Anaerobes
Stomatitis and periodontitis	Gram-positive bacteria Occasionally Gram-negative bacteria Anaerobes Biofilms common
Chronic rhinitis	Gram-negative bacteria *Mycoplasma* spp. *Aspergillus* spp.
Respiratory tract infections	Gram-negative bacteria Gram-positive bacteria Anaerobes (especially in aspiration pneumonia and pyothrorax) *Actinomyces* and *Nocardia* spp. (especially in pyothorax) Viruses
Chronic otitis externa	*Pseudomonas* spp. and occasionally other Gram-negative bacteria Staphylococci and occasionally other Gram-positive bacteria *Malassezia* spp. Biofilms common
Burns and skin wounds	Staphylococci and other Gram-positive bacteria (including enterococci) Gram-negative bacteria (including *Escherichia coli* and *Pseudomonas* spp.) Environmental contaminants (including *Acinetobacter* spp.) Biofilms common
Necrotizing fasciitis	Streptococci and occasionally other Gram-positive bacteria Anaerobes
Urinary tract infections	Gram-negative bacteria (including faecal organisms and *Pseudomonas* spp.) Enterococci Especially with catheters, urolithiasis and/or biofilms
Abscesses and soft-tissue infections	Gram-negative bacteria Gram-positive bacteria Anaerobes Composition influenced by cause (e.g. bite wounds and penetrating injuries compared to surgery)
Osteomyelitis	Gram-negative bacteria Gram-positive bacteria Anaerobes Composition influenced by cause (e.g. compound fracture, post-operative or haematogenous spread) Biofilms common, especially with implants

their likely pathogenicity is invaluable in helping to interpret culture results (Fig. 2.5).

2.8.2 Fungi associated with HAIs

Most fungal HAIs are much less common than bacterial infections (Table 2.10). However, dermatophytosis is frequent and may become endemic, especially with facilities handling cats, guinea pigs and other small mammals (Moriello *et al.*, 2017). *E. cuniculi* is a microsporidian fungal organism that is an emerging HAI in rabbits (Keeble, 2011).

2.8.3 Protozoal HAIs

Relatively few protozoal organisms have been implicated in HAIs. However, while true protozoal HAIs are uncommon, they can be a significant

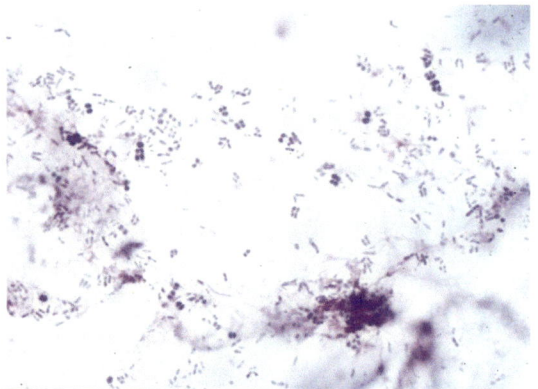

Fig. 2.5. Mixed bacterial overgrowth in a dog with chronic atopic dermatitis; this could be variably reported on culture as *Staphylococcus*, mixed bacterial isolates with different antimicrobial susceptibility, or a mixed growth with no antimicrobial susceptibility testing results. Cytology tells us that this is a mixed predominantly staphylococcal overgrowth, allowing us to make rational decisions about treatment.

source of disease in other animal housing situations. Examples include *Tritrichomonas*, *Giardia* and *Cryptosporidium* spp. (Greene, 2012a). *Giardia* and *Cryptosporidium* are important and common zoonoses. Protozoal oocysts are shed in faeces into the environment where they can become persistent and difficult to eliminate.

2.8.4 Viral HAIs

Viral HAIs are common. There is a very wide range of viruses from many different families that can infect animals (Table 2.11) (Greene, 2012b; Stull and Weese, 2015). Most are highly contagious and readily transmissible in veterinary environments. The concentration of infected and vulnerable animals enhances the risk. Most viral infections result in relatively mild and self-limiting disease that is often underappreciated. However, some viruses can cause more severe and/or zoonotic infections.

2.9 Levels of Disinfection

Disinfection refers to the removal of living organisms capable of causing infection. It is an important part of infection control, although it should never be relied on by itself. In particular, disinfectants must not be used in lieu of effective hand hygiene, surface cleansing, waste disposal and other basic measures. Most disinfectants are ineffective in the presence of organic debris and therefore should only be used on visibly clean hands and surfaces. Levels of disinfection are precisely defined (Stull *et al.*, 2018). This must be understood in terms of the likely HAI risks so that appropriate and effective products are used (Table 2.12).

Table 2.10. Examples of fungi associated with healthcare-acquired infections (HAIs).

Organism	Comments	Suggested classification[a]
Dermatophytes	Common infection, especially in catteries and rodent facilities Highly contagious through direct contact, fomites and environment Readily contaminates environment, and spores difficult to eliminate Zoonotic through direct and indirect contact	Class 4
Sporothrix schenckii complex	Environmental source, so primary HAIs unlikely Highly transmissible and zoonotic by direct contact with infected cases and material	Class 4
Other fungal infections (including *Sporothrix pallida* complex)	Environmental sources, so primary HAIs unlikely Not considered transmissible	Class 1
Encephalitozoon cuniculi	Common in rabbits Spores shed into the environment in urine; resistant to disinfectants and can be difficult to eliminate Potential zoonosis	Class 3

[a]See Table 2.7

Tim Nuttall

Table 2.11. Examples of important viral infections in animals and humans.

Virus	Examples	Suggested classification[a]
Enveloped viruses (require a lipid envelope for survival; less stable in the environment and vulnerable to detergents and 70% alcohol)		
Retroviruses	Feline immunodeficiency virus Feline leukaemia virus	Class 1
Coronaviruses	Feline coronavirus Canine coronavirus Severe acute respiratory syndrome coronavirus 1 and 2 (COVID-19), Middle East respiratory syndrome coronavirus Many other human and animal coronaviruses	Class 2
Rhabdoviruses	Rabies virus	Class 4
Orthomyxoviruses	Influenza viruses Infectious salmon anaemia virus	Class 3/4
Paramyxoviruses	Canine and phocine distemper viruses Cetacean morbillivirus Peste des petits ruminants virus Parainfluenza virus Newcastle disease virus	Class 2/3/4
Herpesviruses	Feline herpesvirus 1 Canine herpesvirus 1 Aujeszky's disease virus Bovine herpesvirus 1 Murine herpesvirus 4 Avian infectious laryngotracheitis virus Many other human and animal herpesviruses	Class 2/3
Poxviruses	Cowpox virus Monkeypox virus Squirrelpox virus Orf virus Bovine papular stomatitis virus Many other animal pox viruses	Class 2/3
Non-enveloped (naked) viruses (tough protein capsule without a lipid envelope; stable in the environment and more resistant to cleansing and disinfection (usually resistant to 70% alcohol))		
Reoviruses	Rotavirus	Class 4
Caliciviruses	Feline calicivirus Rabbit haemorrhagic disease virus Norovirus	Class 3/4
Parvoviruses	Canine and feline parvoviruses Porcine parvovirus (SMEDI) Mink enteritis virus Aleutian disease virus	Class 3/4
Papovaviruses	Papillomaviruses Polyomaviruses	Class 1

Continued

Table 2.11. Continued

Virus	Examples	Suggested classification[a]
Adenoviruses	Canine adenovirus 1 (infectious canine hepatitis) Canine adenovirus 2 Many other animal adenoviruses	Class 1/2

SMEDI, stillbirth, mummification, embryonic death, infertility.
[a]See Table 2.7.

Table 2.12. Levels of disinfection.

Term	Definition
Sterilization	All living organisms Autoclaving, irradiation and ethylene dioxide
High level of disinfection (HLD)	All viruses, vegetative bacteria (i.e. free living), fungi and protozoa Most bacterial, fungal and protozoal spores/oocysts
Intermediate/medium level of disinfection (ILD/MLD)	All vegetative bacteria Most viruses, fungi and protozoa Does not include some non-enveloped viruses (e.g. canine parvovirus), spores and oocysts
Low level of disinfection (LLD; santization (e.g. 70% alcohol gels))	Most vegetative bacteria, fungi and protozoa Enveloped viruses

References

Aksoy, N., Vatansever, C., Zengin Ersoy, G., Adakli Aksoy, B. and Fışgın, T. (2022) The effect of biofilm inhibitor *N-acetylcysteine* on the minimum inhibitory concentration of antibiotics used in Gram-negative bacteria in the biofilm developed on catheters. *International Journal of Artificial Organs* 45(10), 865–870. DOI: 10.1177/03913988221112969.

AVMA (2022) Raw or undercooked animal-source protein in cat and dog diets. American Veterinary Medical Association, Schaumburg, Illinois. Available at: www.avma.org/resources-tools/avma-policies/raw-or-undercooked-animal-source-protein-cat-and-dog-diets (accessed 23 November 2022).

Boerlin, P., Eugster, S., Gaschen, F., Straub, R. and Schawalder, P. (2001) Transmission of opportunistic pathogens in a veterinary teaching hospital. *Veterinary Microbiology* 82(4), 347–359. DOI: 10.1016/s0378-1135(01)00396-0.

BSAVA (2017) Companion animal nutrition. British Small Animal Veterinary Association, Quedgeley, UK. Available at: https://bsava.com/position-statement/companion-animal-nutrition/ (accessed 23 November 2022).

CDC (2022) Pet food safety. Centers for Disease Control and Prevention, Atlanta, Georgia. Available at: www.cdc.gov/healthypets/keeping-pets-and-people-healthy/pet-food-safety.html (accessed 23 November 2022).

CVMA (2018) Raw meat-based diets for pets. Canadian Veterinary Medical Association, Ottawa, Canada. Available at: www.canadianveterinarians.net/policy-and-outreach/position-statements/statements/raw-meat-based-diets-for-pets/ (accessed 4 January 2023).

Dotto, G., Berlanda, M., Pasotto, D., Mondin, A., Zambotto, G. *et al.* (2018) Pets as potential carriers of multidrug-resistant *Enterococcus faecium* of significance to public health. *New Microbiologica* 41(2), 168–172.

Eugster, S., Schawalder, P., Gaschen, F. and Boerlin, P. (2004) A prospective study of postoperative surgical site infections in dogs and cats. *Veterinary Surgery* 33(5), 542–550. DOI: 10.1111/j.1532-950X.2004.04076.x.

Gentilini, F., Turba, M.E., Pasquali, F., Mion, D., Romagnoli, N. *et al.* (2018) Hospitalized pets as a source of carbapenem-resistance. *Frontiers in Microbiology* 9, 2872. DOI: 10.3389/fmicb.2018.02872.

Ghosh, A., Dowd, S.E. and Zurek, L. (2011) Dogs leaving the ICU carry a very large multi-drug resistant enterococcal population with capacity for biofilm formation and horizontal gene transfer. *PloS One* 6(7), e22451. DOI: 10.1371/journal.pone.0022451.

Gibson, J.S., Morton, J.M., Cobbold, R.N., Filippich, L.J. and Trott, D.J. (2011) Risk factors for dogs becoming rectal carriers of multidrug-resistant *Escherichia coli* during hospitalization. *Epidemiology and Infection* 139(10), 1511–1521. DOI: 10.1017/S0950268810002785.

Greene, C.E. (ed.) (2012a) Section IV: protozoal diseases. In: *Infectious Diseases of the Dog and Cat*, 4th edn. Elsevier, St Louis, Missouri, pp. 711–849.

Greene, C.E. (ed.) (2012b) Section I: viral, rickettsial and chlamydial diseases. In: *Infectious Diseases of the Dog and Cat*, 4th edn. Elsevier, St Louis, Missouri, pp. 1–275.

Greene, C.E., Weese, J.S. and Calpin, J.P. (2012) Environmental factors in infectious disease. In: *Infectious Diseases of the Dog and Cat*, 4th edn. Elsevier, St Louis, Missouri, pp. 1078–1097.

Guerini, M., Condrò, G., Friuli, V., Maggi, L. and Perugini, P. (2022) *N-acetylcysteine* (NAC) and its role in clinical practice management of Cystic Fibrosis (CF): a review. *Pharmaceuticals* 15, 217. DOI: 10.3390/ph15020217.

Hall-Stoodley, L., Costerton, J.W. and Stoodley, P. (2004) Bacterial biofilms: from the natural environment to infectious diseases. *Nature Reviews. Microbiology* 2(2), 95–108. DOI: 10.1038/nrmicro821.

Hohenhaus, A.E., Drusin, L.M. and Garvey, M.S. (1997) *Serratia marcescens* contamination of feline whole blood in a hospital blood bank. *Journal of the American Veterinary Medical Association* 210(6), 794–798.

Keeble, E. (2011) Encephalitozoonosis in rabbits – what we do and don't know. *In Practice* 33(9), 426–435. DOI: 10.1136/inp.d6077.

Kessler, R.J., Rankin, S., Young, S., O'Shea, K., Calabrese, M. *et al.* (2010) *Pseudomonas fluorescens* contamination of a feline packed red blood cell unit and studies of canine units. *Veterinary Clinical Pathology* 39(1), 29–38. DOI: 10.1111/j.1939-165X.2009.00190.x.

Kuzi, S., Blum, S.E., Kahane, N., Adler, A., Hussein, O. *et al.* (2016) Multi-drug-resistant *Acinetobacter calcoaceticus-Acinetobacter baumannii* complex infection outbreak in dogs and cats in a veterinary hospital. *Journal of Small Animal Practice* 57(11), 617–625. DOI: 10.1111/jsap.12555.

Langdon, G., Hoet, A.E. and Stull, J.W. (2020) Fluorescent tagging for environmental surface cleaning surveillance in a veterinary hospital. *Journal of Small Animal Practice* 61(2), 121–126. DOI: 10.1111/jsap.13090.

Manoharan, A., Ognenovska, S., Paino, D., Whiteley, G., Glasbey, T. *et al.* (2021) *N-Acetylcysteine* protects bladder epithelial cells from bacterial invasion and displays antibiofilm activity against urinary tract bacterial pathogens. *Antibiotics* 10, 900. DOI: 10.3390/antibiotics10080900.

May, E.R., Ratliff, B.E. and Bemis, D.A. (2019) Antibacterial effect of *N-acetylcysteine* in combination with antimicrobials on common canine otitis externa bacterial isolates. *Veterinary Dermatology* 30(6), 531–e161. DOI: 10.1111/vde.12795.

Moriello, K.A., Coyner, K., Paterson, S. and Mignon, B. (2017) Diagnosis and treatment of dermatophytosis in dogs and cats: clinical consensus guidelines of the world association for veterinary dermatology. *Veterinary Dermatology* 28(3), 266–e68. DOI: 10.1111/vde.12440.

Naziri, Z., Derakhshandeh, A., Firouzi, R., Motamedifar, M. and Shojaee Tabrizi, A. (2016) DNA fingerprinting approaches to trace *Escherichia coli* sharing between dogs and owners. *Journal of Applied Microbiology* 120(2), 460–468. DOI: 10.1111/jam.13003.

Nuttall, T.J., Marsella, R., Rosenbaum, M.R., Gonzales, A.J. and Fadok, V.A. (2019) Update on pathogenesis, diagnosis, and treatment of atopic dermatitis in dogs. *Journal of the American Veterinary Medical Association* 254(11), 1291–1300. DOI: 10.2460/javma.254.11.1291.

Ogeer-Gyles, J.S., Mathews, K.A. and Boerlin, P. (2006) Nosocomial infections and antimicrobial resistance in critical care medicine. *Journal of Veterinary Emergency and Critical Care* 16, 1–18. DOI: 10.1111/j.1476-4431.2005.00162.x.

Oh, Y.I., Baek, J.Y., Kim, S.H., Kang, B.J. and Youn, H.Y. (2018) Antimicrobial susceptibility and distribution of multidrug-resistant organisms isolated from environmental surfaces and hands of healthcare workers in a small animal hospital. *Japanese Journal of Veterinary Research* 66, 193–202.

Pelligand, L., Hammond, R. and Rycroft, A. (2007) An investigation of the bacterial contamination of small animal breathing systems during routine use. *Veterinary Anaesthesia and Analgesia* 34(3), 190–199. DOI: 10.1111/j.1467-2995.2006.00320.x.

Perry, E., Sutton, G.A., Haggag, L., Fleker, M., Blum, S.E. *et al.* (2022) *Pseudomonas aeruginosa* isolation from dog grooming products used by private owners or by professional pet grooming salons: prevalence and risk factors. *Veterinary Dermatology* 33(4), 316–e73. DOI: 10.1111/vde.13072.

PHE (2019) Raw pet foods: handling and preventing infection. Public Health England, London. Available at: www.gov.uk/guidance/raw-pet-foods-handling-and-preventing-infection (accessed 23 November 2022).

Quilling, L.L., Outerbridge, C.A., White, S.D. and Affolter, V.K. (2022) Retrospective case series: necrotising fasciitis in 23 dogs. *Veterinary Dermatology* 33(6), 534–544. DOI: 10.1111/vde.13113.

RCN (2019) *Working with Dogs in Health Care Settings*. Royal College of Nursing, London. Available at: www.rcn.org.uk/Professional-Development/publications/pub-007925 (accessed November 2022).

Sabino, C.V. and Weese, J.S. (2006) Contamination of multiple-dose vials in a veterinary hospital. *Canadian Veterinary Journal* 47, 779–782.

Schmidt, V.M., Williams, N.J., Pinchbeck, G., Corless, C.E., Shaw, S. *et al.* (2014) Antimicrobial resistance and characterisation of staphylococci isolated from healthy Labrador retrievers in the United Kingdom. *BMC Veterinary Research* 10, 17. DOI: 10.1186/1746-6148-10-17.

Singer, A.C., Shaw, H., Rhodes, V. and Hart, A. (2016) Review of antimicrobial resistance in the environment and its relevance to environmental regulators. *Frontiers in Microbiology* 7, 1728. DOI: 10.3389/fmicb.2016.01728.

Siqueira, N.P., Favalessa, O.C., Maruyama, F.H., Dutra, V., Nakazato, L. *et al.* (2022) Domestic birds as source of *Cryptococcus deuterogattii* (AFLP6/VGII): potential risk for cryptococcosis. *Mycopathologia* 187(1), 103–111. DOI: 10.1007/s11046-021-00601-w.

Stull, J.W. and Weese, J.S. (2015) Hospital-associated infections in small animal practice. *Veterinary Clinics of North America. Small Animal Practice* 45(2), 217–233. DOI: 10.1016/j.cvsm.2014.11.009.

Stull, J.W., Bjorvik, E., Bub, J., Dvorak, G., Petersen, C. *et al.* (2018) 2018 AAHA infection control, prevention, and biosecurity guidelines. *Journal of the American Animal Hospital Association* 54(6), 297–326. DOI: 10.5326/JAAHA-MS-6903.

Timofte, D., Maciuca, I.E., Williams, N.J., Wattret, A. and Schmidt, V. (2016) Veterinary hospital dissemination of CTX-M-15 extended-spectrum beta-lactamase-producing *Escherichia coli* ST410 in the United Kingdom. *Microbial Drug Resistance* 22(7), 609–615. DOI: 10.1089/mdr.2016.0036.

Tuerena, I., Williams, N.J., Nuttall, T. and Pinchbeck, G. (2016) Antimicrobial-resistant *Escherichia coli* in hospitalised companion animals and their hospital environment. *Journal of Small Animal Practice* 57(7), 339–347. DOI: 10.1111/jsap.12525.

Van den Bergh, B., Fauvart, M. and Michiels, J. (2017) Formation, physiology, ecology, evolution and clinical importance of bacterial persisters. *FEMS Microbiology Reviews* 41(3), 219–251. DOI: 10.1093/femsre/fux001.

Wales, A., Lawes, J. and Davies, R. (2019) How to advise clients about raw feeding dogs and cats. *BSAVA Companion 2019* 10–15.

Walther, B., Tedin, K. and Lübke-Becker, A. (2017) Multidrug-resistant opportunistic pathogens challenging veterinary infection control. *Veterinary Microbiology* 200, 71–78. DOI: 10.1016/j.vetmic.2016.05.017.

Wardrop, K.J., Birkenheuer, A., Blais, M.C., Callan, M.B., Kohn, B. *et al.* (2016) Update on canine and feline blood donor screening for blood-borne pathogens. *Journal of Veterinary Internal Medicine* 30(1), 15–35. DOI: 10.1111/jvim.13823.

Wieler, L.H., Ewers, C., Guenther, S., Walther, B. and Lübke-Becker, A. (2011) Methicillin-resistant staphylococci (MRS) and extended-spectrum beta-lactamases (ESBL)-producing *Enterobacteriaceae* in companion animals: nosocomial infections as one reason for the rising prevalence of these potential zoonotic pathogens in clinical samples. *International Journal of Medical Microbiology* 301(8), 635–641. DOI: 10.1016/j.ijmm.2011.09.009.

Tim Nuttall

Section 2: Principles of Infection Prevention and Control

This section will outline the evidence for the main principles of infection prevention and control, including suggestions on how to practically implement and maintain improvements in infection-control policies and practices within the veterinary clinic or hospital.

It will cover the following key points:

- *Patient screening* to assess individuals with previously diagnosed multidrug-resistant (MDR) infections. This is an important tool to mitigate the spread of up-and-coming pathogens, but active surveillance through screening of healthy (or targeted) individuals is not yet standard clinical practice in veterinary medicine. Screening may provide significant benefit where MDR pathogens are detected in subclinical individuals, but further research in this field is required.
- *Scrupulous hand hygiene is the cornerstone of infection control practice*, and can be performed by hand washing (using soap and water) or using an alcohol-based hand rub. There are five moments for hand hygiene, illustrated in Fig. 4.1 (Chapter 4, this volume). Techniques are shown in Figs 4.2 and 4.3, which could be installed as posters near hand-cleaning stations.
- Impediments to hand hygiene should be minimised. A 'bare below the elbow' policy should be followed, and nails should be natural, unpolished and less than 2 mm in length.
- Hand hygiene compliance is generally poor and can be improved by *educational campaigns*, providing products/methods to maintain skin health, *surveillance* and *feedback*.
- The use of gloves is not a substitute for excellent hand hygiene.
- To further mitigate transmission of infectious agents, a range of personal protective equipment (PPE) or specialized equipment may be worn by healthcare workers to provide an additional barrier to workwear. Contamination with infectious materials commonly occurs during the donning process due to inappropriate choice of PPE size, or during the doffing process because of incorrect technique. Appropriate training and guidance is important to minimize this risk (see Fig. 6.1, Chapter 6, this volume).
- The importance of *cleaning before disinfection* cannot be overemphasized because organic material can also act as a physical barrier, protecting the microorganisms. Disinfectants should be selected based chiefly on safety and efficacy (summarized in Table 7.2, Chapter 7, this volume), ensuring that application is correct and consistent.

3 Patient Screening

Sian-Marie Frosini* and Rosanne Jepson

Royal Veterinary College, University of London, London, UK

3.1 Introduction

The concept of patient screening is to detect individuals who may have multidrug-resistant (MDR) bacteria residing within their natural microbiota, known as 'carriers'. These animals may have no outward signs of MDR bacterial carriage; however, in the event of disease or veterinary interventions, these bacteria could pose a challenge for successful antimicrobial therapy. Furthermore, carriers may shed these pathogens into the clinic, resulting in healthcare-acquired infections (HAIs) in other patients they are either directly in contact with or with whom they share an environment within the veterinary practice. Consequently, the ability to detect these subclinical carriers is important to mitigate the spread and impact of MDR bacteria.

3.2 The Benefits of Patient Screening

Patient screening is a well-established process for human hospital inpatients and is used prior to elective procedures or planned hospital visits. It has been used to great effect in the control of methicillin-resistant *Staphylococcus aureus* (MRSA) (Cookson *et al.*, 2011), and currently is important in curbing the spread of carbapenem-resistant *Enterobacterales* (CRE) (van Loon *et al.*, 2017). So far, its use in companion animal medicine remains limited; however, this is likely to change in the future as a rising prevalence of MDR bacterial carriage in the pet population results in increased risk for HAIs and further pressure on the veterinary hospital. The use of ever more complicated surgical and medical interventions in companion animals results in animals that may be more vulnerable to bacterial infections. This potentially results in increased morbidity and even fatal consequences, especially if infections are refractory to antimicrobial therapy.

Patient screening is therefore about protecting both the patient, who may be a carrier, and any other animals entering the veterinary hospital at the same time. It is widely believed that most bacterial infections, across all body systems, are endogenous – caused by those bacteria that are carried as part of a healthy microbiome in the gastrointestinal tract or on the skin and are then present in an environment where they should not be found. Thus, the presence of MDR bacteria within the microbiota of these body systems indicates that there is potential for future infections to be complicated by these bacteria. This is not to say that the MDR bacteria are more virulent. In fact, they may have fitness costs associated with their MDR nature, resulting in slower growth than their non-MDR counterparts (Martinez, 2014). However, especially with increasing selective pressure from antimicrobial use, MDR bacteria are likely to become a major player in an infection. Identification of a carrier animal may therefore allow the practitioner to select a suitable empirical antimicrobial, if cytology suggests that the bacterial morphology matches that of previously detected MDR bacteria. Subsequent confirmation through bacterial culture can then allow the veterinarian to continue this antimicrobial therapy or de-escalate if it is not needed. Furthermore, for a practitioner, understanding the local prevalence of MDR pathogens may also guide empirical antimicrobial therapy more generally in other animals under their care. For example, in a region that has an overwhelming prevalence of methicillin-resistant *Staphylococcus pseudintermedius* (MRSP), compared with its susceptible counterpart, it may be rational to assume that when cocci are seen in association with skin disease, they are very likely to be MRSP and so therapy can be guided based on that information, with subsequent treatment de-escalation if MRSP is not identified during bacterial culture.

The veterinary care plan for an animal may be changed if they are confirmed to be MDR carriers

*Corresponding author: sfrosini@rvc.ac.uk

© CAB International 2023. *Infection Control in Small Animal Clinical Practice* (eds F. Allerton and K.L. Bowlt Blacklock)
DOI: 10.1079/9781789244977.0003

when screened. An elective surgical procedure may be postponed in favour of an attempt to decolonize the animal by removing the MDR pathogens from the body. This is the approach taken in human medicine when confronted with people who are MRSA carriers. In humans, there is some evidence to support decolonization as a short-term solution to eliminate MRSA from the skin of an individual (Loeb *et al.*, 2003). However, it does not provide a long-term solution, and careful evaluation is needed before utilizing these methods (Loeb *et al.*, 2003; Cookson *et al.*, 2011). To date, there is little evidence for the utility of decolonization in veterinary medicine (Frosini *et al.*, 2021). However, patient screening may still lead to an amended management plan for the care of an animal, for example using appropriate antimicrobial coverage where animals may be immunosuppressed as part of their disease or treatment, or for those patients where the risk of infection could come with particularly high morbidity or mortality.

Within the veterinary hospital, patient screening may also be an important tool to support appropriate infection-control protocols. By detecting subclinical carriage of MDR pathogens, a chain of events relating to the pathogen can be put into practice to minimize the risk for HAIs originating from a single carrier animal. This is useful both for hospital inpatients, which could be housed in proximity to other pets, and also for an outpatient service where a veterinarian and consulting room may see multiple animals in quick succession, propagating MDR bacterial spread (van Duijkeren *et al.*, 2011; Espadale *et al.*, 2018; Perkins *et al.*, 2020; Schmidt *et al.*, 2020).

3.3 Screening as a Tool for Outbreak Investigation

Patient screening may be employed in the face of a potential outbreak of an HAI. Conventionally, an outbreak is recognized as a similar infection in two or more individuals with both temporal and spatial links (Puleston *et al.*, 2020). Ideally there would also be evidence of transmission between these patients. These outbreaks may be related to MDR bacteria but could also be a result of another communicable disease, such as gastrointestinal disease related to *Salmonella* spp. It is important to note that a single occurrence of a rare pathogen (e.g. CRE in veterinary patients) may be the start

of an unrecognized outbreak if that individual does not have significant risk factors (Puleston *et al.*, 2020). In light of this, it may be necessary for the clinician to be prepared to use active surveillance to minimize the risk of further HAIs.

An individual responsible for infection control within the hospital is needed to communicate the discovery of this pathogen to all clinical staff, and to coordinate active surveillance measures. It may be that specific clinical signs (e.g. unexpected gastrointestinal disease in the case of a *Salmonella* outbreak) should prompt patient screening, or that instead this should be based on physical proximity to the index case. This is seen in human hospitals, where CRE outbreaks within a ward prompt the screening of all individuals sharing that space (CDC, 2009; Puleston *et al.*, 2020). The potential routes for transmission other than patient-to-patient contact are important to consider as well. Screening of the environment, and potentially of staff, may be warranted considering the documented nature of both environment and veterinary staff as vectors for transmission of MDR pathogens (van Duijkeren *et al.*, 2011; Churak *et al.*, 2021; Schmitt *et al.*, 2022). However, this approach should only be undertaken if appropriate actions are taken in the case of a positive sample. This is especially important when considering staff screening, as there may be individual or public health concerns if a carrier of an MDR pathogen, such as CRE, is identified and the infection-control team must be prepared to explain these implications.

When undertaking any patient screening, but especially considering the time pressure related to outbreak investigation and mitigation, dialogue with the diagnostic microbiology laboratory is paramount. This will enable the laboratory to advise on sample types, and allow for rapid, specific methods to be implemented for the pathogens of interest. It will also allow the laboratory to maximize the chance of pathogen detection, such as using enrichment cultures when a low number of the suspected pathogen is expected (Saab *et al.*, 2018).

3.4 Routine Patient Screening

The proportion of healthy animals with detected carriage of MDR pathogens varies greatly across geographical regions and specific animal populations (Hordijk *et al.*, 2013; Pires Dos Santos, 2016; van den Bunt *et al.*, 2020; Börjesson *et al.*,

2020). It does not help that there are no national screening protocols, and in many cases, detection of these pathogens is not notifiable, thus leaving the estimated prevalence to research papers. It is important for a practitioner to put any screening recommendations in the context of both local carriage rates of MDR bacteria (if known) and rates of MDR infections to understand the benefit that screening may potentially bring. In areas of low prevalence in the healthy animal population, the decision to undertake screening remains controversial. As prevalence increases, screening is likely to be a more important part of successful infection control, as has been seen in MRSA in human medicine (Cookson *et al.*, 2011).

In general, those pathogens most considered as worthwhile for patient screening in a veterinary context mirror human medicine: methicillin-resistant staphylococci (MRSP/MRSA), extended-spectrum β-lactamase (ESBL)-producing *Enterobacterales* and CRE.

3.4.1 Methicillin-resistant staphylococci

In animals, there is no literature supporting universal screening for carriage of methicillin-resistant staphylococci, namely MRSA or MRSP (Fig. 3.1). To the authors' knowledge, there are no veterinary hospitals currently instigating an enforced screening recommendation for these (or any) pathogens. Nevertheless, there are many similarities in the epidemiology and microbiological characteristics of MRSA infection and carriage in humans, and that of MRSP in dogs. Thus, when considering screening of dogs in the veterinary practice, mirroring recommendations in human healthcare for MRSA is likely to be of benefit. Common considerations relevant to considering patient screening are that: (i) cats are contaminated 'bystanders' more so than true carriers of these bacteria (Hanselman *et al.*, 2009; Loeffler *et al.*, 2011); and (ii) canine MRSA carriage is probably a result of temporary contamination from a human member of the household (Loeffler *et al.*, 2011). Thus, attention is focused on the links

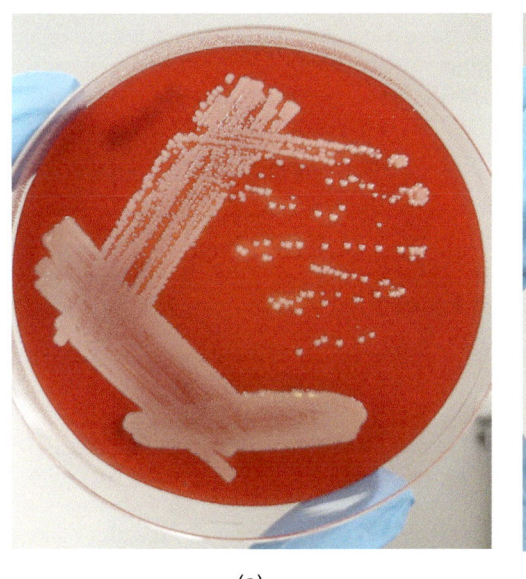
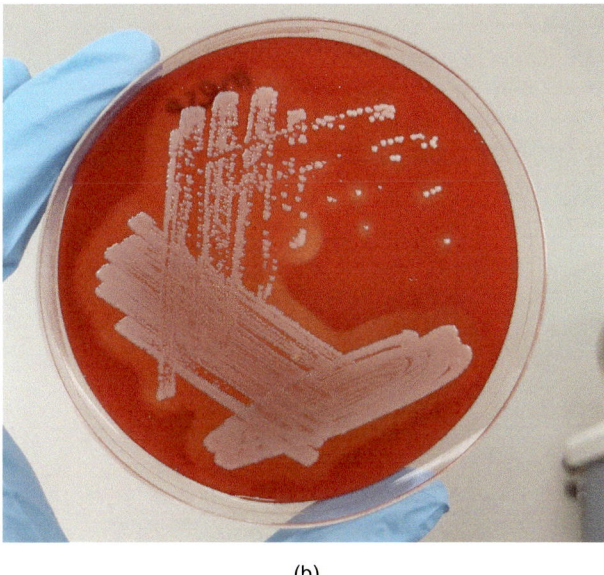

(a)   (b)

Fig. 3.1. Cultures of (a) methicillin-resistant *Staphylococcus aureus* (MRSA) and (b) methicillin-resistant *Staphylococcus pseudintermedius* (MRSP) isolated from healthy canine skin and representing subclinical carriage, grown aerobically on 5% sheep's blood agar. Isolates are from the collections of Dr Anette Loeffler and Dr Sian-Marie Frosini, stored at the Royal Veterinary College, London, UK.

that can be made between MRSA control in human medicine and MRSP in dogs.

MRSA was the first MDR organism to be implicated in large-scale active surveillance programmes in human hospitals. In areas where MRSA is endemic, there remains a strong emphasis on screening patients as part of an overall MRSA control programme, within the limitations of funding and feasibility (Cookson *et al.*, 2011). In 1988, the Netherlands initiated a widely successful 'search and destroy' policy for MRSA, which focused on three main activities: (i) active screening of patients, (ii) pre-emptive isolation of individuals considered 'high risk' for MRSA carriage; and (iii) containment of MRSA-positive individuals (either infected or colonized) in a single room until successful decolonization was performed (Wagenvoort, 2000). All individuals entering the healthcare environment, whether as an in- or outpatient, were screened with throat and nasal swabs, with the addition of perineal swabbing for hospital inpatients. This has been praised as a widely successful protocol, with the Netherlands experiencing low rates of MRSA infection and carriage compared with much of Europe (Wertheim *et al.*, 2004; Souverein *et al.*, 2016). Many countries have shied away from policies of such an intensive nature, especially considering the cost implications, and instead focus on active surveillance through pre-admission assessment and targeted screening of 'high-risk' individuals (Wernitz *et al.*, 2005; Cookson *et al.*, 2011; Deeny *et al.*, 2013; Fuller *et al.*, 2013; DoH, 2014; Kavanagh, 2019; Coia *et al.*, 2021) alongside stringent hand hygiene policies.

The low prevalence of MRSP in the healthy animal population in many areas of the world drives infection-control protocols to consider adopting a similar, targeted approach. In human medicine the targeted individuals usually fall into three groups, for which parallels can be drawn in the canine population:

1. Previously detected carriers. Recommendations for MRSA screening in the UK suggest that once a patient has screened positive, no further screening is necessary, and this individual should be considered an MRSA carrier and treated in isolation (Coia *et al.*, 2021). Repeat screening is only necessary if decolonization is attempted (Coia *et al.*, 2021). The same continuous carriage of MRSP has been described in dogs, lasting in many cases for the entire duration of a longitudinal study (months to years)

(Windahl *et al.*, 2012, 2016; Frosini *et al.*, 2021). Three consecutive sets of swabs at least 48 h apart must be MRSA negative for a patient to be moved out of isolation in a human hospital. Although this is probably robust, a potentially intermittent nature to MRSA carriage has been described in some individuals, probably due to 'hidden' carriage sites (e.g. gastrointestinal tract, throat) that are not sampled (van Belkum, 2016). Thus, a historical negative sample should not be used to predict current carriage status. Again, the same is true for MRSP carriage in dogs. MRSP has been shown to be detected intermittently across carriage sites following resolution of an initial infection (Windahl *et al.*, 2012; Frosini *et al.*, 2021). This intermittent nature means that a negative carriage swab following a previous MRSP-positive status may just be a transient state and so should not be used to 'downgrade' an individual from barrier nursing or isolation in the clinic.

2. Patients with risk factors for potential carriage. In humans, the major risk factors that would trigger patient screening include: previous healthcare admissions, the use of healthcare abroad, occupational risk factors (e.g. healthcare worker, contact with livestock) and indwelling devices (DoH, 2014; van Hout *et al.*, 2021). Typically, in both humans and animals, risk factors for carriage of infection with MRSA/MRSP remain vague and in the most part 'healthcare associated' (e.g. hospitalization, previous antimicrobial therapy) (Huerta *et al.*, 2011; Nienhoff *et al.*, 2011; Lehner *et al.*, 2014; Kasai *et al.*, 2016). As such, it is difficult to pinpoint an optimal targeted approach for screening in veterinary patients. Human guidelines suggest rescreening previously negative patients where there has been a significant exposure risk since the last test. Research in Dutch hospitals has suggested that swabbing at 14-day intervals while patients reside within the hospital may enable increased detection of nosocomial transmission (Bastiaens *et al.*, 2020), although this regular screening remains omitted from the recommendations of many countries. In veterinary medicine, this repeated screening is likely to be of more use in an outbreak investigation than as a routine measure, potentially at cost to the hospital rather than the client.

3. Interventions deemed at risk in the case of complication with methicillin-resistant staphylococci. This is the most well-known intervention; many people may have experienced swabbing for MRSA themselves prior to admission for an elective

procedure (e.g. orthopaedics, dental surgery). If an individual has a positive carriage sample, any subsequent infection with high morbidity or mortality risks (e.g. bloodstream, orthopaedic implant infection) that is associated with Gram-positive cocci on cytology may then be treated empirically with an appropriate antimicrobial for methicillin-resistant staphylococci. Following successful culture, antimicrobial de-escalation can be put in place if MRSA/MRSP was not the cause.

The most sensitive sites determined for MRSA screening are the nares, mouth and perineum (Chipolombwe *et al.*, 2016), with indication that there is a balance between cost and sensitivity for multi-site swabbing. The canine MRSA counterpart, MRSP, is carried in similar skin sites across the body, with predilections for the nostrils, buccal cavity and perineum (Devriese and De Pelsmaecker, 1987; Rubin and Chirino-Trejo, 2011; Bannoehr and Guardabassi, 2012; Windahl *et al.*, 2012; Iverson *et al.*, 2015), but can be detected from all skin and mucosal sites in which it has been investigated. As in humans, multi-site swabbing of dogs has been confirmed as necessary for the highest sensitivity for MRSP detection (Windahl *et al.*, 2012; Frosini *et al.*, 2022). It is widely suggested that finances may be conserved by pooling multiple swabs to be processed simultaneously. This has been shown not to be of detriment for detection of MRSA (Grmek-Kosnik *et al.*, 2018), and is a valuable consideration, as the exact location of these bacteria is not of clinical value in the context of patient screening.

The methicillin-resistant staphylococci represent the most evidence to support the use of targeted patient screening within the veterinary clinic, probably in a hospital or referral setting based on the risk factors for MRSP carriage and infection. However, this should be designed to maximize useful data, such as in the case of early, successful intervention or patient isolation to prevent nosocomial spread.

3.4.2 ESBL-producing *Enterobacterales* and CRE

ESBL-producing *Enterobacterales*, focused predominantly on *Escherichia coli* and *Klebsiella pneumoniae*, are not screened for in human medicine. This is probably due to a multitude of viable antimicrobials remaining open for the treatment of these infections (e.g. carbapenems), thus rendering their detection within the gastrointestinal microbiota of less clinical value. In veterinary medicine, however, these antimicrobials may be considered 'inappropriate' or in some regions be banned for use in companion animals (EMA, 2019). Consequently, ESBL-producing *Enterobacterales* represent an important challenge in veterinary medicine, and so screening may be considered. As they are carried in the gastrointestinal tract, the act of patient screening could mirror that for CRE, which are screened for in human medicine.

CRE, focused largely on *E. coli* and *K. pneumoniae*, are a more recent addition to the barrage of antimicrobial resistance threats in human medicine (Nordmann and Cornaglia, 2012). Recently, they have also started to emerge as pathogens in companion animal medicine, although their description remains sporadic, dependent on geographical location (Köck *et al.*, 2018; Lavigne *et al.*, 2021), and is likely to be a result of 'spillover' from humans into companion animals (Madec *et al.*, 2017; Grönthal *et al.*, 2018). However, the increasing selection of these critical antimicrobials for therapy indicates a need for vigilance in our clinical environment. These pathogens are commonly multi- or even pan-drug resistant (Nordmann and Cornaglia, 2012), and are associated with mortality rates in human bloodstream infections as high as 40–50% (Tumbarello *et al.*, 2012; Logan and Weinstein, 2017). Risk factors for carriage of and infection with CRE are widely similar to other MDR pathogens – antimicrobial use, hospitalization and travel to areas where these bacteria are more prevalent in the population (Madueño *et al.*, 2017; van Loon *et al.*, 2017; Segagni Lusignani *et al.*, 2020; Palacios-Baena *et al.*, 2021). Comparable to the ESBL-producing *Enterobacterales*, these bacteria can also be asymptomatically carried in the lower gastrointestinal tract and shed in faecal material. The detection of CRE from asymptomatic individuals has been shown both in humans (in up to 10% in some populations; Rossini *et al.*, 2016; Yamamoto *et al.*, 2017; Ohno *et al.*, 2020) and infrequently in animals (Grönthal *et al.*, 2018; Köck *et al.*, 2018; Nigg *et al.*, 2019).

Meta-analysis of the top infection-control interventions to control CRE in human hospitals listed active surveillance within the top three measures, alongside isolation procedures and patient cohorting, whereby patients suspected of carriage of these organisms are grouped together within the hospital environment under a single nursing team in the same location (van Loon *et al.*, 2017). Screening for CRE further allows targeted implementation of interventions to stop the spread of CRE, which is of particular importance considering CRE is thought to be acquired primarily within the healthcare environment (Richter and Marchaim, 2017). This is an approach recommended by many national and international groups for CRE control, usually focusing on high-risk individuals rather than blanket policies for all patient admissions (CDC, 2009; PHE, 2020). Screening is undertaken from rectal swabs or stool samples, usually from individuals with a history of colonization or infection with CRE, or who are in long-term acute care facilities, have been hospitalized in a country with high prevalence of CRE (commonly extending to the previous 12 months), or from close contacts of CRE-positive individuals (CDC, 2009; Richter and Marchaim, 2017; Berry *et al.*, 2019; PHE, 2020). Skin, wound or urine cultures (if a urinary catheter is in place) may also be taken. When considering a screening approach for veterinary patients to mirror this, it may be important to consider the animal's link to human healthcare, e.g. owners with an occupational or healthcare-associated risk factor for CRE carriage, as well as the patient risk factors. Repeated periodic screening within facilities for long-term hospitalized patients in high-risk units (e.g. the intensive care unit) is also supported by international groups (CDC, 2009; PHE, 2020). In the UK, repeat screening at 28 days is employed by some hospitals in high-risk units (Tucker *et al.*, 2019; PHE, 2020). Where it is challenging to screen patients based on their length of stay in a busy hospital environment, weekly or monthly screening may be undertaken in some high-risk units of all inpatients (CDC, 2015; Australian Commission on Safety and Quality in Health Care, 2017; PHE, 2020).

In the case of a single negative CRE culture, isolation is continued in the human setting until a further two negative cultures are received more than 48 h apart. For individuals that continue to be CRE negative, clinicians are encouraged to continually consider that these individuals are still high risk and that some medical management, such as antimicrobial use, could promote detectable CRE carriage (PHE, 2020). An individual who has at any time been positive for CRE (either by carriage or infection) is considered a suspected carrier at every new instance of hospitalization, regardless of the time that has elapsed since the positive result. During a single hospitalization episode, repeated screening of a CRE-positive individual is discouraged, as they are likely to remain positive for the duration of their stay (Tacconelli *et al.*, 2019). Effectively, in the case of CRE, a series of negative cultures appears to indicate a low likelihood of CRE shedding at that moment in time, provided that clinical management does not change. However, a negative culture is not considered to 'overwrite' a previous positive culture.

In animals, CRE continue to have a low worldwide prevalence, and so screening of individuals with no defined risk factors for carriage would be likely to have little benefit for the costs incurred. However, the impact of a CRE outbreak in a veterinary hospital would be significant, not least because most veterinarians would not have access to antimicrobials that could treat these infections, which could lead to high morbidity and mortality rates. Thus, veterinarians must remain vigilant for animals entering their premises with risk factors for carriage, predominantly that of owners with occupational risk (e.g. healthcare workers). However, it is likely that this is only discovered after a positive case of infection with a CRE because it is beyond the scope of veterinary work to question owners about their occupation and lifestyle at the time of their pet's hospitalization. Instead, veterinary screening for CRE should focus on individuals with confirmed CRE infections, at the time of detection and in any clinical management subsequently. It is important to note, as in human medicine, that a negative culture does not preclude CRE being detected at a later date (Zimmerman *et al.*, 2013; Tacconelli *et al.*, 2019). Therefore, it may not be considered an appropriate cost to be burdened by the client or the hospital to screen for CRE carriage if it will not change the management of the case in the hospital. Screening may only be suitable in the case of outbreak investigation. Due to the very low prevalence of CRE in veterinary medicine and the risk it poses if it enters our hospitals, it may be prudent to treat all previously confirmed CRE-positive animals as potential carriers in future and treat in isolation. Careful communication with clients of CRE-positive animals is important so that they understand home hygiene precautions, relay carrier status to any future veterinary practices that may care for their pet, and consider their own potential for exposure and carrier status should they require hospital care.

3.5 Practicalities of Screening for MDR Carriage

Screening for carriage of these pathogens is simply a tool for detection; all veterinary hospitals should consider that implementing the correct infrastructure to manage a positive case, when it arises, is paramount to successful infection control.

Cost implications for patient screening render it challenging; individual veterinary hospitals must decide whether these tests are covered by their own infection-control budget or by the client. Where possible, clear notification and discussion of the purpose of screening tests with the diagnostic microbiology laboratory may allow tailored, lower costs. However, it is likely that the reason for testing (surveillance versus clinical management of subsequent infections) may dictate who pays. In cases where active screening will not change case management (e.g. a previously MRSP- or CRE-positive animal may be treated in isolation irrespective of result), it could be argued that screening is only of benefit for local epidemiological purposes. In this case, it remains a valuable tool for outbreak investigation but is yet to become a key part of the infection-control strategy.

In areas with a low prevalence of these pathogens, a targeted surveillance approach, as discussed previously, may be favourable. It may also become prudent as prevalence rates of MDR pathogens rise to screen patients undergoing high-risk procedures, where practical, to pre-empt antimicrobial challenges before they arise (e.g. orthopaedic implants). The potential for catastrophic implications for morbidity and mortality as a result of these MDR pathogens, considering the restrictions in antimicrobial usage in veterinary medicine, drives practitioners to understand a patient's carriage status at the point of treatment. This could prompt changes in management and handling of a patient through the hospital, and may guide rapid, appropriate empirical antimicrobial therapy if bacterial infection occurs down the line.

In veterinary medicine, there is also an extra consideration that is not present for human hospitals. The epidemiological link of many of these pathogens to human medicine indicates the need for clients to be clearly informed of the outcome of patient screening and directed to their own medical practitioner if they feel that detection of these pathogens on their animal may present a risk to themselves.

3.6 Conclusion

In veterinary medicine, active surveillance through screening of healthy (or targeted) individuals is not yet a cornerstone measure for MDR pathogen control. However, it is clear that the use of screening to assess patients with previous MDR infections is an important tool to allow hospitals to mitigate the spread of these up-and-coming pathogens. Clearly, screening only becomes a worthwhile tool if knowledge of an individual's carrier status is used to prompt changes in case management and to guide empirical antimicrobial selection in invasive infections. It is possible that, in time or in regions where these pathogens are already widespread, screening of patients prior to high-risk procedures may be a necessary part of reducing potential morbidity and mortality. Overall, patient screening provides a multitude of epidemiological data for scientific interest, but its use as a clinical infection-control tool remains limited for now, albeit providing significant benefit in those cases where these pathogens are detected in subclinical individuals.

References

Australian Commission on Safety and Quality in Health Care (2017) Recommendations for the control of carbapenemase-producing *Enterobacteriaceae* (CPE): a guide for acute care health facilities: Australian Commission on Safety and Quality in Health Care. *Infection, Disease & Health* 22(4), 159–186. DOI: 10.1016/j.idh.2017.09.001.

Bannoehr, J. and Guardabassi, L. (2012) *Staphylococcus pseudintermedius* in the dog: taxonomy, diagnostics, ecology, epidemiology and pathogenicity. *Veterinary Dermatology* 23(4), 253–266. DOI: 10.1111/j.1365-3164.2012.01046.x.

Bastiaens, G.J.H., Baarslag, T., Pelgrum, C. and Mascini, E.M. (2020) Active surveillance for highly resistant microorganisms in patients with prolonged hospitalization. *Antimicrobial Resistance and Infection Control* 9(1), 8. DOI: 10.1186/s13756-019-0670-8.

Berry, C., Davies, K., Woodford, N., Wilcox, M. and Chilton, C. (2019) Survey of screening methods, rates and policies for the detection of carbapenemase-producing *Enterobacteriaceae* in English hospitals. *Journal of Hospital Infection* 101(2), 158–162. DOI: 10.1016/j.jhin.2018.08.005.

Börjesson, S., Gunnarsson, L., Landén, A. and Grönlund, U. (2020) Low occurrence of extended-spectrum cephalosporinase producing *Enterobacteriaceae* and no detection of methicillin-resistant coagulase-positive staphylococci in healthy dogs in Sweden.

Acta Veterinaria Scandinavica 62(1), 18. DOI: 10.1186/s13028-020-00516-4.

CDC (2009) Guidance for control of infections with carbapenem-resistant or carbapenemase-producing *Enterobacteriaceae* in acute care facilities. *Morbidity and Mortality Weekly Report* 58(10), 256–260.

CDC (2015) *Facility Guidance for Control of Carbapenem-Resistant Enterobacteriaceae (CRE): November 2015 Update – CRE Toolkit*. Centers for Disease Control and Prevention, Atlanta, Georgia. Available at: www.cdc.gov/hai/pdfs/cre/cre-guidance -508.pdf (accessed 17 October 2022).

Chipolombwe, J., Török, M.E., Mbelle, N. and Nyasulu, P. (2016) Methicillin-resistant *Staphylococcus aureus* multiple sites surveillance: a systemic review of the literature. *Infection and Drug Resistance* 9, 35–42. DOI: 10.2147/IDR.S95372.

Churak, A., Poolkhet, C., Tamura, Y., Sato, T., Fukuda, A. *et al.* (2021) Evaluation of nosocomial infections through contact patterns in a small animal hospital using social network analysis and genotyping techniques. *Scientific Reports* 11(1), 1647. DOI: 10.1038/ s41598-021-81301-9.

Coia, J.E., Wilson, J.A., Bak, A., Marsden, G.L., Shimonovich, M. *et al.* (2021) Joint Healthcare Infection Society (HIS) and Infection Prevention Society (IPS) guidelines for the prevention and control of meticillin-resistant *Staphylococcus aureus* (MRSA) in healthcare facilities. *Journal of Hospital Infection* 118S(Suppl), S1–S39. DOI: 10.1016/j. jhin.2021.09.022.

Cookson, B., Bonten, M.J.M., Mackenzie, F.M., Skov, R.L., Verbrugh, H.A. *et al.* (2011) Meticillin-resistant *Staphylococcus aureus* (MRSA): screening and decolonisation. *International Journal of Antimicrobial Agents* 37(3), 195–201. DOI: 10.1016/j. ijantimicag.2010.10.023.

Deeny, S.R., Cooper, B.S., Cookson, B., Hopkins, S. and Robotham, J.V. (2013) Targeted versus universal screening and decolonization to reduce healthcare-associated meticillin-resistant *Staphylococcus aureus* infection. *Journal of Hospital Infection* 85(1), 33–44. DOI: 10.1016/j.jhin.2013.03.011.

Devriese, L.A. and De Pelsmaecker, K. (1987) The anal region as a main carrier site of *Staphylococcus intermedius* and *Streptococcus canis* in dogs. *The Veterinary Record* 121(13), 302–303. DOI: 10.1136/ vr.121.13.302.

DoH (2014) *Implementation of Modified Admission MRSA Screening Guidance for NHS (2014): Department of Health Expert Advisory Committee on Antimicrobial Resistance and Healthcare Associated Infection (ARHAI)*. Department of Health, London. Available at: http://assets.publishing.service.gov.u k/government/uploads/system/uploads/attachment _data/file/345144/Implementation_of_modified_ad mission_MRSA_screening_guidance_for_NHS.pdf (accessed 17 October 2022).

EMA (2019) *Categorisation of Antibiotics in the European Union*. European Medicines Agency, Amsterdam. Available at: www.ema.europa.eu/en/documents/rep ort/categorisation-antibiotics-european-union-answer -request-european-commission-updating-scientific_e n.pdf (accessed 17 October 2022).

Frosini, S.M., Bond, R., King, R.H. and Loeffler, A. (2022) The nose is not enough: Multi-site sampling is best for MRSP detection in dogs and households. *Veterinary Dermatology* 3(6), 576–580. DOI: 10.1111/vde.13118.

Espadale, E., Pinchbeck, G., Williams, N.J., Timofte, D., McIntyre, K.M, *et al.* (2018) Are the hands of veterinary staff a reservoir for antimicrobial-resistant bacteria? A randomized study to evaluate two hand hygiene rubs in a veterinary hospital. *Microbial Drug Resistance* 24(10), 1607–1616. DOI: 10.1089/ mdr.2018.0183.

Frosini, S.M., Bond, R., King, R., Feudi, C., Schwarz, S. *et al.* (2021) Effect of topical antimicrobial therapy and household cleaning on meticillin-resistant *Staphylococcus pseudintermedius* carriage in dogs. *Veterinary Record* 190(8), e937. DOI: 10.1002/ vetr.937.

Fuller, C., Robotham, J., Savage, J., Hopkins, S., Deeny, S.R. *et al.* (2013) The national one week prevalence audit of universal meticillin-resistant *Staphylococcus aureus* (MRSA) admission screening 2012. *PloS One* 8(9), e74219. DOI: 10.1371/journal.pone.0074219.

Grmek-Kosnik, I., Dermota, U., Ribic, H., Storman, A., Petrovic, Z. *et al.* (2018) Evaluation of single vs pooled swab cultures for detecting MRSA colonization. *The Journal of Hospital Infection* 98(2), 149–154. DOI: 10.1016/j.jhin.2017.09.016.

Grönthal, T., Österblad, M., Eklund, M., Jalava, J., Nykäsenoja, S. *et al.* (2018) Sharing more than friendship - transmission of NDM-5 ST167 and CTX-M-9 ST69 *Escherichia coli* between dogs and humans in a family, Finland, 2015. *Euro Surveillance* 23(27), 1700497. DOI: 10.2807/1560-7917. ES.2018.23.27.1700497.

Hanselman, B.A., Kruth, S.A., Rousseau, J. and Weese, J.S. (2009) Coagulase positive staphylococcal colonization of humans and their household pets. *Canadian Veterinary Journal* 50, 954–958.

Hordijk, J., Schoormans, A., Kwakernaak, M., Duim, B., Broens, E. *et al.* (2013) High prevalence of fecal carriage of extended spectrum β-lactamase/AmpC-producing *Enterobacteriaceae* in cats and dogs. *Frontiers in Microbiology* 4, 242. DOI: 10.3389/ fmicb.2013.00242.

Huerta, B., Maldonado, A., Ginel, P.J., Tarradas, C., Gómez-Gascón, L. *et al.* (2011) Risk factors associated with the antimicrobial resistance of staphylococci in canine pyoderma. *Veterinary Microbiology* 150(3–4), 302–308. DOI: 10.1016/j.vetmic.2011.02.002.

Iverson, S.A., Brazil, A.M., Ferguson, J.M., Nelson, K., Lautenbach, E. *et al*. (2015) Anatomical patterns of colonization of pets with staphylococcal species in homes of people with methicillin-resistant *Staphylococcus aureus* (MRSA) skin or soft tissue infection (SSTI). *Veterinary Microbiology* 176(1–2), 202–208. DOI: 10.1016/j.vetmic.2015.01.003.

Kasai, T., Saegusa, S., Shirai, M., Murakami, M. and Kato, Y. (2016) New categories designated as healthcare-associated and community-associated methicillin-resistant *Staphylococcus pseudintermedius* in dogs. *Microbiology and Immunology* 60(8), 540–551. DOI: 10.1111/1348-0421.12401.

Kavanagh, K.T. (2019) Control of MSSA and MRSA in the United States: protocols, policies, risk adjustment and excuses. *Antimicrobial Resistance and Infection Control* 8, 103. DOI: 10.1186/s13756-019-0550-2.

Köck, R., Daniels-Haardt, I., Becker, K., Mellmann, A., Friedrich, A.W. *et al*. (2018) Carbapenem-resistant *Enterobacteriaceae* in wildlife, food-producing, and companion animals: a systematic review. *Clinical Microbiology and Infection* 24(12), 1241–1250. DOI: 10.1016/j.cmi.2018.04.004.

Lavigne, S.H., Cole, S.D., Daidone, C. and Rankin, S.C. (2021) Risk factors for the acquisition of a blaNDM-5 carbapenem-resistant Escherichia coli in a veterinary hospital. *Journal of the American Animal Hospital Association* 57(3), 101–105. DOI: 10.5326/JAAHA-MS-7105.

Lehner, G., Linek, M., Bond, R., Lloyd, D.H., Prenger-Berninghoff, E. *et al*. (2014) Case-control risk factor study of methicillin-resistant *Staphylococcus pseudintermedius* (MRSP) infection in dogs and cats in Germany. *Veterinary Microbiology* 168(1), 154–160. DOI: 10.1016/j.vetmic.2013.10.023.

Loeb, M.B., Main, C., Eady, A. and Walker-Dilks, C. (2003) Antimicrobial drugs for treating methicillin-resistant *Staphylococcus aureus* colonization. *Cochrane Database of Systematic Reviews* 4(4), CD003340. DOI: 10.1002/14651858.CD003340.

Loeffler, A., Pfeiffer, D.U., Lindsay, J.A., Soares Magalhães, R.J. and Lloyd, D.H. (2011) Prevalence of and risk factors for MRSA carriage in companion animals: a survey of dogs, cats and horses. *Epidemiology and Infection* 139(7), 1019–1028. DOI: 10.1017/S095026881000227X.

Logan, L.K. and Weinstein, R.A. (2017) The epidemiology of carbapenem-resistant *Enterobacteriaceae*: the impact and evolution of a global menace. *Journal of Infectious Diseases* 215(suppl.1), S28–S36. DOI: 10.1093/infdis/jiw282.

Madec, J.-Y., Haenni, M., Nordmann, P. and Poirel, L. (2017) Extended-spectrum β-lactamase/AmpC- and carbapenemase-producing *Enterobacteriaceae* in animals: a threat for humans? *Clinical Microbiology and Infection* 23(11), 826–833. DOI: 10.1016/j.cmi.2017.01.013.

Madueño, A., González García, J., Ramos, M.J., Pedroso, Y., Díaz, Z. *et al*. (2017) Risk factors associated with carbapenemase-producing *Klebsiella pneumoniae* fecal carriage: a case-control study in a Spanish tertiary care hospital. *American Journal of Infection Control* 45(1), 77–79. DOI: 10.1016/j.ajic.2016.06.024.

Martinez, J.L. (2014) General principles of antibiotic resistance in bacteria. *Drug Discovery Today: Technologies* 11, 33–39. DOI: 10.1016/j.ddtec.2014.02.001.

Nienhoff, U., Kadlec, K., Chaberny, I.F., Verspohl, J., Gerlach, G.-F. *et al*. (2011) Methicillin-resistant *Staphylococcus pseudintermedius* among dogs admitted to a small animal hospital. *Veterinary Microbiology* 150(1–2), 191–197. DOI: 10.1016/j.vetmic.2010.12.018.

Nigg, A., Brilhante, M., Dazio, V., Clément, M., Collaud, A. *et al*. (2019) Shedding of OXA-181 carbapenemase-producing *Escherichia coli* from companion animals after hospitalisation in Switzerland: an outbreak in 2018. *Euro Surveillance* 24(39), 1900071. DOI: 10.2807/1560-7917.ES.2019.24.39.1900071.

Nordmann, P. and Cornaglia, G. (2012) Carbapenemase-producing *Enterobacteriaceae*: a call for action! *Clinical Microbiology and Infection* 18(5), 411–412. DOI: 10.1111/j.1469-0691.2012.03795.x.

Ohno, Y., Nakamura, A., Hashimoto, E., Noguchi, N., Matsumoto, G. *et al*. (2020) Fecal carriage and molecular epidemiologic characteristics of carbapenemase-producing *Enterobacterales* in primary care hospital in a Japanese city. *Journal of Infection and Chemotherapy* 26(9), 928–932. DOI: 10.1016/j.jiac.2020.04.012.

Palacios-Baena, Z.R., Giannella, M., Manissero, D., Rodríguez-Baño, J., Viale, P. *et al*. (2021) Risk factors for carbapenem-resistant Gram-negative bacterial infections: a systematic review. *Clinical Microbiology and Infection* 27(2), 228–235. DOI: 10.1016/j.cmi.2020.10.016.

Perkins, A.V., Sellon, D.C., Gay, J.M., Lofgren, E.T., Moore, D.A. *et al*. (2020) Prevalence of methicillin-resistant *Staphylococcus pseudintermedius* on hand-contact and animal-contact surfaces in companion animal community hospitals. *Canadian Veterinary Journal* 61(6), 613–620.

PHE (2020) *Framework of Actions to Contain Carbapenemase-Producing Enterobacterales*. Public Health England, London. Available at: https://assets.publishing.service.gov.uk/government/uploads/system/uploads/attachment_data/file/926563/Framework_of_actions_to_contain_CPE-draft.pdf (accessed 17 October 2022).

Pires Dos Santos, T., Damborg, P., Moodley, A. and Guardabassi, L. (2016) Systematic review on global epidemiology of methicillin-resistant Staphylococcus pseudintermedius: inference of population structure from multilocus sequence typing data.

Frontiers in Microbiology 7, 1599. DOI: 10.3389/fmicb.2016.01599.

Puleston, R., Brown, C.S., Patel, B., Fry, C., Singleton, S. *et al.* (2020) Recommendations for detection and rapid management of carbapenemase-producing *Enterobacterales* outbreaks. *Infection Prevention in Practice* 2(3), 100086. DOI: 10.1016/j.infpip.2020.100086.

Richter, S.S. and Marchaim, D. (2017) Screening for carbapenem-resistant *Enterobacteriaceae*: Who, When, and How? *Virulence* 8(4), 417–426. DOI: 10.1080/21505594.2016.1255381.

Rossini, A., Di Santo, S.G., Libori, M.F., Tiracchia, V., Balice, M.P. *et al.* (2016) Risk factors for carbapenemase-producing *Enterobacteriaceae* colonization of asymptomatic carriers on admission to an Italian rehabilitation hospital. *Journal of Hospital Infection* 92(1), 78–81. DOI: 10.1016/j.jhin.2015.10.012.

Rubin, J.E. and Chirino-Trejo, M. (2011) Prevalence, sites of colonization, and antimicrobial resistance among *Staphylococcus pseudintermedius* isolated from healthy dogs in Saskatoon, Canada. *Journal of Veterinary Diagnostic Investigation* 23(2), 351–354. DOI: 10.1177/104063871102300227.

Saab, M.E., Muckle, C.A., Stryhn, H. and McClure, J.T. (2018) Comparison of culture methodology for the detection of methicillin-resistant *Staphylococcus pseudintermedius* in clinical specimens collected from dogs. *Journal of Veterinary Diagnostic Investigation* 30(1), 93–98. DOI: 10.1177/1040638717729396.

Schmidt, J.S., Kuster, S.P., Nigg, A., Dazio, V., Brilhante, M. *et al.* (2020) Poor infection prevention and control standards are associated with environmental contamination with carbapenemase-producing *Enterobacterales* and other multidrug-resistant bacteria in Swiss companion animal clinics. *Antimicrobial Resistance and Infection Control* 9(1), 93. DOI: 10.1186/s13756-020-00742-5.

Schmitt, K., Biggel, M., Stephan, R. and Willi, B. (2022) Massive spread of OXA-48 carbapenemase-producing *Enterobacteriaceae* in the environment of a Swiss companion animal clinic. *Antibiotics* 11(2), 213. DOI: 10.3390/antibiotics11020213.

Segagni Lusignani, L., Presterl, E., Zatorska, B., Van den Nest, M. and Diab-Elschahawi, M. (2020) Infection control and risk factors for acquisition of carbapenemase-producing *Enterobacteriaceae*. A 5 year (2011-2016) case-control study. *Antimicrobial Resistance and Infection Control* 9(1), 18. DOI: 10.1186/s13756-019-0668-2.

Souverein, D., Houtman, P., Euser, S.M., Herpers, B.L., Kluytmans, J. *et al.* (2016) Costs and benefits associated with the MRSA search and destroy policy in a hospital in the region Kennemerland, The Netherlands. *PloS One* 11(2), e0148175. DOI: 10.1371/journal.pone.0148175.

Tacconelli, E., Mazzaferri, F., de Smet, A.M., Bragantini, D., Eggimann, P. *et al.* (2019) ESCMID-EUCIC clinical guidelines on decolonization of multidrug-resistant Gram-negative bacteria carriers. *Clinical Microbiology and Infection* 25(7), 807–817. DOI: 10.1016/j.cmi.2019.01.005.

Tucker, A., George, R., Welfare, W., Cleary, P., Cawthorne, J. *et al.* (2019) Screening for carbapenemase-producing *Enterobacteriaceae* in previous carriers readmitted to hospital: evaluation of a change in screening policy. *Journal of Hospital Infection* 103(2), 156–159. DOI: 10.1016/j.jhin.2019.04.012.

Tumbarello, M., Viale, P., Viscoli, C., Trecarichi, E.M., Tumietto, F. *et al.* (2012) Predictors of mortality in bloodstream infections caused by *Klebsiella pneumoniae* carbapenemase-producing *K. pneumoniae*: importance of combination therapy. *Clinical Infectious Diseases* 55(7), 943–950. DOI: 10.1093/cid/cis588.

van Belkum, A. (2016) Hidden *Staphylococcus aureus* carriage: overrated or underappreciated? *MBio* 7(1), e00079–16. DOI: 10.1128/mBio.00079-16.

van den Bunt, G., Fluit, A.C., Spaninks, M.P., Timmerman, A.J., Geurts, Y. *et al.* (2020) Faecal carriage, risk factors, acquisition and persistence of ESBL-producing *Enterobacteriaceae* in dogs and cats and co-carriage with humans belonging to the same household. *Journal of Antimicrobial Chemotherapy* 75(2), 342–350. DOI: 10.1093/jac/dkz462.

van Duijkeren, E., Kamphuis, M., van der Mije, I.C., Laarhoven, L.M., Duim, B. *et al.* (2011) Transmission of methicillin-resistant *Staphylococcus pseudintermedius* between infected dogs and cats and contact pets, humans and the environment in households and veterinary clinics. *Veterinary Microbiology* 150(3–4), 338–343. DOI: 10.1016/j.vetmic.2011.02.012.

van Hout, D., Bruijning-Verhagen, P.C.J., Blok, H.E.M., Troelstra, A. and Bonten, M.J.M. (2021) Universal risk assessment upon hospital admission for screening of carriage with multidrug-resistant micro-organisms in a Dutch tertiary care centre. *The Journal of Hospital Infection* 109, 32–39. DOI: 10.1016/j.jhin.2020.12.007.

van Loon, K., Voor In 't Holt, A.F. and Vos, M.C. (2017) A systematic review and meta-analyses of the clinical epidemiology of carbapenem-resistant *Enterobacteriaceae*. *Antimicrobial Agents and Chemotherapy* 62(1), e01730-17. DOI: 10.1128/AAC.01730-17.

Wagenvoort, J.H.T. (2000) Dutch measures to control MRSA and the expanding European Union. *Euro Surveillance* 5(3), 26–28. DOI: 10.2807/esm.05.03.00031-en.

Wernitz, M.H., Keck, S., Swidsinski, S., Schulz, S. and Veit, S.K. (2005) Cost analysis of a hospital-wide selective screening programme

Sian-Marie Frosini and Rosanne Jepson

for methicillin-resistant *Staphylococcus aureus* (MRSA) carriers in the context of diagnosis related groups (DRG) payment. *Clinical Microbiology and Infection* 11(6), 466–471. DOI: 10.1111/j.1469-0691.2005.01153.x.

Wertheim, H.F.L., Vos, M.C., Boelens, H.A.M., Voss, A., Vandenbroucke-Grauls, C.M.J.E, *et al.* (2004) Low prevalence of methicillin-resistant *Staphylococcus aureus* (MRSA) at hospital admission in the Netherlands: the value of search and destroy and restrictive antibiotic use. *Journal of Hospital Infection* 56(4), 321–325. DOI: 10.1016/j.jhin.2004.01.026.

Windahl, U., Gren, J., Holst, B.S. and Börjesson, S. (2016) Colonization with methicillin-resistant *Staphylococcus pseudintermedius* in multi-dog households: a longitudinal study using whole genome sequencing. *Veterinary Microbiology* 189, 8–14. DOI: 10.1016/j.vetmic.2016.04.010.

Windahl, U., Reimegård, E., Holst, B.S., Egenvall, A., Fernström, L, *et al.* (2012) Carriage of methicillin-resistant Staphylococcus pseudintermedius in dogs--a longitudinal study. *BMC Veterinary Research* 8, 34. DOI: 10.1186/1746-6148-8-34.

Yamamoto, N., Asada, R., Kawahara, R., Hagiya, H., Akeda, Y. *et al.* (2017) Prevalence of, and risk factors for, carriage of carbapenem-resistant *Enterobacteriaceae* among hospitalized patients in Japan. *Journal of Hospital Infection* 97(3), 212–217. DOI: 10.1016/j.jhin.2017.07.015.

Zimmerman, F.S., Assous, M.V., Bdolah-Abram, T., Lachish, T., Yinnon, A.M. *et al.* (2013) Duration of carriage of carbapenem-resistant *Enterobacteriaceae* following hospital discharge. *American Journal of Infection Control* 41(3), 190–194. DOI: 10.1016/j.ajic.2012.09.020.

4 Hand Hygiene

Steven Murphy[1], Caitlin Forbes[2], Katie Smyth[2] and Kelly L. Bowlt Blacklock[3]*

[1]Southern Counties Veterinary Specialists, Hangersley, Ringwood, UK; [2]Vets Now, Glasgow, UK; [3]Royal (Dick) School of Veterinary Studies, University of Edinburgh, Roslin, UK

4.1 Introduction

For centuries, handwashing with soap and water has been associated with cleanliness, being deeply embedded in religious and cultural habits. However, it was only in the 1800s that the link between hand hygiene and disease transmission was considered. The hero of this story is Hungarian Ignaz Semmelweis, who worked as a house officer in the University of Vienna and observed that the maternal mortality rates secondary to puerperal fever were enormously higher in doctor-led clinics compared with midwife-led clinics. He theorized that this was the result of 'cadaverous particles' that were carried on the hands of doctors and students who spent the morning in the autopsy room and the afternoon in the delivery room. This was a controversial theory at a time when experienced staff attributed the differences in mortality to the mainstream theory of 'miasma' or poisonous air within the doctor-led ward. It remains unclear how the 'miasma' did not reach the adjacent and more crowded midwife-led ward. However, when Jakob Kolletschka, a colleague of Semmelweis, died in 1847 following a scalpel cut during an autopsy, Semmelweis recognized that the lesions on Kolletschka's body mirrored those of his patients with puerperal fever. Convinced of his theory, Semmelweis ordered that all medical staff in the doctor-led ward should wash their hands in chlorinated lime before attending a patient, and within 2 years, the mortality rate plummeted. Semmelweis presented his evidence to the medical profession and came under immediate attack from his contemporaries. Doctors were outraged at the suggestion that their hands might be unclean – an insult to their status as gentlemen.

Semmelweis was ultimately dismissed from his position, but was encouraged to publish his findings by friends and did so in 1861 as a tome entitled *Die Ätiologie, der Begriff und die Prophylaxe des Kindbettfiebers* (*Etiology, Concept and Prophylaxis of Childbed Fever*). Unfortunately, the work was a mass of statistics and almost impossible to read. It was met with hostility and was mocked, leading Semmelweis to compose increasingly irate open letters to his critics, calling them 'murderers'. A lifetime's fight to illuminate the link between hand hygiene and disease transmission took its toll on Semmelweis. He suffered from depression and was tricked into visiting a mental asylum. Once there, he was admitted as a patient and a struggle ensued, during which Semmelweis sustained an injury to his hand. The wound became infected and he died of septicaemia while in the asylum in 1865, aged 47. Few people attended the funeral of this pioneer of infection control.

Fortunately, we now accept that scrupulous hand hygiene is a cornerstone of infection-control practice, being the cheapest and most effective single method to reduce infection risk. However, the Semmelweis reflex (a metaphor for the reflex-like tendency to reject new evidence or new knowledge because it contradicts established norms, beliefs or paradigms) rages on: healthcare workers always believe that it is their peers, never themselves, who are the culprits in poor hand hygiene compliance ratings. To this end, the World Health Organization (WHO) runs an annual *SAVE LIVES: Clean Your Hands* campaign, which aims to progress the goal of maintaining a global profile on the importance of hand hygiene

*Corresponding author: Kelly.blacklock@ed.ac.uk

in healthcare and to 'bring people together' in support of hand hygiene improvement. The authors encourage interested readers to visit the WHO website (WHO, 2022) and access the free Campaign Advocacy Toolkit, which provides a clear, user-friendly framework for advocacy, as well as guidance on how to develop campaign materials at the local level.

This chapter will provide further information on handwashing techniques and surveillance. Further information pertaining to surgical hand hygiene is detailed in Chapter 5 (this volume).

4.2 Hand Hygiene: When and How

Infection prevention and control guidelines were initially developed within human hospital settings after the occurrence of localized healthcare-associated infections (HAIs) involving *Clostridioides difficile*, *Pseudomonas aeruginosa*, *Salmonella* spp. and methicillin-resistant *Staphylococcus aureus* (MRSA). Hand hygiene is at the forefront of these guidelines. The WHO recommends using hand hygiene before and after each point of exposure (WHO, 2022), and promotes the 'five key moments' for hand hygiene surrounding patient interaction (Fig. 4.1).

Hospital staff uniforms were commonly found to be contaminated with MRSA and *C. difficile* (Perry *et al.*, 2001). These findings elicited a change to hospital uniform policies and guidelines to facilitate handwashing and prevent contamination. Protocols now recommend that staff must be uncovered from below the elbows, no jewellery may be worn, and physicians are not allowed to wear long-sleeved white coats (or indeed any other colour if the garment has long sleeves) or ties. This is known as the 'bare below the elbows' approach.

In addition to handwashing being performed at key moments (Fig. 4.1), the method of handwashing used is important to ensure optimal bacterial decontamination. The backs of the hands and fingertips are commonly missed when the hands are cleaned, and therefore an effective and standardized technique has been formulated by the Centres for Disease Control and Prevention (CDC) and WHO (Fig. 4.2).

Alcohol-based hand rub is an effective alternative to soap and water in circumstances when these resources are not available, and where the hands are not visibly soiled but require decontamination

(WHO, 2009a; Hadaway, 2020). When the hands are soiled, hand washing with soap and water is required. The technique involved for effective alcohol hand rub is similar to the handwashing technique (Fig. 4.3).

4.3 Impediments to Hand Hygiene: Fomites

Hands are seen as a vector for infection and could act as potential fomites (Mann, 2016). The recommended 'bare below the elbow' approach aims to encourage and facilitate regular hand hygiene and reduce interpatient contact from sleeves, watches and rings.

4.3.1 Jewellery

Wearing jewellery within the clinical setting has become a controversial subject. Wearing bracelets, rings or watches is thought to reduce the efficacy of hand washing, and therefore current recommendations are that all jewellery is removed from the hands and forearms (Hoffman *et al.*, 1985; Salisbury *et al.*, 1997; Mangram *et al.*, 1999; Hayes *et al.*, 2001; CDC, 2002; Trick *et al.*, 2003; Fagernes and Nord, 2007; Yildirim *et al.*, 2008; Khodavaisy *et al.*, 2011). Additionally, jewellery presents the possibility of causing glove perforations when wearing non-sterile or sterile gloves (Waterman *et al.*, 2006). Importantly, all of the studies used to support these recommendations are small scale, and therefore strong evidence from which to draw robust conclusions is lacking.

In human medicine, wearing rings has been associated with:

- increased risk of hand colonization by Gram-negative bacilli or potentially pathogenic bacteria (Hoffman *et al.*, 1985), despite use of an alcohol-based hand antiseptic solution (Yildirim *et al.*, 2008);
- tenfold higher median skin organism count, contamination with *S. aureus*, Gram-negative bacilli or *Candida* spp., and a stepwise increased risk of contamination with any transient organism as the number of rings worn increased (odds ratio of 2.6 for one ring worn and 4.6 for more than one ring worn) (Trick *et al.*, 2003); and
- increased bacterial counts (representing a danger of infection) on all rings (Khodavaisy *et al.*, 2011), with significantly greater counts

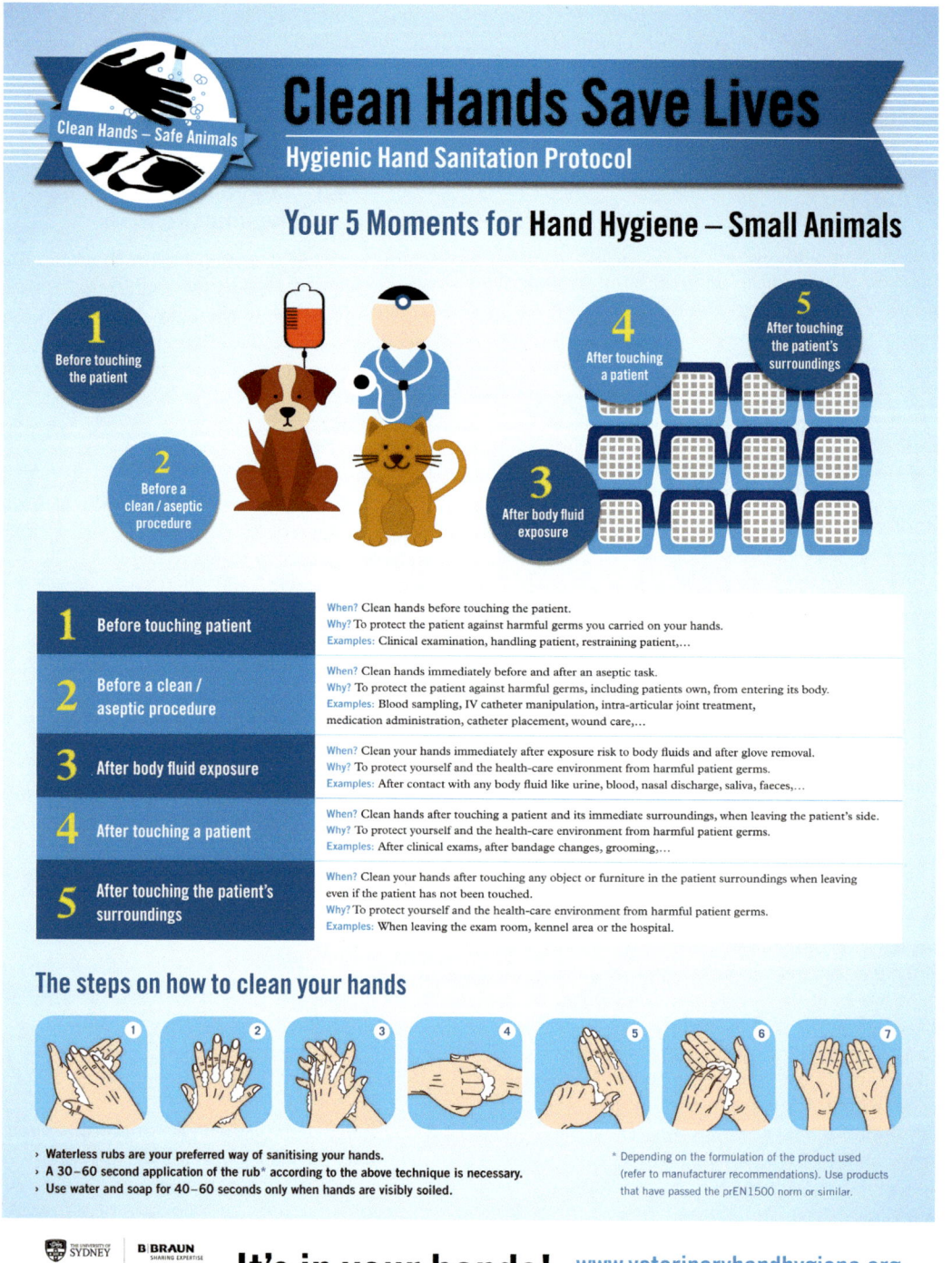

Fig. 4.1. Five key moments for hand hygiene surrounding patient interaction. Adapted from WHO (2022) guidelines. © Denis Verwilghen. Used with permission.

Hand Hygiene

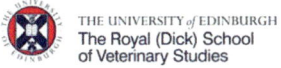
Hand Washing Technique with Soap and Water

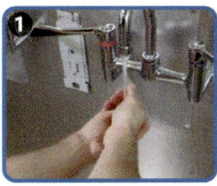

1 Wet hands with water

2 Apply enough soap to cover all hand surfaces

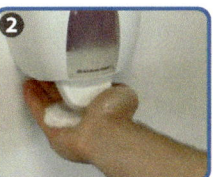

3 Rub hands palm to palm

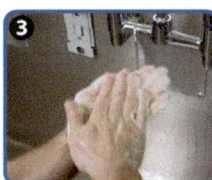

4 Rub back of each hand with the palm of the other hand with fingers interlaced

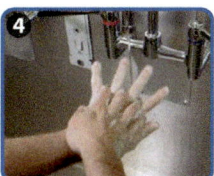

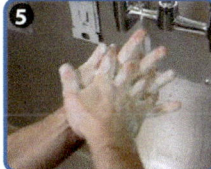

5 Rub palm to palm with fingers interlaced

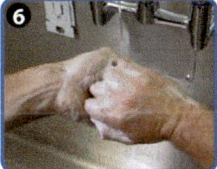

6 Rub with back of fingers to opposing palms with fingers interlocking and vice versa

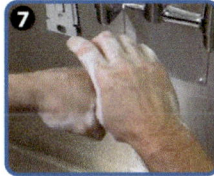

7 Rub each thumb clasped in opposite hand using a rotational movement

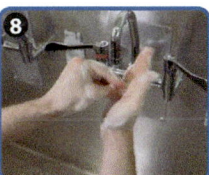

8 Rub tips of fingers in opposite palm in a circular motion

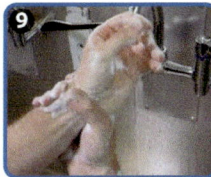

9 Rub each wrist with the opposite hand using a rotational movement

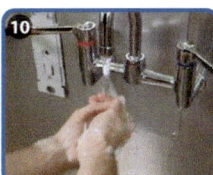

10 Rinse hands with water

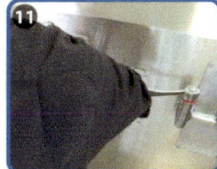

11 Use elbow to turn off tap

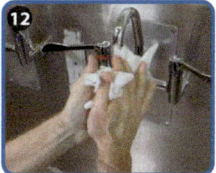

12 Dry thoroughly with disposable paper towel

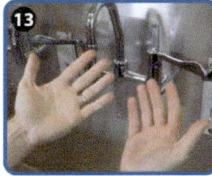

13 Hand washing should take 40-60 seconds

** Steps 3 to 9 require a minimum of 5 repetitions

qrs.ly/cp4u5t7

Digitial Education Unit

Fig. 4.2. Handwashing technique with soap and water. From Mosley and Mather (2019) with permission.

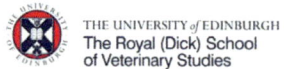
Hand Rub Technique with Alcohol Gel

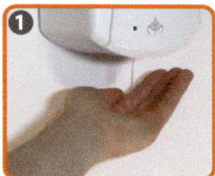

Apply sufficient alcohol gel to a cupped hand to cover all surfaces

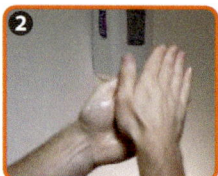

Rub hands palm to palm

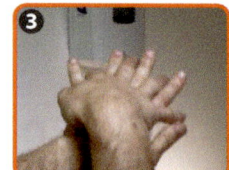

Rub back of each hand with the palm of the other hand with fingers interlaced

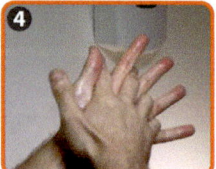

Rub palm to palm with fingers interlaced

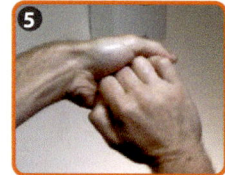

Rub with back of fingers to opposing palms with fingers interlocking and vice versa

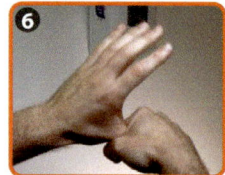

Rub each thumb clasped in opposite hand using a rotational movement

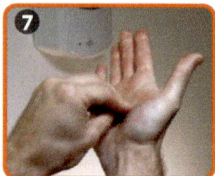

Rub tips of fingers in opposite palm in a circular motion

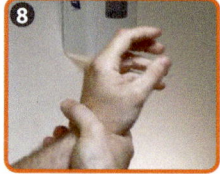

Rub each wrist with the opposite hand using a rotational movement

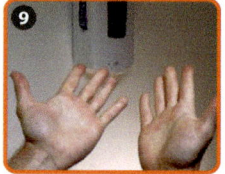

Allow hands to air dry

** Steps 2 to 8 require a minimum of 3 repetitions

qrs.ly/zg4tbjg

Digitial Education Unit

Fig. 4.3. Hand-rub technique with alcohol gel. From Mosley and Mather (2019) with permission.

identified on non-plain rings (Fagernes and Nord, 2007).

In contrast to the above, one study reported no difference in bacterial colonization following a surgical scrub between ring-wearing and non-ring hands of surgeons and anaesthesiologists who wore wedding rings (Al-Allak *et al.*, 2008). These findings were mirrored by a retrospective study showing no increase in surgical-site infections when a wedding ring is or is not worn under the surgical glove, although this study was probably underpowered to determine a difference of this nature as only 2127 patients were enrolled over 4 years (Stein and Pankovich-Wargula, 2009).

The Association of Surgical Technologists have issued *Guidelines for Best Practices for Wearing Jewelry*, based on research published in the Cochrane Database of Systematic Reviews and MEDLINE, the US National Library of Medicine database (AST, 2017). The guidelines contain the following recommendations:

- It is the responsibility of surgical team members to follow CDC standards for recommended operating room attire.
- Non-sterile and sterile surgical team members should remove all jewellery, including facial and oral jewellery prior to entering the operating room.
- The surgery department should review the policy and procedures regarding sterile attire and wearing jewellery on an annual basis.
- Theatre staff should complete continuing education to remain current in their knowledge of hand hygiene practices including the surgical scrub, sterile attire and wearing jewellery.

Evidence pertaining to ring wearing in veterinary staff is scanter than that available for human medicine. Despite this, hand hygiene protocols devised for veterinary use are heavily extrapolated from CDC recommendations and advise that a 'bare below the elbows' approach is maintained, with no jewellery or wristwatches worn (FECAVA, 2019; BEVA, 2022).

4.3.2 Nail polish and nail length

Studies have documented that bacterial growth is most likely to occur along the proximal 1 mm of the nail adjacent to subungual skin (Pottinger *et al.*, 1989; Wynd *et al.*, 1994; McNeil *et al.*, 2001). This site is the most likely region of the

hand to be contaminated with high concentrations of bacteria (especially coagulase-negative staphylococci and Gram-negative rods (including *Pseudomonas* spp.); McGinley *et al.*, 1988; Hedderwick *et al.*, 2000), and can still harbour substantial numbers of potential pathogens after careful handwashing (Gross *et al.*, 1979; Pottinger *et al.*, 1989; McNeil *et al.*, 2001). In human medicine, freshly applied nail polish does not increase the bacterial contamination of the periungual skin, but chipped nail polish may support the growth of larger numbers of organisms on fingernails (Baumgardner *et al.*, 1993; Wynd *et al.*, 1994). In a small veterinary study, professional application of gel nail polish did not seem to affect the ability of surgical scrub to reduce bacterial viability 1 and 14 days after a manicure; however, increasing nail length was correlated with increased bacterial colony-forming units (Anderson *et al.*, 2022). A further study investigated bacterial counts and types of isolates obtained from hands of veterinary surgical personnel, reporting no relationship between the number of colony-forming units and nail biting, staff role, duration of the surgery, whether the nail polish was chipped, duration of nail polish application, type of surgery and handedness. However, higher bacterial counts were isolated from staff with nail lengths greater than 2 mm (Hardy *et al.*, 2017).

Whether or not artificial nails contribute to transmission of HAIs remains unclear. However, research in human medicine has shown that healthcare workers who wear artificial nails are more likely to harbour Gram-negative pathogens than those who have natural nails, both before and after handwashing (Rubin, 1988; Pottinger *et al.*, 1989; McNeil *et al.*, 2001; CDC, 2002). Of particular concern is a report concerning an outbreak of *P. aeruginosa* in a neonatal intensive care unit, which was linked to two nurses (one with long natural nails and one with long artificial nails) who carried the *Pseudomonas* sp. strain on their hands (Moolenaar *et al.*, 2000; CDC, 2002). Personnel wearing artificial nails also have been epidemiologically implicated in several other outbreaks of infection caused by Gram-negative bacilli and yeast (Passaro *et al.*, 1997; Foca *et al.*, 2000; Parry *et al.*, 2001; CDC, 2002).

The CDC *Guideline for Hand Hygiene in Healthcare Settings* (CDC, 2002) states the following:

- Germs can live under artificial fingernails both before and after using an alcohol-based hand sanitizer and handwashing.
- It is recommended that healthcare providers do not wear artificial fingernails or extensions when having direct contact with patients at high risk (e.g. those in intensive care units or operating rooms).

4.4 Maintaining Skin Health

Good hand skin care is essential in optimal infection-control practice. Ensuring good skin health reduces dermatitis, fissures and cracks within the dermis, therefore minimizing sites for bacterial colonization. Factors that can contribute to dermatitis associated with frequent handwashing include using hot water, low relative humidity, failure to use supplementary hand lotion or cream, paper towel quality, allergies to latex gloves and irritant contact dermatitis.

4.4.1 Using hot water

Increased water temperature causes increased skin penetration and irritant capacity of a detergent. In one study, immersion of the arms of healthy volunteers into 40°C water and detergent caused significantly increased transepidermal water loss compared with immersion into 20°C water and detergent (Ohlenschlaeger *et al.*, 1996). Therefore, it is important to choose the right (low) temperature when working with detergent solutions to reduce the risk of developing irritant contact reactions (Emilson *et al.*, 1993).

4.4.2 Low relative humidity (especially during winter or in air-conditioned buildings)

The National Health Service (NHS) recommends that ventilation systems should maintain a temperature of 18–22°C and a relative humidity of 30–70%. In an operating suite, the temperature should be adjustable between 18°C and 25°C by staff, and humidity should fall between 35% and 60% (NHS, 2021). Continuous monitoring of humidity is recommended, because low humidity results in increased risk of skin problems such as dermatitis (Sato *et al.*, 2003; Chou *et al.*, 2007).

4.4.3 Failure to use supplementary hand lotion or cream

Hand lotions and creams contribute to the barrier function of normal skin by replacing skin lipids that may have been lost through handwashing. In human medicine, twice-daily application of hand creams prevents irritant contact dermatitis, improves skin condition and leads to a 50% increase in handwashing frequency (Berndt *et al.*, 2000; McCormick *et al.*, 2000). Interestingly, using hand lotion reduces skin scaling and cracking, which also reduces microbial shedding (Berndt *et al.*, 2000; McCormick *et al.*, 2000). Therefore, the CDC recommends that free skin-care lotion should be provided, and personnel educated regarding the value of regular use of hand-care products (CDC, 2002). Importantly, further research is required to determine whether oil-containing products impact the integrity of gloves (especially latex) (Jones *et al.*, 2000) or the efficacy of antiseptic agents (Larson *et al.*, 1993). However, many companies who manufacture hand hygiene products will also produce a compatible skin-care product.

4.4.4 Paper towel quality

In human medicine, a recent evidence review found that paper towels can dry hands more efficiently, remove bacteria more effectively and cause less contamination of the washroom environment compared with electric air dryers (Huang *et al.*, 2012). Additionally, the use of air dryers may cause the skin on the hands to become irritated and damaged, resulting in poor compliance with hand washing. Therefore, paper towels should preferentially be recommended in locations where hygiene is paramount, such as hospitals and clinics.

Environmental sustainability is a concern in relation to using paper towels: recycled paper can contribute to environmental sustainability, and there is no difference in bacterial reduction when one or two paper towels are used for hand drying (Suen *et al.*, 2019). However, the quality of the paper towel should be considered, and additional research is needed in this regard. Poor-quality towels can be abrasive or ineffective at drying, which damages the skin. Additionally, different absorption characteristics of towels influence their capacity to remove bacteria from washed hands (Gould, 1995; Gustafson *et al.*, 2000; Jumaa, 2005; Huang *et al.*, 2012).

4.4.5 Allergies to latex gloves

Latex products are manufactured using fluid from the rubber tree, *Hevea brasiliensis*. Natural rubber latex contains 15 proven allergens, which can cause a range of hypersensitive immune responses, including coughing, asthma and death from severe anaphylaxis (Wu *et al.*, 2016). Direct skin contact with latex-derived products is the primary route for developing a latex allergy. Studies on health-care workers have suggested that latex sensitivity appears to build up and increase with exposure time (Vangveeravong *et al.*, 2011; Turner *et al.*, 2012). On the skin, latex sensitization can manifest as itchy skin and urticaria, but the chemicals used during the processing and manufacture process have also been associated with skin rashes. Reported data suggest that the average prevalence of latex allergy worldwide is 9.7%, 7.2% and 4.3% among healthcare workers, susceptible patients and the general population, respectively (Wu *et al.*, 2016). Therefore, the use of latex gloves should be avoided wherever possible, and the authors maintain a completely latex-free hospital.

The CDC's National Institute for Occupational Safety and Health raised concerns regarding powdered gloves, including surgical complications related to peritoneal adhesions, aerosolization and inhalation of allergenic latex-coated particles, and non-surgical adverse events such as inflammatory responses to glove powder. As a result, the US Food and Drug Administration (FDA) subsequently banned the use of powdered medical gloves in the USA (FDA, 2016a, b).

4.4.6 Irritant contact dermatitis

Frequent and repeated use of hand hygiene products, especially soaps and detergents, is a primary cause of chronic irritant contact dermatitis among healthcare workers (Tupker, 1996; CDC, 2002). In veterinary studies, the overall prevalence of hand dermatitis is up to 22%, with prevalence being significantly higher in women and those with current allergic disease or a latex allergy (Susitaival *et al.*, 2001; Leggat *et al.*, 2009). Affected individuals complain of dry and/or rough skin, erythema, formation of swellings or blisters, itching, scaling or fissures on the hands, which are caused by the detergent denaturing stratum corneum proteins, altering intracellular lipids, decreasing skin water-binding capacity and decreasing corneocyte cohesion (Wilhelm, 1996; CDC, 2002), As well as causing a decrease in compliance with hand hygiene protocols, the skin damage caused by irritant contact dermatitis alters skin flora, resulting in more frequent colonization and secondary infection by staphylococci and Gram-negative bacilli (Larson *et al.*, 1998; Gallagher and Sunley, 2012). Irritant contact dermatitis is most commonly reported with iodophors and is extremely uncommon with alcohol-based hand rubs (Larson *et al.*, 1986; Widmer, 2000).

Options for minimizing hand hygiene-related irritant contact dermatitis includes replacing products with preparations that cause less damage to the skin (e.g. promoting the use of alcohol-based hand rubs containing emollients instead of soap where appropriate), and using moisturizing skin products or barrier creams.

4.5 Hand Hygiene Products

The appropriate choice of hand hygiene products is key to reducing HAIs in the clinical setting. Several products are available for use as hand hygiene products, and the most commonly utilized products in veterinary medicine are illustrated in Table 4.1. Additional information, and details pertaining to hand hygiene products for surgical hand preparation, is provided in Chapter 5 (this volume).

Importantly, all hand hygiene products can become contaminated with bacteria, including Gram-negative bacilli, which has resulted in outbreaks of HAIs (Marrie and Costerton, 1981; McAllister *et al.*, 1989; Vigeant *et al.*, 1998; Vu-Thien *et al.*, 1998; Hsueh *et al.*, 1999; Sartor *et al.*, 2000; Wong *et al.*, 2018). Of huge concern is the development of bacterial resistance to hand hygiene products, some of which have resulted in HAIs and include chlorhexidine-resistant *Serratia marcescens* (Keck *et al.*, 2020; Allen *et al.*, 2022) and *P. aeruginosa* strains that are pan-resistant to triclosan and chlorhexidine (Beier *et al.*, 2015). Additionally, the widespread use of triclosan, including in many contemporary and personal healthcare products (e.g. soaps and oral products), may represent a public health risk because of the link between triclosan resistance and resistance to other antimicrobials, especially in *Escherichia coli* and *Salmonella* spp. (Yazdankhah *et al.*, 2006).

4.6 Use of Gloves as Personal Protective Equipment

As an item of personal protective equipment, gloves have long been seen as the front line in

Table 4.1. Commonly used products for hand hygiene in veterinary practice (CDC, 2002). Further details regarding surgical hand preparation can be found in Chapter 5 (this volume).

Preparation	Mode of action	Advantages	Disadvantages	Residual activity
Plain (non-antimicrobial) soap	Detergent physically removes dirt and organic matter but has no antimicrobial effect	Cheap and widely available	Can be drying to skin, although emollients can be added	None
Alcohol-based products	Antimicrobial: denatures proteins of microorganisms; 60–95% alcohol is most effective	Excellent activity against bacteria (including multidrug-resistant organisms), fungi and certain enveloped viruses Greater reduction in bacterial counts on hands following use of alcohol-based products compared with antimicrobial soaps or detergents Contact dermatitis is uncommon	Poor activity against bacterial spores, protozoan oocysts and some non-enveloped viruses Not suitable for use when hands are grossly soiled Flammable	None
Chlorhexidine	Antimicrobial: disrupts cytoplasmic membranes, causing the cell to rupture; 4% chlorhexidine is most effective	Good activity against Gram-positive bacteria and enveloped viruses, but less activity against Gram-negative bacteria and fungi Antimicrobial activity only minimally affected by organic material Allergic reactions are uncommon	Minimal activity against tubercle bacilli and non-enveloped viruses, and no activity against spores. Activity reduced by anionic products such as natural soaps, non-ionic surfactants and hand creams containing anionic emulsifying agents Frequency of skin irritation is concentration dependent: use of 4% chlorhexidine for frequent hand hygiene is most likely to cause contact dermatitis	See[a]
Iodine and iodophors	Antimicrobial: rapidly penetrates the cell wall, damaging proteins, nucleotides and fatty acids, leading to rapid cell death Povidone-iodine 5–10% is recommended by the FDA as an antiseptic hand wash (although 7.5–10% is most commonly used)	Good activity against Gram-positive and -negative bacteria, mycobacteria, viruses and fungi Some activity against spore-forming bacteria	No activity against spores. Antimicrobial activity is substantially reduced in the presence of organic material More irritant contact dermatitis is seen with use of iodophor preparations than any other antiseptic hand hygiene products	See[b]

Continued

Table 4.1. Continued

Preparation	Mode of action	Advantages	Disadvantages	Residual activity
Triclosan	Antimicrobial: enters bacterial cells and blocks lipid biosynthesis Concentrations of 0.2–2% have antimicrobial properties	Good activity against Gram-positive bacteria and enveloped viruses Antimicrobial activity only minimally affected by organic material Bacterial counts on hands are lower after triclosan use compared with use of chlorhexidine, iodophors or alcohol-based hand rubs Allergic reactions are uncommon	Less activity against Gram-negative bacteria (especially *P. aeruginosa*) and fungi	Yes; this is affected by pH, the presence of surfactants or emollients, and the ionic nature of the particular formulation

[a]The World Health Organization (WHO) and Centres for Disease Control and Prevention (CDC) describes residual activity of chlorhexidine as 'substantial'. However, authors have questioned whether the study methodology to achieve this recommendation accurately simulates real-world conditions. Specifically, the use of liquid bacterial suspensions to contaminate the skin introduces an unrealistic amount of moisture, which may leave the skin wet for several minutes after application. In clinical situations, hands are typically contaminated by touching dry objects or skin. In one study where participants touched stainless steel discs containing dried *Staphylococcus aureus*, no reduction in bacteria on the chlorhexidine-treated hands was observed for up to 15 min, suggesting that residual chlorhexidine does not offer protection against contamination with transient microorganisms in clinical practice (Rutter *et al.*, 2014). The clinical implications of these findings were challenged subsequently: researchers demonstrated a zone of inhibited growth of *S. aureus* inoculated on to an agar plate where, prior to bacterial inoculation, a fingertip, sanitized 1 h previously with chlorhexidine, touched the agar surface for 15 s (Macias *et al.*, 2015). In the absence of evidence, clinicians should not rely on a residual activity of chlorhexidine to be protective, and frequent use of alcohol-based hand rubs, handwashing and proper glove use in accordance with established guidelines remain the only demonstrably effective means of protecting the hands from transient microorganisms.
[b]Residual activity of iodophors is seen, although the evidence is unclear. Studies have shown that persistent activity has been associated with povidone-iodine for as little as 30–60 min or as long as 6 h, depending on study design (Galle *et al.*, 1978; Peterson *et al.*, 1978; Aly and Maibach, 1983; Pereira *et al.*, 1990; Wade and Casewell, 1991; Hingst *et al.*, 1992; Paulson, 1994; Faoagali *et al.*, 1995; Herruzo-Cabrera *et al.*, 2000).
FDA, US Food and Drug Administration.

protection, for both the wearer and their patients. It was Halsted who first advocated the use of gloves during surgical procedures. Initially, gloves (made by the Goodyear Tire and Rubber Company) were provided to protect the hands of the chief surgical nurse, Caroline Hampton, who suffered from contact dermatitis. However, it was only later that Halstead realized the significance of glove use as a means of avoiding surgical infections: 'It is remarkable that…we could have been so blind as not to have perceived the necessity for wearing them invariably at the operating table.' One of Halsted's assistants is quoted as saying 'Venus came to the aid of Aesculapius' because Halsted and Hampton married in June 1890.

Single-use disposable gloves offer invaluable protection to both the healthcare worker and their patients when used appropriately and in conjunction with effective hand hygiene measures. Gloves

protect the wearer from exposure to any potential pathogens from infected or infectious matter from their patients, as well as protecting their patients from exposure to any pathogens that the healthcare worker may have on their hands.

However, the use of non-sterile gloves still carries a significant potential for cross-contamination and transmission of HAIs, because they are often used when they are not needed, donned too early, doffed too late or not changed at critical points (Loveday *et al.*, 2014). In response to this, Great Ormond Street Hospital NHS Foundation Trust led the 'The gloves are off' education campaign, whereby staff were educated and empowered to only wear gloves when contact with patient bodily fluids was expected, or when they were administering therapeutically active cream, liquid hormones or cytotoxic medication (NHS, 2018). The campaign led to a reduction in staff attending occupational health for hand- or skin-related problems, no adverse rise in HAIs and an 18% reduction in glove use.

It is imperative that clinical staff know that the use of gloves does not replace the requirement for effective hand hygiene. Non-sterile examination gloves should only be worn when there is a risk of contamination from blood or other bodily fluids, or from zoonotic or transmissible diseases (e.g. dermatophytosis), or when administering drugs that may damage or be absorbed through the skin. When performing non-invasive procedures such as taking a pulse or a Doppler blood pressure, gloves should not be worn and hand hygiene alone is sufficient. The WHO recommends the use of alcohol gel before donning and after doffing disposable gloves, which protects against previous hand contamination, as well as from glove defects or cross-contamination. This is essential because bacterial flora that are colonizing patients may be recovered from the hands of up to 30% of healthcare workers who wear gloves during patient contact. In such instances, pathogens presumably gain access to the caregiver's hands via small defects in the gloves or by contamination of the hands during glove removal (WHO, 2009b).

The recommended technique for donning and doffing non-sterile examination gloves is detailed in Fig. 4.4.

Gloves should be removed to perform hand hygiene and should be disposed of safely immediately after use. The reuse or reprocessing of single-use disposable gloves should be avoided as there is not currently an effective way to decontaminate gloves without damaging them. Studies on glove permeability have shown that, after 10 min, alcohol can permeate any type of glove, and some types of gloves are permeated after only 2 min (ECDC, 2020) Other measures of glove decontamination, such as ethylene oxide and peroxide, also showed comparable damage.

Choosing the glove correct size is important: an overly tight glove can influence the wearer's circulation as well as causing damage to the glove's integrity, while an overly loose glove may slip, causing contamination and reducing tactility. Powdered gloves have a slightly higher amount of grip when compared with powder-free gloves and will be absorbent to any residual dampness from hand hygiene products or sweat. However, powdered gloves are more prone to damage and are banned in the American healthcare system (FDA, 2016a, b).

Despite this, powdered gloves are still widely used in many other countries.

When wearing non-sterile examination gloves, it is important that the healthcare worker minimizes their physical interactions outside of the procedure, including touching the patient environment (e.g. bedding, patient chart, bowls), touching their own face/hair or handling additional equipment after the procedure has started. If an interaction with a surface or material outside of the procedure occurs, then the wearer should remove their gloves, perform hand hygiene with an alcohol-based hand rub and don new gloves before resuming the procedure.

Sterile gloves should only be worn to perform aseptic procedures such as surgical procedures, or urinary catheter or central venous catheter placement. Further information about sterile glove use is available in Chapter 5 (this volume).

4.7 Hand Hygiene Auditing and Compliance

4.7.1 Options for monitoring hand hygiene compliance

The most crucial factor in the prevention of transmission of infection is hand hygiene; however, compliance to hand hygiene techniques is often low within both veterinary and human healthcare settings. Monitoring, auditing and providing feedback in relation to hand hygiene compliance has been shown to improve results.

An audit is a process for monitoring and assessing performance with a view to identifying and actioning areas for improvement. The aim of a regular audit in relation to hand hygiene is to provide real-life data about areas where infection control is working well and areas that need improving. This information should improve patient and team safety, outcomes and biosecurity. When undertaking an audit, including that relating to hand hygiene compliance, the Royal College of Veterinary Surgeons (RCVS) Knowledge Clinical Audit defines eight steps, which are illustrated in Table 4.2 in relation to hand hygiene compliance monitoring (RCVS, 2019a). An RCVS Clinical Audit Template is available online free of charge (RCVS, 2019b). Importantly, the audit is repeated regularly to ensure ongoing engagement and a high standard of care. Once completed, these clinical audits can be used as evidence for clinical governance towards the RCVS Practice Standards Scheme.

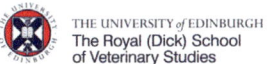

Donning Non-Sterile Gloves

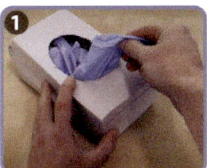

Take the first glove from glove box

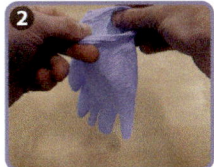

Touch only the edge of the cuff

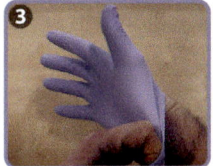

Insert the opposite hand being careful to avoid damage with nails

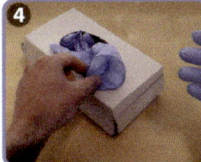

Take a second glove with the the bare hand

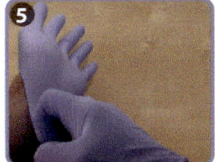

Avoid touching the forearm of the ungloved hand by folding the cuff edge over and pulling on with gloved hand

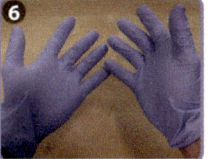

Once gloved, touch only the procedure site and required instruments

Removing Gloves

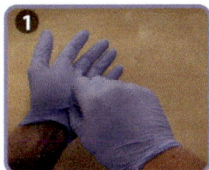

Pinch one glove at wrist level without touching the skin, pull away allowing the glove to turn inside out

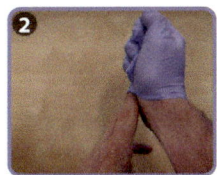

Hold the empty glove in the gloved hand. Slide your bare fingers between the skin and wrist of the remaining glove. Pinch and roll the second glove down over the first

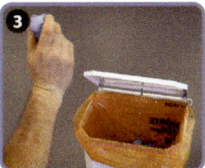

Discard gloves in clinical waste

edin.ac/3xDseIg

Digitial Education Unit

Fig. 4.4. Recommended technique for donning and doffing non-sterile examination gloves. It is imperative that hand hygiene is performed before and after the use of gloves. © Brian Mather, University of Edinburgh, 2022. Used with permission.

Table 4.2. Example steps involved in a clinical audit, following the advice of RCVS Knowledge (RCVS, 2019a).

Step	RCVS Knowledge clinical audit steps	Details
1	Choose a topic	Hand hygiene compliance according to World Health Organization (WHO) guidelines
2	Select criteria	The criteria should be easily understood and measured (e.g. steps during hand washing as illustrated in Fig. 4.2)
3	Set a target	Targets should be set using available evidence and best practice; the first audit will usually obtain a benchmark and should identify areas that are prone to reduced standards
4	Collect data	Hand hygiene compliance can be assessed via direct or indirect methods, or by measuring product consumption
5	Analyse data	Compare the findings with the target; the whole team should work collaboratively to develop an action plan for improvement
6	Implement change	Changes might include a hand hygiene education programme or provision of more alcohol-based hand-rub stations
7	Re-audit	Repeat steps 4 and 5 to ensure the changes are bringing about improvements and address any continued or novel shortfalls
8	Review and reflect	Share findings with employees, managers, clients, or the public (e.g. Fig. 4.7) to promote understanding, teamwork, and compliance

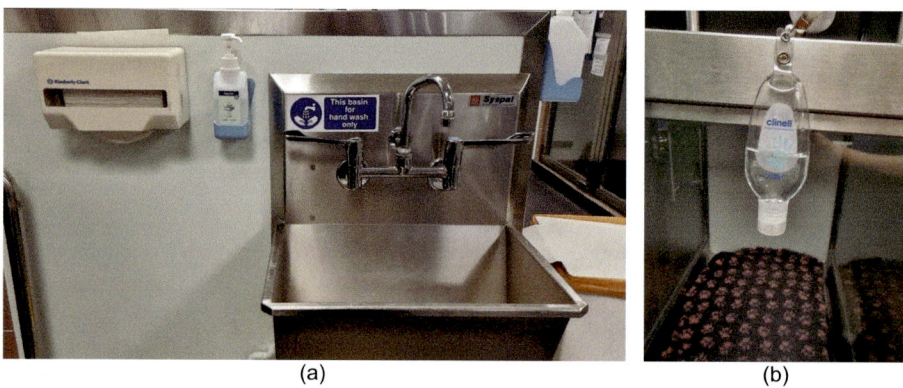
(a)   (b)

Fig. 4.5. (a) To maximize opportunities for hand hygiene, an adequate number of handwashing sinks are required throughout the clinic, and supplies of soap and paper towels should be checked regularly throughout the day. (b) Alcohol rubs should also be provided, either at hand hygiene stations or as individual bottles, which may be clipped on to kennel doors or attached to staff uniforms. Photographs courtesy of Angela MacKay, University of Edinburgh, Edinburgh, UK.

Before auditing can commence, it is imperative that staff are provided with relevant education and opportunities to practice rigorous hand hygiene. This may include seminars, videos and training events to define why, when and how to perform hand hygiene (Figs 4.1–4.3). Visual prompts should be made available at key areas.

For example, a pictorial poster detailing the steps of handwashing could be positioned near handwashing sinks, or a reminder of the 'five key moments for hand hygiene' posted in wards. Plenty of opportunities for hand hygiene should be provided, including sufficient sinks and alcohol hand-rub stations (Fig. 4.5). Additionally, stock levels of soap and paper towels should be checked regularly throughout the day.

Current methods for hand hygiene include direct observation, self-reporting or indirect measurements obtained by measuring the use of hand hygiene products.

Direct observation

Direct observation of hand hygiene provides the most detailed information and can record whether healthcare workers have performed hand hygiene during all of the WHO's five key moments (Fig. 4.1). Additional information that can be gathered is vast and may include the role of the observed healthcare worker, whether gloves are used, the extent to which all surfaces of the hands are cleaned and the time spent performing hand hygiene. The disadvantage of direct observation as an auditing system is that it is time consuming, costly and provides information about only 1–3% of all hand hygiene opportunities in the facility (Boyce, 2011). Finally, direct observation may influence staff behaviour and result in an erroneously elevated compliance rate. Nevertheless, the authors use direct observation in their hospitals (in addition to measuring product consumption; see below) to monitor hand hygiene compliance, and favour the WHO *SAVE LIVES: Clean Your Hands* framework, which is freely available online. In this model, the Hand Hygiene Self-Assessment Framework is a systematic tool with which to obtain a situation analysis of hand hygiene promotion and practices within an individual healthcare facility (WHO, 2010). While this toolkit is designed for use in human healthcare systems, much of the content is relevant to veterinary medicine and is an excellent starting point when clinical staff wish to reflect on existing resources and identify key issues requiring improvement. Based on the results obtained from this framework, a range of tailored template action plans are also available (WHO, 2010).

To monitor hand hygiene compliance, the authors use the WHO's *SAVE LIVES: Clean Your Hands* observation form to record hand hygiene compliance, which is also freely available online (WHO, 2010). Upon first glance, this form appears complicated, but it is accompanied by recommendations for use and in practice is very easy to follow. In short, the observer undertakes a session lasting no more than 20 min during which time the hand hygiene actions performed by the observed healthcare workers are recorded. Data collected include the role of the observed staff member, whether hand hygiene opportunities were observed or missed at each of the WHO's five key moments (Fig. 4.1) and whether gloves were used. Upon completion of this observation session, the data can be entered into a simple Basic Compliance Calculator to give the overall compliance (%) for the observed session. The authors can reassure the reader that the system becomes intuitive and simple after just one session, and cannot recommend the *SAVE LIVES: Clean Your Hands* website highly enough for a wealth of useful, practical and free resources to start monitoring and encouraging hand hygiene in every veterinary clinic (WHO, 2022).

Self-reporting

Self-reporting is simple and quick to perform. Useful platforms that may be beneficial to the veterinary practice include those from the RCVS Knowledge Clinical Audit (RCVS, 2020) and the Bella Moss Foundation Practice Hygiene Self Audit (BMF, 2021), both of which are available free of charge. Hand hygiene compliance is often overestimated by healthcare workers, and therefore this method is not recommended as the sole or major method of evaluating compliance (Boyce, 2011).

Measuring product consumption

Generally, hand hygiene compliance correlates with the use of hand hygiene products, and monitoring product consumption has been used as a surrogate for hand hygiene compliance in a number of hand hygiene campaigns.

Electronic hand hygiene compliance monitoring systems are proliferating in human healthcare settings. Available commercial systems include real-time locating systems or video monitoring for tracking hand hygiene events, and motion sensors that detect patient room entry and exit and correlate this to sensors on sinks or hand-rub dispensers. Individual healthcare workers can also don a badge that records every hand hygiene event around a pre-defined patient zone, providing individual compliance rates. Some systems even provide prompts (e.g. beeps or lights) when hand hygiene is not performed. Currently, electronic hand hygiene monitoring systems are not capable of specifically determining that hand hygiene has been performed at all five of the WHO's key moments (Fig. 4.1) but are likely to capture the key moments 1, 4 and 5, which account for approximately 80% of all hand hygiene opportunities (Boyce, 2011). Electronic hand hygiene set-ups may be more challenging to implement in veterinary medicine because of cost implications, and because patient zones are not as large as in human medicine and do not comprise individual patient rooms. However, further veterinary research is required in relation to the use of automated monitoring systems or simpler methods that might be more applicable to veterinary medicine. For example, a protocol has been reported whereby the volume (ml) of alcohol hand rub and soap products used per patient-day on each ward was calculated. This number is divided by 1.7 (the proposed average mL of product used per hand hygiene episode) to arrive at the estimated number of hand hygiene episodes per patient-day for the ward (Pyrek, 2012).

4.7.2   Maximizing hand hygiene compliance

Hand hygiene compliance in human and veterinary medicine is disturbingly poor. In human medicine, compliance is around 50% (Knepper et al., 2020). However, this is not an unsalvageable statistic, and readers can be heartened by evidence showing that increased compliance is possible. For example, compliance (as measured using an automated hand hygiene monitoring system) in a large university hospital during the COVID-19 pandemic reached 100% in March 2020, although hand hygiene compliance rapidly decreased to baseline subsequently. The authors hypothesized that this compliance surge was driven by fear and increased awareness of the importance of hand hygiene associated with the pandemic, fewer patient visitors, remote rounding by clinicians and nurse batching of tasks while in patient rooms (Makhni et al., 2021). Despite this, there is some evidence that this (transient) improvement in hand hygiene did translate to improved patient care (Bentivegna et al., 2021).

Interestingly, there is a difference in hand hygiene compliance among staff roles and at different time points. Research conducted during the COVID-19 pandemic found that nurses have the highest hand hygiene compliance while auxiliary workers have the lowest (80% and 70%, respectively), and using the WHO's five key moments (Fig. 4.1), compliance is highest after contact with body fluids (91%) and

lowest before touching the patient (68%) (Wang et al., 2021). In similar research completed before the pandemic, nurses had a hand hygiene adherence rate of 63%; allied staff adherence was 86.5%. Compliance was 93% after patient contact versus 63% before patient contact, and compliance of nurses before aseptic procedures was lowest at 39% (Chavali et al., 2014).

In veterinary medicine, recent research has evaluated hand hygiene compliance according to WHO standards. Based on 2056 observations in one study, overall hand hygiene compliance was 32%, being highest in the consultation area (41%) and after contact with body fluids (45%), and lowest in the pre-operating room area (20%) and before clean/aseptic procedures (12%) (Schmidt et al., 2021). Veterinary surgeons showed higher hand hygiene compliance (37%) than nurses (25%) (Schmidt et al., 2021). Encouragingly, initial low rates of hand hygiene practices in veterinary medicine can be improved following a low-cost multi-modal educational campaign, although the improvement following the campaign in this study from 20.6% to 41.7% remains far from ideal (Shea and Shaw, 2012). This is incredibly important, because veterinary staff have been identified as a high-risk group for carrying multidrug-resistant organisms, including MRSA and methicillin-resistant *Streptococcus pseudintermedius*, *Enterobacteriaceae* and *Pseudomonas* spp. (Espadale et al., 2018).

How can we improve hand hygiene compliance?

If we accept that hand hygiene compliance is uniformly abysmal and insufficient to break the transmission chain of pathogens, how can we encourage and improve compliance? There are a number of reasons why hand hygiene compliance is poor. Commonly cited reasons include:

- poor infrastructure (e.g. not enough sinks or alcohol gel, water temperature inadequate, empty soap dispensers, insufficient paper towels);
- skin irritation, including dermatitis;
- lack of education and training;
- lack of role models and peer pressure; and
- busy wards and staff shortages.

Therefore, the role of the whole clinical team is to work together collaboratively to (i) ensure that staff are educated regarding hand hygiene: (ii) provide ample opportunities to perform hand cleaning: (iii) audit team compliance and feedback the results; (iv) monitor progress over time to ensure compliance remains high; and (v) identify and address reasons for non-compliance. The *WHO Guidelines on Hand Hygiene in Health Care* have been developed with the aim of optimizing compliance with hand hygiene by changing healthcare worker behaviour (WHO, 2009a), as described in Box 4.1.

A recent Cochrane review (albeit pre-COVID-19 pandemic) assessed the short- and long-term success of strategies to improve hand hygiene compliance (Gould *et al.*, 2017). The authors found that multimodal interventions, including some or all of the strategies recommended in the WHO guidelines, improved hand hygiene compliance. Additional methods proven to be effective in improving

compliance included performance feedback, education, cues (e.g. signs or scent), placement of alcohol-based hand rub close to the point of use and novel strategies in addition to those recommended by the WHO.

Several researchers have explored novel methods to improve hand hygiene education. Fluorescent or glow gel (Fig. 4.6) can be used in combination with hand hygiene education to obtain a significant improvement in handwashing ability (Fishbein *et al.*, 2011). In human medicine, hand hygiene compliance can be improved with electronic monitoring, direct monitoring and/or video monitoring (Khandelwal *et al.*, 2019; Knepper *et al.*, 2020). In veterinary medicine, the use of automated gesture-recognition software to teach a seven-stage hand hygiene technique to undergraduate students did not improve hand hygiene performance, highlighting the need to

---

Box 4.1. The five essential elements (WHO, 2009a) of an implementation strategy recommended to improve hand hygiene compliance.

1. System change, including availability of alcohol-based hand rub at the point of patient care and/or access to a safe, continuous water supply and soap and towels
2. Training and education of healthcare professionals

3. Monitoring of hand hygiene practices and performance feedback
4. Reminders in the workplace
5. The creation of a hand hygiene safety culture with the participation of both individual healthcare workers and senior hospital managers

---

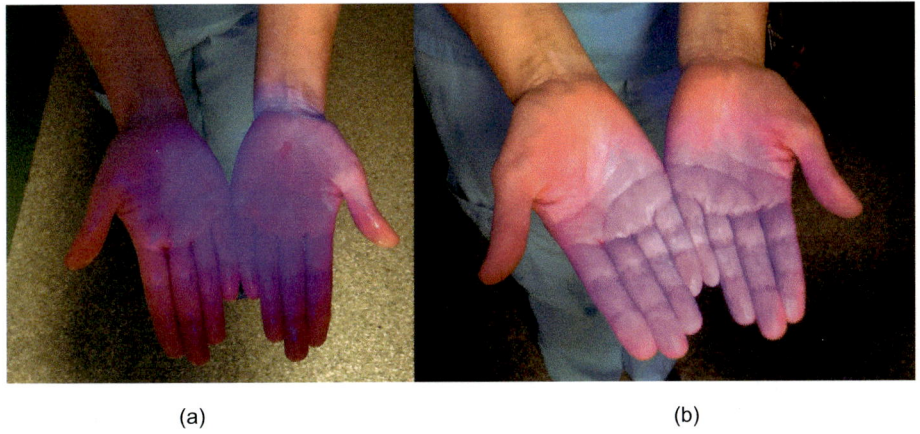

(a)　　　　　　　　　　　　　　　(b)

Fig. 4.6. Fluorescent products can be used as part of an education programme to illustrate sites of bacterial contamination before (a) and after (b) hand hygiene. Images courtesy of Shirley Simpson and Amy Allan, University of Edinburgh, Edinburgh, UK.

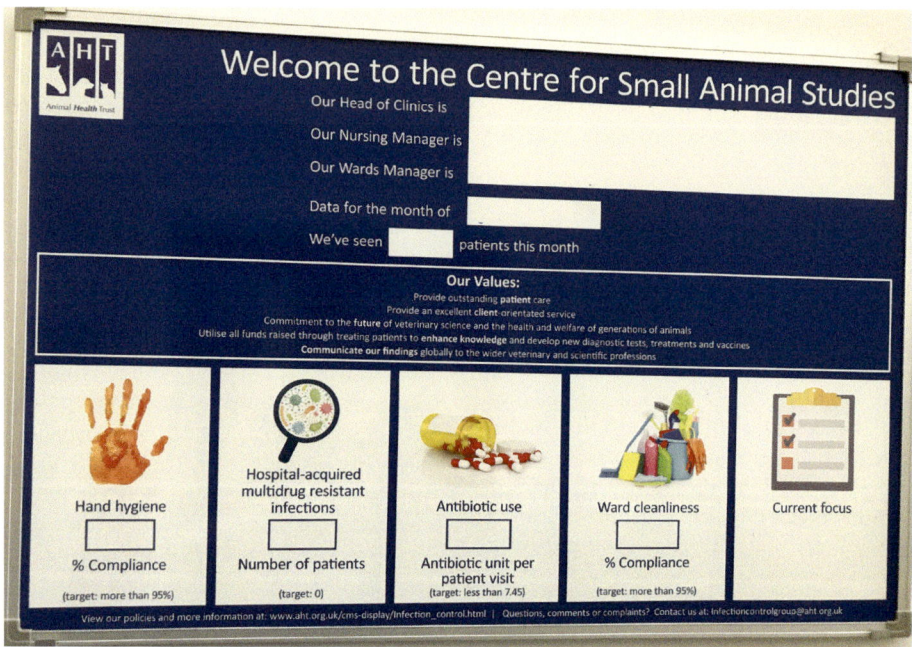

Fig. 4.7. Information boards such as this one, situated in public spaces (e.g. waiting rooms), provide incentives to staff and management to maintain high standards of hygiene within the clinic or hospital. © Kelly L. Bowlt Blacklock.

secure peer buy-in to obtain success (Mosley *et al.*, 2019). Other novel methods of encouraging hand hygiene could include interdepartmental competitions or boards that present up-to-date compliance data (Fig. 4.7). Promotional campaigns might revolve around the CDC's 'Clean Hands Count' campaign on 5 May (World Hand Hygiene Day), which provide opportunities to educate healthcare providers and address the myths and misperceptions surrounding hand hygiene. A large amount of fantastic promotional material is available online for this global campaign (CDC, 2016). Finally, some institutions, including the NHS, have a zero tolerance to non-hand hygiene compliance and follow a disciplinary policy and procedure under the terms of employment, which includes a verbal warning, a final written warning and dismissal.

4.8 Conclusion

It is a well-known fact that hand hygiene decreases disease transmission. Ever since Semmelweis established the link in the 1800s, both human and veterinary medicine has been still dogged by the same issues of non-compliance with hand hygiene, even during a global pandemic, which saw entire countries locked down to prevent transmission. Therefore, there is still a huge way to go to educate healthcare workers (and the public) about the importance of hand hygiene, and effective methods of educating, monitoring and reinforcing compliance are still desperately required. Once sufficient facilities to perform hand hygiene are available, the importance of a cohesive and honest team cannot be underestimated. Excellent hand hygiene compliance can only be created by a healthcare team that owns the task, creates a bespoke action plan and provides feedback to each other to achieve their common goal. The work is continuous and tiring to do well, and therefore generous input and support from management is essential to achieve excellence.

References

Al-Allak, A., Sarasin, S., Key, S. and Morris-Stiff, G. (2008) Wedding rings are not a significant source of bacterial contamination following surgical scrubbing. *Annals of the Royal College of Surgeons of England* 90(2), 133–135. DOI: 10.1308/003588408X242051.

Allen, J.L., Doidge, N.P., Bushell, R.N., Browning, G.F. and Marenda, M.S. (2022) Healthcare-associated infections caused by chlorhexidine-tolerant *Serratia marcescens* carrying a promiscuous IncHI2 multidrug resistance plasmid in a veterinary hospital. *PloS One* 17(3), e0264848. DOI: 10.1371/journal.pone. 0264848.

Aly, R. and Maibach, H.I. (1983) Comparative evaluation of chlorhexidine gluconate (Hibiclens®) and povidone-iodine (E-Z scrub®) sponge/brushes for presurgical hand scrubbing. *Current Therapeutic Research* 34, 740–745.

Anderson, S.L., Wisnieski, L., Achilles, S.L., Wooton, K.E., Shaffer, C.L, *et al*. (2022) The impact of gel fingernail polish application on the reduction of bacterial viability following a surgical hand scrub. *Veterinary Surgery* 50, 1525–1532.

AST (2017) *AST Guideline for Best Practices for Wearing Jewelry*. Association of Surgical Technologists, Littleton, Colorado. Available at: www.ast.org/uploade dFiles/Main_Site/Content/About_Us/Standard%20W earing%20Jewelry.pdf (accessed April 2022).

Baumgardner, C.A., Maragos, C.S. and Larson, E.L. (1993) Effects of nail polish on microbial growth of fingernails: dispelling sacred cows. *AORN Journal* 58, 84–88.

Beier, R.C., Foley, S.L., Davidson, M.K., White, D.G., McDermott, P.F. *et al*. (2015) Characterization of antibiotic and disinfectant susceptibility profiles among *Pseudomonas aeruginosa* veterinary isolates recovered during 1994–2003. *Journal of Applied Microbiology* 118, 326–342.

Bentivegna, E., Allesio, G., Spuntarelli, V., Luciani, M., Santina, I. *et al*. (2021) Impact of COVID-19 prevention measures on risk of health care-associated *Clostridium difficile* infection. *American Journal of Infection Control* 49, 640–642. DOI: 10.1016/j. ajic.2020.09.010.

Berndt, U., Wigger-Alberti, W., Gabard, B. and Elsner, P. (2000) Efficacy of a barrier cream and its vehicle as protective measures against occupational irritant contact dermatitis. *Contact Dermatitis* 42, 77–80. DOI: 10.1034/j.1600-0536.2000.042002077.x.

BEVA (2022) Hand hygiene. British Equine Veterinary Association, Ely, UK. Available at: www.beva.org.uk/ Guidance-and-Resources/Practice-Managers/workpl ace-safety/Hand-Hygiene (accessed October 2022).

BMF (2021) BMF practice hygiene self audit. Bella Moss Foundation, Edgware, UK. Available at: https://bella mossselfaudit.co.uk/introduction (accessed October 2022).

Boyce, J.M. (2011) Measuring healthcare worker hand hygiene activity: current practices and emerging technologies. *Infection Control and Hospital Epidemiology* 32(10), 1016–1028. DOI: 10.1086/662015.

CDC (2002) Guideline for hand hygiene in health-care settings: recommendations of the healthcare infection control practices advisory committee and the HICPAC/ SHEA/APIC/IDSA hand hygiene task force. *Morbidity and Mortality Weekly Report* 51, 1–45.

CDC (2016) Hand hygiene in healthcare settings. Clean Hands Count Campaign. Centers for Disease Control and Prevention, Atlanta, Georgia. Available at: www.c dc.gov/handhygiene/campaign/index.html (accessed 18 October 2022).

Chavali, S., Menon, V. and Shukla, U. (2014) Hand hygiene compliance among healthcare workers in an accredited tertiary care hospital. *Indian Journal of Critical Care Medicine* 18(10), 689–693. DOI: 10.4103/0972-5229.142179.

Chou, T.-C., Lin, K.-H., Sheu, H.-M., Su, S.-B., Lee, C.-W. *et al*. (2007) Alterations in health examination items and skin symptoms from exposure to ultra-low humidity. *International Archives of Occupational and Environmental Health* 80(4), 290–297. DOI: 10.1007/ s00420-006-0133-4.

ECDC (2020) Use of gloves in healthcare and non-healthcare settings in the context of the COVID 19 pandemic. European Centre for Disease Prevention and Control, Stockholm. Available at: www.ecdc.euro pa.eu/en/publications-data/gloves-healthcare-and-no n-healthcare-settings-covid-19 (accessed 18 October 2022).

Emilson, A., Lindberg, M. and Forslind, B. (1993) The temperature effect on in vitro penetration of sodium lauryl sulfate and nickel chloride through human skin. *Acta Dermato-Venereologica* 73(3), 203–207. DOI: 10.2340/0001555573203207.

Espadale, E., Pinchbeck, G., Williams, N.J., Timofte, D., McIntyre, K.M, *et al*. (2018) Are the hands of veterinary staff a reservoir forantimicrobial-resistant bacteria? A randomized study to evaluate two handhygiene rubs in a veterinary hospital. *Microbial Drug Resistance* 24(10), 1607–1616. DOI: 10.1089/mdr.2018.0183.

Fagernes, M. and Nord, R. (2007) A study of microbial load of different types of finger rings worn by healthcare personnel. *Nordic Journal of Nursing Research* 27(2), 21–24. DOI: 10.1177/010740830702700206.

Faoagali, J., Fong, J., George, N., Mahoney, P. and O'Rourke, V. (1995) Comparison of the immediate, residual, and cumulative antibacterial effects of Novaderm R,* Novascrub R,* Betadine Surgical Scrub, Hibiclens, and liquid soap. *American Journal of Infection Control* 23(6), 337–343. DOI: 10.1016/0196-6553(95)90263-5.

FDA (2016a) Medical device bans. US Food and Drug Administration, Silver Spring, Maryland. Available at: www.fda.gov/medical-devices/medical-device-safety/ medical-device-bans (accessed October 2022).

FDA (2016b) Banned devices; powdered surgeon's gloves, powdered patient examination gloves, and absorbable powder for lubricating a surgeon's glove. US Food and Drug Administration, Silver Spring, Maryland. Available at: www.federalregister.gov/doc

uments/2016/12/19/2016-30382/banned-devices-po wdered-surgeons-gloves-powdered-patient-examin ation-gloves-and-absorbable-powder (accessed 18 October 2022).

FECAVA (2019) FECAVA key recommendations for hygiene and infection control in veterinary practice. Federation of European Companion Animal Veterinary Associations, Brussels. Available at: www.fecava.org/wp-content/uploads/2019/03/FECAVA_ Infectioncontrol_2018_LR.pdf (accessed 18 October 2022).

Fishbein, A.B., Tellez, I., Lin, H., Sullivan, C. and Groll, M.E. (2011) Glow gel hand washing in the waiting room: a novel approach to improving hand hygiene education. *Infection Control and Hospital Epidemiology* 32(7), 661–666. DOI: 10.1086/660359.

Foca, M., Jakob, K., Whittier, S., Della Latta, P., Factor, S. et al. (2000) Endemic *Pseudomonas aeruginosa* infection in a neonatal intensive care unit. *New England Journal of Medicine* 343(10), 695–700. DOI: 10.1056/NEJM200009073431004.

Gallagher, R. and Sunley, K. (2012) Appropriate glove use in dermatitis prevention. *Nursing Times* 108(37), 12–14.

Galle, P.C., Homesley, H.D. and Rhyne, A.L. (1978) Reassessment of the surgical scrub. *Surgery, Gynecology & Obstetrics* 147(2), 215–218.

Gould, D. (1995) Hand decontamination: nurses' opinions and practices. *Nursing Times* 91(17), 42–45.

Gould, D.J., Moralejo, D., Drey, N., Chudleigh, J.H. and Taljaard, M. (2017) Interventions to improve hand hygiene compliance in patient care. *Cochrane Database of Systematic Reviews* 9(9), CD005186. DOI: 10.1002/14651858.CD005186.pub4.

Gross, A., Cutright, D.E. and D'Alessandro, S.M. (1979) Effect of surgical scrub on microbial population under the fingernails. *American Journal of Surgery* 138(3), 463–467. DOI: 10.1016/0002-9610(79)90288-5.

Gustafson, D.R., Vetter, E.A., Larson, D.R., Ilstrup, D.M., Maker, M.D. et al. (2000) Effects of 4 hand-drying methods for removing bacteria from washed hands: a randomized trial. *Mayo Clinic Proceedings* 75(7), 705–708. DOI: 10.4065/75.7.705.

Hadaway, A. (2020) Handwashing: clean hands save lives. *Journal of Consumer Health on the Internet* 24(1), 43–49. DOI: 10.1080/15398285.2019.1710981.

Hardy, J.M., Owen, T.J., Martinez, S.A., Jones, L.P. and Davis, M.A. (2017) The effect of nail characteristics on surface bacterial counts of surgical personnel before and after scrubbing. *Veterinary Surgery* 46(7), 952–961. DOI: 10.1111/vsu.12685.

Hayes, R.A., Trick, W.E., Vernon, M.O., Nathan, C., Peterson, B.J, et al. (2001) Ring use as a risk factor (RF) for hand colonization in a surgical intensive care unit (SICU). In: *41st the Interscience Conference Antimicrobial Agents and Chemotherapy*, 16–19, December, Chicago, IL, Abstract K-1333.

Hedderwick, S.A., McNeil, S.A., Lyons, M.J. and Kauffman, C.A. (2000) Pathogenic organisms associated with artificial fingernails worn by healthcare workers. *Infection Control and Hospital Epidemiology* 21(8), 505–509. DOI: 10.1086/501794.

Herruzo-Cabrera, R., Vizcaino-Alcaide, M.J. and Fdez-Aciñero, M.J. (2000) Usefulness of an alcohol solution of N-duopropenide for the surgical antisepsis of the hands compared with handwashing with iodine-povidone and chlorhexidine: clinical essay. *Journal of Surgical Research* 94(1), 6–12. DOI: 10.1006/jsre.2000.5931.

Hingst, V., Juditzki, I., Heeg, P. and Sonntag, H.G. (1992) Evaluation of the efficacy of surgical hand disinfection following a reduced application time of 3 instead of 5 min. *The Journal of Hospital Infection* 20(2), 79–86. DOI: 10.1016/0195-6701(92)90109-y.

Hoffman, P.N., Cooke, E.M., McCarville, M.R. and Emmerson, A.M. (1985) Micro-organisms isolated from skin under wedding rings worn by hospital staff. *British Medical Journal* 290, 206–207. DOI: 10.1136/bmj.290.6463.206.

Hsueh, P.R., Teng, L.J., Yang, P.C., Pan, H.L., Ho, S.W. et al. (1999) Nosocomial pseudoepidemic caused by *Bacillus cereus* traced to contaminated ethyl alcohol from a liquor factory. *Journal of Clinical Microbiology* 37(7), 2280–2284. DOI: 10.1128/JCM.37.7.2280-2284.1999.

Huang, C., Ma, W. and Stack, S. (2012) The hygienic efficacy of different hand-drying methods: a review of the evidence. *Mayo Clinic Proceedings* 87(8), 791–798. DOI: 10.1016/j.mayocp.2012.02.019.

Jones, R.D., Jampani, H., Mulberry, G. and Rizer, R.L. (2000) Moisturizing alcohol hand gels for surgical hand preparation. *AORN Journal* 71(3), 584–587. DOI: 10.1016/s0001-2092(06)61580-9.

Jumaa, P.A. (2005) Hand hygiene: simple and complex. *International Journal of Infectious Diseases* 9(1), 3–14. DOI: 10.1016/j.ijid.2004.05.005.

Keck, N., Dunie-Merigot, A., Dazas, M., Hirchaud, E., Laurence, S. et al. (2020) Long-lasting nosocomial persistence of chlorhexidine-resistant *Serratia marcescens* in a veterinary hospital. *Veterinary Microbiology* 245, 108686. DOI: 10.1016/j.vetmic.2020.108686.

Khandelwal, V., Mishra, G. and Sharma, S. (2019) Video surveillance of hand hygiene: a better tool for monitoring and ensuring hand hygiene adherence surveillance of hand hygiene: a better tool for monitoring and ensuring hand hygiene adherence. *Indian Journal of Critical Care Medicine* 23(5), 224–226. DOI: 10.5005/jp-journals-10071-23165.

Khodavaisy, S., Nabili, M., Davari, B. and Vahedi, M. (2011) Evaluation of bacterial and fungal contamination in the health care workers' hands and rings in the intensive care unit. *Journal of Preventive Medicine and Hygiene* 52(4), 215–218.

Knepper, B.C., Miller, A.M. and Young, H.L. (2020) Impact of an automated hand hygiene monitoring system combined with a performance improvement intervention on hospital-acquired infections. *Infection Control and Hospital Epidemiology* 41(8), 931–937. DOI: 10.1017/ice.2020.182.

Larson, E., Leyden, J.J., McGinley, K.J., Grove, G.L. and Talbot, G.H. (1986) Physiologic and microbiologic changes in skin related to frequent handwashing. *Infection Control* 7(2), 59–63. DOI: 10.1017/s019594170006389x.

Larson, E., Anderson, J.K., Baxendale, L. and Bobo, L. (1993) Effects of a protective foam on scrubbing and gloving. *American Journal of Infection Control* 21(6), 297–301. DOI: 10.1016/0196-6553(93)90386-i.

Larson, E.L., Norton Hughes, C.A., Pyrek, J.D., Sparks, S.M., Cagatay, E.U. *et al.* (1998) Changes in bacterial flora associated with skin damage on hands of health care personnel. *American Journal of Infection Control* 26(5), 513–521. DOI: 10.1016/s0196-6553(98)70025-2.

Leggat, P.A., Smith, D.R. and Speare, R. (2009) Hand dermatitis among veterinarians from Queensland, Australia. *Contact Dermatitis* 60(6), 336–338. DOI: 10.1111/j.1600-0536.2009.01562.x.

Loveday, H.P., Wilson, J.A., Pratt, R.J., Golsorkhi, M., Tingle, A. *et al.* (2014) epic3: national evidence-based guidelines for preventing healthcare-associated infections in NHS hospitals in England. *Journal of Hospital Infection* 86(Suppl. 1), S1–S70. DOI: 10.1016/S0195-6701(13)60012-2.

Macias, J.H., Ruiz, S., Macias, A.E. and Alvarez, J.A. (2015) Substantive effect of chlorhexidine. *Journal of Hospital Infection* 90(1), 82–83. DOI: 10.1016/j.jhin.2015.01.016.

Makhni, S., Umscheid, C.A., Soo, J., Chu, V., Bartlett, A. *et al.* (2021) Hand hygiene compliance rate during the COVID-19 pandemic. *JAMA Internal Medicine* 181(7), 1006–1008. DOI: 10.1001/jamainternmed.2021.1429.

Mangram, A.J., Horan, T.C., Pearson, M.L., Silver, L.C., Jarvis, W.R. *et al.* (1999) Guideline for prevention of surgical site infection. *Infection Control & Hospital Epidemiology* 20, 250–278. DOI: 10.1086/501620.

Mann, A. (2016) Bare below the elbows — is there any evidence? *The Veterinary Nurse* 7(2), 60–66. DOI: 10.12968/vetn.2016.7.2.60.

Marrie, T.J. and Costerton, J.W. (1981) Prolonged survival of *Serratia marcescens* in chlorhexidine. *Applied and Environmental Microbiology* 42(6), 1093–1102. DOI: 10.1128/aem.42.6.1093-1102.1981.

McAllister, T.A., Lucas, C.E., Mocan, H., Liddell, R.H., Gibson, B.E. *et al.* (1989) *Serratia marcescens* outbreak in a paediatric oncology unit traced to contaminated chlorhexidine. *Scottish Medical Journal* 34(5), 525–528. DOI: 10.1177/003693308903400506.

McCormick, R.D., Buchman, T.L. and Maki, D.G. (2000) Double-blind, randomized trial of scheduled use of a novel barrier cream and an oil-containing lotion for protecting the hands of health care workers. *American Journal of Infection Control* 28(4), 302–310. DOI: 10.1067/mic.2000.107425.

McGinley, K.J., Larson, E.L. and Leyden, J.J. (1988) Composition and density of microflora in the subungual space of the hand. *Journal of Clinical Microbiology* 26(5), 950–953. DOI: 10.1128/jcm.26.5.950-953.1988.

McNeil, S.A., Foster, C.L., Hedderwick, S.A. and Kauffman, C.A. (2001) Effect of hand cleansing with antimicrobial soap or alcohol-based gel on microbial colonization of artificial fingernails worn by health care workers. *Clinical Infectious Diseases* 32(3), 367–372. DOI: 10.1086/318488.

Moolenaar, R.L., Crutcher, J.M., Joaquin, V.H.S., Sewell, L.V., Hutwagner, L.C, *et al.* (2000) A prolonged outbreak of *Pseudomonas Aeruginosa* in a neonatal intensive care unit did staff fingernails play a role in disease transmission? *Infection Control & Hospital Epidemiology* 21(2), 80–85. DOI: 10.1086/501739.

Mosley, C. and Mather, B. (2019) *Hand Washing Technique with Soap and Water, and Hand Rub Technique with Alcohol Gel*. RCVS Knowledge, The Royal (Dick) School of Veterinary Studies, Edinburgh, UK. Available at: https://knowledge.rcvs.org.uk/document-library/covid-19-resources-from-university-of-edinburgh-royal-dick/ (accessed October 2022).

Mosley, C., Mosley, J.R., Bell, C., Aitchison, K., Rhind, S.M. *et al.* (2019) Teaching best practice in hand hygiene: student use and performance with a gamified gesture recognition system. *Veterinary Record* 185(14), 444. DOI: 10.1136/vr.105338.

NHS (2018) 'The Gloves Are Off' campaign. National Health Service, London. Available at: www.england.nhs.uk/atlas_case_study/the-gloves-are-off-campaign/ (accessed 18 October 2022).

NHS (2021) *Health Technical Memorandum 03-01 Specialised Ventilation for Healthcare Premises. Part A: The Concept, Design, Specification, Installation and Acceptance Testing of Healthcare Ventilation Systems*. National Health Service, London. Available at: www.england.nhs.uk/wp-content/uploads/2021/05/HTM0301-PartA-accessible-F6.pdf (accessed 18 October 2022).

Ohlenschlaeger, J., Friberg, J., Ramsing, D. and Agner, T. (1996) Temperature dependency of skin susceptibility to water and detergents. *Acta Dermato-Venereologica* 76(4), 274–276. DOI: 10.2340/0001555576274276.

Parry, M.F., Grant, B., Yukna, M., Adler-Klein, D., McLeod, G.X. *et al.* (2001) Candida osteomyelitis and diskitis after spinal surgery: an outbreak that implicates artificial nail use. *Clinical Infectious Diseases* 32(3), 352–357. DOI: 10.1086/318487.

Passaro, D.J., Waring, L., Armstrong, R., Bolding, F., Bouvier, B. *et al.* (1997) Postoperative *Serratia marcescens* wound infections traced to an out-of-hospital source. *Journal of Infectious Diseases* 175(4), 992–995. DOI: 10.1086/514008.

Paulson, D.S. (1994) Comparative evaluation of five surgical hand scrub preparations. *AORN Journal* 60(2), 246. DOI: 10.1016/s0001-2092(07)62743-4.

Pereira, L.J., Lee, G.M. and Wade, K.J. (1990) The effect of surgical handwashing routines on the microbial counts of operating room nurses. *American Journal of Infection Control* 18(6), 354–364. DOI: 10.1016/0196-6553(90)90249-r.

Perry, C., Marshall, R. and Jones, E. (2001) Bacterial contamination of uniforms. *Journal of Hospital Infection* 48(3), 238–241. DOI: 10.1053/jhin.2001.0962.

Peterson, A.F., Rosenberg, A. and Alatary, S.D. (1978) Comparative evaluation of surgical scrub preparations. *Surgery, Gynecology & Obstetrics* 146(1), 63–65.

Pottinger, J., Burns, S. and Manske, C. (1989) Bacterial carriage by artificial versus natural nails. *American Journal of Infection Control* 17(6), 340–344. DOI: 10.1016/0196-6553(89)90003-5.

Pyrek, K.M. (2012) *Hand hygiene monitoring goes high-tech*. Infection Control Today. Available at: www.england.nhs.uk/wp-content/uploads/2016/03/ge3-hand-hygient-tchnlgy-evidnc-manufctr.pdf (accessed 5 January 2023).

RCVS (2019a) *Clinical Audit Case Example: Handwashing Audit by Vets Now Glasgow*. RCVS Knowledge, London. Available at: https://knowledge.rcvs.org.uk/document-library/vets-now-referrals-glasgow-case-example/ (accessed 18 October 2022).

RCVS (2019b) Clinical audit template. Royal College of Veterinary Surgeons, London. Available at: https://knowledge.rcvs.org.uk/document-library/clinical-audit-template/ (accessed 22 April 2022).

RCVS (2020) *Clinical Audit Case Example: Hand Hygiene Audit by Vale Vets*. Royal College of Veterinary Surgeons Knowledge, London. Available at: https://knowledge.rcvs.org.uk/document-library/knowledge-award-2020-champion-practice-hygiene-audit-at-vale/ (accessed 18 October 2022).

Rubin, D.M. (1988) Prosthetic fingernails in the OR: a research study. *AORN Journal* 47(4), 944–955. DOI: 10.1016/s0001-2092(07)66549-1.

Rutter, J.D., Angiulo, K. and Macinga, D.R. (2014) Measuring residual activity of topical antimicrobials: is the residual activity of chlorhexidine an artefact of laboratory methods? *Journal of Hospital Infection* 88(2), 113–115. DOI: 10.1016/j.jhin.2014.06.010.

Salisbury, D.M., Hutfilz, P., Treen, L.M., Bollin, G.E. and Gautam, S. (1997) The effect of rings on microbial load of health care workers' hands. *American Journal of Infection Control* 25(1), 24–27. DOI: 10.1016/s0196-6553(97)90049-3.

Sartor, C., Jacomo, V., Duvivier, C., Tissot-Dupont, H., Sambuc, R. *et al.* (2000) Nosocomial *Serratia marcescens* infections associated with extrinsic contamination of a liquid nonmedicated soap. *Infection Control and Hospital Epidemiology* 21(3), 196–199. DOI: 10.1086/501743.

Sato, M., Fukayo, S. and Yano, E. (2003) Adverse environmental health effects of ultra-low relative humidity indoor air. *Journal of Occupational Health* 45(2), 133–136. DOI: 10.1539/joh.45.133.

Schmidt, J.S., Hartnack, S., Schuller, S., Kuster, S.P. and Willi, B. (2021) Hand hygiene compliance in companion animal clinics and practices in Switzerland: an observational study. *Veterinary Record* 189(1), e307. DOI: 10.1002/vetr.307.

Shea, A. and Shaw, S. (2012) Evaluation of an educational campaign to increase hand hygiene at a small animal veterinary teaching hospital. *Journal of the American Veterinary Medical Association* 240(1), 61–64. DOI: 10.2460/javma.240.1.61.

Stein, D.T. and Pankovich-Wargula, A.L. (2009) The dilemma of the wedding band. *Orthopedics* 32(2), 86. DOI: 10.3928/01477447-20090201-10.

Suen, L.K.P., Lung, V.Y.T., Boost, M.V., Au-Yeung, C.H. and Siu, G.K.H. (2019) Microbiological evaluation of different hand drying methods for removing bacteria from washed hands. *Scientific Reports* 9(1), 13754. DOI: 10.1038/s41598-019-50239-4.

Susitaival, P., Kirk, J. and Schenker, M.B. (2001) Self-reported hand dermatitis in California veterinarians. *American Journal of Contact Dermatitis* 12, 103–108.

Trick, W.E., Vernon, M.O., Hayes, R.A., Nathan, C., Rice, T.W. *et al.* (2003) Impact of ring wearing on hand contamination and comparison of hand hygiene agents in a hospital. *Clinical Infectious Diseases* 36(11), 1383–1390. DOI: 10.1086/374852.

Tupker, R.A. (1996) Detergents and cleansers. In: van der Valk, P.G.M. and Maibach, H.I. (eds) *The Irritant Contact Dermatitis Syndrome*. CRC Press, New York, pp. 71–76.

Turner, S., McNamee, R., Agius, R., Wilkinson, S.M., Carder, M., *et al.* (2012) Evaluating interventions aimed at reducing occupational exposure to latex and rubber glove allergens. *Occupational and Environmental Medicine* 69(12), 925–931. DOI: 10.1136/oemed-2012-100754.

Vangveeravong, M., Sirikul, J. and Daengsuwan, T. (2011) Latex allergy in dental students: a cross-sectional study. *Journal of the Medical Association of Thailand* 94(Suppl. 3), S1–8.

Vigeant, P., Loo, V.G., Bertrand, C., Dixon, C., Hollis, R. *et al.* (1998) An outbreak of *Serratia marcescens* infections related to contaminated chlorhexidine. *Infection Control and Hospital Epidemiology* 19(10), 791–794. DOI: 10.2307/30141429.

Vu-Thien, H., Darbord, J.C., Moissenet, D., Dulot, C., Dufourcq, J.B. *et al.* (1998) Investigation of an outbreak of wound infections due to *Alcaligenes xylosoxidans* transmitted by chlorhexidine in a burns unit. *European Journal of Clinical Microbiology &*

Infectious Diseases 17(10), 724–726. DOI: 10.1007/s100960050168.

Wade, J.J. and Casewell, M.W. (1991) The evaluation of residual antimicrobial activity on hands and its clinical relevance. *Journal of Hospital Infection* 18, 23–28. DOI: 10.1016/0195-6701(91)90259-B.

Wang, Y., Yang, J., Qiao, F., Feng, B., Hu, F. *et al.* (2021) Compared hand hygiene compliance among healthcare providers before and after the COVID-19 pandemic: a rapid review and meta-analysis. *American Journal of Infection Control* 50(5), 563–571. DOI: 10.1016/j.ajic.2021.11.030.

Waterman, T.R., Smeak, D.D., Kowalski, J. and Hade, E.M. (2006) Comparison of bacterial counts in glove juice of surgeons wearing smooth band rings versus those without rings. *American Journal of Infection Control* 34(7), 421–425. DOI: 10.1016/j.ajic.2005.11.007.

WHO (2009b) *Glove Use Information Leaflet*. World Health Organization, Geneva, Switzerland. Available at: www.who.int/gpsc/5may/Glove_Use_Information_Leaflet.pdf (accessed October 2022).

WHO (2010) *Hand Hygiene Self-Assessment Framework 2010*. World Health Organization, Geneva, Switzerland. Available at: https://cdn.who.int/media/docs/default-source/integrated-health-services-(ihs)/hand-hygiene/monitoring/hhsa-framework-october-2010.pdf (accessed October 2022).

WHO (2022) SAVE LIVES – clean your hands. World Health Organization, Geneva, Switzerland. Available at: www.who.int/campaigns/world-hand-hygiene-day (accessed 18 October 2022).

WHO (World Health Organization) (2009a) *WHO guidelines on hand hygiene in health care: first global patient safety challenge clean care is safer care*, Vol. 21. The WHO Multimodal Hand Hygiene Improvement Strategy, World Health Organization, Geneva.

Widmer, A.F. (2000) Replace hand washing with use of a waterless alcohol hand rub? *Clinical Infectious Diseases* 31(1), 136–143. DOI: 10.1086/313888.

Wilhelm, K.P. (1996) Prevention of surfactant-induced irritant contact dermatitis. *Current Problems in Dermatology* 25, 78–85. DOI: 10.1159/000425517.

Wong, J.K., Chambers, L.C., Elsmo, E.J., Jenkins, T.L., Howerth, E.W. *et al.* (2018) Cellulitis caused by the *Burkholderia cepacia* complex associated with contaminated chlorhexidine 2% scrub in five domestic cats. *Journal of Veterinary Diagnostic Investigation* 30(5), 763–769. DOI: 10.1177/1040638718782333.

Wu, M., McIntosh, J. and Liu, J. (2016) Current prevalence rate of latex allergy: why it remains a problem? *Journal of Occupational Health* 58(2), 138–144. DOI: 10.1539/joh.15-0275-RA.

Wynd, C.A., Samstag, D.E. and Lapp, A.M. (1994) Bacterial carriage on the fingernails of OR nurses. *AORN Journal* 60(5), 796. DOI: 10.1016/s0001-2092(07)63328-6.

Yazdankhah, S.P., Scheie, A.A., Høiby, E.A., Lunestad, B.-T., Heir, E. *et al.* (2006) Triclosan and antimicrobial resistance in bacteria: an overview. *Microbial Drug Resistance* 12(2), 83–90. DOI: 10.1089/mdr.2006.12.83.

Yildirim, I., Ceyhan, M., Cengiz, A.B., Bagdat, A., Barin, C. *et al.* (2008) A prospective comparative study of the relationship between different types of ring and microbial hand colonization among pediatric intensive care unit nurses. *International Journal of Nursing Studies* 45(11), 1572–1576. DOI: 10.1016/j.ijnurstu.2008.02.010.

5 Surgical Hand Preparation

ALISON YOUNG*

Royal Veterinary College, Hawkshead Lane, North Mymms, Hertfordshire, UK

5.1 Aseptic Hand Preparation: Where Did It All Begin?

During the 1840s, a Hungarian physician called Ignaz Semmelweis (Fig. 5.1) was an early pioneer of antiseptic procedures. Some ridiculed him for his work linking hand washing to better medical care. Semmelweis had been led to this conclusion when he noticed that maternity wards where women were giving birth under the supervision of midwives had far fewer deaths than those on a doctor-led ward. During these times, it was standard practice for doctors to assist and observe their students training using cadavers during morning sessions. They then went to work on the delivery ward in the afternoon with little or no hand washing in between the two sessions.

Further investigations showed that the cause was the transfer of 'cadaverous particles' from the hands of the doctors on to the women they treated. Midwives only worked on delivery wards and so were not exposing their patients to the same transfer. At this point, the transferred particles were not known as germs, as this discovery was yet to come.

In 1847, Semmelweis introduced mandatory hand washing for the students and doctors who worked for him in Vienna General Hospital. With this practice, the mortality rate in the doctor-led unit plummeted. Semmelweis attempted to introduce this concept to other hospitals but was dismissed again. This was partly because the doctors felt aggrieved that Semmelweis was directly implicating them in the higher death rate.

Semmelweis published articles detailing his findings in 1858 and 1860, but these, along with a book written later, were all condemned by his peers.

In 1867, Joseph Lister worked on the idea of sanitizing hands and surgical instruments prior to

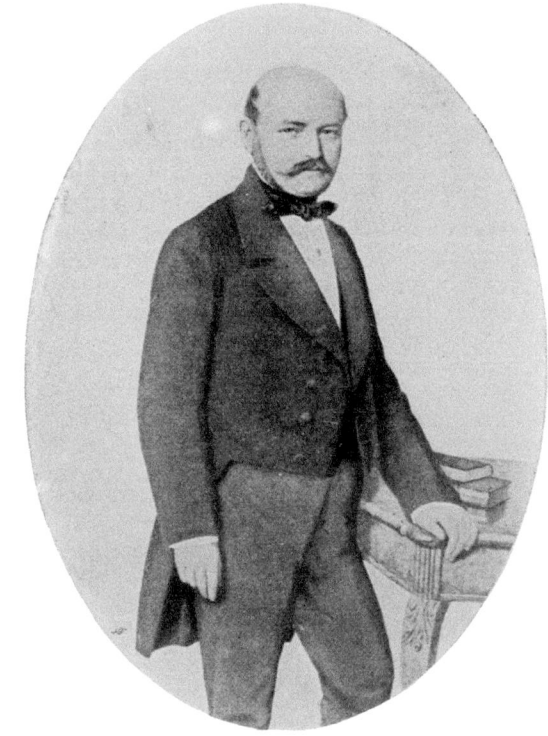

Ignaz Philipp Semmelweis (1818–65)

Fig. 5.1. The father of hand hygiene, Ignaz Semmelweis. The Wellcome Collection. Public Domain mark.

surgery, and published an article in *The Lancet* that fundamentally changed medicine. 'An address on the antiseptic system of treatment in surgery' described the positive outcomes when using antiseptic sprays on wounds, dressings and surgical tools, as well as hand-washing techniques (Lister,

*ayoung@RVC.AC.UK

1867). This theory also had its critics, but by the 1870s more surgeons had incorporated scrubbing up into their routine prior to surgery.

Scrubbing up during the 19th century usually consisted of washing hands with antimicrobial soap and warm water, and often used a brush. In 1894, three steps were suggested (Reinicke, 1894):

1. Wash hands with hot water, medicated soap and a brush for 5 min.
2. Apply 90% ethanol for 3–5 min with a brush.
3. Rinse with an antiseptic liquid.

In 1939, a 7-min hand wash was suggested, with surgeons using soap, water and a brush. After drying the hands, this protocol was followed by applying 70% ethanol for 3 min (Price, 1938). By the 20th century, the recommendation for hand preparation was reduced from upwards of 10 min to the 5-min procedure we commonly see today.

Although surgeons routinely scrubbed for surgery from the 1870s, it was not until the 1980s that hand hygiene in healthcare became more standardized. The American healthcare system incorporated the first national hand hygiene guidelines (Simmons and CDC, 1981; Garner and Favero, 1986). Many more have been introduced in the years since, and similar guidelines are widespread in countries including the USA, Canada and parts of Europe (WHO, 2005, 2009). The National Health Service in the UK has adopted this policy throughout the majority of its trusts (NHS, 2022).

5.2   Objectives of Surgical Hand Preparation

Our veterinary patients are likely to have a higher risk of contamination than human patients (Verwilghen *et al.*, 2011). This leads to a higher contamination load on the hands of a veterinary surgeon compared with our human counterparts.

Surgical hand preparation should reduce the release of skin bacteria from the hands of the surgical team for the duration of the procedure in case of an unnoticed puncture of the surgical glove releasing bacteria to the open wound (Kampf *et al.*, 2005a).

Surgical hand preparation differs from the hygiene hand wash. The World Health Organization (WHO) *Guidelines on Hand Hygiene in Health Care* state that the product used for surgical hand preparation should continue to inhibit the growth of bacteria under the surgical gloves (WHO, 2009). Rapid multiplication of skin bacteria occurs under surgical gloves if hands are washed with a non-antimicrobial soap, whereas it occurs more slowly following pre-operative hand preparation with a medicated soap (WHO, 2009).

5.3   Hand Hygiene for Healthcare Workers

It is not just the surgical team that need to be aware of the importance of hand hygiene. For healthcare workers, hand hygiene is the primary measure proven to be effective in the reduction of healthcare-associated infections (HAIs). Further information on hand hygiene can be found in Chapter 4 (this volume).

To ensure the vocabulary used remains standard the WHO have provided terminology to define each technique and the products available:

- *Surgical hand antisepsis/surgical hand preparation*: antiseptic hand wash or antiseptic hand rub performed pre-operatively by the surgical team to eliminate transient and reduce resident skin flora. Such antiseptics often have persistent antimicrobial activity.
- *Surgical hand scrub(bing)/pre-surgical scrub*: surgical hand preparation with antimicrobial soap and water.
- *Hand rub(bing)*: a treatment that involves rubbing the hands without the addition of water:
- *Surgical hand rubbing*: surgical hand preparation with an alcohol-based hand rub, as per surgical hand preparation described above.
- *Hygienic hand rubbing*: using an alcohol-based hand rub to reduce the transient flora without necessarily affecting the resident skin flora. It is broad spectrum and fast acting.

Several professional organizations have defined requirements for surgical hand preparation. The WHO advises that this should be performed using either a suitable antimicrobial soap and water or a suitable alcohol-based hand rub, preferably with a product ensuring sustained activity, before donning sterile gloves (WHO, 2016).

The National Institute for Health and Care Excellence (NICE) has created guidelines and recommendations on hand decontamination (NICE, 2008). According to these recommendations, the operating team should wash their hands prior to the first operation on the list using an aqueous antiseptic surgical solution, using a single-use brush or pick for the nails to ensure that hands and nails are visibly clean. Before subsequent operations, hands should be cleaned using either an alcohol hand rub or an antiseptic surgical solution. If hands are soiled, then they should be washed again with an antiseptic surgical solution. There is now more evidence available regarding the use of brushes and nail picks, which will be discussed later in this chapter.

5.4 Is Hand Preparation for Surgery Necessary?

Semmelweis's and Lister's early works linked contamination from the healthcare worker to the patient. Patients developed puerperal fever, commonly known as childbed fever, with haemolytic *Streptococcus* being the most common organism introduced into the reproductive tract. This led to pyrexia, pus emanating from the birth canal, and abscessation of the abdomen and chest, culminating in sepsis and death.

There is more recent evidence to show the transfer of microorganisms from surgeons to their patient, which could lead to catastrophic consequences for that patient. Many studies have documented that healthcare workers can contaminate their hands or gloves with pathogens such as Gram-negative bacilli, *Staphylococcos aureus*, enterococci or *Clostridioides difficile* when performing 'clean' procedures (Coello *et al.*, 1994; Pittet *et al.*, 1999)

The efficacy of surgical hand preparation in reducing surgical-site infection (SSI) and decreasing morbidity/mortality has never been proven using a randomized controlled clinical trial due to the ethical questions the trial would pose by including a cohort in which surgical hand preparation was not performed.

Although there is a need for aseptic hand preparation before surgery, it is not the only factor implicated in achieving aseptic conditions to minimize SSI risk. Other factors that must be considered include the wearing of surgical gloves, maintaining an appropriate operating environment, and adequate preparation of the patient and surgical team. Further details can be found in Chapters 6–8 (this volume).

5.5 Surgical Hand Preparation Products

Options for agents used in surgical hand preparation are described in Table 5.1.

Table 5.1. Definitions for hand preparation products. Data from WHO (2009).

Product	Definition
Alcohol-based (hand) rub	An alcohol-containing preparation (liquid, gel or foam) designed for application to the hands to reduce the growth of microorganisms. Such preparations may contain one or more types of alcohol with excipients, other active ingredients and humectants
Antimicrobial (medicated) soap	Soap (detergent) containing an antiseptic agent at a concentration that is sufficient to reduce or inhibit the growth of microorganisms
Antiseptic agent	An antimicrobial substance that reduces or inhibits the growth of microorganisms on living tissues. Examples include alcohols, chlorhexidine gluconate, chlorine derivatives, iodine, chloroxylenol (PCMX), quaternary ammonium compounds and triclosan
Detergent (surfactant)	Compounds that possess a cleaning action. They are composed of a hydrophilic and a lipophilic part and can be divided into four groups: anionic, cationic, amphoteric and non-ionic. Although products used for hand washing or antiseptic hand wash in healthcare represent various types of detergents, the term 'soap' is used to refer to such detergents in WHO guidelines and the remainder of this chapter
Plain soap	Detergents that do not contain antimicrobial agents, or that contain very low concentrations of antimicrobial agents that are effective solely as preservatives

WHO, World Health Organization.

Alison Young

The ideal surgical scrub solution includes a detergent or soap to remove surface dirt and oils, as well as some surface bacteria. Antimicrobial solutions are chosen to destroy the microorganisms found on the hands. Aqueous solutions containing povidone-iodine, chlorhexidine gluconate and triclosan have become standard over the past few decades.

The products used for surgical hand preparation include:

- aqueous solutions containing a medicated soap;
- alcohol-based hand rubs; and
- alcohol-based rubs containing additional non-volatile active ingredients

Each of these options will be discussed in further detail below.

5.5.1 Aqueous solutions containing a medicated soap

Chlorhexidine gluconate

Chlorhexidine gluconate 4.0% is the active ingredient in chlorhexidine hand scrub (Fig. 5.2). It is effective against a wide range of Gram-positive

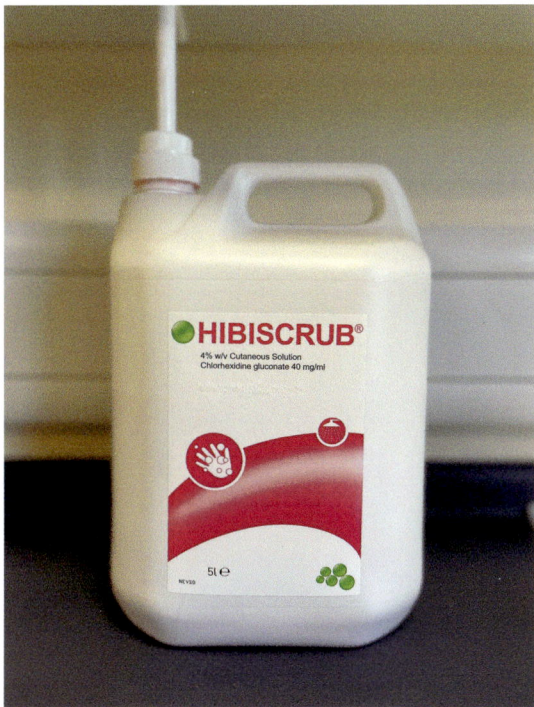

Fig. 5.2. Chlorhexidine gluconate.

and -negative bacteria, lipophilic viruses and yeasts (Hibbard *et al.*, 2002). Although its immediate antimicrobial activity is slower than that of alcohols, it is more persistent because it binds to the outermost layer of skin, the stratum corneum (Larson *et al.*, 1990). Over time, repeated exposure can lead to a cumulative effect where both transient and resident organisms are reduced (Larson *et al.*, 1990). Chlorhexidine is positively charged and reacts with the negatively charged microbial cell surface, thereby destroying the integrity of the cell membrane. Subsequently, chlorhexidine penetrates the cell and causes leakage of intracellular components, leading to cell death. As Gram-positive bacteria are more negatively charged, they are more sensitive to this agent.

Povidone-iodine

Povidone-iodine 5% (0.5% available iodine) is the active ingredient in povidone-based hand scrub (Fig. 5.3). An iodophor is a complex of iodine and a carrier molecule, which increases the solubility of iodine and slows down the release of iodine, thereby prolonging its effect. Povidone-iodine is the most used iodophor.

Iodophors are effective against a wide range of Gram-positive and -negative bacteria, *Mycobacterium tuberculosis*, fungi and viruses (Joress, 1962). Iodophors rapidly reduce the numbers of transient and colonizing bacteria but have little or no residual effect (Larson *et al.*, 1990).

Triclosan

Triclosan is an antibacterial and antifungal agent that is found in several products including soaps, suture material, detergents and toothpaste. It inhibits staphylococci, coliforms, *Enterobacteriaceae* and a wide range of Gram-negative intestinal and skin flora (Bartzokas *et al.*, 1983).

Because of concerns regarding the possibility of antimicrobial resistance, endocrine disruption and environmental pollution, the US Food and Drug Administration (FDA) ruled in 2016 that triclosan, along with some other active ingredients, are not generally recognized as safe and effective for hand preparation. It is therefore rarely used, and there are far superior products available.

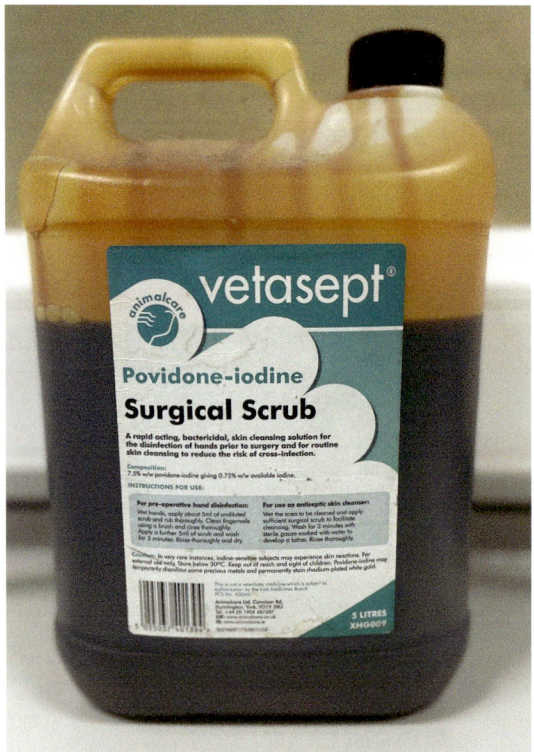

Fig. 5.3. Povidone-iodine surgical scrub.

5.5.2 Alcohol-based products

Alcohol hand preparations are available as both liquids and gels. Not every alcohol hand rub solution is appropriate for use in surgical hand preparation as they may contain different alcohol concentrations. The concentration rather than the type of alcohol is thought to be most important in determining its effectiveness (Larson, 1995). In gels designed for hygienic hand disinfection (i.e. not surgical hand preparation), there is no more than 75% alcohol.

All products must have passed European or American regulatory agencies testing. EN 1500 is the standard that specifies a test method simulating practical conditions for establishing a product for hygienic hand rub. Currently, there is no alcohol-based gel that meets EN 1500 within 30 s of product application; all require longer skin contact times to achieve effective hand hygiene, which is disadvantageous for their use in the healthcare setting.

EN 12791 specifies a test method that simulates practical conditions to determine whether a product intended for surgical hand rubbing or washing effectively reduces the resident and possibly transient microbial flora detected on the hands. The same techniques are used for both test methods. The EN12791 specification includes the forearms, which is not required for a hygienic hand rub.

Alcohol-based hand rubs

Although often viewed as a relatively recent introduction, alcohol-based products have been used in infection control for over 100 years (Fig. 5.4) (Kampf and Kramer, 2004).

Alcohol-based hand rubs are usually available in preparations of 60–90% strength and are effective against a wide range of Gram-positive and -negative bacteria, *Mycobacterium tuberculosis*, and many fungi and viruses.

The three main alcohols used are ethanol, isopropanol and *n*-propanol, and some rubs may contain a mixture of these. Compared with other common antiseptic products, alcohol is associated with the

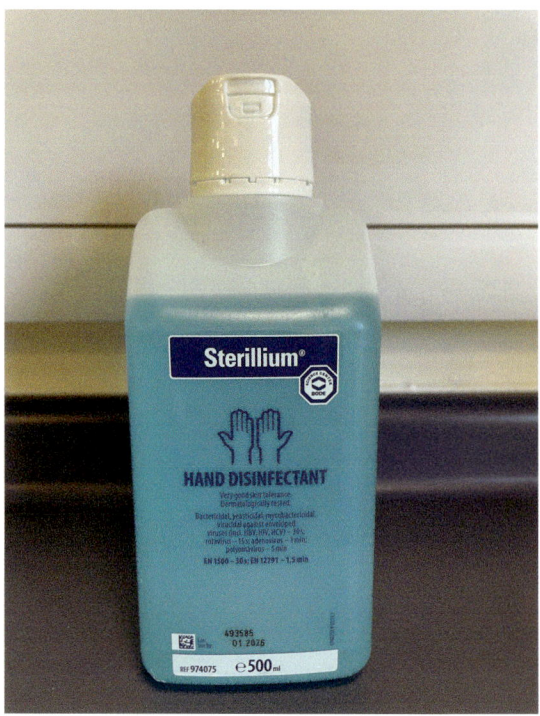

Fig. 5.4. Alcohol-based hand rub (e.g. Sterillium).

Alison Young

most rapid and greatest reduction in microbial counts (Lowbury *et al.*, 1974) but does not remove surface dirt because it does not contain surfactants or have a foaming action (Hobson *et al.*, 1998). A Cochrane review noted that alcohol-based solutions usually, but not always, contain additional active ingredients to combine the rapid bactericidal effect of alcohol with more persistent antimicrobial activity (Tanner *et al.*, 2016).

The WHO (2009) states that the antibacterial efficacy of products containing high concentrations of alcohol far surpasses that of any medicated soap presently available.

Alcohol has such a rapid and effective initial reduction of skin flora that bacterial regrowth to baseline on the gloved hand takes more than 6 h (Rotter *et al.*, 2007).

Alcohol-based rubs containing additional non-volatile active ingredients

Hand rubs with additional active ingredients are recommended by the WHO (2009). Some alcohol-based rubs contain a non-volatile 'active ingredient' such as chlorhexidine gluconate. More recently, it has been demonstrated that these products have no benefits over using an alcohol rub alone, and formulations containing 'active' substances without a clear benefit but with potential risks should be avoided when alternative formulations with the same level of antimicrobial activity, dermal tolerance and user acceptability are available (Kampf *et al.*, 2017).

5.5.3 Which product to choose for surgical hand preparation?

Product comparisons

Many studies have compared the products available for surgical hand preparation, including the use of alcohol-based hand rubs and scrubbing with medicated soap products (Marchetti *et al.*, 2003). Studies have aimed to investigate activity levels pre- and post-application, residual activity, dermal tolerance of the user, cost and availability of the product (Pietsch, 2001; Widmer, 2013)

Both chlorhexidine and povidone-iodine have been shown to cause an immediate reduction in bacteria, with the biggest reduction seen when using chlorhexidine (Tanner *et al.*, 2008; Verwilghen *et al.*, 2011). Povidone-iodine has shown a lack of

cumulative and residual activity: 6 h after scrubbing, all bacterial counts exceeded the baseline counts (Aly and Maibach, 1988). Chlorhexidine gluconate and alcohol-based products have comparable activity initially, but the residual activity of alcohol-based products has been shown to be far superior after 3 h (Verwilghen *et al.*, 2011).

Most of the evidence available regarding surgical hand preparation products is based on studies from human medicine, with the information extrapolated to veterinary patients. One study in a veterinary setting compared chlorhexidine gluconate, povidone-iodine and an alcohol-based hand rub (Verwilghen *et al.*, 2011). Preliminary studies showed significant differences between immediate and sustained activities of the different products tested: reduction in colony-forming units (CFU) after hand asepsis with povidone-iodine was significantly less than chlorhexidine or alcohol-based hand rub, even after gloving was carried out. Therefore, the inclusion of povidone in the latter parts of this study was not continued. The authors concluded that alcohol-based hand rub showed good efficiency in the clinical trial and could be considered as a useful alternative method for veterinary surgical hand antisepsis. However, they also found that 80% of respondents still used disinfectant soaps, mainly chlorhexidine gluconate, and scrubbing brushes as their pre-surgical hand preparation choice (Verwilghen *et al.*, 2011).

All of these product comparisons showed the superiority of an alcohol-based product or chlorhexidine over povidone-iodine when comparing the number of CFU on the hands of the user (Marchetti *et al.*, 2003; Verwilghen *et al.*, 2011). There are also valid reasons, including dermal tolerance and cost, to choose an alcohol-based hand rub over chlorhexidine. However, there has been no statistically significant difference found between the two hand decontamination techniques and the prevention of SSI. A 2016 Cochrane review concluded that there was no firm evidence that one type of hand antisepsis is better than another in reducing SSIs (Tanner *et al.*, 2016). The Centers for Disease Control and Prevention (CDC) does not specifically recommend one product over another for surgical hand preparation (CDC, 2002).

Surgical hand preparation using scrub (chlorhexidine) or rub (alcohol-based hand rub) techniques are both suitable for preparation of the hands prior to surgery. Despite this, several factors favour the use of alcohol-based hand rub, including rapid action, time savings, fewer side-effects and no risk of recontamination by rinsing the hands with water (WHO, 2009). Hand rub does not depend on high-quality drinking water, an issue particularly important in countries with limited resources (Widmer, 2013).

Effects on the skin of the user

A product with better dermal tolerance for the surgical team means improved compliance with hygiene guidelines (Parienti et al., 2002). Healthier hands, without abrasions from traditional scrubbing, makes hands less likely to harbour bacteria (WHO, 2009; Verwilghen et al., 2011).

If the skin on the user's hands becomes damaged and broken, then the likelihood of performing an effective hand hygiene protocol or surgical hand preparation technique is reduced. This would have consequences on the health of the patients they are treating because of increased risk of HAIs.

The effects of chlorhexidine on the hands of users have caused some concerns. A comparison of an alcohol-based hand rub and chlorhexidine was carried out to review dermal tolerance of the user. This study showed that alcohol-based hand rub resulted in less skin roughness and transepidermal water loss, and superior skin hydration and clinical assessment by a dermatologist. A high number of participants removed themselves from the study for reasons related to the use of the chlorhexidine on their skin, such as skin hydration. In conclusion, this study suggested that alcohol-based products are superior to chlorhexidine in terms of skin compatibility and efficacy (Pietsch, 2001).

Economics

Studies have shown that aseptic preparation with an alcohol hand rub was equivalent to surgical hand scrubbing in preventing SSIs after clean and clean-contaminated surgery (Parienti et al., 2002). It also showed that surgical hand rub was cost saving, by 67%, in comparison with surgical hand scrubbing (Tavolacci et al., 2006). This was mainly due to the additional cost of water filters and sterile towels used in the hand scrub technique. Without the requirement for water filters within the UK, there is very little economic difference between performing a surgical hand preparation with alcohol rub or an antiseptic soap product. There may be differences identified if future studies include groups involving

procedures other than clean or clean-contaminated surgeries (Tavolacci et al., 2006).

Conclusion

The advantages and disadvantages of each product and technique described above show that alcohol-based hand rubs are preferable for surgical hand preparation. This conclusion uses information covering a broad range of criteria – product efficacy (Marchetti et al., 2003; Verwilghen et al., 2011), dermal tolerance of the user (Parienti et al., 2002) and potential cost saving (Tavolacci et al., 2006).

If a surgical scrub using a medicated soap product is preferred by a surgeon, then chlorhexidine gluconate is the product of choice (Marchetti et al., 2003; Verwilghen et al., 2011).

5.6 Jewellery, Nail Polish and Artificial Nails

Current NICE guidelines recommend that the operating team should remove hand jewellery, artificial nails, and nail polish before operations, and WHO guidelines prohibit the wearing of such items by the surgical team or in the operating theatre (NICE, 2008; WHO, 2009).

There is limited data on the impact of wearing nail polish or artificial nails in the operating theatre with respect to infection control. There have been various studies examining nail length, native versus artificial nails and the presence of nail polish and their effect on hand hygiene but these often involve very small group numbers.

One small randomized controlled trial evaluated the effect of nail polish on the number of bacterial CFU left on hands after pre-operative surgical scrubbing. Nail polish did not influence bacterial counts and types of isolates, but nail length was a risk factor for increased bacterial counts. Based on the results, the authors recommended that nail length be kept under 2 mm (Hardy et al., 2017).

A study compared the effectiveness of hand hygiene performed by healthcare workers with native nails versus artificial nails. The baseline presence of pathogens from those with native nails was 41% less than from those with artificial nails. Antimicrobial soaps were less effective in removing contamination from the hands of healthcare workers with artificial nails, whereas alcohol hand rubs were more successful in both groups. The length of the nails varied between the two cohorts, and so nail length and the presence of nail polish could not be analysed. This study supports the opinion of the Association of Operating Room Nurses (AORN) that the use of artificial fingernails by healthcare workers might contribute to the transmission of pathogens to patients and that artificial nails should not be worn in the operating room (McNeil *et al.*, 2001). A more recent study looking at gel nail polish, rather than artificial nails, showed no association between the gel nail polish and the reduction of viable bacterial counts. However, it did show that increasing nail length was correlated with increased CFU ml^{-1} after hand preparation (Anderson *et al.*, 2021).

Higher microbial counts have been found on the hands of healthcare workers who wear rings (Hoffman *et al.*, 1985; Jacobson *et al.*, 1985). However, a Cochrane review in 2011 concluded that there was insufficient evidence to remove rings, based on subsequent SSI rate (Manley and McNamara, 2010). A further Cochrane review in 2014 found no recent randomized controlled trials that compared wearing of rings with the removal of rings, and no trials of nail polish versus no nail polish that measured surgical infection rates (Arrowsmith and Taylor, 2014).

5.7 Equipment: Scrub Brushes and Nail Picks

For many years, it was routine practice for surgical hand preparation to be performed with a soap-based product, such as chlorhexidine gluconate or povidone-iodine, and a scrubbing brush with running water.

The two common methods to perform hand preparation with a scrubbing brush are as follows:

- The timed method: a specified time (3–5 min) scrub is performed, ensuring that equal time is taken on each surface of the hand and forearm.
- The counted brush stroke method: a certain number of brush strokes are designated for each finger, palm, back of hand and arm.

Almost all studies now discourage the use of brushes because no additional antimicrobial effect has been seen when using a brush (McBride *et al.*, 1973; Loeb *et al.*, 1997). Surgical hand preparation using a scrubbing brush has been shown to cause damage to the skin of the user due to the abrasive nature of the brushes (Kikuchi-Numagami *et al.*, 1999).

The use of nail picks has been evaluated and comparisons made between groups using them and those that did not. Bacterial numbers isolated immediately post-scrub and then 1 h later were compared in both groups. There were no statistically significant differences in bacterial numbers between the groups that used nail picks and those that did not, and therefore their use was deemed unnecessary (Tanner *et al.*, 2009).

5.8 Scrubbing with Products that Require Water

Water cannot remove fats, oils and proteins that are commonly found in organic soiling and is not suitable for cleaning soiled hands when used in isolation. Soaps and detergents are therefore required in addition to water so that organic soiling is removed effectively. Aseptic hand preparations with antimicrobial products often require a flow of water, and there are some considerations when designing the area in which this procedure will take place.

Running water is required to flush away any contamination and the soap-based product at the end of the surgical scrub. To prevent contamination, specifically allocated scrub sinks should be available (Fig. 5.5). These sinks are separate from, and should not be used as, general hand wash sinks. They are not an area where cleaning buckets are disposed of.

Scrub sinks are still required within the theatre area even with the introduction of alcohol-based products for aseptic hand preparation of the surgical team. A general hand wash is always required at least once at the beginning of a surgical list, and more often if there is gross contamination of the hands.

Large scrub sinks are suitable for use by the surgical team. Specially designed scrub sinks have smooth welds and coved corners for easy cleaning and are made from rust-free materials such as stainless steel. Provision must be made to allow the water to be turned on or off without the use of the operator's hands. Elbow or knee leavers, foot switches and infrared sensors are options commonly available.

The temperature of the water used for the surgical hand preparation is important. Warm water makes antiseptics and soap work more effectively,

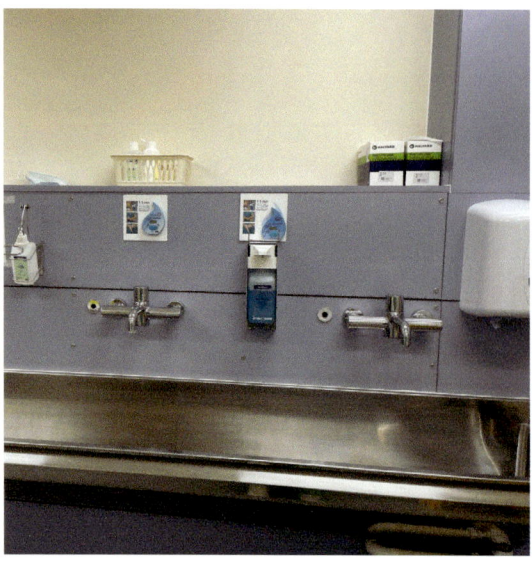

Fig. 5.5. To prevent contamination, specifically allocated scrub sinks should be available, with taps operated by foot/knee pedals or sensors (as shown here).

while cold water prevents the soap from lathering properly, meaning that any contamination or bacteria may not be washed away. Water that is too hot removes more of the protective fatty acids from the skin of the user, which may cause it to become dry and damaged. Additionally, water that is too hot may be too uncomfortable to wash for the recommended time. Therefore, washing with hot water should be avoided (WHO, 2009).

Some healthcare facilities do not have sufficient quality water. Such water would be classed as contaminated, and the use of antibacterial soap alone may not be adequate to achieve a satisfactory surgical hand preparation.

Contamination of the water supply within a healthcare setting can occur. *Pseudomonas* spp., specifically *P. aeruginosa*, are frequently isolated from taps/faucets in hospitals and have been linked to a variety of infections in clinical settings, including intensive care units (Griffith *et al.*, 2003). It is very concerning that *P. aeruginosa* and *Enterobacteriaceae* (*Enterobacter*, *Klebsiella* and *Citrobacter* spp.) were the most frequently isolated pathogens (Franco *et al.*, 2020). Biofilms can build up on any surfaces exposed to water and bacteria. The hand-washing sink design brings potentially high concentrations of healthcare pathogens into close proximity to patients, healthcare workers

and fomites, which provide easy transfer. Bacterial biofilms are usually pathogenic in nature and can cause nosocomial infections. The National Institutes of Health (NIH) revealed that among all microbial and chronic infections, 65% and 80%, respectively, are associated with biofilm formation (Jamal *et al.*, 2018).

In some areas of the world, water is a limited resource. It is estimated that one surgical hand preparation with traditional agents uses approximately 20 l of warm water, or 60 l or more for the entire surgical team (WHO, 2009). In both instances, a method of hand preparation that requires less water may be necessary, such as the use of alcohol-based hand rubs.

5.9   Drying Hands

After the surgical hand scrub using water, the hands are dried using sterile cloths or sterile disposable paper towels. Several methods of drying have been evaluated outside the surgical hand preparation with no sterility constraints. There were no significant differences in bacterial load identified among techniques, such as warm air drying, waving hands, etc. (Gustafson *et al.*, 2000).

Ideally, a towel would be available for each arm to allow the hand to be dried first, followed by the arm. Thereafter, the towel would be discarded to prevent recontamination. If this is not possible, the towel could be mentally divided into four quarters – one for each hand and arm – to prevent the same area being used twice.

If the user is applying an alcohol-based hand rub after a surgical hand scrub/wash, it is important that the hands are fully dry before application. If the hands are not dry, then the activity of the alcohol-based rub may be reduced.

5.10   Methods for Surgical Hand Preparation

5.10.1   Antimicrobial soap

Information relating to hand scrubbing can be found in Fig. 4.2 (see Chapter 4, this volume). Current WHO (2006) guidelines advise the following protocol (WHO, 2006):

- Start timing. Scrub each side of each finger, between the fingers, and the back and front of the hand for 2 min.

Alison Young

- Proceed to scrub the arms, always keeping the hand higher than the arm. This helps to avoid recontamination of the hands by water from the elbows and prevents bacteria-laden soap and water from contaminating the hands.
- Wash each side of the arm from wrist to elbow for 1 min.
- Repeat the process on the other hand and arm, always keeping hands above elbows. If the hand touches anything at any time, the scrub must be lengthened by 1 min for the area that has been contaminated.
- Rinse hands and arms by passing them through the water in one direction only, from fingertips to elbow. Do not move the arm back and forth through the water.
- Proceed to the operating theatre holding hands above elbows.
- At all times during the scrub procedure, care should be taken not to splash water on to surgical attire.
- Once in the operating theatre, hands and arms should be dried using a sterile towel and aseptic technique before donning gown and gloves.

Most guidelines available are derived from the WHO guidelines (Section 13.4. Surgical hand antisepsis using medicated soap; WHO, 2009). From the evidence discussed within this chapter, there are now elements of this protocol that should be updated secondary to more recent evidence updates.

Key points that require updating include:

- Use of scrubbing brushes. Should they be abandoned?
- Washing hands first and then washing the arms to the elbows. Should the hands be washed last to ensure there is no chance of contamination from the elbows?

5.10.2   Alcohol-based hand rub

The surgical team should routinely wash their hands with a pH-neutral soap prior to the first scrub of the day, and at any point thereafter should gross contamination of the hands occur. The nature of the work of the veterinary team often includes a mix of physical examinations and surgical procedures, and so this wash prior to surgical hand preparation is likely to be required each time.

The aim of the pre-surgical hand wash is to remove transient bacterial flora and any foreign material. After washing with a pH-neutral soap, the hands should be rinsed under running tap water and dried with paper towels before the alcohol-based hand preparation is used. It is essential that hands are dry before application of the alcohol-based product.

The application of alcohol-based hand rubs as a surgical hand preparation has not been standardized throughout the world. The WHO recommends that users follow the six basic steps for hygienic hand asepsis (Fig. 4.3, see Chapter 4, this volume), plus additional steps to rub the forearms (WHO, 2009).

The key points/tips are as follows (WHO, 2009):

- The hands should be wet with alcohol-based rub throughout the whole procedure:
- Use enough product (approximately 15 ml, depending on size of hands).
- One study showed that hands being wet was more significant than the volume of product used (Kampf and Ostermeyer, 2004).
- Forearms and hands are covered with alcohol-based rub for the first minute, while the second part focuses on the hands only.
- Hands are always to be kept above the elbows.

Surgical hand preparation using an alcohol-based hand rub requires 3 min, as outlined in the European Standard EN 12791. More recently, a 90 s application time has been shown to be equivalent to a 3 min rub with a propanol-based hand rub; at 1 min, the hand rub was found to be significantly less effective, whereas at 2 and 3 min, there was no additional effect (Kampf et al., 2005b). Historically, it was thought that training was unnecessary to use alcohol-based hand rubs successfully. Two studies have now shown that training in alcohol-based hand-rub use significantly improves bacterial killing (Labadie et al., 2002; Widmer and Dangel, 2004). Newer members of the team, or those who have not used an alcohol-based product before, should be shown and given time to learn the technique for its use.

5.11   Gloving

5.11.1   History of gloves in surgery

Sterile gloves are free from all microorganisms. They are required for any invasive procedure and when contact with any sterile site, tissue or body cavity is expected (PIDAC, 2012).

Gloves were first introduced for surgery in the 1890s. William Halsted commissioned the first pair by the Goodyear Tire and Rubber Company because they were needed to protect the hands of the surgical teams from the harsh effects of carbolic acid, which was being used as a disinfecting agent. A secondary, and revolutionary, outcome was the reduction in the post-operative infection rate and decreased mortality for the patient.

In the early 1900s, the use of surgical gloves was routine across Europe and the USA. The 1980s saw the introduction of standard precautions as the healthcare practices changed with the increased concern regarding HIV and hepatitis transmission in human medicine.

Today, sterile surgical gloves are worn as a protective barrier in surgery to reduce the risk of pathogen transmission, and in veterinary medicine, this is primarily for the benefit of the patient.

In human healthcare, in addition to protecting the patients, gloves reduce the risk to the healthcare worker of being exposed to blood-borne pathogens. In some surgical procedures, wearing two pairs of gloves ('double gloving') has become increasingly common to reduce the risk of cross-contamination after glove punctures during surgery. It may be mandatory depending on the status of the patient with a blood-borne disease (Tanner and Parkinson, 2006). However, this is not usually relevant in veterinary medicine.

In Europe, surgical gloves must receive approval under the Medical Device Directive (MDD) to receive a CE mark and be eligible for sale on the market. MDD testing prioritizes patient safety. Personal protective equipment certification focuses on keeping the wearer of the glove safe and is not mandatory. Neither type of certification takes the risks of perforations in gloves into account when approving.

5.11.2 Types of glove materials

Gloves are provided as sterile, single use and disposable. Most commonly, they are made from latex, although there are several other material options available for those allergic to latex. They are considered as Class IIa medical devices.

Latex gloves are made from natural rubber that fits comfortably and protects against viruses and bacteria. The nature of the material means that the fit provides comfort for the user and allows the maintenance of fine hand movement. This is the most common type of material for single-use, sterile surgical gloves.

Latex-free gloves are made from synthetic, non-natural rubber latex; synthetic polyisoprene and polychloroprene are commonly used materials. Latex-free gloves are used in surgical procedures when the user has a latex allergy or a latex-free environment is required for the benefit of the patient or surgical team. There are environmental issues with disposal of latex-free gloves because hydrogen chloride is released on incineration of polychloroprene.

Nitrile (acrylonitrile) gloves are made from synthetic rubber that resists punctures and harsh cleaning chemicals. Nitrile gloves are a suitable alternative to latex gloves or when a latex-free environment is required.

Vinyl gloves are made from polyvinyl chloride, a petroleum-based film. Vinyl gloves are suitable for non-aseptic procedures and tasks with a low risk of contact with body fluid. They are often used as disposable gloves because they are inexpensive to manufacture. They are less durable than latex and nitrile, are permeable to blood-borne viruses and are prone to leakage because they have a low tensile strength. They are available as single-use sterile gloves, but due to their lack of durability, they are not suitable for surgery.

The outside of gloves is smooth with a microtextured finish. Some are available with a heavy textured finish for superior grip, which may be useful for some procedures such as orthopaedic surgeries.

5.11.3 Glove performance

Punctures/damage to gloves

Significant differences in the glove defect rate depend on the wearer's role during the surgical procedure. Many of these damages are not noticed until the end of the procedure when the gloves are removed and blood is noticed on the surgeon's hands. Perforation principally occurs on the index finger of the non-dominant hand and occurs in up to 67% of surgical interventions (Dodds *et al.*, 1990; Eklund *et al.*, 2002; Yinusa *et al.*, 2004).

The cause of damage to surgical gloves is not always clear; however, several practices seem to increase the number of glove perforations (Thomas-Copeland, 2009), including:

- retracting tissue with the fingers;
- using dull instruments;

- blindly feeling for needle placement with the tip of the finger; and
- loading and unloading the needle holder by hand.

Length of wear

Glove performance decreases with the length of time the gloves are worn. Glove defects can be as high as 56% for surgeries that last more than 2 h compared with 20% for surgeries that last less than 2 h (St Germaine *et al.*, 2003). See section 5.11.7 for further information on changing gloves.

Double gloving

The potential breakdown of the barrier provided by the glove has led to 'double gloving' becoming more commonplace. Furthermore, a number of additional products have been developed to try and prevent or alert the wearer to any potential defect.

The evidence for wearing two pairs of gloves to prevent hand contamination is convincing. A Cochrane review in 2006 concluded that two layers of surgical gloves can reduce the number of breaks to the innermost glove that might allow cross-infection between the surgical team and patient (Tanner and Parkinson, 2006). A second pair of gloves does protect the first set, without apparently lessening the surgical skill (Mischke *et al.*, 2014).

This review led to several professional organizations issuing guidelines or statements incorporating the Cochrane recommendations for practice. These organizations included the Royal College of Surgeons of England (Rainsworth, 2005), the National Association of Theatre Nurses (Beesley and Pirie, 2005) and the Association of PeriOperative Nurses (AORN, 2005).

Wearing of two pairs of surgical gloves has been shown to provide increased protection for the surgical team. NICE advise that there is no available evidence that double gloving reduces the risk of SSIs or that glove perforation increases the risk of SSIs. They do recognize current practices for double gloving in certain circumstances when the risk of glove perforation and its consequences for contamination of the operative field (e.g. in prosthetic surgery) is high. They also recommend considering wearing two pairs of sterile gloves when there is a high risk of glove perforation and the consequences of contamination may be serious.

Double gloving is becoming more popular in veterinary medicine, especially during procedures where sharp instruments, bone or teeth are commonly encountered, such as dentistry and orthopaedic procedures.

5.11.4 Options to reduce glove damage

Undergloves

Coloured undergloves are available for surgical use, with the aim of providing an increased awareness and more visual prompt to the occurrence of damage in the outer pair (Fig. 5.6). The technique is the same as wearing two pairs of standard gloves, known as 'double gloving'. Some undergloves contain moisturizing agents to help retain moisture and rehydrate the skin, and some have an interlocking beaded cuff design to help reduce roll down (Wigmore and Rainey, 1994). Use of these gloves has shown an increase in the recognition of glove perforation by the surgeon (Meakin *et al.*, 2016).

Glove-in-glove

A glove-in-glove product consists of two pairs of gloves that are already combined to allow both pairs to be applied in one 'don', which reduces the time taken to glove and the packaging required. The outer glove can be removed during surgery and replaced if required.

Heavy-duty gloves

Some surgical gloves are marketed as having increased durability because they are around 50% thicker than standard surgical gloves. Such products are promoted for use in orthopaedics.

Knitted cotton gloves

Knitted cotton gloves are provided as a sterile product, and are worn over the top of standard surgical gloves. They are often used to offer protection against perforation of surgical gloves by instruments, sharp bone fragments or when tying sutures. They also absorb blood and other fluids during surgery. Concerns have been raised regarding the potential accumulation of bacteria

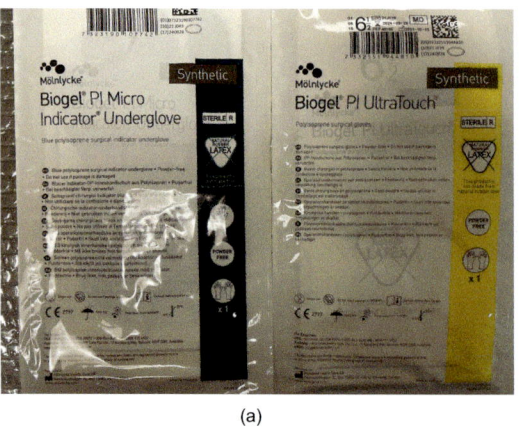 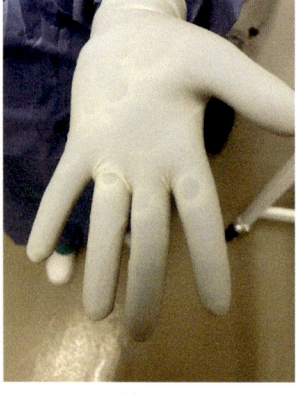 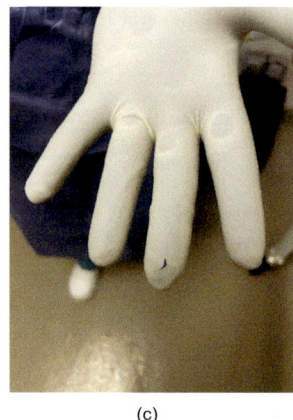

(a)   (b)   (c)

Fig. 5.6. (a) Coloured undergloves are available for surgical use, with the aim of providing an increased awareness and more visual prompt to the occurrence of damage in the outer pair. (b) Gloves pre-damage. (c) Gloves post-damage.

through contamination of the gloves (Wichmann *et al.*, 2019).

Knit fabric glove liners

Glove liners are designed to be worn between two powder-free surgical gloves to provide additional protection during rigorous procedures. They are available as single-use and reusable products. The reusable gloves have a cuff with a grid to enable wearers to monitor the number of times the glove has been rewashed and resterilized.

Glove hole detection systems

Over the years, research has attempted to define methods to facilitate the surgeon in quickly noticing a breach in surgical gloves. An example of a product developed to detect glove damage is an indicator glove, which comprises an inner glove coloured by green dye and an outer glove. Both gloves are donned simultaneously in a double-gloving technique. When a breach in the outer glove occurs, the inner glove develops a dark patch around the puncture hole, generating a visible indicator to signal the need for an immediate glove change. This is an optical change effect and does not involve release of dye or any other material. Some studies have shown this to be an unreliable system in a dry clinical setting because it requires the ingress of fluid by capillary action between the two gloves to cause a colour change

in the inner glove, which signals the presence of a hole (Fisher *et al.*, 1999).

5.11.5   Other glove options
Sensitive gloves

Sensitive gloves are, on average, 20% thinner than standard latex surgical gloves. They allow the wearer a more sensitive touch and are recommended for delicate procedures such as ophthalmology, microsurgery and cardiovascular procedures.

Gloves containing additional coatings

ANTIMICROBIAL TECHNOLOGY. Gloves with antimicrobial technology contain a proprietary antimicrobial coating, chlorhexidine gluconate, to provide an additional level of protection to surgical staff against viruses and bacteria in the event of a breach during surgery. The product is proposed to suppress the regrowth of bacteria on the surgeon's hands to help prevent bacterial contamination of the surgical site in the event of damage to the glove. If double gloving, gloves with antimicrobial technology are worn as the outer glove (Assadian *et al.*, 2014; Suchomel *et al.*, 2018).

There may be contraindications in using this type of glove after surgical hand preparation with alcohol-based hand rubs as the dermal tolerance of the user with prolonged exposure to chlorhexidine gluconate may be an issue. Further work investigating this interaction is required.

Alison Young

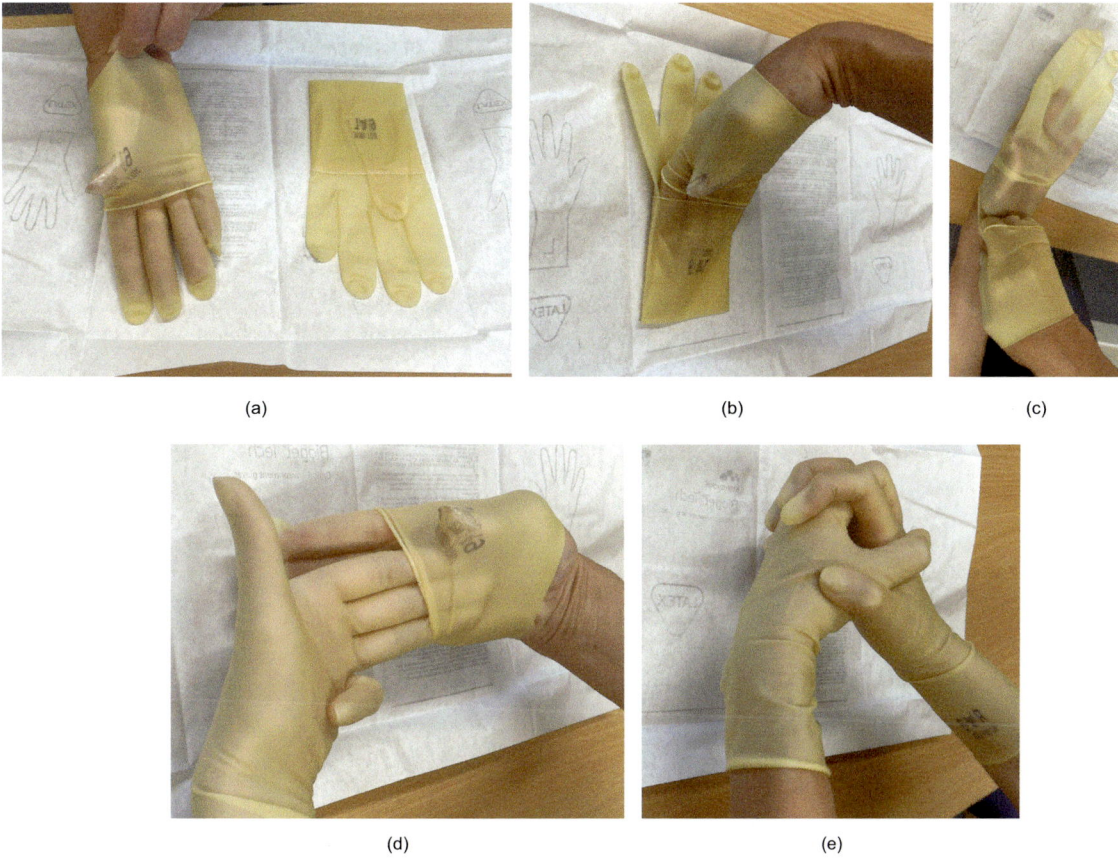

(a) (b) (c)

(d) (e)

Fig. 5.7. (a) Open gloving is performed on a clean surface, which does not have to be sterile. (b) To don the gloves, the cuff of the left glove is picked up with the right hand. The left hand is slid into the glove until there is a snug fit over the thumb joints and knuckles. Importantly, the right hand only touches the folded cuff. (c) The fingertips of the left hand are slid into the folded cuff of the right glove, and the glove pulled up and over the wrist. (d) The fingers of the gloved leftt hand are placed under the cuff of the partially gloved rightt hand and the cuff unfolded over the wrist. Importantly, the gloved finger tips must not touch the bare forearms or wrists. (e) Fully gloved hands.

EMOLLIENT COATING. An emollient coating helps the surgical team to don surgical gloves and promotes moisturization of the skin during use. One small study asked healthcare workers to self-evaluate their skin health after wearing a dermal therapy formula in gloves: 81% of the peri-operative nurses and healthcare workers rated the skin on the hand that had worn the glove as less dry than it had been at baseline, while 65% rated their skin as more hydrated, and 58% rated their skin as smoother and more supple after wearing a surgical glove coated with a dermal therapy formulation (Davis and Harper, 2005). Importantly, moisturizing products must be compatible with the glove and not contain components that may weaken or degrade the glove or interact with the hand preparation product. Further information would be required regarding the interaction of the emollient with the skin preparation product and may be more suitable for use in non-sterile gloves.

5.11.6 Methods of donning sterile gloves

Open gloving

An open gloving technique is used when donning a pair of gloves for minor procedures where only the hands need to be covered and a gown is not

---

being worn. Examples of situations where open gloving is indicated include patient skin preparation for surgery, bone marrow biopsy, and urinary or long-stay catheter placement. Open gloving is performed on a clean surface, which does not have to be sterile (Fig. 5.7).

Closed gloving

Closed gloving is the recommended method for donning gloves for surgical procedures when a long-sleeved gown is worn. It prevents contamination when gloving because the fingers, hands and wrists are not exposed. Fingers, hands and wrists should not be extended beyond the cuff of the gown until the gloves are being pulled on (Fig. 5.8; AST, 2008).

Assisted gloving

The assisted gloving method is used to don gloves on another member of the surgical team, and is a preferred method of gloving when replacing a glove while maintaining a sterile field.

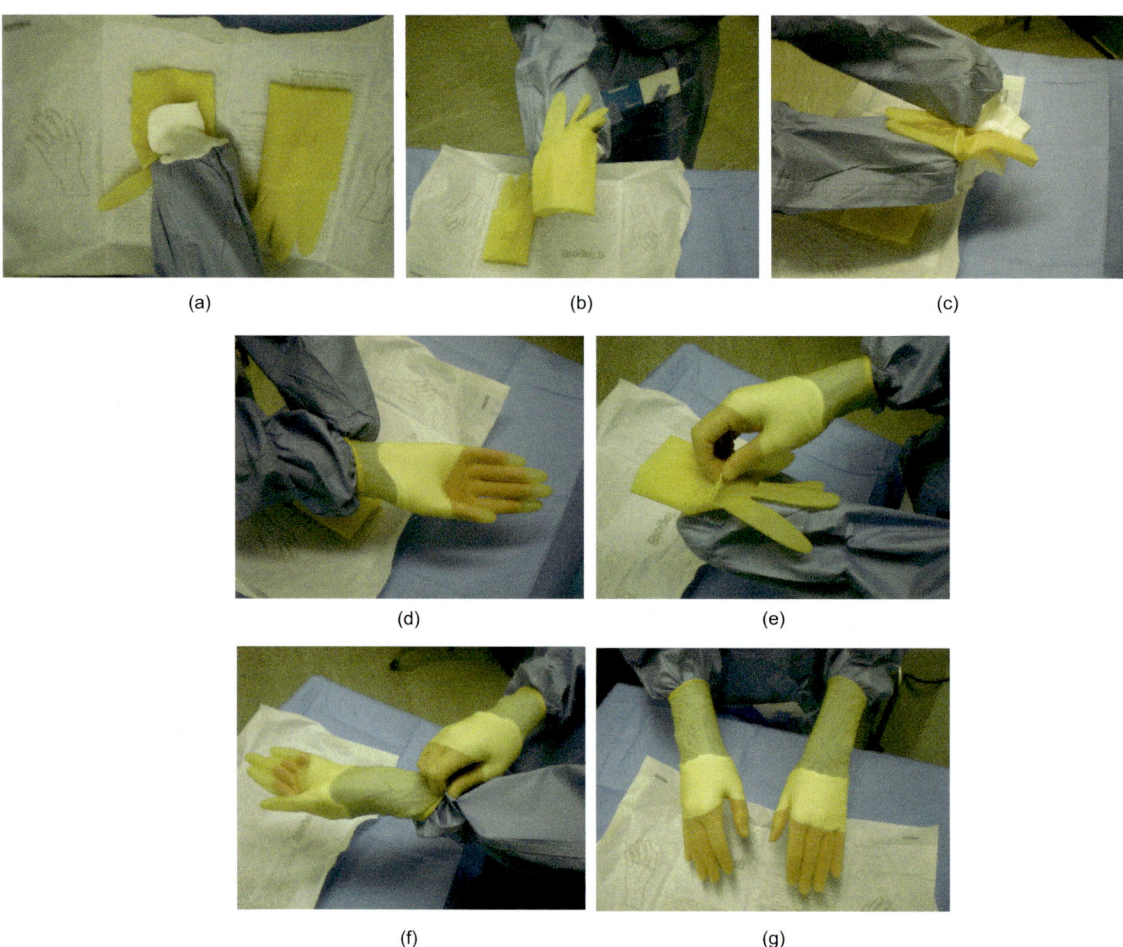

(a) (b) (c)

(d) (e)

(f) (g)

Fig. 5.8. Closed gloving is the recommended method for donning gloves for surgical procedures when a long-sleeved gown is worn. (a) Keeping the fingers inside the gown cuff, the glove pack is opened to display the gloves upside down. (b) The right thumb is placed inside the top cuff edge of the right glove (with the glove and hand in a thumb-to-thumb orientation). (c) The glove is picked up and laid flat on the right hand. (d) The left thumb (while still in the gown) is placed under the cuff on the right glove and the glove stretched over the right hand. Importantly, the white cuff must remain inside the glove. (e–f) The procedure is then repeated with the left glove. (g) Fully gloved hands.

Alison Young

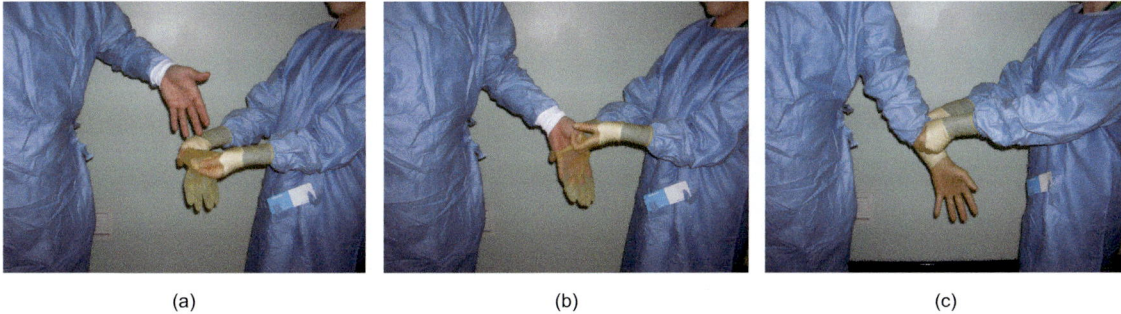

Fig. 5.9. The assisted gloving method is the preferred method of gloving when replacing a glove while maintaining a sterile field. (a) The scrubbed assistant picks up the glove with their fingers under the cuff and holds the palm of the glove towards the person being gloved. (b) The scrubbed assistant stretches the cuff to open the glove, keeping their thumbs away from the bare hands. (c) The glove cuff is unfolded over the cuff of the gown.

5.11.7 Changing gloves

Due to the commonality of intraoperative defects in surgical gloves, several studies have looked at the optimal times to change gloves during longer surgical procedures.

In all surgeries, team members should change their gloves when they suspect any potential contamination, if they see or suspect a visible glove defect or perforation, or after touching a non-sterile surface. It is best practice, and is recommended, to change both gloves (left and right) when an obvious incident occurs. When double gloving is used, both pairs should be changed if concerns are raised regarding the integrity of the outer glove. Gloves should also be changed after direct contact with methyl methacrylate (Waegemaekers *et al.*, 1983).

The time interval of surgical glove changes has been investigated and various imprecise recommendations (ranging from 30 to 180 min) identified (Harnoss *et al.*, 2010). In visceral surgery, glove perforation rates have been correlated with the duration of glove wearing, and therefore it is recommended that gloves are changed every 90 min by the surgeon and first assistant, and every 150 min by the scrub nurses and second assistants (Harnoss *et al.*, 2010).

Additional studies have also shown an increase in glove micro-perforations over time but did not show any significant difference in the rates between the separate roles of the surgical team; therefore, the authors recommended that surgeons, first assistants and surgical nurses directly assisting in the operating field change gloves after 90 min of surgery (Partecke *et al.*, 2009).

In reality, the surgeon and assistant change gloves routinely without a timed reminder. For example, in oncological surgery and gastrointestinal surgery, gloves are often changed to prevent seeding or contamination. In orthopaedic surgery, gloves are changed after cement is handled. A timed method to change gloves is not routinely carried out in all human surgical procedures.

There is a potential risk of contamination of the surgeon's gloves after draping of the patient (Makki *et al.*, 2014). Although this study showed relatively low numbers of isolates on gloves, it may be a sensible option to routinely change gloves, or the outer glove if double gloved, after draping.

The effect of gown cuff contamination was investigated in a prospective veterinary-based study. Bacterial load of the cuff was assessed at the beginning and end of surgery when the gloves were removed by a non-sterile assistant and replaced using a closed gloving technique. It concluded that closed glove exchange does not appear to be a risk factor for bacterial contamination for new gloves donned; however, further studies are warranted evaluating SSI rates with closed regloving in clean soft-tissue surgeries (Sidhu *et al.*, 2021).

Technique for changing gloves

During closed gloving, the cuff of the gown moves from over the fingertips to midway between the back of the hand and the wrist (Fig. 5.10). Once the cuff has risen to the wrist, it should never be pulled down over the hand again, because drawing the cuff over the hand may result in contamination by

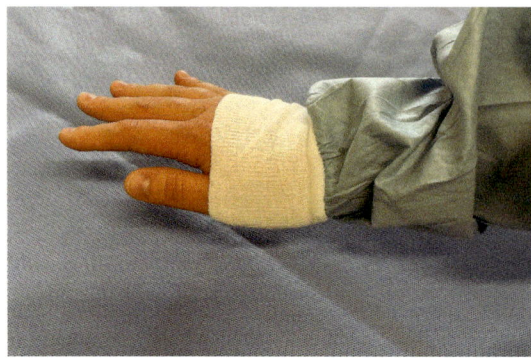

Fig. 5.10. During closed gloving, the cuff of the gown moves from over the fingertips to midway between the back of the hand and the wrist. It should not be pulled down over the hand again.

the cuff. Open assisted gloving should then be used to don a clean pair of gloves (Fig. 5.9) (AST, 2014).

If necessary, the gloves and gown should be removed, and an additional surgical hand preparation performed before donning a new sterile gown and gloves. With the introduction of alcohol-based hand rubs for aseptic hand preparation, this is a very quick and easy process, and eliminates risk.

5.12   Conclusion

There is much information available for all of the topics covered in this chapter. Looking back through the history of surgical hand preparation, it can be seen that previous products and techniques have been superseded as more research and development has taken place. The surgical team should be aware of all of the products available, the correct usage and potential disadvantages in order to make an informed decision.

References

Aly, R. and Maibach, H.I. (1988) Comparative antibacterial efficacy of a 2-minute surgical scrub with chlorhexidine gluconate, povidone-iodine, and chloroxylenol sponge-brushes. *American Journal of Infection Control* 16(4), 173–177. DOI: 10.1016/0196-6553(88)90029-6.

Anderson, S.L., Wisnieski, L., Achilles, S.L., Wooton, K.E., Shaffer, C.L. *et al.* (2021) The impact of gel fingernail polish application on the reduction of bacterial viability following a surgical hand scrub. *Veterinary Surgery* 50(7), 1525–1532. DOI: 10.1111/vsu.13703.

AORN (2005) *Standards, Recommended Practices and Guidelines*. Association of periOperative Registered Nurses, Denver, CO.

Arrowsmith, V.A. and Taylor, R. (2014) Removal of nail polish and finger rings to prevent surgical infection. *Cochrane Database of Systematic Reviews* 2014(8), CD003325. DOI: 10.1002/14651858.CD003325.pub3.

Assadian, O., Kramer, A., Ouriel, K., Suchomel, M., McLaws, M.L. *et al.* (2014) Suppression of surgeons' bacterial hand flora during surgical procedures with a new antimicrobial surgical glove. *Surgical Infections (Larchmt)* 15(1), 43–49. DOI: 10.1089/sur.2012.230.

AST (2008) *AST Standards of Practice for Surgical Attire, Surgical Scrub, Hand Hygiene and Hand Washing*. Association of Surgical Technologists, Littleton, CO. Available at: www.ast.org/uploadedFiles/Main_Site/Content/About_Us/Standard_Surgical_Attire_Surgical_Scrub.pdf (accessed 6 January 2023).

AST (2014) *Standards of Practice for Gowning and Gloving*. Revised 2014. Association of Surgical Technologists, Littleton, CO. Available at: https://www.ast.org/uploadedFiles/Main_Site/Content/About_Us/Standard_%20Gowning_and_Gloving.pdf (accessed 18 October 2022).

Bartzokas, C.A., Gibson, M.F., Graham, R. and Pinder, D.C. (1983) A comparison of triclosan and chlorhexidine preparations with 60 per cent isopropyl alcohol for hygienic hand disinfection. *Journal of Hospital Infection* 4(3), 245–255. DOI: 10.1016/0195-6701(83)90025-7.

Beesley, J. and Pirie, S. (eds) (2005) *NATN Standards and Recommendations for Safe Perioperative Practice*. National Association of Theatre Nurses, Harrogate, UK.

CDC (2002) Guideline for hand hygiene in health care settings. *Morbidity and Mortality Weekly Report* 51, 17–25.

Coello, R., Jiménez, J., García, M., Arroyo, P., Minguez, D. *et al.* (1994) Prospective study of infection, colonization and carriage of methicillin-resistant *Staphylococcus aureus* in an outbreak affecting 990 patients. *European Journal of Clinical Microbiology & Infectious Diseases* 13(1), 74–81. DOI: 10.1007/BF02026130.

Davis, D.D. and Harper, R.A. (2005) Using gloves coated with a dermal therapy formula to improve skin condition. *AORN Journal* 81(1), 157–162. DOI: 10.1016/s0001-2092(06)60068-9.

Dodds, R.D.A., Barker, S.G.E., Morgan, N.H., Donaldson, D.R. and Thomas, M.H. (1990) Self protection in surgery: the use of double gloves. *British Journal of Surgery* 77(2), 219–220. DOI: 10.1002/bjs.1800770228.

Eklund, A.M., Ojajärvi, J., Laitinen, K., Valtonen, M. and Werkkala, K.A. (2002) Glove punctures and postoperative skin flora of hands in cardiac surgery. *Annals* of Thoracic Surgery 74(1), 149–153. DOI: 10.1016/s0003-4975(02)03690-1.

Fisher, M.D., O'Keefe, J.S., Williams, F.M., Neal, J.G., Syverud, S.A. et al. (1999) Failure of a new double glove hole detection system in the emergency department. Journal of Biomedical Materials Research 48(2), 199–201. DOI: 10.1002/(sici)1097-4636(1999)48:2<199::aid-jbm15>3.0.co;2-b.

Franco, L.C., Tanner, W., Ganim, C., Davy, T., Edwards, J. et al. (2020) A microbiological survey of handwashing sinks in the hospital built environment reveals differences in patient room and healthcare personnel sinks. Scientific Reports 10(1), 8234. DOI: 10.1038/s41598-020-65052-7.

Garner, J.S. and Favero, M.S. (1986) CDC guideline for handwashing and hospital environmental control, 1985. Infection Control 7(4), 231–243. DOI: 10.1017/s0195941700084022.

Griffith, C.J., Malik, R., Cooper, R.A., Looker, N. and Michaels, B. (2003) Environmental surface cleanliness and the potential for contamination during handwashing. American Journal of Infection Control 31(2), 93–96. DOI: 10.1067/mic.2003.62.

Gustafson, D.R., Vetter, E.A., Larson, D.R., Ilstrup, D.M., Maker, M.D. et al. (2000) Effects of 4 hand-drying methods for removing bacteria from washed hands: a randomized trial. Mayo Clinic Proceedings 75(7), 705–708. DOI: 10.4065/75.7.705.

Hardy, J.M., Owen, T.J., Martinez, S.A., Jones, L.P. and Davis, M.A. (2017) The effect of nail characteristics on surface bacterial counts of surgical personnel before and after scrubbing. Veterinary Surgery 46(7), 952–961. DOI: 10.1111/vsu.12685.

Harnoss, J.C., Kramer, A., Heidecke, C.D. and Assadian, O. (2010) Wann sollte in operationsräumen ein wechsel chirurgischer handschuhe erfolgen? Zentralblatt Fur Chirurgie 135(1), 25–27. DOI: 10.1055/s-0029-1224684.

Hibbard, J.S., Mulberry, G.K. and Brady, A.R. (2002) A clinical study comparing the skin antisepsis and safety of chloraprep, 70% isopropyl alcohol, and 2% aqueous chlorhexidine. Journal of Infusion Nursing 25(4), 244–249. DOI: 10.1097/00129804-200207000-00007.

Hobson, D.W., Woller, W., Anderson, L. and Guthery, E. (1998) Development and evaluation of a new alcohol-based surgical hand scrub formulation with persistent antimicrobial characteristics and brushless application. American Journal of Infection Control 26(5), 507–512. DOI: 10.1016/s0196-6553(98)70024-0.

Hoffman, P.N., Cooke, E.M., McCarville, M.R. and Emmerson, A.M. (1985) Micro-organisms isolated from skin under wedding rings worn by hospital staff. British Medical Journal 290, 206–207. DOI: 10.1136/bmj.290.6463.206.

Jacobson, G., Thiele, J.E., McCune, J.H. and Farrell, L.D. (1985) Handwashing: ring-wearing and number of microorganisms. Nursing Research 34(3), 186–188.

Jamal, M., Ahmad, W., Andleeb, S., Jalil, F., Imran, M. et al. (2018) Bacterial biofilm and associated infections. Journal of the Chinese Medical Association 81(1), 7–11. DOI: 10.1016/j.jcma.2017.07.012.

Joress, S.M. (1962) A study of disinfection of the skin. Annals of Surgery 155(2), 296–304. DOI: 10.1097/00000658-196200000-00020.

Kampf, G. and Kramer, A. (2004) Epidemiologic background of hand hygiene and evaluation of the most important agents for scrubs and rubs. Clinical Microbiology Reviews 17(4), 863–893. DOI: 10.1128/CMR.17.4.863-893.2004.

Kampf, G. and Ostermeyer, C. (2004) Influence of applied volume on efficacy of 3-minute surgical reference disinfection method prEN 12791. Applied and Environmental Microbiology 70(12), 7066–7069. DOI: 10.1128/AEM.70.12.7066-7069.2004.

Kampf, G., Goroncy-Bermes, P., Fraise, A. and Rotter, M. (2005a) Terminology in surgical hand disinfection--a new Tower of Babel in infection control. Journal of Hospital Infection 59(3), 269–271. DOI: 10.1016/j.jhin.2004.09.020.

Kampf, G., Ostermeyer, C. and Heeg, P. (2005b) Surgical hand disinfection with a propanol-based hand rub: equivalence of shorter application times. Journal of Hospital Infection 59(4), 304–310. DOI: 10.1016/j.jhin.2004.09.022.

Kampf, G., Kramer, A. and Suchomel, M. (2017) Lack of sustained efficacy for alcohol-based surgical hand rubs containing "residual active ingredients" according to EN 12791. Journal of Hospital Infection 95(2), 163–168. DOI: 10.1016/j.jhin.2016.11.001.

Kikuchi-Numagami, K., Saishu, T., Fukaya, M., Kanazawa, E. and Tagami, H. (1999) Irritancy of scrubbing up for surgery with or without a brush. Acta Dermato-Venereologica 79(3), 230–232. DOI: 10.1080/000155599750011057.

Labadie, J.C., Kampf, G., Lejeune, B., Exner, M., Cottron, O. et al. (2002) Recommendations for surgical hand disinfection -- requirements, implementation and need for research. A proposal by representatives of the SFHH, DGHM and DGKH for a European discussion. The Journal of Hospital Infection 51(4), 312–315. DOI: 10.1053/jhin.2002.1243.

Larson, E.L. (1995) APIC guideline for handwashing and hand antisepsis in health care settings. American Journal of Infection Control 23(4), 251–269. DOI: 10.1016/0196-6553(95)90070-5.

Larson, E.L., Butz, A.M., Gullette, D.L. and Laughon, B.A. (1990) Alcohol for surgical scrubbing? Infection Control and Hospital Epidemiology 11(3), 139–143. DOI: 10.1086/646137.

Lister, J. (1867) Illustrations of the antiseptic system of treatment in surgery. Lancet 90, 668–669. DOI: 10.1016/S0140-6736(02)58116-2.

Loeb, M.B., Wilcox, L., Smaill, F., Walter, S. and Duff, Z. (1997) A randomized trial of surgical scrubbing with a brush compared to antiseptic soap alone. *American Journal of Infection Control* 25(1), 11–15. DOI: 10.1016/s0196-6553(97)90047-x.

Lowbury, E.J.L., Lilly, H.A. and Ayliffe, G.A.J. (1974) Preoperative disinfection of surgeons' hands: use of alcoholic solutions and effects of gloves on skin flora. *British Medical Journal* 4(5941), 369–372. DOI: 10.1136/bmj.4.5941.369.

Makki, D., Deierl, K., Pandit, A. and Trakru, S. (2014) A prospective study on the risk of glove fingertip contamination during draping in joint replacement surgery. *Annals of the Royal College of Surgeons of England* 96(6), 434–436. DOI: 10.1308/003588414X 13946184902046.

Manley, K. and McNamara, I. (2010) Theatre etiquette, sterile technique and surgical site preparation. *Surgery* 29, 55–58.

Marchetti, M.G., Kampf, G., Finzi, G. and Salvatorelli, G. (2003) Evaluation of the bactericidal effect of five products for surgical hand disinfection according to prEN 12054 and prEN 12791. *Journal of Hospital Infection* 54(1), 63–67. DOI: 10.1016/s0195-6701(03)00039-2.

McBride, M.E., Duncan, W.C. and Knox, J.M. (1973) An evaluation of surgical scrub brushes. *Surgery, Gynecology & Obstetrics* 137, 934–936.

McNeil, S.A., Foster, C.L., Hedderwick, S.A. and Kauffman, C.A. (2001) Effect of hand cleansing with antimicrobial soap or alcohol-based gel on microbial colonization of artificial fingernails worn by health care workers. *Clinical Infectious Diseases* 32(3), 367–372. DOI: 10.1086/318488.

Meakin, L.B., Gilman, O.P., Parsons, K.J., Burton, N.J. and Langley-Hobbs, S.J. (2016) Colored indicator undergloves increase the detection of glove perforations by surgeons during small animal orthopedic surgery: a randomized controlled trial. *Veterinary Surgery* 45(6), 709–714. DOI: 10.1111/vsu.12519.

Mischke, C., Verbeek, J.H., Saarto, A., Lavoie, M.-C., Pahwa, M. *et al.* (2014) Gloves, extra gloves or special types of gloves for preventing percutaneous exposure injuries in healthcare personnel. *Cochrane Database of Systematic Reviews* 3, CD009573.

NHS (2022) *National Infection Prevention and Control Manual for England*. National Health Service, London. Available at: www.england.nhs.uk/publication/national-infection-prevention-and-control/ (accessed 19 October 2022).

NICE (2008) Surgical site infections: prevention and treatment. NICE Guidance NG125. National Institute for Health and Care Excellence, London. Available at: www.nice.org.uk/guidance/ng125/chapter/recommendations (accessed 6 January 2023).

Parienti, J.J., Thibon, P., Heller, R., Le Roux, Y., von Theobald, P. *et al.* (2002) Hand-rubbing with an aqueous alcoholic solution vs traditional surgical hand-scrubbing and 30-day surgical site infection

rates: a randomized equivalence study. *Journal of the American Medical Association* 288, 722–727.

Partecke, L.I., Goerdt, A.M., Langner, I., Jaeger, B., Assadian, O. *et al.* (2009) Incidence of microperforation for surgical gloves depends on duration of wear. *Infection Control & Hospital Epidemiology* 30, 409–414.

PIDAC (2012) *Routine Practices and Additional Precautions In All Health Care Settings*, 3rd edn. Provincial Infectious Diseases Advisory Committee, Queen's Printer for Ontario, Toronto, ON. Available at: www.publichealthontario.ca/-/media/documents/B/2012/bp-rpap-healthcare-settings.pdf (accessed 19 October 2022).

Pietsch, H. (2001) Hand antiseptics: rubs versus scrubs, alcoholic solutions versus alcoholic gels. *Journal of Hospital Infection* 48(Suppl. A), S33–S36. DOI: 10.1016/S0195-6701(01)90010-6.

Pittet, D., Dharan, S., Touveneau, S., Sauvan, V. and Perneger, T.V. (1999) Bacterial contamination of the hands of hospital staff during routine patient care. *Archives of Internal Medicine* 159, 821–826.

Price, P.B. (1938) The bacteriology of normal skin: a new quantitative test applied to a study of the bacterial flora and the disinfectant action of mechanical cleansing. *Journal of Infectious Diseases* 63, 301–318.

Rainsworth, R. (2005) RCS supports double gloving. Available at: http://regentmedical.com/global/news-andevents.aspx?information id=49.

Reinicke, E.A. (1894) Bakteriologische untersuchungen über die desinfektion der hände. *Zentralblatt Fur Gynäkology* 47, 1189–1199.

Rotter, M.L., Kampf, G., Suchomel, M. and Kundi, M. (2007) Population kinetics of the skin flora on gloved hands following surgical hand disinfection with 3 propanol-based hand rubs: a prospective, randomized, double-blind trial. *Infection Control and Hospital Epidemiology* 28(3), 346–350. DOI: 10.1086/510865.

Sidhu, D.S., Gull, T. and Skinner, O.T. (2021) Influence of intraoperative closed glove exchange on glove contamination during clean soft tissue surgeries. *Veterinary Surgery* 50, 1510–1517. DOI: 10.1111/vsu.13688.

Simmons, B.P. and CDC (Centers for Disease Control and Prevention) (eds) (1981) CDC Hospital Infections Program (HIP). Guidelines for prevention and control of nosocomial infections. CDC, Atlanta, GA, pp. 6–10. Available at: https://wonder.cdc.gov/wonder/prevguid/p0000107/p0000107.asp#head002000000000000 (accessed 19 October 2022).

St Germaine, R.L., Hanson, J. and de Gara, C.J. (2003) Double gloving and practice attitudes among surgeons. *American Journal of Surgery* 185, 141–145. DOI: 10.1016/S0002-9610(02)01217-5.

Suchomel, M., Brillmann, M., Assadian, O., Ousey, K.J. and Presterl, E. (2018) Chlorhexidine-coated surgical gloves influence the bacterial flora of hands over a period of 3 hours. *Antimicrobial Resistance and Infection Control* 7, 108. DOI: 10.1186/s13756-018-0395-0.

Tanner, J. and Parkinson, H. (2006) Double gloving to reduce surgical cross-infection. *Cochrane Database of Systematic Reviews* 3, CD003087.

Tanner, J., Swarbrook, S. and Stuart, J. (2008) Surgical hand antisepsis to reduce surgical site infection. *Cochrane Database of Systematic Reviews* 1, CD004288.

Tanner, J., Khan, D., Walsh, S., Chernova, J., Lamont, S. *et al.* (2009) Brushes and picks used on nails during the surgical scrub to reduce bacteria: a randomised trial. *Journal of Hospital Infection* 71, 234–238.

Tanner, J., Dumville, J.C., Norman, G. and Fortnam, M. (2016) Surgical hand antisepsis to reduce surgical site infection. *Cochrane Database of Systematic Reviews* 1, CD004288.

Tavolacci, M.P., Pitrou, I., Merle, V., Haghighat, S., Thillard, D. *et al.* (2006) Surgical hand rubbing compared with surgical hand scrubbing: comparison of efficacy and costs. *Journal of Hospital Infection* 63, 55–59. DOI: 10.1016/j.jhin.2005.11.012.

Thomas-Copeland, J. (2009) Do surgical personnel really need to double-glove? *AORN Journal* 89, 322–328.

Verwilghen, D.R., Mainil, J., Mastrocicco, E., Hamaide, A., Detilleux, J. *et al.* (2011) Surgical hand antisepsis in veterinary practice: evaluation of soap scrubs and alcohol based rub techniques. *Veterinary Journal* 190, 372–377. DOI: 10.1016/j.tvjl.2010.12.020.

Waegemaekers, T.H., Seutter, E., den Arend, J.A. and Malten, K.E. (1983) Permeability of surgeons' gloves to methyl methacrylate. *Acta Orthopaedica Scandinavica* 54, 790–795.

WHO (2005) Clean care is safer care. World Health Organization, Geneva, Switzerland. Available at: www.who.int/news-room/events/detail/2005/10/13/default-calendar/clean-care-is-safer-care (accessed 22 November 2022).

WHO (2006) *WHO Guidelines on Hand Hygiene in Health Care (Advanced Draft): Global Safety Challenge 2005–2006: Clean Care Is Safer Care.* World Health Organization, Geneva, Switzerland. Available at: https://apps.who.int/iris/handle/10665/69323 (accessed 18 November 2022).

WHO (2009) *WHO Guidelines on Hand Hygiene in Health Care.* World Health Organization, Geneva, Switzerland. Available at: http://apps.who.int/iris/bitstream/10665/44102/1/9789241597906_eng.pdf (accessed 19 October 2022).

WHO (2016) Surgical handrubbing technique. World Health Organization, Geneva, Switzerland. Available at: https://cdn.who.int/media/docs/default-source/integrated-health-services-(ihs)/clean-hands-2016/hh-surgicala3.pdf?sfvrsn=1b5e2929_3 (accessed 18 November 2022).

Wichmann, T., Moriarty, T.F., Keller, I., Pfister, S., Deggim-Messmer, V. *et al.* (2019) Prevalence and quantification of contamination of knitted cotton outer gloves during hip and knee arthroplasty surgery. *Archives of Orthopaedic and Trauma Surgery* 139, 451–459. DOI: 10.1007/s00402-018-3061-3.

Widmer, A.F. and Dangel, M. (2004) The alcohol handrub: evaluation of technique and microbiological efficacy with international infection control professionals. *Infection Control & Hospital Epidemiology* 25, 207–209.

Widmer, A.F. (2013) Surgical hand hygiene: scrub or rub? *Journal of Hospital Infection* 83, S35–S39. DOI: 10.1016/S0195-6701(13)60008-0.

Wigmore, S.J. and Rainey, J.B. (1994) Use of coloured undergloves to detect glove puncture. *British Journal of Surgery* 81, 1480.

Yinusa, W., Li, Y.H., Chow, W., Ho, W.Y. and Leong, J.C. (2004) Glove punctures in orthopaedic surgery. *International Orthopaedics* 28, 36–39. DOI: 10.1007/s00264-003-0510-5.

6 Personal Protective Equipment

MELLORA SHARMAN[1] AND HELEN SILVER-MACMAHON[2]*

[1]VeCT, Broers Building, 21 JJ Thomson Avenue, Cambridge, CB3 0FA, UK; [2]VetLed, Sunnybank Cottage Bullocks Farm Lane, Wheeler End, High Wycombe, HP14 3NQ, UK

6.1 Introduction

Regular exposure to infectious materials places healthcare workers at particular risk for healthcare-acquired infections (HAIs), which can result in significant health implications, as well as subsequent absenteeism during treatment and recovery. Personal protective equipment (PPE) encompasses a range of specialized equipment worn by healthcare workers that provides a barrier and protects against contamination, therefore mitigating transmission of infectious agents between the patient, the healthcare worker and the environment. Poor infection-control practices, including insufficient or inappropriate use of PPE, increases risk to healthcare personnel and patients alike. Up to 30–40% of veterinarians report exposure to zoonotic diseases in practice (Schnurrenberger et al., 1978; Lipton et al., 2008). This might include relatively minor individual risk, such as exposure to dermatophytes, but more serious and larger zoonotic outbreaks in animal care workers have also been documented (Weese et al., 2002; Koopmans et al., 2004; Chollet et al., 2015). Furthermore, exposure to some zoonotic agents such as rabies or Hendra virus, carry a significant risk of death (Weese et al., 2002; Field et al., 2010; Playford et al., 2010; Jackson, 2013).

Non-zoonotic HAIs, especially those involving multidrug-resistant (MDR) organisms, pose a significant risk of impacting individual patients, extending hospitalization, increasing morbidity and contributing to mortality (Cornejo-Juárez et al., 2015; Serra-Burriel et al., 2020). Within the last decade, there have been several examples of nosocomial outbreaks within the veterinary or animal care sector including methicillin-resistant *Staphylococcus pseudintermedius* (MRSP), virulent calicivirus and equine herpesvirus 1 (Reynolds et al., 2009; Grönthal et al., 2014). Of course, the consequences of such HAIs extend beyond individual morbidity and mortality, and can result in restriction of hospital admissions or even temporary ward or hospital closures, causing substantial economic impact (Klevens et al., 2007; Scott, 2009; Marchetti and Rossiter, 2013; Grönthal et al., 2014; Stull and Weese, 2015; Haque et al., 2018). In previous decades, annual financial losses due to the direct costs of HAIs in European and US human healthcare systems have been estimated at €7 billion and US$6.5 billion per annum, respectively. Updated estimates and inclusion of both direct and indirect costs are, in reality, likely to place this figure much higher (Scott, 2009; Arefian et al., 2016). Potential financial losses to pet owners, or veterinary clinics and hospitals, as a result of HAIs may be largely unknown, but are equally relevant given that pet treatments are largely client financed and the majority of veterinary facilities maintain profitability within very narrow margins.

Implementation of robust and cost-effective infection-control measures helps reduce the transmission risk of zoonoses and other HAIs. Ultimately, an ideal infection-control programme includes adequate development of policies and procedures, specific training of personnel, incorporation of environmental controls such as negative-pressure rooms, the development of appropriate workflow practices, and appropriate access to and use of PPE (as will be discussed in this chapter). Regular audits and compliance assessments play an important role in determining the effectiveness of policies and practices. Understanding the variety of barriers that limit implementation of PPE use policies

*Corresponding author: helen@vetled.co.uk

DOI: 10.1079/9781789244977.0006

is also crucial when appropriately executing and monitoring the effectiveness of these policies and procedures.

It is important to note that one of the single most important and basic control measures any individual can undertake in managing infection control risks remains hand hygiene (see Chapters 4 and 5, this volume), and PPE should only ever be used to complement this basic practice where needed (Aiello *et al.*, 2008; WHO and WHO Patient Safety, 2009).

6.2 Apparel and Personal Protective Equipment

All personnel involved in patient interactions have a responsibility to be cognisant of risks, to be aware of policies and procedures, and to actively engage in minimizing contamination and transmission of infectious agents to themselves or to other patients.

6.2.1 Apparel policies

Before considering additional PPE implementation, it is important to ensure that a robust baseline apparel policy is in place. Workwear and uniform policies within medical and veterinary healthcare should consider patient safety, public confidence and staff comfort, as well as ensuring effective hygiene, and prevention of infection transmission remains of paramount importance (NHS, 2020).

Good practice takes into account the following key points:

- A 'bare below the elbows' policy should be adopted, as cuffs at the wrist become heavily contaminated and are likely to come into contact with patients.
- A uniform policy (see *Scrubs and uniforms* section below).
- Fingernails should be clean, short and unvarnished. Long nails are harder to clean and are therefore a potential hazard. False nails should not be worn because they harbour microorganisms and make effective hand hygiene more difficult.
- Long hair should be tied back behind the collar.
- No jewellery. This includes wristwatches, which may harbour microorganisms and make hand hygiene more difficult. Necklaces, hoop or loop earrings and rings can also present possible hazards for patients and staff.

- Neck ties (except bow ties) and lanyards should not be worn during patient care activities because they become contaminated by pathogens and are rarely laundered (NHS, 2020).
- Soft-soled shoes with enclosed toes should be worn to protect the wearer from spills, dropped objects, injury or contamination.

Scrubs and uniforms

Uniforms or scrubs are routinely worn within veterinary healthcare to remove the risks associated with, or to protect personal clothing from, contamination. Although no conclusive evidence exists that uniforms and workwear play a direct role in spreading infection, it is widely acknowledged that contamination occurs during clinical shifts from a variety of sources (Sanon and Watkins, 2012; Kokkinos *et al.*, 2020; NHS, 2020). Therefore, several important considerations should be taken into account when formulating an infection-control policy relating to workwear. This is likely to encompass factors such as purpose, when and where workwear should be worn, and particularly laundering requirements.

The Royal College of Nursing and Midwifery outlines the importance of workwear being fit for purpose, easy to clean and able to withstand regular laundering. NHS England also mandates that staff are provided with sufficient apparel to wear a clean complete uniform every day, with an additional spare uniform available should contamination occur (NHS, 2020). Some controversy exists regarding when scrubs or uniforms are donned: documented evidence of infection risk from travelling in uniform is limited; however, wearing of scrubs and uniforms during transit is generally regarded as unhygienic, and therefore within human healthcare settings it is advised that workwear be donned upon arrival at the workplace (AORN, 2009; NHS, 2020). This is worthy of consideration given that The Workplace (Health, Safety and Welfare) Regulations (1992) state that if special clothing is required for the purpose of work, sufficient suitable facilities must be provided for clothing changes.

How and where uniforms and scrubs will be laundered is also an important consideration. The available literature shows that washing at a temperature of 60°C removes almost all microorganisms (NHS, 2020). Central laundry services more reliably ensure that washing is undertaken in a manner that is effective for infection-control purposes (Wilson *et al.*, 2007). However, logistics or cost may mean that workwear is ultimately laundered within the home environment, in which case specific guidance should be provided. Recent studies within veterinary care settings support NHS literature indicating that home laundering at 30°C with detergent is efficacious at reducing the bacterial load of Gram-positive microorganisms, including methicillin-resistant *Staphylococcus aureus* (MRSA) (Wilson *et al.*, 2007; Kokkinos *et al.*, 2020). As some fabric types may have a maximum laundering temperature below 30°C, it is sensible to take this into account when selecting material or making workwear purchases.

Additional novel technologies have been explored to determine their benefit in reducing uniform contamination rates and transmission risk. One study examined the efficacy of antimicrobial-impregnated scrubs in preventing acquisition of pathogens on healthcare providers' clothing, but found that there was no decrease in bacterial contamination (Anderson *et al.*, 2017). In contrast, copper-coated paramide and copper-coated polyester textiles demonstrated significant antimicrobial activity against a variety of nosocomial MDR pathogens, and therefore could be useful in reducing the transmission of pathogens between patients, healthcare workers and the environment (Irene *et al.*, 2016).

6.2.2 PPE

To further mitigate transmission of infectious agents, a range of PPE or specialized equipment may be worn by healthcare workers to provide an additional barrier to workwear. For any individual situation, PPE selection will be determined by a range of factors including the following:

- *Type of risk.* For example, will the caregiver encounter open wounds, large volumes of body fluid that might penetrate clothing, and/or tissue or fluid with a contagious potential?
- *Durability and appropriateness of PPE for a task.* For example, is a gown/coverall or apron preferable, and is the PPE fluid-proof (e.g. plastic apron) or made of absorbable material (e.g. fabric gown)?
- *Fit.* A range of appropriate sizes should be available for gowns/gloves/coveralls and fit tests should be undertaken for respiratory PPE.

Development of an algorithm to aid risk determination and PPE selection may be of benefit for reference within a ward setting. An example of such an algorithm is provided in Fig. 6.1 and further guidance on PPE use in certain settings is provided in Table 6.1. An overview of pertinent points of consideration for various types of PPE will follow.

Donning and doffing

Contamination with infectious materials commonly occurs during the donning process due to inappropriate choice of PPE size, or during the doffing process because of incorrect technique. To prevent contamination during use of PPE, it is recommended that appropriate training and guidance are provided on selection of PPE, as well as donning and doffing protocols, and that appropriate sizes are also available.

Beam *et al.* (2011) reported the most common breaches while donning PPE were failing to tie the gown at the neck and waist, not conducting a seal check on the respirator, and donning the equipment in an improper sequence. Breaches reported when doffing PPE related to the sequence of removal and personnel removing contaminated items from the room. Common errors reported in both veterinary and human healthcare PPE simulation studies include incorrect removal of gloves, unnecessary touching of surfaces in the room and unprotected areas of the wearer's body (Beam *et al.*, 2011; Casanova *et al.*, 2012; Christmann *et al.*, 2019).

It is imperative that particular attention is paid to the donning and doffing protocols (Figs 6.2 and 6.3). Various resources are available to remind healthcare workers of the required protocol, including video- or illustration-based training, or formal observation and instruction (Christmann *et al.*, 2019; Verbeek *et al.*, 2020). Success, or otherwise, of some of these strategies will be discussed in more detail later. Broadly speaking, active training reduces errors compared with folder-based training (Verbeek *et al.*, 2020). Unsurprisingly, complex PPE protocols, or those that include items that are more difficult to don and doff, increase the risk of errors and contamination (Verbeek *et al.*, 2020). Use of a one-step glove and gown removal doffing protocol might decrease the rate of contamination (Verbeek *et al.*, 2020).

The importance of correct glove size has been demonstrated in several studies (Sax *et al.*, 2007; Christmann *et al.*, 2019). Christmann *et al.* (2019) found that inappropriate glove size selection resulted in an overall contamination rate of 15%

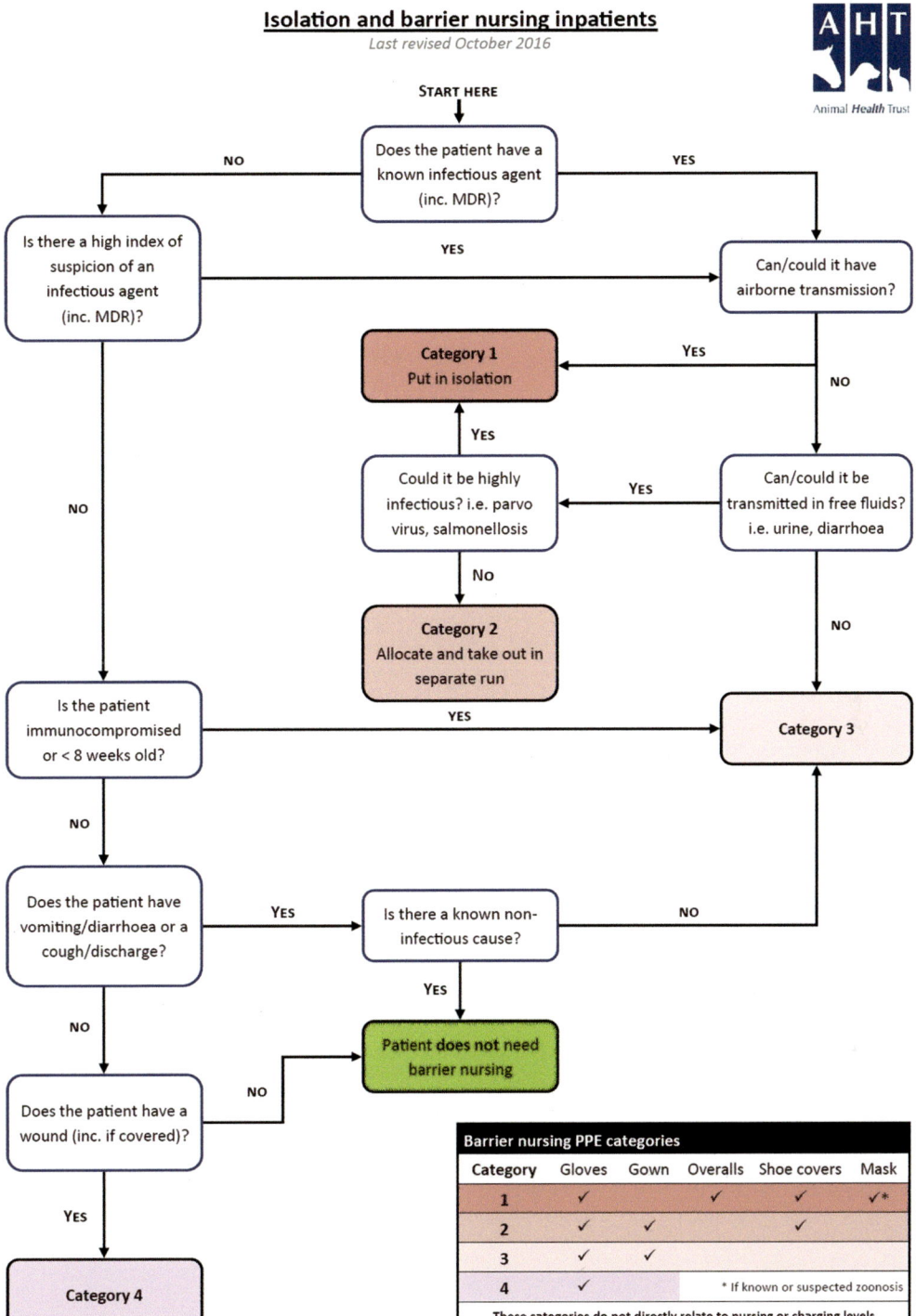

Fig. 6.1. An algorithm for personal protective equipment use in an isolation and barrier nursing setting. Courtesy of The Animal Health Trust, Newmarket, UK.

Table 6.1. Guidance on appropriate use of aprons, gowns, and face and eye/mouth protection.

Activity	Aprons/gowns/coveralls	Face and eye/mouth protection
Sterile procedures	Yes	Risk assessment
Contact with wounds or skin lesions	Yes	Risk assessment
Cleaning up incontinence	Yes	Risk assessment
Potential exposure to blood/other body fluids, e.g. cleaning up spillages, taking specimens, non-sterile procedures	Yes	Risk assessment
Touching patients with unidentified skin rashes	Risk assessment	Risk assessment
Emptying/changing urinary catheter bags	Yes	Risk assessment
Using disinfectants or cleaning agents	Yes	Risk assessment
General cleaning of clinical areas	Risk assessment	NA
Bed making, dressing patients/clients	Yes	NA
Oral care	Risk assessment	Risk assessment
Feeding patients	Risk assessment	NA
Handling waste	Risk assessment	Risk assessment

NA, not applicable.

due to development of a gap between coverall sleeves and gloves. A Cochrane review concluded low-certainty evidence that gowns that provided a better fit around the neck, wrists and hands, and better coverage of the gown–glove interface led to lower contamination rates (Verbeek *et al.*, 2020). Fit-testing of respirators (i.e. N95 masks) or other medical mask types is a commonly accepted prerequisite to ensure appropriate respiratory protection (see further discussion later).

Appropriate use of aprons

Disposable plastic aprons can offer good protection during a multitude of activities where close contact with patients, materials or equipment may result in contamination of clothing. Aprons may be appropriate when restraining patients or changing bedding; however, it is important to consider whether sufficient coverage will be provided, or whether a gown or coverall would be more desirable. For example, the use of aprons is not recommended for nursing patients with open wounds and infection with MDR organisms (Fig. 6.1) because an apron will not cover (and thereby protect) all areas, such as the arms.

Appropriate use of gowns

When exposure to significant amounts of body fluids is anticipated, gowns provide better protection than

aprons to reduce cross-contamination of workwear or exposed body areas (e.g. the lower arms) (Caveney *et al.*, 2011; Verbeek *et al.*, 2020; Siegel *et al.*, 2007). One might argue that all fluids, secretions and excretions pose a potential risk until proved otherwise, and therefore some component of PPE use is reasonable in the majority of clinical settings.

Gowns should be disposable, impermeable, single use and readily available in a variety of sizes to ensure that all areas of the body are covered. Gown material should also be of adequate strength to avoid easily tearing or puncturing, be comfortable to wear for long periods and be affordable. As stated previously, gowns that fit well around the neck and wrists reduce contamination risk (Verbeek *et al.*, 2020).

Combined use of gowns with gloves is recommended (CDC, 2004), and gowns should always be donned first. Gowns should cover the arms and front of the body, from neck to below mid-thigh (Siegel *et al.*, 2007). Contamination of the glove–gown interface is exacerbated by inappropriate sizing of gowns or gloves, or poor technique when donning or doffing. Therefore, particular care should be taken when removing gowns and gloves to prevent contamination of the skin (particularly of the wrists), the wearer's clothes and the environment:

● Gowns should always be removed before leaving the patient care area to prevent environmental contamination (Siegel *et al.*, 2007).

The type of PPE used will vary based on the level of precautions required, such as standard and contact, droplet or airborne infection isolation precautions. The procedure for putting on and removing PPE should be tailored to the specific type of PPE.

1. GOWN

- Fully cover torso from neck to knees, arms to end of wrists, and wrap around the back
- Fasten in back of neck and waist

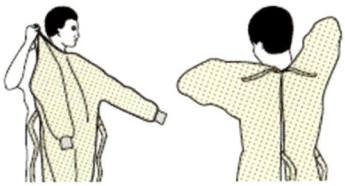

2. MASK OR RESPIRATOR

- Secure ties or elastic bands at middle of head and neck
- Fit flexible band to nose bridge
- Fit snug to face and below chin
- Fit-check respirator

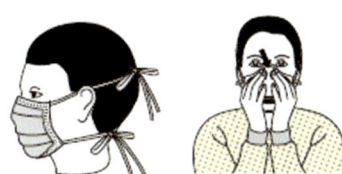

3. GOGGLES OR FACE SHIELD

- Place over face and eyes and adjust to fit

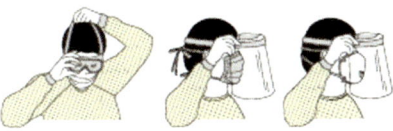

4. GLOVES

- Extend to cover wrist of isolation gown

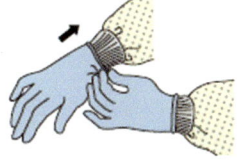

USE SAFE WORK PRACTICES TO PROTECT YOURSELF AND LIMIT THE SPREAD OF CONTAMINATION

- Keep hands away from face
- Limit surfaces touched
- Change gloves when torn or heavily contaminated
- Perform hand hygiene

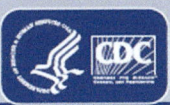

Fig. 6.2. Donning sequence as outlined by the Centers for Disease Control and Prevention (CDC). From: www.cdc.gov/hai/pdfs/ppe/PPE-Sequence.pdf (accessed 20 October 2022).

- Gowns should be untied, or ties broken by pulling the front of the gown with a gloved hand (Caveney *et al.*, 2011).
- The outer side of the gown (which has been exposed to the patient or other materials and is therefore more contaminated) should be turned inward and rolled into a bundle, taking care to keep the contaminated surface on the inside (Caveney *et al.*, 2011; Siegel *et al.*, 2007).
- Gown and gloves should be peeled off the wrists and hands and disposed of in an appropriate bin (Caveney *et al.*, 2011).

SEQUENCE FOR REMOVING PERSONAL PROTECTIVE EQUIPMENT (PPE)

Except for respirator, remove PPE at doorway or in anteroom. Remove respirator after leaving patient room and closing door.

1. GLOVES

- Outside of gloves is contaminated!
- Grasp outside of glove with opposite gloved hand; peel off
- Hold removed glove in gloved hand
- Slide fingers of ungloved hand under remaining glove at wrist
- Peel glove off over first glovet
- Discard gloves in waste container

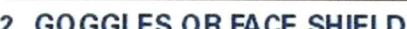

2. GOGGLES OR FACE SHIELD

- Outside of goggles or face shield is contaminated!
- To remove, handle by head band or ear pieces
- Place in designated receptacle for reprocessing or in waste container

3. GOWN

- Gown front and sleeves are contaminated!
- Unfasten ties
- Pull away from neck and shoulders, touching inside of gown only
- Turn gown inside out
- Fold or roll into a bundle and discard

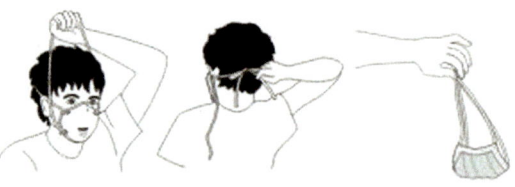

4. MASK OR RESPIRATOR

- Front of mask/respirator is contaminated — DO NOT TOUCH!
- Grasp bottom, then top ties or elastics and remove
- Discard in waste container

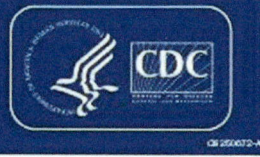

PERFORM HAND HYGIENE BETWEEN STEPS IF HANDS BECOME CONTAMINATED AND IMMEDIATELY AFTER REMOVING ALL PPE

CDC

Fig. 6.3. Doffing sequence, as outlined by the Centers for Disease Control and Prevention (CDC). From: www.cdc.gov/hai/pdfs/ppe/PPE-Sequence.pdf (accessed 20 October 2022).

Mellora Sharman and Helen Silver-MacMahon

- Hands should be washed immediately.
- Where contamination of clothes underneath the gown is suspected, they should be changed immediately and laundered.

Additional reduction in contamination can be achieved by doffing using a gown-and-sealed-glove combination, and/or by incorporating an additional decontamination step using quaternary ammonium or bleach prior to glove removal (Verbeek *et al.*, 2020).

Appropriate use of coveralls

If highly infectious (e.g. parvovirus, salmonellosis) or airborne (e.g. kennel cough) diseases are suspected, then impermeable coveralls are preferable to a gown because coveralls will better prevent contamination of clothing and transmission of the disease. While no clinical studies have been undertaken to compare the efficacy of gowns versus coveralls in preventing contamination, the latter are designed to offer better overall protection in comparison with gowns, which have openings at the back and only provide coverage to the mid-calf region (Fig. 6.4) (CDC, 2020). Coveralls generally offer head and feet protection and should be chosen if it is expected that animals will require handling or restraint on the floor of their kennel. Removal of coveralls is otherwise the same as for gowns, taking care not to contaminate underlying clothing or the environment. Compared with gowns and aprons, coveralls are harder to don and doff, and can add to heat stress. Training is therefore essential to ensure compliance and to reduce contamination.

Appropriate use of gloves

It cannot be overstated that hand hygiene remains the most important measure to protect patients (discussed in Chapters 4 and 5, this volume). It is fundamental to understand that glove use should not modify or replace hand hygiene practices: washing hands with soap and water or using an alcohol-based hand rub should always be performed prior to donning gloves (WHO, 2009). One of the primary benefits of wearing gloves is that the risk of pathogen dissemination within the clinical environment and transmission between patients is additionally reduced, therefore promoting patient protection (WHO, 2009).

Guidance on when to use gloves in human healthcare and what type of glove should be selected can be found in the World Health Organization (WHO) Glove Pyramid (Fig. 6.5). This pyramid offers a helpful guide, although some differences between risks in human *vs* veterinary healthcare are likely to change some of these recommendations. For example, the risk of exposure to HIV in human medicine means glove use with IV catheter placement may be considered necessary, but the same risk does not apply to a veterinary setting. The Centres for Disease Control and Prevention (Siegel *et al.*, 2007) recommends that disposable medical gloves should be worn to prevent contamination of healthcare personnel's hands when:

- direct contact with blood, body fluids, mucous membranes, non-intact skin and other infectious materials such as excretions is anticipated;

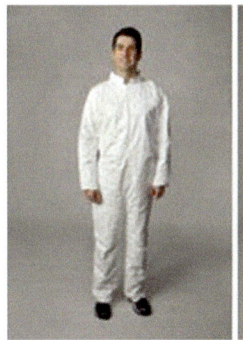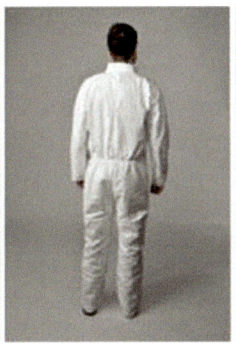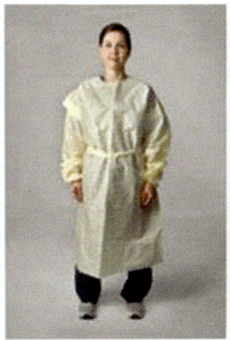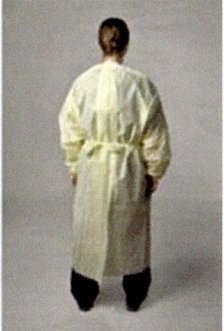

Fig. 6.4. Examples of use of a typical coverall and isolation gown. From: www.cdc.gov/niosh/npptl/topics/protectiveclothing/ (accessed 20 October 2022).

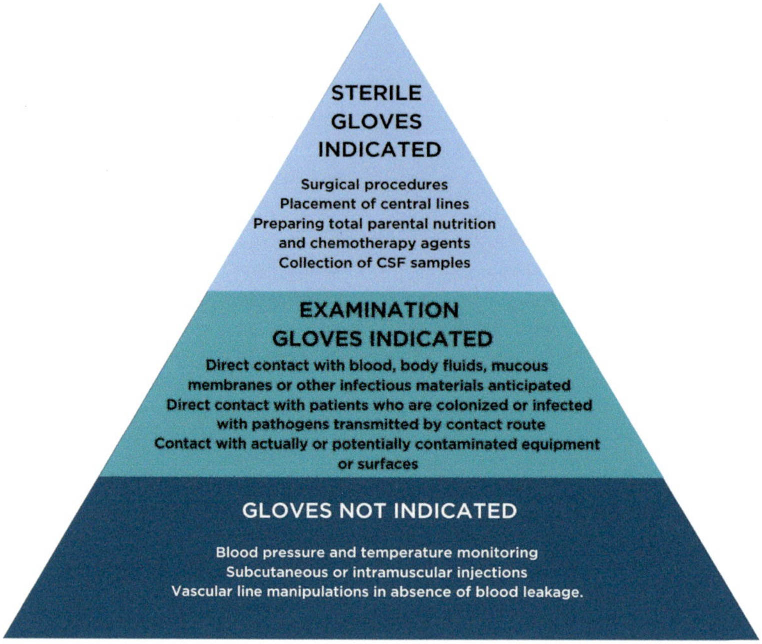

Fig. 6.5. The WHO Glove Pyramid provides guidance on when to use gloves, and what type of glove to choose. Adapted from the WHO Glove Pyramid for Veterinary Healthcare.

- direct contact is made with patients who are colonized or infected with pathogens transmitted by the contact route (e.g. MRSA); or
- there is contact with actually or potentially contaminated patient care equipment and environmental surfaces (e.g. during endoscopy or when changing bedding).

It is important to remember that the use of gloves in situations where they are not indicated is a waste of resources, and therefore any individual should rationalize glove use according to the criteria listed above. Within human healthcare, nurses report skin issues and contact dermatitis, which have been attributed to glove use. The NHS Gloves Off campaign (NHS, 2018) highlights core initiatives of balancing environmental and dermatological impact against routinely integrating risk assessment into decision making around glove use when interacting with patients or medications, and aims to reduce unnecessary glove use, improve staff and patient well-being and reduce the environmental impact of plastic use.

Growing evidence suggests that the misuse of gloves due to peer pressure, organizational influence or emotion is a growing concern in clinical human practice (Wilson and Loveday, 2014). Gloves are not indicated in a human medical setting where procedures are being undertaken that pose minimal risk. This is similar to expectations in veterinary medicine and would include such procedures as blood pressure and temperature monitoring, administration of subcutaneous or intramuscular injections, and vascular line manipulations in the absence of blood leakage (Fig. 6.5). Furthermore, continuous wearing of gloves (universal gloving) is unacceptable because it significantly increases device-related contamination (WHO and WHO Patient Safety, 2009).

Disposable, non-sterile medical gloves are available in a range of materials and should be selected according to the planned task. This might include anticipated contact with mucous membranes or non-intact skin, exposure to blood, intravenous catheter placement or removal, or the potential presence of infectious agents. Sterile gloves are indicated for surgical procedures when performing vascular access, such as for central lines, for invasive radiological procedures and, among other tasks, when preparing intravenous solutions such as chemotherapy or total parenteral nutrition

Mellora Sharman and Helen Silver-MacMahon

(Fig. 6.5). Sterile gloves should be donned using appropriate closed or open gloving techniques. Heavier, reusable utility gloves are indicated for non-patient care activities, such as handling or cleaning of contaminated equipment or surfaces (Siegel *et al.*, 2007).

Nitrile gloves are preferable for most clinical procedures: there is evidence that vinyl gloves have higher failure rates than latex or nitrile gloves, and latex gloves are renowned for causing sensitivities in the wearer. Gloves should be donned immediately before patient contact to ensure that other microorganisms are not transferred to susceptible sites on the patient (Wilson and Loveday, 2014), and a range of sizes should be available to ensure the correct fit (Sax *et al.*, 2007).

When gloves are worn in combination with other PPE, they should be donned last. To ensure a continuous and reliable barrier between the elbows and fingertips, gloves that fit snugly around the wrist are used with a long-sleeved gown (Siegel *et al.*, 2007). Double gloving may reduce risk during exposure-prone, high-risk situations (Casanova *et al.*, 2012).

Gloves should always be removed where damage to their integrity is noted, before touching mobile devices or keyboards, and when contact with the patient or their surroundings is completed (WHO, 2009). To remove gloves, the wrist of the glove should be grasped and pulled gently over the hand, turning the contaminated surface inward; the second glove should then be pulled over the first such that they are wrapped together, and they should immediately be placed in the appropriate waste disposal. Hand hygiene should be performed immediately after doffing and disposal of gloves to further ensure that any infectious material that may have penetrated the gloves is removed, as well as to decontaminate high-risk areas such as the wrists.

There is no evidence basis to support the reprocessing or reuse of medical gloves (WHO, 2009), and gloves should therefore be treated as single use and appropriately disposed of immediately after removal.

Appropriate use of face protection: masks, goggles and face shields

The main indications for use of face protection within the veterinary healthcare setting are:

1. Risk of contamination from blood, body fluids, secretions or excretions being splashed into the face and eyes, or that may be aerosolized and inhaled. This is especially pertinent when there is a zoonotic risk.
2. Protection for patients during sterile procedures from infectious agents that may be found in the mouth or nose of treating personnel (e.g. MRSA).

When selecting face protection, the manufacturer's guidance should be followed together with assessment of the indications and purpose for use. Two types of facemask are available for use in veterinary healthcare settings: surgical masks and respirator masks (i.e. N95 masks), which will be discussed further.

SURGICAL MASKS. Surgical masks are fluid resistant and protect the wearer from splashes, large droplets or sprays of bodily or other hazardous fluids. Surgical masks also protect patients from the wearer's respiratory emissions (OSHA, 2015). Surgical masks do not provide the wearer with protection from inhaling smaller airborne particles as they are not designed for a close fit and are therefore not considered respiratory protection (OSHA, 2015; Wilson, 2019). As with other items of PPE, fit is an important consideration: masks should be closely fitted and comfortable. Loose-fitting masks will result in inhalation and exhalation of air around the edges rather than through the mask and therefore air filtration will be compromised. When worn for an extended period, the mask may become moist, which has been shown to disrupt the passage of air through the mask and increase the flow around the outside (Wilson, 2019). Face masks should not be touched when being worn. Masks should not be worn around the neck when not in use but instead removed and disposed of immediately and appropriately. The manufacturer's instructions should be followed when removing face masks: handling the front of the mask directly must be avoided; rather, the mask should be removed by loosening the straps or ear loops. Following removal, masks should be folded in on themselves and disposed of. Importantly, having removed face protection, hand hygiene should be performed immediately and before touching other surfaces.

RESPIRATOR MASKS. Where the wearer may be exposed to smaller particles that may represent a contagious or zoonotic risk (e.g. Hendra virus, or respiratory tuberculosis), a respirator mask is preferable because it filters particles of less than 1 µm in diameter with 95% efficiency through a process of layering and electrostatic filtration (Wilson, 2019; Minutephysics, 2020). Particulate respirator masks are face-fit tested to ensure an effective seal to the face and are discarded when deformed or damaged. Discarding the respirator mask immediately after use is advisable, although recent shortages secondary to increased demand with COVID-19 has meant that respirator masks have been subjected to resterilization for repeated use where necessary (Su-Velez *et al.*, 2020).

CONTROVERSIES. There is limited and somewhat conflicting evidence that fit-tested respirator masks provide better protection against some respiratory viruses than other medical masks, despite a clear difference in fit between the two styles of mask (Loeb *et al.*, 2009; MacIntyre *et al.*, 2011; Radonovich *et al.*, 2019). In non-aerosol-generating care of COVID-19 patients, low-certainty evidence concluded that medical masks and respirators offer a similar level of protection (Bartoszko *et al.*, 2020). However, a properly fit-tested N95 mask may remain preferable in situations where exposure risk carries the possibility of significant morbidity or mortality, such as with Ebola or Hendra virus.

FACE SHIELDS. Face shields or goggles may be chosen in addition to masks in some situations where the risk of eyes being splashed is high. Face shields are not an effective alternative to a mask because particles may enter the visor due to its loose-fitting nature.

Hair and hair coverings

Hair is a significant carrier of bacteria. Long hair should always be tied back, but hair coverings should also be used when there is a risk that blood, body fluids or secretions may be encountered, and when reverse barrier nursing is undertaken.

Appropriate use of footwear

Use of correct footwear aids infection-control and -prevention practice. Closed-toe shoes should be worn to avoid contamination with body fluids or potential injury from sharps. Footwear should be kept clean. Even where gross contamination is not evident, hand hygiene should be performed following the handling of footwear.

Shoe covers provide additional protection for footwear in situations with a high risk of contamination, and are also used during certain barrier nursing situations, or within isolation rooms. Shoe covers should be donned just prior to entering the potentially contaminated zone and should be removed immediately after exiting. Foot baths or floor mats containing appropriate disinfectant solutions might also be implemented in barrier nursing or isolation settings to reduce footwear contamination and subsequent transmission of infectious materials throughout the hospital (Morley *et al.*, 2005). It should be noted that the reduction in infectious material load associated with the use of foot mats is only modest, and therefore this should not be solely relied upon (Hornig *et al.*, 2016). Both footbaths and foot mats do, however, prove useful as a visual reminder that an isolation area is being entered or exited, and therefore can prompt personnel to additionally observe and implement other infection-control protocols (Hornig *et al.*, 2016).

Dedicated shoes are sensible for use in operating theatres to avoid tracking contaminants into a sterile environment. If dedicated theatre shoes are not available, then using shoe covers may be a reasonable alternative. In this setting, shoe covers are donned when entering the operating theatre, and removed immediately after exiting, when they would be classified as contaminated. For this reason, new shoe covers should always be applied when re-entering the surgical suite.

6.3 Stethoscopes and Infection Risk

Stethoscopes are in regular contact with the unsanitized skin and hair of human and veterinary patients. Therefore, it is not surprising they are potential fomites for pathogen transmission, including MDR bacteria (Jones *et al.*, 1995; Marinella *et al.*, 1997; McCord *et al.*, 2010; KuKanich *et al.*, 2012; Fujita *et al.*, 2013; O'Flaherty and Fenelon, 2015; Jeyakumari *et al.*, 2017). On average, 85% of stethoscopes are contaminated (range 47% to 100% in humans; 67–100% in veterinary species) (Jones *et al.*, 1995; Marinella *et al.*, 1997; O'Flaherty and Fenelon, 2015; Jeyakumari *et al.*, 2017). Importantly, bacteria isolated from stethoscopes include a variety of known or opportunistic pathogens (Fujita *et al.*, 2013; Marcos *et al.*, 2020). In one veterinary study, stethoscopes routinely cultured MDR bacteria, with a high frequency

Mellora Sharman and Helen Silver-MacMahon

of enterococcal contamination (KuKanich *et al.*, 2012). Isolation of MRSA (2%) and MRSP (5%) from veterinary stethoscopes has also been reported (McCord *et al.*, 2010).

Although stethoscopes demonstrate a risk for bacterial transmission, no well-established guidelines on optimal cleaning methods exist (Ali *et al.*, 2016). Alcohol-based disinfectants effectively reduced bacterial contamination in some studies (Núñez *et al.*, 2000; Raghubanshi *et al.*, 2017). However, evidence suggests that antiseptics may provide better residual activity from short-term recontamination (Álvarez *et al.*, 2016). Novel and innovative approaches have also been developed, with one research group evaluating a prototype wearable ultraviolet germicidal irradiation (UV-GI) pocket device, which demonstrated a 94.8% reduction in bacterial counts on the stethoscope membrane compared with untreated stethoscopes (Messina *et al.*, 2015, 2018). Given limited comparative data on the effectiveness of stethoscope decontamination protocols, one recent veterinary study aimed to compare three methods to reduce bacterial contamination, comprising two easily available and topically applied agents and the use of a novel UV-GI approach (Marcos *et al.*, 2020). In this study, no overall difference was observed among cleaning protocols, all of which resulted in a significant and adequate reduction in contamination rates. However, where higher rates of contamination were present, UV-GI underperformed when compared with the topical liquid treatments (Marcos *et al.*, 2020).

The study by Marcos *et al.* (2020) also highlighted that rapid bacterial recolonization of the stethoscope occurred, regardless of the cleaning technique used and despite stethoscopes remaining out of clinical circulation. This was considered to be a result of bacterial survival within protected niches, and occurred to a similar degree among the different cleaning protocols, despite the inclusion of a disinfectant with proposed residual activity (Marcos *et al.*, 2020). These findings highlight that daily cleaning of stethoscopes insufficiently removed the risk posed by stethoscopes in transferring bacterial populations between patients. Assessment of veterinarians' attitude towards stethoscope hygiene in this study also highlighted a need for educational or other strategies to actively improve cleaning habits (Marcos *et al.*, 2020).

6.4 Policy Implementation and Adherence

Despite inherent risks for animal care workers, there is a casual indifference to implementation of infection-control policies relating to PPE within the veterinary sector. As a reflection of this, evaluation of PPE use within veterinary settings is limited, with a recently published systematic review identifying only four studies that adequately assessed PPE use (Willemsen *et al.*, 2019). Overall, studies reported that PPE use was either inadequate or inappropriate (Wright *et al.*, 2008; Murphy *et al.*, 2010; Dowd *et al.*, 2013; Mendez *et al.*, 2014; Anderson and Weese, 2015). Wright *et al.* (2008) concluded that most veterinarians surveyed were unaware of appropriate PPE use and did not actively engage in practices to help reduce zoonotic disease transmission. The use of PPE was often undermined by concurrent non-compliant clothing, including open laboratory coats or the wearing of long sleeves that extended beyond those of laboratory coats (Anderson and Weese, 2015). Only 37% of veterinarians reported wearing PPE when handling clinically ill animals (Venkat *et al.*, 2019).

Perception of risk to self is a commonly cited reason for generally improved PPE use; however, disparities exist between risk perception and the use of PPE (Wright *et al.*, 2008; Dowd *et al.*, 2013; Mendez *et al.*, 2014). In the study by Wright *et al.* (2008), despite 71.2% of small animal veterinarians indicating concern regarding dermatophytosis, 80.6% of those concerned did not utilize PPE when examining patients with dermatological signs. Similarly, 43.4% and 90% of large animal and equine veterinarians, respectively, failed to use appropriate PPE when involved in the examination of patients with dermatological changes. One-third (32.3%) of large animal veterinarians did not use PPE when undertaking a neurological examination, despite indicating their concerns regarding the risk of rabies, and 99.1% of large animal veterinarians failed to use respiratory or eye protection when aiding parturition or handling products of conception, despite their worries about the risk of brucellosis (Wright *et al.*, 2008). A reasonable explanation for this apparent disparity between risk perception and PPE use is likely to lie in the index for suspicion for a given infectious agent as a differential. However, although the index of suspicion may be low, the consequences can be significant. For example, it is worrying that in an endemic Hendra virus region of Australia, reported PPE usage by veterinarians was variable, given that 57.1% of humans die after contracting the infection (Mendez *et al.*, 2014).

Under some circumstances, risk perception appears to impact implementation of PPE practices: PPE use generally increases when certain procedures are being undertaken, such as post-mortems and surgical and dentistry procedures (Dowd *et al.*, 2013; Willemsen *et al.*, 2019; Venkat *et al.*, 2019). Veterinary staff are also more likely to utilize PPE when patients are unwell, or when high-risk products are being handled (Wright *et al.*, 2008; Mendez *et al.*, 2014; Willemsen *et al.*, 2019). In a Hendra virus endemic area, the frequency and type of PPE used increased as the health of the horse declined and the index of suspicion or risk for Hendra virus therefore increased (Mendez *et al.*, 2014). The authors of this study reported a striking increase in PPE usage from 32.4% to 84.8% when veterinarians were examining a healthy versus a sick horse, respectively (Mendez *et al.*, 2014).

Several studies have explored the potential barriers to PPE usage and determined that concerns regarding the cost of PPE, lack of availability, and worry about heat stress and negative client perception were frequently cited barriers to PPE use (Dowd *et al.*, 2013; Willemsen *et al.*, 2019). Improved utilization of PPE was associated with prior experience with zoonoses, concern regarding liability, knowledge of industry standards and guidelines, postgraduate qualifications, or employment within government, research or laboratory environments (Wright *et al.*, 2008; Dowd *et al.*, 2013; Mendez *et al.*, 2014; Willemsen *et al.*, 2019). Interestingly, one study described male veterinarians as being less likely to utilize PPE (Wright *et al.*, 2008). These findings are reflected in other studies investigating PPE use and compliance with infection-control practices in human healthcare (Yassi *et al.*, 2007), and perhaps highlight a machoistic tendency towards a sense of invincibility, and/or that the utilization of PPE might challenge one's own perception of masculinity.

6.4.1 Interventions to improve PPE implementation

Extrapolating evidence from human medicine that evaluates the effectiveness of other infection-control procedures (e.g. hand hygiene) demonstrates that proactive initiatives reduce HAI rates. Multi-modal

interventions are recommended by the WHO to improve compliance with hand hygiene (Ducel *et al.*, 2002; Gould *et al.*, 2017). These approaches include ensuring adequate availability of necessary materials, staff education and training, as well as providing reminders and performance feedback (Ducel *et al.*, 2002; Gould *et al.*, 2017). Robust studies that evaluate interventions to improve compliance with PPE in human healthcare remain somewhat limited, with the majority of data coming from small studies or studies that were considered low-certainty evidence in a recent Cochrane systematic review (Burch and Bunt, 2020; Verbeek *et al.*, 2020). In one of the larger studies, both active (face-to-face) and passive (video or written instruction) training methods appeared to improve compliance with the use of PPE, with no statistically significant difference between training methodologies (Shigayeva *et al.*, 2007; Verbeek *et al.*, 2020). Active training appeared to improve compliance when considering a safe doffing sequence, particularly when compared with no instruction or the use of folder or video information only, although this evidence was of low certainty (Shigayeva *et al.*, 2007; Casalino *et al.*, 2015; Verbeek *et al.*, 2020). Training via computer simulations, repeated training sessions and training sessions that involved performance feedback are reported to yield lower error rates (Casalino *et al.*, 2015; Hung *et al.*, 2015; Verbeek *et al.*, 2020).

Evidence of interventions aimed at improving PPE use in a veterinary setting is even more limited. A study of veterinary students demonstrated that video instruction alone resulted in higher contamination rates during a simulated isolation procedure compared with those students who received instruction via video and who also had access to a wall chart, or those who received instruction via the wall chart alone (Christmann *et al.*, 2019). Longer-term studies evaluating the retention of skills training relating to PPE use are not readily available in either human or veterinary health.

Education and instruction might improve skillsets and standards, but still do not consistently appear to improve compliance with infection-control interventions in healthcare workers (Rosenthal *et al.*, 2003; Dramowski *et al.*, 2015). The WHO's evidence-based toolkit for improving compliance to standard hygiene precautions outlines a multi-modal approach, and highlights the importance of coupling education and training together with evaluation and performance feedback (WHO and

Mellora Sharman and Helen Silver-MacMahon

WHO Patient Safety, 2009). Elsewhere, there is agreement that incorporation of regular auditing, provision of regular performance feedback and implementation of systems that make staff more accountable appear to be more effective than education alone in improving compliance (Rosenthal *et al.*, 2003; Cromer *et al.*, 2004). Key components have been identified in the sustained success of a programme designed to improve PPE compliance in association with chemotherapeutic handling, which include education, ownership over required changes, peer-performance monitoring, leadership support, and continuous monitoring and performance feedback (Hennessy and Dynan, 2014). It is reasonable to assume that similar approaches will be beneficial in improving compliance of PPE usage in a range of infection-control settings.

Improved infection-control education and policy development within veterinary practices is likely to be a key step in shifting from indifference. A recent survey of veterinarians in Arizona found that only 42% of respondents were aware of a written infection-control manual or policy within their practice (Venkat *et al.*, 2019). Further support for improving the overall knowledge and implementation of infection-control policies within the veterinary sector is also given by the finding that frequency and adequacy of PPE use was positively correlated with the existence of infection-control policies within individual practices surveyed (Wright *et al.*, 2008; Mendez *et al.*, 2014). Furthermore, for veterinarians in an endemic Hendra virus region of Australia, a positive association was seen between PPE use and an individual's involvement in infection-control or Hendra virus training programmes within the prior 12 months (Mendez *et al.*, 2014). Use also improved where there was a dedicated Hendra virus training programme within the practice, or where there had been experience dealing with a suspected or known case (Mendez *et al.*, 2014). In the study by Venkat *et al.* (2019), 85% of veterinarians agreed or strongly agreed that they would benefit from receiving further education and training on infection-control practices and zoonotic disease, or by having better access to guidelines on infection-control practices (e.g. Fig. 6.1) (Venkat *et al.*, 2019). More widespread adoption and implementation of infection-control practices in veterinary healthcare might further be aided by provision of easy and open access to existing policies of larger private or academic centres, or

by providing templates to aid practice development of protocols for their own individual needs.

6.5 Conclusion

Veterinarians, veterinary nurses and animal care workers have an important and unique role in infection control. Personnel must be cognisant of the risk for transmitting HAIs between patients, and should remain vigilant and mindful of the personal risks that regular interaction can pose to contracting zoonotic disease. Overall, significant work is still required to inform and improve infection-control policy development in line with that of human health to mitigate some of the unique risks that veterinary staff face.

References

Workplace (Health, Safety and Welfare) Regulations (1992). Available at: https://www.legislation.gov.uk/uksi/1992/3004/regulation/24/made (accessed 23 February 2023).

Aiello, A.E., Coulborn, R.M., Perez, V. and Larson, E.L. (2008) Effect of hand hygiene on infectious disease risk in the community setting: a meta-analysis. *American Journal of Public Health* 98(8), 1372–1381. DOI: 10.2105/AJPH.2007.124610.

Ali, S., Goryaeva, M., Kotronias, R.A., Sheriff, I.H.N., Cereceda-Monteoliva, N. *et al.* (2016) Have you cleaned your stethoscope today? *Journal of Hospital Infection* 94(3), 281–282. DOI: 10.1016/j.jhin.2016.07.024.

Álvarez, J.A., Ruíz, S.R., Mosqueda, J.L., León, X., Arreguín, V. *et al.* (2016) Decontamination of stethoscope membranes with chlorhexidine: should it be recommended? *American Journal of Infection Control* 44(11), e205–e209. DOI: 10.1016/j.ajic.2016.07.012.

Anderson, D.J., Addison, R., Lokhnygina, Y., Warren, B., Sharma-Kuinkel, B. *et al.* (2017) The Antimicrobial Scrub Contamination and Transmission (ASCOT) trial: a three-arm, blinded, randomized controlled trial with crossover design to determine the efficacy of antimicrobial-impregnated scrubs in preventing healthcare provider contamination. *Infection Control and Hospital Epidemiology* 38(10), 1147–1154. DOI: 10.1017/ice.2017.181.

Anderson, M.E.C. and Weese, J.S. (2015) Video observation of sharps handling and infection control practices during routine companion animal appointments. *BMC Veterinary Research* 11, 185. DOI: 10.1186/s12917-015-0503-9.

AORN (2009) Uniforms and workwear: guidance for NHS employers. Association of periOperative Registered Nurses, Denver, Colorado. Available at: www.

england.nhs.uk/coronavirus/documents/uniforms-and-workwear-guidance-for-nhs-employers/#good-practice (accessed 25 October 2020).

Arefian, H., Vogel, M., Kwetkat, A. and Hartmann, M. (2016) Economic evaluation of interventions for prevention of hospital acquired infections: a systematic review. *PloS One* 11(1), e0146381. DOI: 10.1371/journal.pone.0146381.

Bartoszko, J.J., Farooqi, M.A.M., Alhazzani, W. and Loeb, M. (2020) Medical masks vs N95 respirators for preventing COVID-19 in healthcare workers: a systematic review and meta-analysis of randomized trials. *Influenza and Other Respiratory Viruses* 14(4), 365–373. DOI: 10.1111/irv.12745.

Beam, E.L., Gibbs, S.G., Boulter, K.C., Beckerdite, M.E. and Smith, P.W. (2011) A method for evaluating health care workers' personal protective equipment technique. *American Journal of Infection Control* 39(5), 415–420. DOI: 10.1016/j.ajic.2010.07.009.

Burch, J. and Bunt, C. (2020) Which type of personal protective equipment (PPE), and which interventions to increase PPE use by healthcare workers, help reduce the spread of highly infectious diseases? *Cochrane Clinical Answers*. Available at: www.cochranelibrary.com/cca/doi/10.1002/cca.3056/full (accessed 19 October 2022).

Casalino, E., Astocondor, E., Sanchez, J.C., Díaz-Santana, D.E., Del Aguila, C. *et al.* (2015) Personal protective equipment for the Ebola virus disease: a comparison of 2 training programs. *American Journal of Infection Control* 43(12), 1281–1287. DOI: 10.1016/j.ajic.2015.07.007.

Casanova, L.M., Rutala, W.A., Weber, D.J. and Sobsey, M.D. (2012) Effect of single- versus double-gloving on virus transfer to health care workers' skin and clothing during removal of personal protective equipment. *American Journal of Infection Control* 40(4), 369–374. DOI: 10.1016/j.ajic.2011.04.324.

Caveney, L., Jones, B. and Ellis, K. (eds) (2011) *Veterinary Infection Prevention and Control*. Wiley, Chichester, UK.

CDC (2004) Guidance for the selection and use of Personal Protective Equipment (PPE) in healthcare settings. Centers for Disease Control and Prevention: Atlanta, Georgia. Available at: www.cdc.gov/hai/pdfs/ppe/ppeslides6-29-04.pdf (accessed 14 November 2022).

CDC (2020) Considerations for selecting protective clothing used in healthcare for protection against microorganisms in blood and body fluids. Centers for Disease Control and Prevention, Atlanta, Georgia. Available at: www.cdc.gov/niosh/npptl/topics/protectiveclothing/ (accessed 19 October 2022).

Chollet, A., Wespi, B., Roosje, P., Unger, L., Venner, M. *et al.* (2015) An outbreak of *Arthroderma vanbreuseghemii* dermatophytosis at a veterinary school associated with an infected horse. *Mycoses* 58(4), 233–238. DOI: 10.1111/myc.12301.

Christmann, U., Vroegindewey, G., Rice, M., Williamson, J.A., Johnson, J.W. *et al.* (2019) Effect of different instructional methods on contamination and personal protective equipment protocol adherence among veterinary students. *Journal of Veterinary Medical Education* 46(1), 81–90. DOI: 10.3138/jvme.0417-053r.

Cornejo-Juárez, P., Vilar-Compte, D., Pérez-Jiménez, C., Ñamendys-Silva, S.A., Sandoval-Hernández, S. *et al.* (2015) The impact of hospital-acquired infections with multidrug-resistant bacteria in an oncology intensive care unit. *International Journal of Infectious Diseases* 31, 31–34. DOI: 10.1016/j.ijid.2014.12.022.

Cromer, A.L., Hutsell, S.O., Latham, S.C., Bryant, K.G., Wacker, B.B. *et al.* (2004) Impact of implementing a method of feedback and accountability related to contact precautions compliance. *American Journal of Infection Control* 32(8), 451–455. DOI: 10.1016/j.ajic.2004.06.003.

Dowd, K., Taylor, M., Toribio, J.-A.L.M.L., Hooker, C. and Dhand, N.K. (2013) Zoonotic disease risk perceptions and infection control practices of Australian veterinarians: call for change in work culture. *Preventive Veterinary Medicine* 111(1–2), 17–24. DOI: 10.1016/j.prevetmed.2013.04.002.

Dramowski, A., Marais, F., Goliath, C. and Mehtar, S. (2015) Impact of a quality improvement project to strengthen infection prevention and control training at rural healthcare facilities. *African Journal of Health Professions Education* 7, 73–75.

Ducel, G., Fabry, J. and Nicolle, L. (eds) (2002) *Prevention of Hospital-Acquired Infections: A Practical Guide*, 2nd edn. WHO, Geneva.

Field, H., Schaaf, K., Kung, N., Simon, C., Waltisbuhl, D. *et al.* (2010) Hendra virus outbreak with novel clinical features, Australia. *Emerging Infectious Diseases* 16(2), 338–340. DOI: 10.3201/eid1602.090780.

Fujita, H., Hansen, B. and Hanel, R. (2013) Bacterial contamination of stethoscope chest pieces and the effect of daily cleaning. *Journal of Veterinary Internal Medicine* 27(2), 354–358. DOI: 10.1111/jvim.12032.

Gould, D.J., Moralejo, D., Drey, N., Chudleigh, J.H. and Taljaard, M. (2017) Interventions to improve hand hygiene compliance in patient care. *Cochrane Database of Systematic Reviews* 9(9), CD005186. DOI: 10.1002/14651858.CD005186.pub4.

Grönthal, T., Moodley, A., Nykäsenoja, S., Junnila, J., Guardabassi, L. *et al.* (2014) Large outbreak caused by methicillin resistant *Staphylococcus pseudintermedius* ST71 in a Finnish veterinary teaching hospital--from outbreak control to outbreak prevention. *PloS One* 9(10), e110084. DOI: 10.1371/journal.pone.0110084.

Haque, M., Sartelli, M., McKimm, J. and Abu Bakar, M. (2018) Health care-associated infections - an

Mellora Sharman and Helen Silver-MacMahon

overview. *Infection and Drug Resistance* 11, 2321–2333. DOI: 10.2147/IDR.S177247.

Hennessy, K.A. and Dynan, J. (2014) Improving compliance with personal protective equipment use through the model for improvement and staff champions. *Clinical Journal of Oncology Nursing* 18(5), 497–500. DOI: 10.1188/14.CJON.497-500.

Hornig, K.J., Burgess, B.A., Saklou, N.T., Johnson, V., Malmlov, A. *et al.* (2016) Evaluation of the efficacy of disinfectant footmats for the reduction of bacterial contamination on footwear in a large animal veterinary hospital. *Journal of Veterinary Internal Medicine* 30(6), 1882–1886. DOI: 10.1111/jvim.14576.

Hung, P.-P., Choi, K.-S. and Chiang, V.C.-L. (2015) Using interactive computer simulation for teaching the proper use of personal protective equipment. *Computers, Informatics, Nursing* 33(2), 49–57. DOI: 10.1097/CIN.0000000000000125.

Irene, G., Georgios, P., Ioannis, C., Anastasios, T., Diamantis, P. *et al.* (2016) Copper-coated textiles: armor against MDR nosocomial pathogens. *Diagnostic Microbiology and Infectious Disease* 85(2), 205–209. DOI: 10.1016/j.diagmicrobio.2016.02.015.

Jackson, A.C. (2013) Current and future approaches to the therapy of human rabies. *Antiviral Research* 99(1), 61–67. DOI: 10.1016/j.antiviral.2013.01.003.

Jeyakumari, D., Nagajothi, S., Kumar, P., Ilayaperumal, G. and Vigneshwaran, S. (2017) Bacterial colonization of stethoscope used in the tertiary care teaching hospital: a potential source of nosocomial infection. *International Journal of Research in Medical Sciences* 5, 142–145.

Jones, J.S., Hoerle, D. and Riekse, R. (1995) Stethoscopes: a potential vector of infection? *Annals of Emergency Medicine* 26(3), 296–299. DOI: 10.1016/s0196-0644(95)70075-7.

Klevens, R.M., Edwards, J.R., Richards, C.L., Horan, T.C., Gaynes, R.P. *et al.* (2007) Estimating health care-associated infections and deaths in U.S. hospitals, 2002. *Public Health Reports* 122(2), 160–166. DOI: 10.1177/003335490712200205.

Kokkinos, P., Morgan, L., Hughes, K., Pollard, D., Gasson, J. *et al.* (2020) Scrubs contamination, domestic laundry effect and workwear habits of clinical staff at a referral hospital. *Journal of Small Animal Practice* 61(5), 272–277. DOI: 10.1111/jsap.13114.

Koopmans, M., Wilbrink, B., Conyn, M., Natrop, G., van der Nat, H. *et al.* (2004) Transmission of H7N7 avian influenza A virus to human beings during a large outbreak in commercial poultry farms in the Netherlands. *Lancet* 363(9409), 587–593. DOI: 10.1016/S0140-6736(04)15589-X.

KuKanich, K.S., Ghosh, A., Skarbek, J.V., Lothamer, K.M. and Zurek, L. (2012) Surveillance of bacterial contamination in small animal veterinary hospitals with special focus on antimicrobial resistance and virulence traits of enterococci. *Journal of the*

American Veterinary Medical Association 240(4), 437–445. DOI: 10.2460/javma.240.4.437.

Lipton, B.A., Hopkins, S.G., Koehler, J.E. and DiGiacomo, R.F. (2008) A survey of veterinarian involvement in zoonotic disease prevention practices. *Journal of the American Veterinary Medical Association* 233(8), 1242–1249. DOI: 10.2460/javma.233.8.1242.

Loeb, M., Dafoe, N., Mahony, J., John, M., Sarabia, A. *et al.* (2009) Surgical mask vs N95 respirator for preventing influenza among health care workers: a randomized trial. *Journal the American Medical Association* 302(17), 1865–1871. DOI: 10.1001/jama.2009.1466.

MacIntyre, C.R., Wang, Q., Cauchemez, S., Seale, H., Dwyer, D.E. *et al.* (2011) A cluster randomized clinical trial comparing fit-tested and non-fit-tested N95 respirators to medical masks to prevent respiratory virus infection in health care workers. *Influenza and Other Respiratory Viruses* 5(3), 170–179. DOI: 10.1111/j.1750-2659.2011.00198.x.

Marchetti, A. and Rossiter, R. (2013) Economic burden of healthcare-associated infection in US acute care hospitals: societal perspective. *Journal of Medical Economics* 16(12), 1399–1404. DOI: 10.3111/13696998.2013.842922.

Marcos, P.S., Hermes, D. and Sharman, M. (2020) Comparative assessment of the effectiveness of three disinfection protocols for reducing bacterial contamination of stethoscopes. *Infection Control and Hospital Epidemiology* 41(1), 120–123. DOI: 10.1017/ice.2019.308.

Marinella, M.A., Pierson, C. and Chenoweth, C. (1997) The stethoscope: a potential source of nosocomial infection? *Archives of Internal Medicine* 157(7), 786–790. DOI: 10.1001/archinte.157.7.786.

McCord, K., Stanton, K., Bolte, D., Hyatt, D. and Lunn, K. (2010) Methicillin-resistant *Staphylococcus* spp. contamination of stethoscopes in a small animal veterinary teaching hospital. *Journal of Veterinary Internal Medicine* 24, 762.

Mendez, D., Buttner, P. and Speare, R. (2014) Hendra virus in Queensland, Australia, during the winter of 2011: veterinarians on the path to better management strategies. *Preventive Veterinary Medicine* 117(1), 40–51. DOI: 10.1016/j.prevetmed.2014.08.002.

Messina, G., Burgassi, S., Messina, D., Montagnani, V. and Cevenini, G. (2015) A new UV-LED device for automatic disinfection of stethoscope membranes. *American Journal of Infection Control* 43(10), e61–6. DOI: 10.1016/j.ajic.2015.06.019.

Messina, G., Spataro, G., Rosadini, D., Burgassi, S., Mariani, L. *et al.* (2018) A novel approach to stethoscope hygiene: a coat-pocket innovation. *Infection, Disease & Health* 23(4), 211–216. DOI: 10.1016/j.idh.2018.06.002.

Minutephysics (2020) The astounding physics of N95 masks. Available at: https://youtu.be/eAdanPfQdCA (accessed 20 October 2020).

Morley, P.S., Morris, S.N., Hyatt, D.R. and Van Metre, D.C. (2005) Evaluation of the efficacy of disinfectant footbaths as used in veterinary hospitals. *Journal of the American Veterinary Medical Association* 226(12), 2053–2058. DOI: 10.2460/javma.2005.226.2053.

Murphy, C.P., Reid-Smith, R.J., Weese, J.S. and McEwen, S.A. (2010) Evaluation of specific infection control practices used by companion animal veterinarians in community veterinary practices in southern Ontario. *Zoonoses and Public Health* 57(6), 429–438. DOI: 10.1111/j.1863-2378.2009.01244.x.

NHS (2018) The gloves are off' campaign. National Health Service, London. Available at: www.england.nhs. uk/atlas_case_study/the-gloves-are-off-campaign/ (accessed 20 October 2022).

NHS (2020) *Uniforms and Workwear: Guidance for NHS Employers.* National Health Service, London. Available at: www.england.nhs.uk/wp-content/uploads/2020/04/Uniforms-and-Workwear-Guidance-2-April-2020.pdf (accessed 20 October 2022).

Núñez, S., Moreno, A., Green, K. and Villar, J. (2000) The stethoscope in the emergency department: a vector of infection? *Epidemiology and Infection* 124(2), 233–237. DOI: 10.1017/s0950268800003563.

O'Flaherty, N. and Fenelon, L. (2015) The stethoscope and healthcare-associated infection: a snake in the grass or innocent bystander? *Journal of Hospital Infection* 91(1), 1–7. DOI: 10.1016/j.jhin.2015.04.010.

OSHA (2015) *Hospital Respiratory Protection Program Toolkit: Resources for Respirator Program Administrators.* Occupational Safety and Health Administration, Washington, DC. Available at: www.osha.gov/sites/default/files/publications/OSHA3767.pdf (accessed 20 October 2022).

Playford, E.G., McCall, B., Smith, G., Slinko, V., Allen, G. *et al.* (2010) Human Hendra virus encephalitis associated with equine outbreak, Australia, 2008. *Emerging Infectious Diseases* 16, 219–223.

Radonovich, L.J.Jr., Simberkoff, M.S., Bessesen, M.T., Brown, A.C., Cummings, D.A.T, *et al.* (2019) N95 vs medical masks for preventing influenza among health care personnel: a randomized clinical trial. *Journal of the American Medical Association* 322, 824–833.

Raghubanshi, B.R., Sapkota, S., Adhikari, A., Dutta, A., Bhattarai, U. and Bhandarui, R. (2017) Use of 90% ethanol to decontaminate stethoscopes in resource limited settings. *Antimicrobial Resistance and Infection Control* 6: 68.

Reynolds, B.S., Poulet, H., Pingret, J.-L., Jas, D., Brunet, S. *et al.* (2009) A nosocomial outbreak of feline calicivirus associated virulent systemic disease in France. *Journal of Feline Medicine and Surgery* 11, 633–644.

Rosenthal, V.D., Guzman, S., Pezzotto, S.M. and Crnich, C.J. (2003) Effect of an infection control program using education and performance feedback on rates of intravascular device-associated bloodstream infections in intensive care units in Argentina. *American Journal of Infection Control* 31, 405–409.

Sanon, M.-A. and Watkins, S. (2012) Nurses' uniforms: how many bacteria do they carry after one shift? *Journal of Public Health and Epidemiology* 4, 311–315.

Sax, H., Allegranzi, B., Uçkay, I., Larson, E., Boyce, J. and Pittet, D. (2007) 'My five moments for hand hygiene': a user-centred design approach to understand, train, monitor and report hand hygiene. *Journal of Hospital Infection* 67, 9–21.

Schnurrenberger, P.R., Grogor, J.K., Walker, J.F. and Martin, R.J. (1978) The zoonosis-prone veterinarian. *Journal of the American Veterinary Medical Association* 173, 373–376.

Scott, R.D. (2009) The direct medical costs of healthcare-associated infections in U.S. hospitals and the benefits of prevention. CDC, Atlanta, Georgia. Available at: www.cdc.gov/hai/pdfs/hai/scott_costpaper.pdf (accessed 20 October 2022).

Serra-Burriel, M., Keys, M., Campillo-Artero, C., Agodi, A., Barchitta, M. *et al.* (2020) Impact of multi-drug resistant bacteria on economic and clinical outcomes of healthcare-associated infections in adults: systematic review and meta-analysis. *PLoS One* 15, e0227139. DOI: 10.1371/journal.pone.0227139.

Shigayeva, A., Green, K., Raboud, J.M., Henry, B., Simor, A.E, *et al.* (2007) Factors associated with critical-care healthcare workers' adherence to recommended barrier precautions during the toronto severe acute respiratory syndrome outbreak. *Infection Control & Hospital Epidemiology* 28, 1275–1283.

Siegel, J.D., Rhinehart, E., Jackson, M., Chiarello, L. and and Health Care Infection Control Practices Advisory Committee (2007) 2007 Guideline for Isolation Precautions: Preventing Transmission of Infectious Agents in Health Care Settings. *American Journal of Infection Control* 35(10 Suppl 2), S65–S164. Available at: https://www.cdc.gov/infectioncontrol/guidelines/isolation/index.html/isolation2007.pdf

Stull, J.W. and Weese, J.S. (2015) Hospital-associated infections in small animal practice. *Veterinary Clinics of North America – Small Animal Practice* 45, 217–233.

Su-Velez, B.M., Maxim, T., Long, J.L., St John, M.A. and Holliday, M.A. (2020) Decontamination methods for reuse of filtering facepiece respirators. *JAMA Otolaryngology – Head and Neck Surgery* 146, 734–740.

Venkat, H., Yaglom, H.D. and Adams, L. (2019) Knowledge, attitudes, and practices relevant to zoonotic disease reporting and infection prevention practices among veterinarians – Arizona, 2015. *Preventive Veterinary Medicine* 169, 104711.

Verbeek, J.H., Rajamaki, B., Ijaz, S., Sauni, R., Toomey, E. *et al.* (2020) Personal protective equipment for preventing highly infectious diseases due to exposure to contaminated body fluids in healthcare staff. *Cochrane Database of Systematic Reviews* 4, CD011621.

Weese, J.S., Peregrine, A.S. and Armstrong, J. (2002) Occupational health and safety in small animal veterinary practice: Part I – nonparasitic zoonotic diseases. *Canadian Veterinary Journal* 43, 631–636.

WHO (2009) *Glove Use Information Leaflet*. World Health Organization, Geneva, Switzerland. Available at: https://cdn.who.int/media/docs/default-source/integrated-health-services-(ihs)/infection-prevention-and-control/hand-hygiene/tools/glove-use-information-leaflet.pdf (accessed 20 October 2022).

WHO and WHO Patient Safety (2009) *Guide to Implementation: A Guide to the Implementation of the WHO Multimodal Hand Hygiene Improvement Strategy*. World Health Organization, Geneva, Switzerland. Available at: https://apps.who.int/iris/handle/10665/70030 (accessed 7 January 2023).

Wilson, J. (2019) *Infection Control in Clinical Practice Updated Edition*, 3rd edn. Elsevier Health Sciences.

Wilson, J.A., Loveday, H.P., Hoffman, P.N. and Pratt, R.J. (2007) Uniform: an evidence review of the microbiological significance of uniforms and uniform policy in the prevention and control of healthcare-associated infections. report to the Department of Health (england). *Journal of Hospital Infection* 66, 301–307. DOI: 10.1016/j.jhin.2007.03.026.

Willemsen, A., Cobbold, R., Gibson, J., Wilks, K., Lawler, S. *et al.* (2019) Infection control practices employed within small animal veterinary practices – a systematic review. *Zoonoses and Public Health* 66, 439–457.

Wilson, J. and Loveday, H. (2014) Does glove use increase the risk of infection? *Nursing Times*. Available at: www.nursingtimes.net/clinical-archive/infection-control/does-glove-use-increase-the-risk-of-infection-19-09-2014/ (accessed October 2022).

Wright, J.G., Jung, S., Holman, R., Marano, N. and McQuiston, J. (2008) Infection control practices and zoonotic disease risks among veterinarians in the United States. *Journal of the American Veterinary Medical Association* 232, 1863–1872.

Yassi, A., Lockhart, K., Copes, R., Kerr, M., Corbiere, M. *et al.* (2007) Determinants of healthcare workers' compliance with infection control procedures. *Healthcare Quarterly* 10, 44–52.

7 Environmental Cleaning and Disinfection

Lucas Pantaleon*

DVM One Health, Versailles, KY, USA

7.1 Infection Control, Prevention and Biosecurity

From the One Health perspective, infection control, prevention and biosecurity (ICPB) could be defined as the implementation of strategies to protect human, animal and environmental health against pathogenic microorganisms. The ultimate goal is to improve the quality of patient care by reducing infection rates, morbidity and mortality while improving personnel safety and reducing costs. Biosecurity focuses on the implementation of measures to prevent the entry of pathogens into a population or facility (e.g. an animal shelter or breeding kennels). The objective of infection prevention and control is to limit the impact that the introduction of a pathogen would have on a population (e.g. inpatients within a small animal hospital) (Weese, 2014). In the latter scenario, exposure to pathogens is largely inevitable, as small animal hospitals are 'open populations' with animals from different sources coming and going. Therefore, measures must be in place to identify and contain threats (infection control) in conjunction with biosecurity activities aimed at reducing the risk of pathogen introduction (Weese, 2014). The three pillars of ICPB (human, animal and environment) are shared by the One Health concept and should be implemented with One Health in mind, especially when it comes to collaboration and cross-learning from different disciplines to control the spread of pathogenic microorganisms.

The importance of the interrelation between animals (colonized or infected), people and environment, and their intricate interaction with microbes, is an important aspect of ICPB in veterinary hospitals. Animals that are clinically affected with a contagious disease have the potential to spread it to other patients within the hospital. Subclinical carriers may pass undetected and will always pose a disease challenge to every veterinary hospital independent of size or specialty (Traverse and Aceto, 2015).

ICPB practices, antibiotic stewardship, and innovation of drugs and therapies are important to combat and control the emergence of microorganism resistance and prevent the spread of contagious infectious diseases (Spellberg et al., 2013). However the limited prospect for newer, safer and affordable antimicrobials and vaccines to cure and prevent disease, along with the emergence of multidrug-resistant microbes, makes cleaning and disinfection strategies absolutely vital (Sattar, 2006; Spellberg et al., 2013). The veterinary care team should strive to implement adequate cleaning and disinfection protocols as part of a broad ICPB plan. At every veterinary facility, the standard of care should include a high level of environmental cleaning and disinfection (Traverse and Aceto, 2015). Leadership and team work will improve collaboration and increase successes, ultimately improving the quality of care and personnel safety, reducing the need for antibiotics use, avoiding unnecessary costs and saving lives.

Infectious disease outbreaks can have devastating short- and long-term effects for veterinarians and animal care facilities. Animals that are under stress are more vulnerable to developing illness. Furthermore, stressed animals that are not showing clinical signs of a disease (carriers) can shed infectious microorganisms into their environment, putting other animals at risk, especially those that are immunosuppressed. It is also important to know that some diseases can be spread from animals to

---

*lucaspantaleon@gmail.com

DOI: 10.1079/9781789244977.0007

people (zoonotic diseases), and thus animal care givers (veterinarians, staff and clients) need to be educated about the risks and how to protect themselves to minimize exposure to zoonotic diseases. Similarly, animal care givers must also be aware that reverse zoonosis can occur, whereby disease is transmitted from humans to animals.

7.2 Healthcare-Associated Infections

The financial impact of an infectious disease outbreak is considerable and can be divided into direct fixed costs (remodelling of the facility, labour, equipment, utilities), direct variable costs (medications, treatments, procedures, supplies, diagnostic testing), indirect costs (morbidity, mortality, affected athletic performance potential, decreased worker productivity, liability) and intangible costs (bad publicity, loss of clients, loss of teaching opportunities, decreased morale) (Morley, 2002; Scott, 2009).

Healthcare-associated infections (HAIs) in human hospitals can prove very costly to the healthcare system (Scott, 2009). In the USA alone, over 1.7 million patients per year suffer from HAIs, with more than one-third of these believed to be preventable infections (Roberts, 2010). The annual direct hospital costs of treating HAIs in the USA ranges from US$28.4 billion to US$45 billion (Scott, 2009). Prevention of HAIs is therefore a prime example of value-based medicine, where the goals of improving outcomes and decreasing cost are synergistic (Roberts, 2010; Porter and Lee, 2013). In the US healthcare system, HAIs are subject to mandatory reporting and are linked to reimbursement: providers receive reduced payment for patients who succumb to an HAI, which incentivizes providers to improve infection prevention measures (Roberts, 2010). Furthermore, prevention of HAIs may also contribute to the reduction of antimicrobial-resistant infections (Roberts, 2010).

The prevalence of HAIs in privately owned veterinary hospitals is less well understood (KuKanich et al., 2012). Outbreaks of HAIs in veterinary teaching hospitals has resulted in reported loses that vary between thousands of dollars up to US$4.12 million per outbreak, although these costs were probably conservative and potentially greater in the long term (Morley, 2002; Dallap Schaer et al., 2010)

A study that investigated HAIs in companion animals revealed that 16.3% of 1535 dogs and 12% of 416 cats had at least one nosocomial event, with the most common reported clinical sign being surgical-site inflammation (Ruple-Czerniak et al., 2013). A survey of veterinary teaching hospitals revealed that 82% of the institutions had reported an outbreak of an infectious disease, with most commonly detected agents being *Salmonella enterica* (65%), followed by methicillin-resistant *Staphylococcus aureus* (MRSA) (42%) and *Escherichia coli* (16%). Fifty-eight per cent of these institutions had to restrict patient admissions, while 32% had to close in order to control the outbreak. *S. enterica* has been the pathogen most often (77%) involved in restricting admissions, followed by equine herpesvirus 1 (14%), MRSA (9%) and *Clostridioides difficile* (9%) (Benedict, 2008). In large animal hospitals, the importance of nosocomial salmonellosis is demonstrated by a mortality rate of 30–60% (Morley, 2013).

Contagious infectious diseases in a hospital and livestock environment are not only a risk for the animal resident population; some zoonotic diseases pose a risk for the human caregivers. In a study of veterinary hospitals, 50% of the surveyed institutions reported a zoonotic infection, with attack rates during the outbreak as high as 20–50% (Benedict, 2008; Morley, 2013) The three microorganisms most commonly involved as zoonoses were *Cryptosporidium parvum* (68%), MRSA (16%) and *S. enterica* (16%) (Benedict, 2008).

In human and veterinary medicine, HAIs are common, which highlights the importance of cleaning and disinfection as a critical element of an ICPB protocol. A recent report highlighted the fact that human and animal relationships will continue to intensify due to animal husbandry practices, growth of the companion animal market, climate change and ecosystem disruption, anthropogenic development of habitats, and global travel and commerce (Messenger et al., 2014). Thus, as the number of animal–human interactions rises, so does the potential for zoonosis and reverse zoonosis to occur.

7.3 Infection Prevention *Status Quo*

Correctly performing cleaning and disinfection tasks is paramount for a successful ICPB programme in veterinary hospitals. Nevertheless, these duties are normally placed on the 'back burner' and decisions are delegated without first educating and training the team members in charge of cleaning and disinfecting. The animal care team must understand that cleaning and disinfection are vitally important in providing high standards of care to veterinary patients.

Implementing and improving infectious disease prevention strategies in order to challenge the status quo requires an organizational cultural change. Decreasing the number of infectious diseases among the patient population would have a direct positive impact on the value provided and to patient outcomes, thus providing a strong incentive for shifting the mentality away from the 'way things get done'. Leaders who understand the direction to be followed, are vested in the process and are strong proponents for change are paramount for a cultural change to 'stick'. Implementing ICPB needs leadership support and a teamwork approach where people from different areas (multi-disciplinary teams) collaborate and cooperate with ideas on how best to implement it in a way tailored to the individual hospital.

Education at all levels of the organization about the importance of infection prevention and feedback given to personnel are paramount for success. Education and feedback lead to increased compliance, thus making for a successful programme implementation. High compliance (>80%) of housekeeping personnel was shown to be a key factor for lowering HAIs in human hospitals (Alfa *et al.*, 2015).

It has been shown that only half of veterinary hospitals have a written protocol for cleaning and disinfection. Furthermore, the wide variety of disinfectants used in the veterinary healthcare sector makes the examination of a relationship between cleaning and contamination difficult to establish. Cleaning and disinfection of cage doors, thermometers and mouth gags was found to be deficient at some veterinary hospitals (Traverse and Aceto, 2015).

Shifting the status quo will mean moving away from the current reactive way of managing infectious diseases towards the implementation of proactive measures (Traverse and Aceto, 2015). As zoonotic disease is an inherent risk factor in veterinary medicine, ICPB programmes must address measures to protect the health of the animal care team. As we will discuss, the hospital environment is an important target for the implementation of

Table 7.1. Environmental survival time ranges for pathogens of concern to veterinary and human medicine.

Pathogen	Environmental survival time
Staphylococcus aureus (including MRSA)	7 days to >12 months
Enterococcus spp. (including VRE)	5 days to >46 months
Acinetobacter spp.	3 days to 11 months
Clostridioides difficile spores	>5 months
Pseudomonas aeruginosa	6 h to 16 months
Klebsiella spp.	2 h to >30 months
Salmonella spp.	Months to years

VRE, vancomycin-resistant enterococci.

proactive ICPB measures (Traverse and Aceto, 2015).

7.4 Environment

The hospital environment and fomites (equipment used within the hospital) can harbour and propagate the transmission of pathogenic microorganisms, which can survive on surfaces for prolonged periods of time (Burgess *et al.*, 2004; Dallap Schaer *et al.*, 2010; KuKanich *et al.*, 2012; Weber *et al.*, 2013). Some veterinary equipment (e.g. stethoscopes, thermometers) are routinely used to examine multiple animals and can become contaminated. Table 7.1 describes pathogen survival time on human and veterinary hospital surfaces (Traub-Dargatz, 2007; Rutala, 2012).

Environmental persistence varies among microorganisms because microbiological factors that favour surface environment-mediated transmission are variable. Several microbiological factors need to be considered (Weber *et al.*, 2013), including:

- the pathogen's capacity to survive for prolonged time periods on surfaces;
- the ability to conserve virulence factors such that it can infect a viable host if exposed;
- the frequency of environmental contamination;
- the ability to colonize patients or to transiently colonize caregivers' hands;
- the size of the inoculating dose; and
- the degree of resistance to surface disinfectants.

In human hospitals, admitting a patient to a room previously occupied by an individual infected with MRSA or vancomycin-resistant *Enterococcus* (VRE) significantly increases the risk of the patient acquiring those pathogens (Weber *et al.*, 2013). In large veterinary hospitals, *Salmonella* spp. is a potentially serious environmental contaminant. The sharing of common instruments and animal housing are risk factors for healthcare-acquired salmonellosis (Burgess *et al.*, 2004). Viral pathogens such as feline calicivirus have been shown to survive in a dried state for 21–28 days at room temperature, 8–12 h on computer keyboards, 1–2 days on a computer mouse and up to 3 days on telephone buttons and receivers (Weber *et al.*, 2013). This highlights the importance that environmental surfaces can play in harbouring and disseminating microbes.

In healthcare situations, the patient's endogenous flora and the hands of healthcare workers represent the most critical sources of environmental contamination (Morley, 2002; Weber *et al.*, 2013; Rutala and Weber, 2014). This is especially true for gastrointestinal and respiratory pathogens, as they can be very contagious, especially where indirect transmission via fomites is not well controlled in the hospital environment (Morley, 2002).

As outlined in Chapter 4 (this volume), hand hygiene is the most effective means to limit contamination from either direct patient contact or indirectly from touching contaminated environmental surfaces and fomites (Morley, 2002; Weber *et al.*, 2013; Alfa *et al.*, 2015).

Contact with contaminated environmental surfaces is just as likely to contaminate hands as direct contact with a patient (Rutala and Weber, 2014). Personnel using improper ICPB practices can further the dissemination of environmental pathogens across the hospital. In human healthcare, hand/glove contamination is strongly correlated with the degree of environmental contamination: the more contaminated the environment, the higher the likelihood that hands become contaminated, spreading pathogens to other patients and surfaces (Weber *et al.*, 2013). In the veterinary setting, proper footwear hygiene is important, especially in high-risk and high-traffic areas. Thus, proper use of a foot bath with a disinfectant solution is common practice in veterinary hospitals (Morley, 2002).

7.5 Environment and Pathogens

Substandard cleaning and disinfection processes increase the risk to animals subsequently occupying that environment (e.g. a contaminated kennel or examination table) of acquiring the microorganism from the environment. Cleaning and disinfection practices, including the use of daily cleaning disinfectants, reduce HAIs, while improper cleaning and disinfecting is likely to aid the spread of pathogenic microorganisms (Donskey, 2013; Rutala and Weber, 2014; Alfa *et al.*, 2015). Studies in human healthcare have shown that less than 50% of hospital room surfaces were adequately cleaned and disinfected (Weber *et al.*, 2013). *Enterococcus* spp., a frequent gastrointestinal tract commensal, has virulence factors (gelatinase, which contributes to biofilm formation), carries intrinsic and acquired resistance mechanisms to multiple antibiotics, and can survive in clean hospital environments for prolonged periods, all of which provokes disease and infections that can be difficult to treat (Sava *et al.*, 2010; KuKanich *et al.*, 2012). *Enterococcus faecalis* can form a biofilm on surfaces such as cage doors. Biofilms reduce disinfectant efficacy, promoting bacterial persistence on environmental surfaces (KuKanich *et al.*, 2012). In a recent small animal study, bacteria of the family *Enterobacteriaceae* were eliminated by routine cleaning and disinfection practices, but *Enterococcus* spp. were not eliminated by these practices (KuKanich *et al.*, 2012).

In human medicine, tools such as improved education and training, checklists to assure that all surfaces and equipment and devices are treated, and provision of feedback to the cleaning team have been shown to improve the frequency of adequate cleaning from 71% to 77% (Weber *et al.*, 2013). These tools can also be adapted to and implemented in veterinary hospitals, because a better trained and educated animal care team will be more compliant in putting ICPB protocols into practice.

7.6 Cleaning, Disinfection and Sterilization

Cleaning is defined as the removal of visible soiling (e.g. organic and inorganic material) from objects and surfaces, and is normally accomplished manually or mechanically using water with detergents or enzymatic products. Thorough cleaning is essential before high-level disinfection and sterilization, because inorganic and organic materials that remain on the surfaces of instruments interfere with the effectiveness of these processes (Rutala and Weber, 2019).

The microbiocidal efficacy of disinfectants is inversely proportional to the degree of soiling on the targeted surface (Sattar, 2010). It has been shown experimentally that efficient cleaning alone can eliminate approximately 90% of bacteria from concrete surfaces, demonstrating the value of the initial step of physically removing pathogens from surfaces prior to disinfection (Dwyer, 2004). This step is key for preventing and eliminating biofilm formation on environmental surfaces and instruments.

Sterilization is the process that destroys all forms of microbial life (including spores) and can be done by physical or chemical methods. Some examples of sterilization methods are steam under pressure, dry heat, ethylene oxide gas, hydrogen peroxide gas plasma, and liquid chemicals (Rutala and Weber, 2019). Disinfection is a process that eliminates many or all pathogenic microorganisms, except bacterial spores, from surfaces or devices. As in human health care, chemical disinfection (liquid disinfectants) is most commonly used in veterinary hospitals. Some disinfectants (chemical sterilants) have the ability to inactivate bacterial spores when used with a prolonged contact time.

Fig. 7.1 depicts the activities of different disinfectants (high-, intermediate- and low-level products)

against different classes of microorganism (vegetative bacteria, fungi, mycobacteria, enveloped and non-enveloped viruses, and bacterial spores). It can be seen that none of these products has a complete spectrum of activity, and bacterial spores can persist in the environment despite the use of all of the available disinfectants. Routine use of a disinfectant applied to a cleaned non-porous surface (low risk for environmental microbial persistence) would require a low-level disinfectant. In contrast, disinfecting an area contaminated with a more resilient pathogen would require a higher-level disinfectant. The disinfection level varies in direct proportion to the concentration of the disinfectant and the contact time needed for the surface to remain wet (Traverse and Aceto, 2015).

Some microorganisms are much harder to kill than others. For example, small non-enveloped viruses such as canine parvovirus are able to survive in the environment and show resistance to many disinfectants. Understanding the pathogens involved and adjusting the disinfection protocol is an important aspect of a hospital's infection-control policy. Reflecting this, the products used will be different for areas of high disease risk (e.g. isolation units) compared with those of low disease risk (e.g. staff office). Additionally, the larger the number of microorganisms, the longer the time required by the disinfectant to kill them (Rutala and Weber, 2019). Therefore, by reducing the number of pathogens with thorough cleaning, the

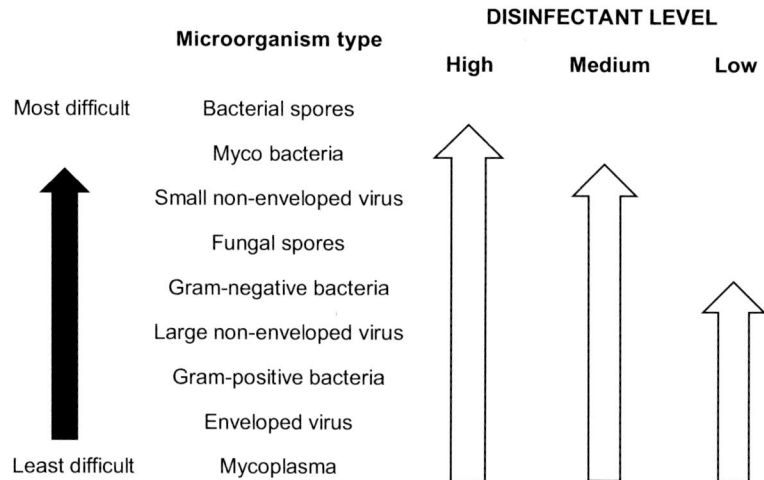

Fig. 7.1. The disinfectant level required, according to the type of microorganism (from least to most difficult to kill). Modified from Rutala and Weber (2014).

Lucas Pantaleon

safety of the disinfectant is improved and the time to kill the microbial load on a surface is shortened (Rutala and Weber, 2019).

Several factors can affect the disinfection and sterilization process, all of which impact on the efficacy for inactivating microorganisms. These include: the completeness of prior cleaning of a surface, the type and level of microbial contamination, the concentration and contact time of the disinfectant, the physical nature of the surface, the presence of biofilm, and the temperature and pH of the product (Rutala and Weber, 2019).

7.6.1 Completeness of prior cleaning

Serum, blood and faeces interfere with the microbicidal activity of disinfectants by producing a complex that is less active. Organic material can also act as a physical barrier, protecting the microorganisms. This, once again, highlights the importance of cleaning before disinfection (Rutala and Weber, 2019).

7.6.2 Type and level of microbial contamination

Some microorganisms, such as bacterial spores, are innately resistant to chemical disinfectants due to their spore coat and cortex that act as a protective barrier. It is important to keep in mind that the most resistant microorganism present in any environment should dictate the time required for a surface or device to be disinfected or sterilized (Rutala and Weber, 2019).

7.6.3 Concentration and contact time of the disinfectant

An important concept in disinfection is the disinfectant contact time: the time surfaces or devices need to remain exposed to the disinfectant solution to achieve an effective outcome (Rutala and Weber, 2019). Depending on the ambient temperature (high temperature will evaporate the disinfectant faster) and the contact time on the disinfectant label, disinfectants may have to be reapplied in order to meet the required contact time.

7.6.4 Presence of biofilm

A biofilm is a mass of bacterial cells encapsulated with extracellular matrix materials that confers protection from disinfectants. The bacterial communities contained in a biofilm attach to surfaces very tightly and are difficult to remove. Bacteria organized in biofilms may be resistant to disinfectants by multiple mechanisms, including the physical characteristics of biofilms, genotypic variation of the bacteria, microbial production of neutralizing enzymes, and physiological gradients within the biofilm (pH) (Rutala and Weber, 2019). Some commercial products contain enzymes or detergents that can degrade biofilms or decrease the numbers of viable bacteria within the biofilm, but there are currently no US Environmental Protection Agency (EPA)- or US Food and Drug Administration (FDA)-cleared products that are registered for this purpose (Rutala and Weber, 2019).

7.6.5 Product temperature and pH

Generally, the higher the temperature, the greater the disinfectant activity. An acidic pH also improves the disinfectant activity for some classes of disinfectants. Areas of the world that have hard water (high concentration of divalent cations) may experience a decreased rate of kill for some disinfectants because divalent cations can form insoluble precipitates within the disinfecting solution, reducing their potency (Rutala and Weber, 2019).

For cleaning, disinfection and sterilization processes to be effective, it is paramount that the healthcare team is appropriately trained and strictly follows the procedures in the practice infection-control policy. Where possible, this should be regularly updated so that it incorporates new evidence-based recommendations and adheres to product label instructions.

Selecting the right cleaning product and disinfectant can ensure the overall success of the programme and can have a dramatic impact on facility maintenance costs. There are many EPA-registered disinfectants available, which makes the selection of a single product for all purposes very difficult. It is important to identify an agent that kills all relevant pathogens of concern quickly and effectively, without presenting a health hazard to humans or animals, and without damaging equipment and environmental surfaces. Ninety per cent of the disinfectant market is composed of approximately 14 different types of disinfectants and combinations thereof (Table 7.2) (Omidbakhsh and Sattar, 2006).

Table 7.2. Summary of the most important characteristic of some commonly used disinfectant classes in veterinary medicine. Adapted from The Center for Food Security and Public Health (n.d.).

Characteristic	Alcohols	Aldehydes	Oxidizing agents	Phenols	Quaternary ammonium
Active ingredients	Ethanol Isopropanol	Formaldehyde Glutaraldehyde	Peroxygen: Hydrogen peroxide, Paracetic acid, Potassium peroxymonosulfate. Halogens: chlorine: Sodium hypochlorite (bleach), Chlorine dioxide	Ortho-phenylphenol, Orthobenzylparachlorophenol	Benzalkonium chloride, Alkyldimethyl ammonium chloride
Brand names[a]			Clorox Wysiwash Rescue Virkon S	One Stroke Tek-Trol Lysol	Roccal-D
Mechanism of action	Precipitates proteins Denatures lipids	Denatures proteins Damages nucleic acid	Denatures proteins / Denature proteins and lipids	Denatures proteins Disrupts cell wall	Denatures proteins, Disrupts cell wall
Attributes	Fast acting Fast evaporation No residue Damage to rubber	Slow acting Affected by pH Irritant Non-corrosive	Fast acting Affected by pH Corrosive Irritant / Fast acting Damages copper, brass and zinc Powdered form can be irritating Low toxicity Environmentally safe	Can leave residual film on surfaces Damages rubber Non-corrosive Irritant	Best at neutral or basic pH Can be corrosive Irritant
Precautions	Flammable	Carcinogenic	Forms toxic gases if mixed with acids or ammonia / Toxic to cats and pigs		
Bactericidal	+	+	+	+	+
Virucidal	+/–[b]	+/–	+	+	+ (enveloped)
Fungicidal	+	+	+/–	+	+
TB-cidal	+	+	+/–	+	–
Sporocidal	–	+	+	–	+

Continued

Lucas Pantaleon

Table 7.2. Continued

Characteristic	Alcohols	Aldehydes	Oxidizing agents	Phenols	Quaternary ammonium
Efficacy	Inactivated by OM	Inactivated by OM, hard water, soaps and detergents	Inactivated by UV light and OM	Effective with OM, hard water, soaps and detergents	Effective with OM, hard water, soaps and detergents	Inactivated by OM, hard water, soaps and anionic detergents

+, effective; +/−, variable or limited activity; −, not effective; OM, organic matter; TB, tuberculosis.

[a]Disclaimer: The use of trade names serves only as examples and does not in any way signify endorsement of a particular product.

[b]Inability of isopropyl alcohol to inactivate hydrophilic viruses (e.g. parvovirus) (Rutala and Weber, 2019).

7.7 Toxic and Environmental Effects

Toxicity varies among disinfectants, but it is important that all products be used with the appropriated safety precautions and only for the intended purposes (Rutala and Weber, 2019). Three important factors are associated with specific health risks from chemical exposure: (i) exposure duration; (ii) intensity (how much chemical is involved); and (iii) route (skin, mucous membranes and inhalation) (Rutala and Weber, 2019). Acute toxicity can occur following an accidental spill and a single exposure event, but repeated exposures at low concentrations over a prolonged time can also lead to chronic toxicity (Rutala and Weber, 2019).

There may be country-specific exclusions or maximum limits imposed on the concentration of certain chemicals (e.g. glutaraldehyde, formaldehyde and some phenols) which may be disposed via the sewer system, with the aim being to minimize harm to the environment (Rutala and Weber, 2019).

Sodium hypochlorite, quaternary ammonium, chlorine gas and glutaraldehyde (all active ingredients in veterinary disinfectants) can cause occupational illnesses (Sattar, 2006). Quaternary ammonium has been shown to induce occupational asthma, most likely due to the induction of immunoglobulin E sensitization to aeroallergens (Sattar, 2006). Glutaraldehyde is commonly used for endoscope disinfection but is a skin irritant, and can cause occupational asthma or rhinitis, as well as being mutagenic (Omidbakhsh, 2006).

There is also some concern about the residues and long-term environmental impact of disinfectants, especially on surface and ground water (Sattar, 2006). Evidence exists that, with repeated use of chemical disinfectants, the tolerance of microorganisms to the disinfectant could increase, as well as promoting the emergence of cross-resistance to clinically important antibiotics (Condell et al., 2012). There are currently no data suggesting that multidrug-resistant bacteria are any less sensitive to liquid disinfectants compared with antibiotic-sensitive bacteria, provided the correct contact times and concentrations are used (Rutala and Weber, 2019). Antibiotics have a specific target on the bacterium that defines their mechanism of action (see Chapter 16, this volume), but disinfectants do not have a distinct bacterial cell target upon which to act (Condell et al., 2012). While resistance to antibiotics can emerge from targeted gene mutations, tolerance to disinfectants is mediated by less well-characterized mechanisms. Bacterial resistance to disinfectant may be afforded by an upregulation of efflux pumps or alterations in the cell-wall structure that impacts permeability (Condell et al., 2012). Prolonged exposure to quaternary ammonium disinfectants could theoretically increase the co-selection of antibiotic resistance within environmental bacteria (Gaze et al., 2005). Downstream from the intended point of application, sublethal concentrations of disinfectants may exert a selective pressure on bacteria, favouring the growth of resistant strains (Gaze et al., 2005). However, it is thought that the higher disinfectant concentrations used, and the targeting of several different bacterial cell structures, makes the emergence of tolerance less likely. For example, oxygen-releasing biocides, such as hydrogen peroxide, cause indiscriminate oxidative damage to multiple microorganism structures (cellular proteins and nucleic acid), ultimately causing cell death (Alfa and Jackson, 2001; Finnegan et al., 2010; Condell et al., 2012). As such, oxidation is less likely to induce resistance to the disinfectant (Dunowska et al., 2005).

In summary, important steps to prevent or minimize the emergence of bacterial tolerance include proper surface cleaning to remove organic matter and biofilm, assurance of an adequate disinfectant contact time and recommended concentrations, and allowing surfaces to be properly dried before applying the disinfectant to avoid an additional dilution effect (Condell et al., 2012). The rotational use of disinfectants has been suggested in some settings in order to prevent the development of bacterial resistance (Rutala and Weber, 2019).

7.8 Surface Disinfection

The combination of cleaning and disinfection, when done properly, is critical for breaking the transmission of infectious disease. In human hospitals, the removal of floor microbes is a component for controlling HAIs. It was shown that cleaning hospital floors with soap and water yielded an 80% reduction in the bacterial numbers; this was less effective than use of a phenol-based disinfectant, which reduced bacterial counts by 94–99.9%. Despite this, the bacterial count on the floors had returned to pre-disinfection levels within a few hours of applying the disinfectant (Rutala and Weber, 2019). Using mops to clean floors is a common practice in veterinary hospitals. It has been shown that the detergent water in mop buckets becomes contaminated as time passes, which can lead to seeding of bacteria in different areas where the mop is used (Rutala and Weber, 2019). Bacterial contamination of soap and water increased significantly after cleaning, while the contamination of a disinfectant solution did not change (Rutala and Weber, 2019). Further studies have found that improperly cleaned surfaces in hospitals can harbour bacteria that can later be transferred to other surfaces by the use of a shared mop or cloth or by touch (Rutala and Weber, 2019).

Disinfectant selection should be an important part of the decision-making process when ICPB protocols are put into practice. The development of rational approaches for the selection and use of disinfectants will optimize its application, improve safety for people and animals, and reduce the discharge of potentially harmful chemicals into the environment (Sattar, 2006). Disinfectants should be selected based chiefly on safety and efficacy, as the use of the wrong formulation for an inappropriate contact time generates a false sense of security, risking the spread of pathogenic organisms over a wider area during the process. Selecting the optimal disinfectant should be based on five key criteria, as outlined in Table 7.3 (Rutala and Weber, 2014).

Selecting a disinfectant is one component for effective disinfection. The second component is the practice, which encompasses correct product application covering all surfaces to be disinfected, training personnel and following the manufacturer's label instructions (Rutala and Weber, 2014).

7.9 Application of Disinfectants: Wiping or Mopping?

Provided an effective surface disinfectant is applied to surfaces in sufficient amounts with adherence to the appropriate contact time, the mechanical action of wiping could further improve the process of surface decontamination (Sattar, 2010). However, if the necessary contact time is not respected or the disinfectant is not applied at the correct concentration, wiping will be ineffective and could serve simply to spread the microorganisms over a wider area (Sattar, 2010).

The material used for wiping is also significant, as some products can have a deleterious effect on the disinfectant action. In the author's experience, products of the same formulation can have different microbicidal effects when tested in a laboratory setting using a liquid or wipe method of application.

A study has shown that the interaction between the wipe material and the disinfectant is complex (Ahmadpour, 2014). This study revealed that the type of wipe substrate (cotton, microfibre or disposable wipe) has a significant effect on the saturation of the wipe with disinfectant and on the release of the disinfectant on to the surface. This interaction can have a direct impact on the speed at which the surface dries, thus affecting contact time. A wipe

Table 7.3. The five key criteria used to select the optimal disinfectant

Property	Questions to ask
Kill claims	Is the product effective against the most prevalent pathogens, including those that: (i) cause hospital infections; (ii) cause outbreaks; and (iii) are of concern in your facility?
Kill and wet contact times	How fast does the product kill the pathogens of concern? Does the product keep surfaces wet for the required kill time?
Safety	Does the product have an acceptable toxicity rating? Does the product have an acceptable flammability rating? What is the personal protection equipment required? Is the product compatible with the surfaces at your facility?
Ease of use	Is its odour acceptable? Does it have an acceptable shelf life? Does the product come in formats that meet your facility's needs (i.e. liquids, concentrate, wipes and multiple sizes)? Does the product work in the presence of organic matter? Does the product clean and disinfect in a single step? Are the directions for use simple and easy to understand?
Other factors	Does the supplier offer training and education? What type of customer support is offered? Is the overall cost acceptable? Can the product be the standardized disinfectant used in your facility?

that is able to release the disinfectant evenly over a large surface area will have a positive effect on disinfection.

Cotton towels bind 83% of quaternary ammonium disinfectants after just 30 s, hence negatively impacting disinfectant efficacy and failing to pass bactericidal testing (Engelbrecht *et al.*, 2013). Other studies have also shown a negative interaction between cotton and quaternary ammonium disinfectants (Rutala *et al.*, 2007; Rutala and Weber, 2019). This is an important finding, as application of quaternary ammonium disinfectants using cotton mops or cotton towels in animal settings is widespread.

Another study has shown that the wetness of the wipe could negatively affect its ability to clean a surface (Gold and Hitchins, 2013). Wipes that were oversaturated with a disinfectant solution had a decreased cleaning efficacy. Furthermore, wipes that are too wet can lead to excessive disinfectant deposition on to a surface, causing corrosion over time or damage to electronics. Thus, proper wipe saturation is an important determinant on how the disinfectant wipe performs in field situations.

There is work required to develop reliable and standardized testing protocols to simulate the wiping action in order to support accurate label claims.

Microfibre-based fabrics are gaining popularity as wiping disinfectants. Microfibres are densely constructed, polyester and polyamide (nylon) fibres that are approximately 1/16 the thickness of a human hair. The microfibres are positively charged to attract negatively charged dust and are more absorbent than a cotton-loop mop (Rutala and Weber, 2019). Good-quality, reusable microfibre cloths or mops, when used correctly, can remove surface contamination more effectively than other materials, and retain microorganisms within the material to lower the risk of pathogens being spread while wiping contaminated surfaces (Sattar, 2010). Furthermore, the use of microfibre cloths may lower the required concentration of disinfectants, therefore reducing environmental chemical load (Sattar, 2010). Table 7.4 highlights some of the advantages and disadvantage of microfibre cloths (Sattar, 2010).

7.10 Challenges

There are some challenges encountered when using different disinfectants in a 'real-world' situation, such as the complex environment of a veterinary hospital. Some of the issues facing the hospital team when selecting cleaning and disinfecting products are as follows:

- The environmental pathogens are often unknown.
- There is a mixture of microorganisms, some of which may persist as biofilms.
- Organic material and other residues could render the disinfectant inactive.
- Disinfectants are labelled to work on non-porous surfaces. In veterinary hospitals, there are a multitude of surface types, some of which may not be receptive to disinfection (e.g. untreated wood or porous floor material). Furthermore, the disinfectant could damage the surfaces or devices. Damaged surfaces will make those surfaces more difficult to clean and disinfect because microorganisms could 'hide' within the defects.

An additional challenge is that label claims are reached under laboratory conditions using different

Table 7.4. Advantages and limitations of microfibre cloths.

Advantages	Limitations
Light in weight and flexible	Higher initial cost
Effective pick-up and retention of microbes	Higher surface contact and resistance to gliding
Hypoallergenic	Dry moping suitable only for dust removal
Washable and reusable	Less efficient when fully saturated
Lower disinfectant use	May trap lint when washed with other fabrics
Require less water for use	Fabric is softer and quaternary ammonium compounds clog the microfibre pores
	Not suitable for use with bleach of certain types (e.g. polyamide)

Lucas Pantaleon

Table 7.5. The properties of an ideal disinfectant. Modified from Rutala and Weber (2019).

Broad spectrum	Soluble
Fast acting	Stable
Not affected by environmental factors	Good cleaning properties
Non-toxic	Environmentally friendly
Surface compatibility	Economical
Odourless	Easy to use

protocols and different levels of stringency that may not be replicable in a hospital environment. Laboratory testing of disinfectant products only provides a rough indication of the manner in which a disinfectant would be expected to perform under field conditions (Sattar, 2010).

7.11 The Ideal Disinfectant

Selecting the ideal disinfectant requires more than just focusing on what the product kills. The Centers for Disease Control and Prevention (CDC) has described the properties of an ideal disinfectant (Table 7.5). Some of the key considerations for choosing a proper disinfectant are: cleaning ability, microbicidal spectrum, disinfection contact time, compatibility with surfaces and materials, and overall toxicity profile. These properties should be taken into account when faced with the task of deciding among the different disinfectants available.

7.12 Proper Use of Disinfectants According to Risk Level

There are different levels of biosecurity required throughout any veterinary hospital. The level of infection risk will depend on the nature of the patients and care offered in different zones. It is ideal to consider separation of different areas within the facility depending on biosecurity/infectious disease control. As an example, a graded number system may be complemented with a colour-coded system (Fig. 7.2). A colour-coded system portrays a clear visual message to everyone involved with the care of animals within the hospital and to personnel involved with the cleaning and disinfection process of the different areas. For example, a kennel with a red tag hanging on the door will tell the personnel cleaning that kennel that an animal with an infectious contagious disease was housed and that the cleaning/disinfection process must be more stringent.

It is also important to keep in mind that the movement of equipment and/or personnel between a Biosecurity Level 3 area and lower-tier areas must be minimized or restricted.

The level of any area may need to be altered, depending on the status of the patients being treated.

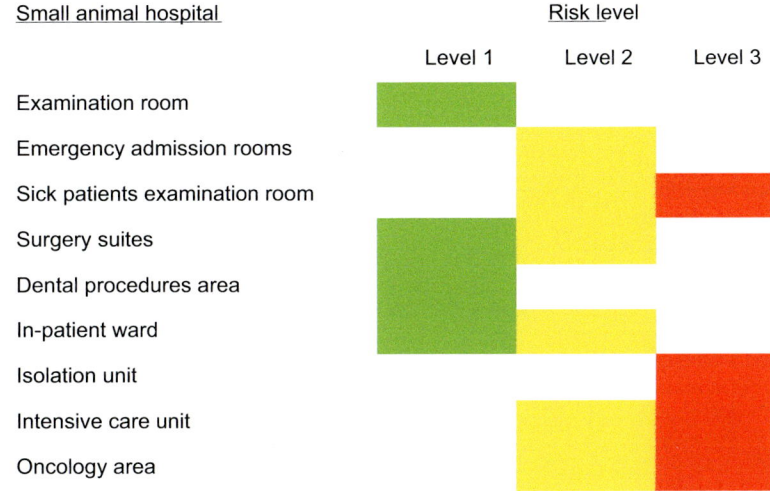

Fig. 7.2. Suggested graded number system, complemented with a colour-coded system, which could be implemented in various zones throughout the hospital.

It is important to keep in mind that the area allocation is not 'set in stone'. On the contrary, it should be a dynamic process, changing with the risk. For example, if a puppy is examined in an outpatient examination room and physical examination findings suggest the possibility of canine parvovirus infection, then the risk level of that room will be increased from level 1/green to level 3/red. No other animals should be examined in that room until it has been properly cleaned and disinfected.

7.13 Transmission-Based Precautions

In small animal hospitals, transmission-based precautions are instituted to prevent the spread of important transmissible pathogens from infected or colonized animals. There are three types of transmission-based precautions: airborne, droplet and contact. Table 7.6 below describes transmission precautions for dogs and cats (Sykes and Weese, 2014).

7.14 New Technologies

New technologies and methods for enhancing environmental surface cleaning and disinfection have the potential to improve infection control within the practice.

7.14.1 Chemical-free cleaning

An innovative methodology based on ultra-microfibre cloths and steam technology has been implemented in an Australian healthcare system. The materials are used for cleaning and micro-organism removal via ultra-microfibre cloths (a combination of polyester and polyamide), removing particles by absorption and static attraction (Gillespie *et al.*, 2013). The microfibres trap dirt and microbes, which are not transferred to other surfaces during the wiping process (Gillespie *et al.*, 2013). Steam technology involves the application of hot gas (maintained at temperatures of 140°C) under pressure (97% dry steam). This loosens surface dirt and microorganisms, including norovirus and vegetative and spores of *C. difficile*, facilitating their removal by the microfibre cloths (Gillespie *et al.*, 2013). The cloths and mops used for daily cleaning are dampened with water, used for a single patient room, and laundered for reprocessing. Disposable microfibre cloths are used for cleaning equipment and reusable microfibre cloths are used to clean surfaces; both are effective in removing bacteria (Gillespie, 2019).

This method of cleaning and disinfection has the advantages of reducing water usage (90% less is used for cleaning), being environmentally friendly, eliminating the need for detergents and disinfectants, shortening the time needed for cleaning and disinfection, and improving surface cleanliness (Gillespie *et al.*, 2013; Gillespie, 2019). Safety and risk of injury due to lifting buckets or slipping is also reduced. Additionally, the initial capital investment in steam machines and ultra-microfibre cloths and mops was offset by eliminating liquid chemicals and replacing them with dry cleaning

Table 7.6. Transmission precautions for dogs and cats. Modified from Sykes and Weese (2014).

Transmission route	Pathogen	Transmission precautions
Airborne	*Mycobacterium tuberculosis* *Yersinia pestis* *Francisella tularensis*	Isolation; ideally negative-pressure room Wearing N95 respirator mask Barrier nursing
Droplet	Canine infectious respiratory disease complex Infectious feline upper respiratory tract disease	Isolation Space animals four feet apart or more Barrier nursing

Contact	Multidrug-resistant bacteria
	 Dermatophytes *Leptospira* spp.
	 Salmonella spp.
	 Parvovirus
		Warning signage on the cage
		 Barrier nursing
		 Dedicated equipment Isolation for
		    certain pathogens
		 Limit movement of affected animals
		 Hand hygiene precautions
		 Proper cleaning, disinfection and
		    disposal

Lucas Pantaleon

(Gillespie *et al.*, 2013). Another benefit is that as microfibre cloths are only dampened with water, not saturated, they are appropriate for cleaning delicate items such as keyboards, electrical leads or screens without the use of chemicals or scrubbing (Gillespie *et al.*, 2016).

Human norovirus is a non-enveloped RNA virus belonging to the same family as feline calicivirus and is similarly recognized for its virulence and environmental persistence (Abernethy *et al.*, 2013). Norovirus can survive for up to 28 days on environmental surfaces and hands (Chiu, 2015). A study showed that using an ultra-microfibre cloth and steam technology was as effective in containing a norovirus outbreak as the classic two-step process that used bleach (Abernethy *et al.*, 2013).

Ultra-microfibre cloth and steam technology has been used in different settings from operating room environments to containment of outbreaks. To the author's knowledge, it has not been used in the veterinary healthcare setting, but its implementation could uncover many potential advantages. However, careful testing and evaluation would be recommended before implementing it widely.

7.14.2 Self-sanitizing surfaces

Prevention of HAIs calls for disinfection of high-touch surfaces, because these surfaces contribute to pathogen transmission and hand contamination (Tamimi *et al.*, 2014). Commonly used disinfectants are effective at removing pathogens from high-touch objects; however, they provide no residual activity (Tamimi *et al.*, 2014). Additionally, the application of disinfectants needs to be closely monitored, because cleaning cloths could reduce the effective concentration of the produce, and human error is common (Tamimi *et al.*, 2014). Self-disinfecting surfaces would help to address these pitfalls, as they act against microbes on a continuing basis (Tamimi *et al.*, 2014).

To achieve self-sanitization, a disinfectant can be chemically bound to a surface or it can be made from a material that incorporates the disinfectant (Sattar, 2010). Titanium dioxide-containing coatings can release microbicidal ions when exposed to UV light, killing microbes via an oxidizing process (Sattar, 2010). The EPA has approved registration for copper and other alloys on antimicrobial hard surfaces (Sattar, 2010). Copper surfaces have been shown to reduce the rate of MRSA and VRE colonization of intensive care unit rooms, as well as the number of organisms on surfaces (Tamimi *et al.*, 2014).

Some concerns exist regarding some types of self-sanitizing surfaces. For example, a time-related decay of the active chemical potentially could render surfaces at a sublethal level for nosocomial pathogens. Furthermore, the continuous exposure of pathogens to these types of surfaces could lead to the development of microbicide-resistant strains (Sattar, 2010).

7.15 Conclusion

The three pillars of ICPB (human, animal and environment) are shared by the One Health concept and should be implemented with One Health in mind. The importance of cleaning before disinfection cannot be overemphasized, because organic material can also act as a physical barrier, protecting the microorganisms. Disinfectants should chiefly be selected on safety and efficacy, ensuring that application is correct and consistent. A holistic team approach, including education and feedback, is essential in improving buy-in and maximizing compliance.

References

Abernethy, M., Gillespie, E., Snook, K. and Stuart, R.L. (2013) Microfiber and steam for environmental cleaning during an outbreak. *American Journal of Infection Control* 41(11), 1134–1135. DOI: 10.1016/j.ajic.2013.02.011.

Ahmadpour, F.E.A. (2014) *Is a wipe a wipe? implications of various wipe substrate materials on proper disinfection of surfaces using commonly used disinfectant chemistries.* Virox Technologies. Available at: http://cdn2.hubspot.net/hub/241248/file-627172614-pdf/SHEA_Poster/Wipe_Study_Poster_1.pdf (accessed 20 October 2020).

Alfa, M.J. and Jackson, M. (2001) A new hydrogen peroxide-based medical-device detergent with germicidal properties: comparison with enzymatic cleaners. *American Journal of Infection Control* 29(3), 168–177. DOI: 10.1067/mic.2001.113616.

Alfa, M.J., Lo, E., Olson, N., MacRae, M. and Buelow-Smith, L. (2015) Use of a daily disinfectant cleaner instead of a daily cleaner reduced hospital-acquired infection rates. *American Journal of Infection Control* 43(2), 141–146. DOI: 10.1016/j.ajic.2014.10.016.

Benedict, K.M. (2008) Characteristics of biosecurity and infection control programs at veterinary teaching hospitals. *Journal of the American Veterinary*

Medical Association 233(5), 767–773. DOI: 10.2460/javma.233.5.767.

Burgess, B.A., Morley, P.S. and Hyatt, D.R. (2004) Environmental surveillance for *Salmonella enterica* in a veterinary teaching hospital. *Journal of the American Veterinary Medical Association* 225(9), 1344–1348. DOI: 10.2460/javma.2004.225.1344.

Chiu, S. (2015) Efficacy of common disinfectant/cleaning agents in inactivating murine norovirus and feline calicivirus as surrogate viruses for human norovirus. *American Journal of Infection Control* 43(11), 1208–1212. DOI: 10.1016/j.ajic.2015.06.021.

Condell, O., Iversen, C., Cooney, S., Power, K.A., Walsh, C. *et al.* (2012) Efficacy of biocides used in the modern food industry to control salmonella enterica, and links between biocide tolerance and resistance to clinically relevant antimicrobial compounds. *Applied and Environmental Microbiology* 78(9), 3087–3097. DOI: 10.1128/AEM.07534-11.

Dallap Schaer, B.L., Aceto, H. and Rankin, S.C. (2010) Outbreak of salmonellosis caused by *Salmonella enterica* serovar Newport MDR-AmpC in a large animal veterinary teaching hospital. *Journal of Veterinary Internal Medicine* 24(5), 1138–1146. DOI: 10.1111/j.1939-1676.2010.0546.x.

Donskey, C.J. (2013) Does improving surface cleaning and disinfection reduce health care-associated infections? *American Journal of Infection Control* 41(5 Suppl), S12–9. DOI: 10.1016/j.ajic.2012.12.010.

Dunowska, M., Morley, P.S. and Hyatt, D.R. (2005) The effect of Virkon S fogging on survival of *Salmonella enterica* and *Staphylococcus aureus* on surfaces in a veterinary teaching hospital. *Veterinary Microbiology* 105(3–4), 281–289. DOI: 10.1016/j.vetmic.2004.11.011.

Dwyer, R.M. (2004) Environmental disinfection to control equine infectious diseases. *Veterinary Clinics of North America: Equine Practice* 20(3), 531–542. DOI: 10.1016/j.cveq.2004.07.001.

Engelbrecht, K., Ambrose, D., Sifuentes, L., Gerba, C., Weart, I. *et al.* (2013) Decreased activity of commercially available disinfectants containing quaternary ammonium compounds when exposed to cotton towels. *American Journal of Infection Control* 41(10), 908–911. DOI: 10.1016/j.ajic.2013.01.017.

Finnegan, M., Linley, E., Denyer, S.P., McDonnell, G., Simons, C, *et al.* (2010) Mode of action of hydrogen peroxide and other oxidizing agents: differences between liquid and gas forms. *Journal of Antimicrobial Chemotherapy* 65(10), 2108–2115. DOI: 10.1093/jac/dkq308.

Gaze, W.H., Abdouslam, N., Hawkey, P.M. and Wellington, E.M.H. (2005) Incidence of class 1 integrons in a quaternary ammonium compound-polluted environment. *Antimicrobial Agents and Chemotherapy* 49(5), 1802–1807. DOI: 10.1128/AAC.49.5.1802-1807.2005.

Gillespie, E.E. (2019) Smarter cleaning is safer for health. *Infection Control and Hospital Epidemiology* 40(8), 947. DOI: 10.1017/ice.2019.144.

Gillespie, E., Wilson, J., Lovegrove, A., Scott, C., Abernethy, M, *et al.* (2013) Environment cleaning without chemicals in clinical settings. *American Journal of Infection Control* 41(5), 461–463. DOI: 10.1016/j.ajic.2012.07.003.

Gillespie, E., Brown, R., Treagus, D., James, A. and Jackson, C. (2016) Improving operating room cleaning results with microfiber and steam technology. *American Journal of Infection Control* 44(1), 120–122. DOI: 10.1016/j.ajic.2015.08.016.

Gold, K.M. and Hitchins, V.M. (2013) Cleaning assessment of disinfectant cleaning wipes on an external surface of a medical device contaminated with artificial blood or *Streptococcus pneumoniae. American Journal of Infection Control* 41(10), 901–907. DOI: 10.1016/j.ajic.2013.01.029.

KuKanich, K.S., Ghosh, A., Skarbek, J.V., Lothamer, K.M. and Zurek, L. (2012) Surveillance of bacterial contamination in small animal veterinary hospitals with special focus on antimicrobial resistance and virulence traits of enterococci. *Journal of the American Veterinary Medical Association* 240(4), 437–445. DOI: 10.2460/javma.240.4.437.

Messenger, A.M., Barnes, A.N. and Gray, G.C. (2014) Reverse zoonotic disease transmission (zooanthroponosis): a systematic review of seldom-documented human biological threats to animals. *PloS One* 9(2), e89055. DOI: 10.1371/journal.pone.0089055.

Morley, P.S. (2002) Biosecurity of veterinary practices. *Veterinary Clinics of North America. Food Animal Practice* 18(1), 133–155. DOI: 10.1016/s0749-0720(02)00009-9.

Morley, P.S. (2013) Evidence-based infection control in clinical practice: if you buy clothes for the emperor, will he wear them? *Journal of Veterinary Internal Medicine* 27(3), 430–438. DOI: 10.1111/jvim.12060.

Omidbakhsh, N. (2006) A new peroxide-based flexible endoscope-compatible high-level disinfectant. *American Journal of Infection Control* 34(9), 571–577. DOI: 10.1016/j.ajic.2006.02.003.

Omidbakhsh, N. and Sattar, S.A. (2006) Broad-spectrum microbicidal activity, toxicologic assessment, and materials compatibility of a new generation of accelerated hydrogen peroxide-based environmental surface disinfectant. *American Journal of Infection Control* 34(5), 251–257. DOI: 10.1016/j.ajic.2005.06.002.

Porter, M. and Lee, T.H. (2013) The strategy that will fix health care. *Harvard Business Review* October, 1–19.

Roberts, R.R. (2010) Costs attributable to healthcare-acquired infection in hospitalized adults and a comparison of economic methods. *Medical Care* 48(11), 1026–1035. DOI: 10.1097/MLR.0b013e3181ef60a2.

Ruple-Czerniak, A., Aceto, H.W., Bender, J.B., Paradis, M.R., Shaw, S.P. *et al.* (2013) Using syndromic surveillance to estimate baseline rates for healthcare-associated infections in critical care units of small animal referral hospitals. *Journal of Veterinary Internal Medicine* 27(6), 1392–1399. DOI: 10.1111/jvim.12190.

Rutala, W.A. (2012) Does improving surface cleaning and disinfection reduce HAI? Webber Training Teleclass. Available at: https://webbertraining.com/files/library/docs/442.pdf (accessed 20 October 2022).

Rutala, W.A. and Weber, D.J. (2019) Guideline for disinfection and sterilization in healthcare facilities, 2008. CDC, Atlanta, Georgia. Available at: www.cdc.gov/infectioncontrol/guidelines/disinfection/ (accessed 20 October 2022).

Rutala, W.A. and Weber, D.J. (2014) Selection of the ideal disinfectant. *Infection Control and Hospital Epidemiology* 35(7), 855–865. DOI: 10.1086/676877.

Rutala, W.A., Gergen, M.F. and Weber, D.J. (2007) Microbiologic evaluation of microfiber mops for surface disinfection. *American Journal of Infection Control* 35(9), 569–573. DOI: 10.1016/j.ajic.2007.02.009.

Sattar, S.A. (2006) Allen Denver Russell memorial lecture, 2006. *Journal of Applied Microbiology* 101(4), 743–753. DOI: 10.1111/j.1365-2672.2006.03128.x.

Sattar, S.A. (2010) Promises and pitfalls of recent advances in chemical means of preventing the spread of nosocomial infections by environmental surfaces. *American Journal of Infection Control* 38(5 Suppl 1), S34–40. DOI: 10.1016/j.ajic.2010.04.207.

Sava, I.G., Heikens, E. and Huebner, J. (2010) Pathogenesis and immunity in enterococcal infections. *Clinical Microbiology and Infection* 16(6), 533–540. DOI: 10.1111/j.1469-0691.2010.03213.x.

Scott, R.D. (2009) The direct medical costs of healthcare-associated infections in the US hospitals and the benefits of prevention. CDC, Atlanta, Georgia. Available at: www.cdc.gov/HAI/pdfs/hai/Scott_CostPaper.pdf (accessed 20 October 2022).

Spellberg, B., Bartlett, J.G. and Gilbert, D.N. (2013) The future of antibiotics and resistance. *New England Journal of Medicine* 368(4), 299–302. DOI: 10.1056/NEJMp1215093.

Sykes, J. and Weese, J.S. (2014) Infection control programs for dogs and cats. In: Sykes, J. (ed.) *Canine and Feline Infectious Diseases*. Elsevier, St Louis, Missouri, pp. 105–118.

Tamimi, A.H., Carlino, S. and Gerba, C.P. (2014) Long-term efficacy of a self-disinfecting coating in an intensive care unit. *American Journal of Infection Control* 42(11), 1178–1181. DOI: 10.1016/j.ajic.2014.07.005.

The Center for Food Security and Public Health (n.d.) *Characteristics of Selected Disinfectants*. Ames, Iowa: Iowa State University. Available at: www.cfsph.iastate.edu/Disinfection/Assets/CharacteristicsSelectedDisinfectants.pdf (accessed 20 October 2022).

Traub-Dargatz, J.L. (2007) Salmonellosis. In: Sellon, D.C. and Long, M.T. (eds) *Equine Infectious Diseases*. Saunders, Elsevier, St Louis, MO.

Traverse, M. and Aceto, H. (2015) Environmental cleaning and disinfection. *Veterinary Clinics: Small Animal Practice* 45(2), 299–330. DOI: 10.1016/j.cvsm.2014.11.011.

Weber, D.J., Anderson, D. and Rutala, W.A. (2013) The role of the surface environment in healthcare-associated infections. *Current Opinion in Infectious Diseases* 26(4), 338–344. DOI: 10.1097/QCO.0b013e3283630f04.

Weese, J.S. (2014) Infection control and biosecurity in equine disease control. *Equine Veterinary Journal* 46(6), 654–660. DOI: 10.1111/evj.12295.

Section 3: Infection Control of the Surgical Patient

The emotional costs of surgical care remain understudied in both human and veterinary medicine. René Leriche spoke for us all in 1951 when he said: 'Every surgeon carries within himself a small cemetery, where from time to time he goes to pray – a place of bitterness and regret, where he must look for an explanation for his failures.' To think that those who paved the way for us carried the same problems we do today is both disheartening and comforting. This section details the evidence and recommendations for infection control of the surgical patient. Anyone who has picked up a scalpel will have encountered a surgical-site infection (SSI), and therefore we hope that the guidance contained herein will be helpful, easy to implement and empathetic.

This section covers the following key points:

- Thorough and efficient *preparation of the patient's skin* is an essential step prior to any surgical intervention. Suitable antiseptics are illustrated in Table 8.1 (Chapter 8, this volume).
- Theatre staff, surgeons and anaesthetists should be encouraged to *disinfect* mobile phones and tablets on a regular basis to reduce the risk of introducing contamination.
- Clinical signs of an SSI typically appear within 3–7 days but can occur at any time following a surgical procedure.
- *Emergence of resistant bacteria* has reinforced the requirement for antimicrobial stewardship.

Staphylococcus pseudintermedius is one of the most commonly cultured bacteria in SSIs, with methicillin-resistant species prevalent.

- SSIs are multifactorial in origin and achieving *0% infection rates is unrealistic*.
- SSI rates should be *actively and passively monitored*, which will inform the need for proactive (rather than reactive) interventions
- Treatment of SSIs includes addressing and reducing contamination, removing implants (wherever possible), obtaining samples for bacteriological analysis, open-wound management, antimicrobial therapy and wound closure. Generous multi-modal analgesia, adequate nutrition and excellent nursing are central to success in caring for patients with SSIs.
- A variety of dressings are available to treat open wounds, which is often daunting. *Understanding the phases of healing will often help in decision making.*
- It is important that those caring for the patient are aware at the onset that the wound-healing journey may be long, tiring and costly (both financially and emotionally), but not without reward.
- *Recent advances in open wound management* such as negative-pressure wound therapy (or vacuum-assisted closure) offer huge improvements in wound care and are suitable for use in dogs and cats.

8 Infection Prevention and Control in Theatre

KATHRYN PRATSCHKE*

Royal (Dick) School of Veterinary Studies, University of Edinburgh, Roslin, UK

8.1 Introduction

Surgical-site infections (SSIs) remain a significant complication in both human and veterinary surgery. Negative consequences for the patient include increased morbidity with a consequent impact on quality of life, prolonged hospital stays and sometimes a requirement for further treatment. In a veterinary context, there are financial implications for clients in addition to the increased stress and worry of coping with their pet having a post-operative infection. The occurrence and impact of SSIs are still poorly quantified in veterinary surgery, and there is limited objective information available in the literature regarding the various components of infection-control policies.

An important reality to bear in mind is that not all SSIs can be prevented, regardless of the quality and rigour of an infection-control policy. However, a proportion of SSIs are preventable, so the goal is to reduce or eliminate this preventable fraction of cases. Surgery by its very nature breaches the intact skin barrier and can thus allow access to deeper tissues. Trauma is caused to tissues and blood vessels through handling, dissection and use of retractors, and the tendency of tissues to dry through exposure compounds the problem. Foreign material is introduced in the form of suture material and surgical implants (Fig. 8.1). Taken together, these factors create an environment that can favour microbial survival. A key part of infection control therefore is to minimize the potential for endogenous and exogenous bacterial contamination of the surgical wound. Most SSIs are thought to develop from skin flora, with other conventionally accepted sources of contamination being surgical staff and the operating room environment (Brown *et al.*, 1997; Reichman and Greenberg, 2009; Andrade *et al.*, 2016; Hayes *et al.*, 2017; Pelosi, 2018; Roesler *et al.*, 2018; Birgand *et al.*, 2019; Jolivet and Lucet, 2019).

8.2 Patient Preparation

8.2.1 Terminology

The following terms are commonly used:

- *Antisepsis* refers to a reduction or inhibition of the growth of microorganisms on the skin or mucus membranes. Antiseptics are the products used to achieve this aim.
- An *antiseptic* prevents the growth and action of pathogenic organisms on living tissue, and is used for patient preparation and surgical hand hygiene (Pelosi, 2018).
- *Disinfectants* are usually chemical agents and are designed to destroy the majority of pathogens found on inanimate objects (Pelosi, 2018).
- *Asepsis* means freedom from pathogenic microorganisms to an extent that prevents the possibility of infection (Jolivet and Lucet, 2019).
- *Surgical asepsis* means the complete avoidance of contamination by pathogenic organisms that might originate from the operating theatre, theatre personnel or patient. Surgical asepsis is a shared responsibility, relying on commitment and compliance from all theatre staff, whether nurses, technicians or veterinarians.

Table 8.1 lists commonly used antiseptics and disinfectants, with their efficacies, advantages and disadvantages.

*Kathryn.Pratschke@ed.ac.uk

© CAB International 2023. *Infection Control in Small Animal Clinical Practice* (eds F. Allerton and K.L. Bowlt Blacklock)
DOI: 10.1079/9781789244977.0008

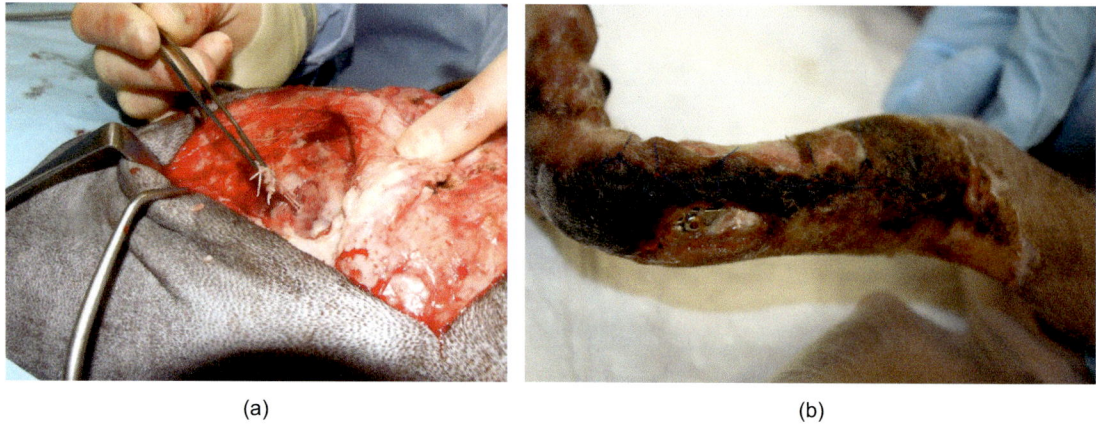

(a)   (b)

Fig. 8.1. Foreign material is introduced during surgery in the form of suture material and surgical implants. In the presence of infection, foreign material can act as a surface for biofilm formation, thereby facilitating both superficial and deep surgical-site infections. (a) A deep-seated body wall abscess linked to non-absorbable suture material. (b) A fracture repair that has subsequently developed a surgical-site infection with exposure of the orthopaedic implant and devitalization of the overlying skin.

8.2.2 General considerations

Thorough and efficient preparation of the patient's skin is an essential step prior to any surgical intervention. In clean surgery, the commensal microbiota of the patient at and around the surgical site are the main source of contamination (Preston Stubbs *et al.*, 1996; Dumville *et al.*, 2015; Boucher *et al.*, 2018; Pelosi, 2018; Jolivet and Lucet, 2019). In contaminated surgeries, the flora from the intestinal, urogenital and respiratory tracts may also become involved. The most common bacteria isolated from SSIs in dogs are reportedly staphylococci, with *Staphylococcus pseudintermedius* being the most frequently seen (Singh *et al.*, 2013; Belo *et al.*, 2018). If *Staphylococcus aureus* is identified on veterinary patients, then it is considered likely to be of human origin as *S. aureus* is a human commensal but not canine or feline (Belo *et al.*, 2018). Over the course of the past decade or so in veterinary patients, there has been a worrying emergence of antibiotic-resistant bacteria, including methicillin-resistant *S. pseudintermedius* in both dogs and cats. The high antimicrobial resistance levels associated with this bacterium are a cause for concern not just for veterinary but also for human health. A recent case report described *S. pseudintermedius* bacteraemia in a lung transplant patient, a potentially very serious condition, where the authors speculated that

the patient's canine companion was the most likely source of infection (Somayaji *et al.*, 2016; Grönthal *et al.*, 2017; Belo *et al.*, 2018; Small *et al.*, 2021).

Preparation of the skin for aseptic surgery in veterinary patients is more challenging than in human patients due to the thick hair coat, a more contaminated living environment and less frequent bathing that is characteristic of veterinary patients. Much of the available information that provides the evidence base for how we prepare veterinary patients for surgery is extrapolated from published work in the human literature, and the difference in patient populations needs to be remembered when considering the recommendations.

Prior to commencing skin preparation for elective surgery, the patient's skin should be checked for any evidence of conditions such as eczema or pyoderma, particularly adjacent to the proposed surgical site. If there are questions over skin health, and a surgery is elective in nature, then it is better postponed until the skin condition is under control. This is particularly important for routine elective orthopaedic procedures that will require the use of an orthopaedic implant with consequent risk of implant biofilm formation and deep-seated infection (Andrade *et al.*, 2016; Hayes *et al.*, 2017; Stine *et al.*, 2018).

  Kathyrn Pratschke

Table 8.1. Characteristics of antiseptics in common use in veterinary clinical practice for patient skin preparation prior to surgery.

Antiseptic	Mode of action	Action against:							Speed of action	Duration
		Gram-positive	Gram-negative	Mycobacteria	Fungi	Viruses	Spores			
Iodine and iodophors	Oxidation and substitution by free iodine	E	G	G	G	G	P to M	Rapid in alcohol-based, otherwise moderate	2 h
Chlorhexidine	Cell-membrane disruption	E	G	P	M	G	P	Rapid in alcohol-based, otherwise moderate	6 h
Alcohol (isopropyl and ethyl alcohol)	Denaturation of proteins	E	E	G	G	V	P	Very rapid	0 h

E, excellent; G, good; M, moderate; P, poor; V, variable.

8.2.3 Pre-operative bathing

Classically, pre-operative showers starting the day prior to admission were advised for human patients, the aim being to eliminate transient flora and reduce the level of commensal residents (Reichman and Greenberg, 2009; Graling and Vasaly, 2013; Webster and Osborne, 2015; Edmiston and Leaper, 2017; Makhni et al., 2018; Lucero and Dryden, 2019). Bathing with an antiseptic soap such as 4% chlorhexidine was typically advised. However, the impact this practice has on the occurrence of SSIs remains unproven and a number of studies, including a Cochrane meta-analysis from 2015 that considered 10,157 patients, found no strong or compelling evidence to support pre-operative antiseptic showers (Reichman and Greenberg, 2009; Webster and Osborne, 2015; Makhni et al., 2018; Huang et al., 2019).

We have no evidence specific to veterinary patients regarding whether there is a benefit to pre-operative bathing the day prior to surgery, and on a practical level this would often be hard, if not impossible, to ensure. The pragmatic compromise is that a patient with gross contamination of the coat and skin from mud, faeces or similar should be bathed in advance of surgery, the aim being to remove gross dirt and contamination. Either a neutral non-medicated soap or a medicated soap such as 4% chlorhexidine can be used in the absence of any compelling evidence for one over the other (Pelosi, 2018).

8.2.4 Hair removal

In people, current guidelines suggest that hair should only be removed if it will interfere with the planned surgery, as there is no proven benefit to pre-operative hair removal per se (Jolivet and Lucet, 2019). The situation is clearly different with veterinary patients that have a dense hair coat covering the body compared with the sparsely haired nature of people. Hair removal can potentially cause microabrasions to the skin leading to exudative rashes, both of which compromise the protective skin barrier (Clayton et al., 2017). It is logical therefore that the least traumatic method possible should be used for hair removal to minimize such trauma, i.e. clipping rather than shaving (Rosewell, 2015; Pelosi, 2018; Jolivet and Lucet, 2019; Lucero and Dryden, 2019; Reynolds and Nichols, 2019). Depilatory creams are occasionally but infrequently used in people; they are considered suboptimal due to the risk of allergic reactions and reactive skin rashes. In any case, it is questionable how effective they would be on a typical veterinary patient.

In people, the timing of hair removal has uncertain impact on the incidence of infection. A recent Cochrane systematic review found low-level evidence that there may be a small reduction in SSI risk with hair removal on the day of surgery compared with 24 h prior to surgery (Tanner and Melen, 2021). For veterinary patients, removal of hair within a 4-h pre-operative window is thought to be associated with a lower incidence of SSI than when hair is removed further in advance of surgery. However, the available veterinary evidence is limited and in terms of the 'pyramid of evidence', the evidence is of low quality and therefore of uncertain reliability (Brown et al., 1997; Mayhew et al., 2012). Although the mechanism is not clear, it has been suggested that advance clipping allows more time for recolonization with environmental contaminants prior to surgery.

Theatre staff should wear disposable gloves and an apron while clipping patients for surgery. The hair coat should be clipped with clean, sharp, no. 40 clipper blades to minimize the potential for skin trauma, with clipper blades checked before each use for any wear and tear that might increase the risk of skin abrasions. Blade sharpness can be assessed by the ease with which it cuts the patient's coat, and blunt blades should be changed immediately to avoid causing skin abrasions. Clippers can be cleaned during use by spraying with pressurized air to remove loose fur and then spraying with a suitable clipper spray to disinfect, cool and lubricate the blades. Blades should be thoroughly cleaned once weekly using a bactericidal blade-wash solution. If blades are used on a patient that may be infectious or carrying zoonotic pathogens, then the blade should be removed from the clippers immediately after use and soaked for 30 min in a solution such as Anigene HLD4V, which is bactericidal, fungicidal, virucidal, mycobactericidal and sporicidal. They can then be dried before being sterilized using ethylene oxide. Steam sterilization blunts sharp implements and is not recommended for clipper blades. Although it has been suggested that patient hair should only be clipped in the direction of natural growth to reduce the risk of skin trauma (Rosewell, 2015), the validity of this recommendation is unclear, and the condition of the clipper blades and degree of care taken by the

Kathyrn Pratschke

operator are likely to have a greater impact on skin trauma.

8.3 Antiseptics and Surgical Skin Preparation

Staff should wear clean disposable gloves and aprons to reduce the risk of iatrogenic contamination during skin preparation. Skin preparation involves two key components: (i) using an appropriate antiseptic solution; and (ii) an effective method of application that adheres to the manufacturer's recommendations regarding optimal application and contact times. The aim is to reduce the number of resident and transient microbes on the skin at the site of the planned surgical incision and the surrounding skin. Skin preparation protocols (including details of antiseptic to be used, concentration, any preparation required and any site-specific caveats) should be detailed in writing as a standard operating procedure (SOP) and the contents regularly reviewed to take account of any new evidence or information. Different SOPs may be required for different areas of the body; for example, preparation for ear surgery in the presence of a ruptured tympanic membrane will not be the same as a total hip replacement surgery or preparation for an ophthalmic procedure.

Any staff who will be involved in patient preparation for surgery should be trained appropriately in line with the written SOPs. Where specific contact times or minimum contact times are specified in the manufacturer's recommendations, a stopwatch or timer should be used to ensure the necessary contact time is adhered to as this is an element of antisepsis that is particularly prone to poor compliance (Anderson et al., 2013).

The ideal skin antiseptic would have a broad spectrum of action against bacteria, fungi and viruses, including efficacy against spore-forming and vegetative bacteria. It would be minimally irritant, non-toxic and have good residual activity. It would not have any long-term teratogenic or carcinogenic risks for either patient or theatre staff (Boucher et al., 2018; Pelosi, 2018). The most commonly used substances currently for pre-operative skin preparation in veterinary surgery are chlorhexidine, povidone-iodine and 70% isopropyl alcohol (Pelosi, 2018). Skin preparation solutions such as electrochemically activated water, F10 Skin Prep Solution and chloroxylenol have been mentioned

in individual, small-scale clinical studies, but they uniformly performed more poorly than either chlorhexidine or povidone-iodine and cannot be recommended for routine use (Preston Stubbs et al., 1996; Boucher et al., 2018).

8.3.1 Iodine/iodophors

Iodine/iodophors are iodine solutions that are effective against fungi, viruses, Gram-positive and -negative bacteria and *Mycobacterium tuberculosis*. They penetrate cell walls and then oxidize and substitute the microbial contents with free iodine (Durani and Leaper, 2008; Pelosi, 2018; Jolivet and Lucet, 2019; Chen et al., 2020). Iodophor has largely replaced iodine as the active ingredient in antiseptics; it comprises free iodine molecules bound to a polymer such as povidone (polyvinylpyrrolidone), hence the widespread use of the term 'povidone-iodine' (Durani and Leaper, 2008). Iodophors contain a surfactant or stabilizing agent that will liberate free iodine, and typically a 10% povidone-iodine formulation will provide 1% free iodine (Berkelman et al., 1982; Durani and Leaper, 2008; Reichman and Greenberg, 2009). The literature reporting the use and efficacy of povidone-iodine includes a wide variety of concentrations depending on the study and the surgical site. Concentrations ranging from 0.5% to 10% have been reported, and this lack of uniformity makes it difficult to draw definitive conclusions regarding the optimum concentration for surgical skin preparation (Dumville et al., 2015; Belo et al., 2018; Pelosi, 2018). Certain sites, such as the eye, require lower concentrations be used for safety reasons, and for large open wounds, concentrations as low as 0.5% are suggested due to the risk of systemic absorption (Pelosi, 2018).

8.3.2 Chlorhexidine

Chlorhexidine is a cationic biguanide that combines with anions on bacterial cell surfaces, altering cell-wall permeability, and leading to apoptosis and cell death (Chen et al., 2020). Chlorhexidine has good efficacy against Gram-positive and -negative bacteria, yeasts and some viruses (Dumville et al., 2015). It has greater efficacy in the presence of organic matter and body fluids than povidone-iodine, and is also suggested to have better residual activity (Dumville et al., 2015; Jolivet and Lucet, 2019; Chen et al., 2020). For surgical scrub solutions concentrations of 2–4% are generally used, although there is limited evidence to show improved efficacy with higher concentrations (Lucero and Dryden, 2019).

8.3.3 Alcohol

Alcohol denatures bacterial cell walls, can disrupt bacterial metabolism and has efficacy against Gram-positive and -negative bacteria, *M. tuberculosis*, fungi and viruses (Dumville *et al.*, 2015; Jolivet and Lucet, 2019). The concentration of the alcohol is important; typically, 70% isopropyl alcohol is used, and reduced efficacy is seen with lower concentrations. Although there is excellent immediate efficacy, alcohol loses its antimicrobial effect once it evaporates, so the effect is short-lived.

8.3.4 Choice of antiseptic and antiseptic formulation

Chlorhexidine and povidone-iodine are available in both aqueous and alcohol-based forms. Alcohol-based antiseptics have been associated with lower SSI rates in randomized controlled trials (RCTs) and meta-analyses in the human literature (Dumville *et al.*, 2015; Jolivet and Lucet, 2019; NICE Guideline Updates Team, 2019); similar RCTs with large patient numbers are not available for veterinary patients, but it seems likely the findings would be similar given the known additional benefits to an alcohol-based formulation of antiseptic. It is important to remember that where diathermy will be used, the potentially flammable nature of alcohol-based antiseptics means they must be allowed to fully air dry with no residual pools that might soak the patient or the surgical drapes (Pelosi, 2018; NICE Guideline Updates Team, 2019; Chen *et al.*, 2020).

There is a large body of literature comparing various skin disinfectants with each other, but the degree of variability within and between studies makes it difficult to draw the information together into a coherent narrative. Different concentrations of antiseptics have been used in different studies, different application protocols have been used, some studies compare aqueous-based antiseptics to alcohol-based giving an unequal comparison, and in some veterinary studies, solutions that are not in routine validated clinical use have been used for comparison groups (Preston Stubbs *et al.*, 1996; Dumville *et al.*, 2015; Charles *et al.*, 2017; Belo *et al.*, 2018; Boucher *et al.*, 2018; Melekwe

et al., 2018; Jolivet and Lucet, 2019; Lucero and Dryden, 2019; Reynolds and Nichols, 2019; Chen *et al.*, 2020). Another problem specific to many of the veterinary studies is that they involve only small numbers of patients, and even when prospective in nature and described as an RCT by the authors, in truth they do not fulfil the necessary criteria for RCT classification (Akobeng, 2005). To be an RCT means that a sample of the population of interest is randomly allocated to one or another of two or more interventions and the groups are followed up for a specified period of time during which – apart from the interventions being compared – the two groups are treated and observed in an identical manner. Participants, staff and study personnel should ideally be blinded to minimize bias, and a power calculation is necessary before starting to confirm minimum numbers required for a statistically significant result. Applying these criteria, we do not have any RCT studies in the veterinary literature on which to base decisions regarding pre-operative skin preparation (Evans, 2003; Murad *et al.*, 2016).

Overall, the current balance of evidence favours using an alcohol-based form of either chlorhexidine or povidone-iodine for pre-surgical skin preparation (Osuna *et al.*, 1990a, b; Jolivet and Lucet, 2019). Within that recommendation, however, there are some site-specific and condition-specific antiseptic requirements, and there are also contraindications of which surgeons and theatre staff need to be aware. Chlorhexidine is potentially both neurotoxic and ototoxic, and should not be used where the tympanic membrane may not be intact (Boothe and Boothe, 2015; Singh and Blakley, 2018; Epstein, 2021). Chlorhexidine is potentially harmful to the cornea, with the potential to cause irritation, abrasions and even blindness, so great care should be taken when using chlorhexidine-based scrub solutions anywhere near the eyes (Chen *et al.*, 2020; Epstein, 2021). Alcohol can similarly cause damage to the cornea and nerves, and is also best avoided on mucus membranes due to its drying effect (Pelosi, 2018; Jolivet and Lucet, 2019). These limitations mean that iodine-based, non-alcoholic, non-detergent solutions are considered the safest option for pre-operative preparations involving the eyes, ears and mouth, ensuring the appropriate concentration of povidone-iodine is used for each site (Boothe and Boothe, 2015; Pelosi, 2018; Epstein, 2021). Care is typically advised when using povidone-iodine for prepping large skin wounds as

Kathyrn Pratschke

there is a risk of iodine absorption, although there is little information regarding this occurrence in clinical veterinary patients (Boothe and Boothe, 2015; Pelosi, 2018).

In recent years, there has been a trend towards using single-use products such as individual pre-prepared sachets of antiseptic solution or single-use antiseptic applicators. This approach reduces the risk of errors in making up scrub solution to the correct concentration required, saves time and reduces the risk of contamination via multi-use bottles. Despite these advantages, financial limitations and a move towards increased sustainability mean that the use of multi-dose bottles to make up skin preparation solutions is likely to continue in veterinary practices and hospitals. Great care needs to be taken to ensure that these multi-dose bottles are used and stored in line with the manufacturer's recommendations, that they do not become contaminated during use, and that skin preparation solutions are made up appropriately and to the correct concentration every time. In the event of any increase in SSI rate, multi-dose bottles should be checked for contamination.

Single-use applicators are particularly useful for the final skin preparation performed in theatre prior to surgery. The correct dose of antiseptic is provided with an attached sponge as a sterile, single-use item (Fig. 8.2). Whatever skin preparation option is used, it is crucial that sufficient time is allowed for the skin to fully dry before the patient is draped. As a guide, minimum drying time for a

2% chlorhexidine in 70% isopropyl alcohol solution is 3 min. Of note, it can take hair up to an hour to fully dry, and during this time it will continue to pose a flammable risk so when performing skin preparation with an alcohol-based solution, it is advisable to minimize runoff into surrounding hair. If an alcohol-based skin preparation solution does soak into surrounding hair, then every effort should be made to dry the patient's coat with sterile swabs or towels. Any puddles of preparation solution that form (e.g. in flank folds or the inguinum following an abdominal preparation) should be soaked up and removed with sterile swabs as they will not dry in the requisite 3 min period and can therefore pose a flammable risk during surgery.

8.3.5 Potential side effects of antiseptics

For chlorhexidine, contact dermatitis, hypersensitivity and anaphylactic shock have been reported as potential side effects for the patient, while for povidone-iodine, allergic contact dermatitis, urticaria and anaphylactic shock have been described (Jolivet and Lucet, 2019). To date, the more severe adverse reactions such as anaphylactic shock are only reported for people. Despite the lack of current evidence for these severe reactions in veterinary patients, it would be prudent for staff performing surgical skin preparation to exercise due caution.

The veterinary literature typically comments on a high risk of skin reaction, erythema and moist dermatitis with povidone-iodine use in dogs; this is

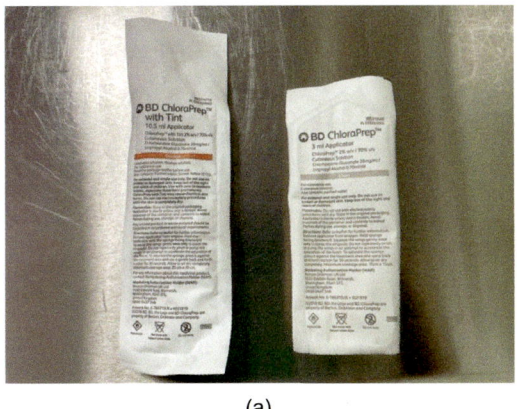
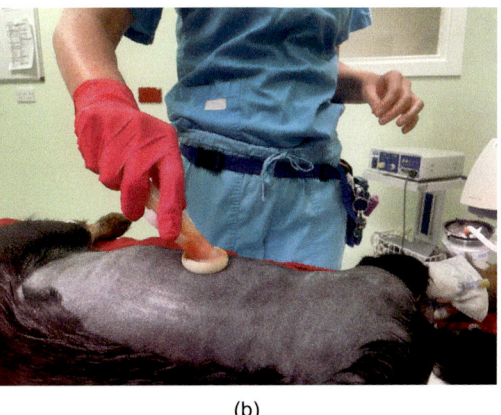

(a)   (b)

Fig. 8.2. (a) Single-use applicators are particularly useful for the final skin preparation performed in theatre prior to surgery. The correct dose of antiseptic is provided with an attached sponge as a sterile single-use item. (b) A 10.5 ml Chloraprep applicator with tint, which facilitates visual confirmation that the entire surgical site has been covered.

largely based on a series of three studies performed in the 1990s (Osuna *et al.*, 1990a, b, 1992). These three studies found an almost 50% incidence in acute contact dermatitis with povidone-iodine compared with chlorhexidine-based scrub solutions. The reactions were characterized by erythema, oedema, papules, wheals and serum weeping. This extent of reaction has not, however, been reported in subsequent veterinary studies, nor is it in keeping with anecdotal and clinical experience (Darouiche *et al.*, 2010; Dumville *et al.*, 2015; Belo *et al.*, 2018; Jolivet and Lucet, 2019; NICE Guideline Updates Team, 2019; Chen *et al.*, 2020). In one of these studies, the dogs had two 3 min scrubs with residual antiseptic removed using alcohol-soaked swabs, followed by a final paint or spray application of antiseptic, while in another they had up to three scrubs with a final alcohol wipe (Osuna *et al.*, 1990a, b). These skin preparation protocols are stronger than current practice, and may potentially have increased the damage to superficial skin layers and inadvertently predisposed to inflammation mediated via Langerhans cells (Silberberg-Sinakin and Thorbecke, 1980; Clayton *et al.*, 2017; Nikolić *et al.*, 2019).

There are situations where povidone-iodine should be used in preference to chlorhexidine, and concern over potential adverse skin reactions should not preclude its use. In people, tolerance for both chlorhexidine and povidone-iodine is very good, with only exceedingly rare confirmed cases of significant adverse reactions (Dumville *et al.*, 2015; Almond, 2017; Jolivet and Lucet, 2019).

8.3.6 Chlorhexidine 'resistance'

Chlorhexidine is the only one of the commonly used antiseptics for which resistance has been identified. Resistance is mediated predominantly by *qac* genes and can readily be transferred between bacterial species via plasmids (Kampf, 2016; Jolivet and Lucet, 2019). Chlorhexidine will retain its antiseptic efficacy in the face of resistance but potentially with reduced reliability. Outbreaks caused by contaminated chlorhexidine solutions at 0.05% concentration have been reported for *Pseudomonas aeruginosa*, *Serratia marcescens*, *Burkholderia cepacia*, *Ralsonia pickettii* and *Achromobacter xylosoxidans* (Kampf, 2016). The bacterial species that are of greatest concern for chlorhexidine resistance to date include *Pseudomonas*, *Proteus*, *Enterobacter* and *Enterococcus* spp. and

multidrug-resistant *Klebsiella pneumoniae* (Kampf, 2016). Chlorhexidine resistance has mainly been a feature in intensive care unit patients in human healthcare, where daily use of chlorhexidine can be very high: in addition to staff hand hygiene with chlorhexidine-based soaps there may also be routine daily patient bathing with chlorhexidine gluconate as well as daily oral rinses and use at catheter insertion sites for daily cleansing and dressing changes (Kampf, 2016; Huang *et al.*, 2019; Jolivet and Lucet, 2019). None the less, evidence exists to show that *P. aeruginosa* can readily develop stable resistance to chlorhexidine with repeated exposure, and this has been confirmed in veterinary isolates as well as at the *in vitro* level (Thomas *et al.*, 2000; Beier *et al.*, 2015). The jury is still out regarding whether there is potential for cross-resistance to antibiotics, but the possibility cannot be excluded (Kampf, 2016).

8.3.7 Which is better, a circular or a back-and-forth skin preparation technique?

Historically, the circular or bulls-eye technique has been used in veterinary patients, whereby the scrub starts at the centre of the clipped area where the surgical incision will be located and then moves out in a circular motion towards the periphery (Rosewell, 2015; Reynolds and Nichols, 2019). In recent years, however, there has been a trend towards using a back-and-forth technique, which is the most common technique used in human medicine. With this approach, the scrub starts at the site of the proposed incision and works outwards but in a to-and-fro motion applying gentle pressure and friction; this is suggested to allow deeper cleaning through dermal layers than the single-direction concentric method (Stonecypher, 2009). A recent review of National Institute for Health and Care Excellence (NICE) guidelines in 2019 came to the non-committal conclusion that there is insufficient information available regarding evaluation of different methods of application of surgical scrub solutions in human healthcare to draw any firm conclusions, but that it is an area that warrants further study (NICE Guideline Updates Team, 2019). One veterinary study found no significant difference between the concentric and the back-and-forth techniques, but this study had only five patients in each group, so it can only be considered weak evidence and likely to have been statistically underpowered (Reynolds and Nichols, 2019). Until

Kathyrn Pratschke

such time as more specific objective data become available, there is no compelling evidence to support one technique over the other.

8.3.8 How many applications of antiseptic are required?

As with the technique for application, we lack objective randomized data to provide an evidence-based answer to this question. The review of NICE guidelines in 2019 concluded that there was no strong evidence to demonstrate an advantage of two applications of antiseptic compared with one, but of course this is based on information gained from surgical skin preparation in people and the same may not automatically be true for veterinary patients with their dense hair coats and different living environments and habits (NICE Guideline Updates Team, 2019). Veterinary studies from the 1990s and 2000s used up to three applications of antiseptic, but the standard approach nowadays is removal of all dirt and gross contamination through washing with either a non-medicated soap or antiseptic soap, followed by a single antiseptic application (Osuna *et al.*, 1990a, b; Belo *et al.*, 2018; Boucher *et al.*, 2018; Pelosi, 2018).

8.3.9 Quality control and monitoring of surgical preparation protocols

There is limited literature in the veterinary field regarding the clinical audit or monitoring of adherence to recommended guidelines in patient preparation for surgery. However, an observational study from 2013 that involved both first-opinion and referral practices suggested frequent poor compliance with many of the fundamental steps in patient preparation (Anderson *et al.*, 2013). These included non-sterile contact with the surgical site after the final skin preparation in 11% of observed cases, and less time and attention paid to adequate preparation in cats compared with dogs and in neutering operations than other types of surgery. There was also inadequate contact time with antiseptic skin preparation solutions in most of the patients and practices surveyed, with some allowing less than 30 s of contact time rather than the recommended 3 min minimum (Anderson *et al.*, 2013). This study also identified a surprising lack of awareness of what was considered current best practice for surgical preparation of the patient and surgeon, despite

this information being readily available in standard veterinary surgical textbooks.

If adherence to infection-control policies and quality of pre-surgical patient preparation are to be monitored or audited for compliance and quality, then regular monitoring is likely to be more accurate than occasional observation because the Hawthorne effect may lead to altered behaviour in some individuals if they are aware of observation (Anderson *et al.*, 2013; Rezk *et al.*, 2021).

8.4 Theatre Ventilation

Ventilation systems are crucial in operating theatres as they are the primary method of eliminating airborne pathogenic particles. During surgery, particles can arise from dust, textiles, skin scale shedding and respiratory aerosols from both the patient and the theatre team; many of these particles will be bacteria-carrying particles. The role of ventilation is to remove these particles, which may be loaded with viable microorganisms (Diab-Elschahawi *et al.*, 2011; Bischoff *et al.*, 2017; Gaines *et al.*, 2017).

The two most common types of ventilation system found in operating theatres are laminar airflow and conventional/turbulent airflow (Theodorou *et al.*, 2021). Laminar ventilation or airflow is sometimes also referred to as ultraclean airflow. It requires installation of either vertical or horizontal air filters that provide unidirectional, clean air via high-efficiency particulate airflow (HEPA) filters. In vertical laminar airflow, continuous filtered air is provided directly on to the operating table, giving a continuous column of air moving from the operative field outwards. Horizontal laminar airflow requires that filters are installed in one of the walls of the operating room, and airflow is then provided in a horizontal manner in the direction of the patient (Sadrizadeh *et al.*, 2021). Regardless of whether a vertical or horizontal system is used, airflow should move under positive pressure from the operative field to the periphery of the room in a one-way manner (Bischoff *et al.*, 2017; Sadrizadeh *et al.*, 2021; Theodorou *et al.*, 2021). Laminar airflow systems can have air changes up to 300 times h^{-1}, and should be capable of supplying air that contains fewer than ten colony-forming units (CFU) m^{-3} (Theodorou *et al.*, 2021). A minimum size of 320 × 320 cm is needed for the ceiling distribution system in a vertical laminar flow system, and anything smaller than this compromises the efficiency of the system (Diab-Elschahawi *et al.*, 2011). As horizontal systems can use either wall-mounted units or mobile units, similar figures are not available. Both vertical and horizontal systems can be affected – sometimes quite significantly – by the positions and movements of theatre staff, theatre lights and items of theatre equipment that might be in the path of the airflow (Diab-Elschahawi *et al.*, 2011; Sadrizadeh *et al.*, 2014, 2021; Gaines *et al.*, 2017; Kai *et al.*, 2019; Liu *et al.*, 2021). They are also impacted by the frequency of door opening during surgery.

Conventional or turbulent airflow ventilation uses a supply of clean air provided via either ceiling or wall diffusers to the operating room. Extraction is usually at floor level, via pressure-release dampers and also any gaps (e.g. doors, panels) (Theodorou *et al.*, 2021). These systems rely on positive pressure to move air out of the operating room, but there is no control over the direction of airflow and thus turbulent airflow results. Conventional/turbulent airflow systems largely rely on dilution of airborne contaminants and positive-pressure ventilation preventing the introduction of additional contaminants to the operating room, such as when doors are opened (Sadrizadeh *et al.*, 2021; Theodorou *et al.*, 2021). These systems are capable of up to 25 air changes h^{-1} with a minimum recommended number of 15 air changes h^{-1}. They typically supply air containing up to 180 CFU m^{-3}. The layout and size of the operating room and the location of inflow/outflow points can all impact the efficiency of these systems.

For many years, it was believed that a reduction in airborne contamination would translate into a reduced incidence and risk of SSIs (Diab-Elschahawi *et al.*, 2011; Bischoff *et al.*, 2017; Pelosi, 2018; Liu *et al.*, 2021; Lv *et al.*, 2021). One of the cornerstone studies underpinning the role of ultraclean ventilation in reducing airborne contamination and therefore SSI rate was carried out between 1974 and 1979 in the UK and Sweden, and focused on deep sepsis following joint surgery (Lidwell *et al.*, 1982). However, there are several issues with this study, including inconsistent use of body exhaust suits by operating staff, no randomization of patients, and the fact that the study did not control for important confounding factors such as administration of peri-operative antibiotics (only given in approximately 60% of patients). A study subsequently published in 2003 that assessed the impact of operating room ventilation *after* controlling for antibiotic prophylaxis in 22,170 hip replacements found no significant difference in SSI rates between laminar air flow and conventional air flow theatres (Engesaeter *et al.*, 2003). In recent years, several meta-analyses have also failed to find an advantage to laminar airflow compared with conventional mixing airflow systems (Diab-Elschahawi *et al.*, 2011; Pada and Perl, 2015; Bischoff *et al.*, 2017; Sadrizadeh *et al.*, 2021). Despite these uncertainties and conflicting research findings, both the NICE and the British Orthopaedic Association currently recommend that laminar airflow be used for orthopaedic procedures involving prostheses (Theodorou *et al.*, 2021). Evidence for the use of laminar airflow in general surgery in human healthcare settings is less robust, being based largely on retrospective studies rather than on RCTs, and there are no specific current recommendations available (Theodorou *et al.*, 2021).

Reducing the microbial bioburden in an operating theatre is a logical aim and will continue to be an important part of maintaining a suitable environment for aseptic surgery, while accepting that complete elimination of all bacteria from the operating room is not a realistic aim (Hoffman *et al.*, 2002; Gaines *et al.*, 2017; Dallolio *et al.*, 2018). However, increasing evidence suggests that this approach is insufficient on its own. It does not take account of the interaction between such factors as the number of bacteria-carrying particles, peri-operative antibiosis, peri-operative hypothermia, human microbial status and the patient's microbiome, all of which are of key importance in determining whether an SSI develops or not (Gaines *et al.*, 2017; Alverdy *et al.*, 2021). We also do not truly know whether the number of potential bacteria-carrying particles in an operating theatre is directly related to the incidence and risk of SSI. This has not been demonstrated comprehensively and we currently lack definitive evidence of a correlation between airborne bacterial counts and SSIs.

8.5 Operating Room Traffic and Personnel

It has been long believed that increased traffic through the theatre, frequent door openings during surgery, higher numbers of people present in the operating theatre and increased conversation during surgery are all risk factors for SSIs (Birgand *et al.*, 2014, 2015; Almond, 2017; de Oliveira and Sarmento Gama, 2017; Gaines *et al.*, 2017; Pelosi, 2018; Roesler *et al.*, 2018). The frequency of door opening in particular is often viewed as a surrogate marker for good infection control and adherence to good theatre etiquette (Al-Benna, 2012; Andersson *et al.*, 2012; Birgand *et al.*, 2014; Troughton *et al.*, 2019). Although there are several studies that describe a relationship between the number of door openings during surgery and increased airborne bioburden in operating theatres, there are also studies that contradict this finding and show no impact on airborne particulate count or bacteria-carrying particles. (Ritter *et al.*, 1975; Scaltriti *et al.*, 2007; Stocks *et al.*, 2010; Andersson *et al.*, 2012; Birgand *et al.*, 2015). On balance, it seems reasonable to conclude that increased frequency and number of door openings are likely to increase airborne dust and the numbers of particles and microbes (Scaltriti *et al.*, 2007; Andersson *et al.*, 2012; Pada and Perl, 2015), but exactly how this impacts either wound contamination or SSI rate is unknown at present (Birgand *et al.*, 2015). In a similar vein, although the available evidence supports people as a source of airborne contamination within a theatre, there is a lack of agreement in the literature regarding whether the number of personnel in an operating theatre has a direct impact on the risk of wound infection, with several studies documenting no effect on either SSI or general surgical complication rates (Ritter *et al.*, 1975; Birgand *et al.*, 2014; Sadrizadeh *et al.*, 2014; Montiel *et al.*, 2021).

8.6 Peri-operative Hypothermia and Forced-Air Warming Devices

It is perhaps worth highlighting at the start of this section that almost all the available information regarding peri-operative hypothermia and infection risks are based on studies performed on people in human healthcare settings. Whether it is entirely appropriate to directly extrapolate the findings and recommendations to veterinary patients in a veterinary healthcare setting is not clear. It seems reasonable to use the information to inform our decision making, while maintaining an open mind regarding the possibility that not all the facts as they apply to human patients will automatically apply to veterinary patients.

Hypothermia is generally described in the medical literature as being the point where the patient's body temperature drops 2°C below normal (Wood *et al.*, 2014; Baucom *et al.*, 2015; Bu *et al.*, 2019; de Simone *et al.*, 2020; Siddiqiui *et al.*, 2020). Body temperature under normal conditions is kept in a tightly regulated range through both heat genesis and thermal insulation (largely vaso-dilation and vasoconstriction) (de Simone *et al.*, 2020). The combination of surgery and anaesthesia challenges these normal physiological regulators of temperature, such that hypothermia is thought to occur in up to 70% of human patients (Burger and Fitzpatrick, 2009; Bu *et al.*, 2019). Several studies, including anaesthesiology and animal model studies, have suggested adverse effects from peri-operative hypothermia that include myocardial ischaemia, prolonged recovery, increased risk of bleeding, impaired immune responses, delayed wound healing and increased risk of SSIs (Sessler, 2008; Bu *et al.*, 2019; de Simone *et al.*, 2020; Hu *et al.*, 2020; Siddiqiui *et al.*, 2020). In 2009, the World Health Organization (WHO) published its *Guidelines for Safe Surgery* in which it specified 'maintenance of normothermia' as one of ten objectives formulated with the intention of reducing SSI risks. In recent years, however, several studies have been published, including systematic reviews and meta-analyses, that have not found any statistically significant link between peri-operative hypothermia and increased risk of infection (Baucom *et al.*, 2015; Bu *et al.*, 2019; de Simone *et al.*, 2020; Xu *et al.*, 2020). A consideration, discussed in some more recent studies, is that potential confounding factors that might increase risk of SSI have not been accounted for in earlier reports, such as patient body mass index, duration of anaesthesia, type of surgery, intraoperative blood loss, patient age and comorbidities (Baucom *et al.*, 2015; Madrid *et al.*, 2016; Xu *et al.*, 2020). Based on currently available evidence, it is reasonable to say that peri-operative normothermia is desirable from the point of view of minimizing physiological disruption, and may also help to reduce the risk of SSIs, but further strong objective evidence is desirable (Baucom *et al.*, 2015; Madrid *et al.*, 2016; de Simone *et al.*, 2020).

Forced-air warming (FAW) is the most common method in use for maintaining peri-operative patient temperatures, and such systems are in routine use in veterinary hospitals and practices. FAW systems transfer heat through air convection; the blower unit is typically connected via a rubber hose to a perforated air blanket (both single-use and reusable options are available). Concerns have been raised that FAW systems may increase the risk of wound infection through disruption of laminar air flow/clean air and also through direct contamination of operating room air (Albrecht *et al.*, 2011; Reed *et al.*, 2013; Wood *et al.*, 2014). An evaluation of filtration adequacy and operating room airborne contamination in one study found that 58% of the FAW blowers evaluated in one hospital internally generated and emitted airborne contaminants (Albrecht *et al.*, 2011). Microorganisms were identified on internal air path surfaces in 92.3% of the units tested; *S. aureus* was present in 13.5%, coagulase-negative staphylococci in 3.9% and methicillin-resistant *S. aureus* (MRSA) in 1.9% of FAW units. These investigators found that the 0.2 μm-rated intake filter provided as standard on some of the FAW units was inadequate for preventing microbial build-up and emissions; they advocated a more stringent filter system be used. Another recent study using 23 Bair Hugger Model 750 units in daily clinical use in a hospital identified a filtration efficiency of only 63.8% on average. All machines had microorganisms on internal air paths beyond the filter, and of the 23 machines, 74% grew coagulase-negative staphylococci and 26% had moulds (Reed *et al.*, 2013). However, what has not been documented is whether contamination of FAW units, or even increased contamination of operating room air linked to these units, translates to an increased risk of SSIs. Based on currently available evidence, there is no reason to avoid using FAW units during surgery, and the physiological benefits of maintaining normothermia are significant (Baucom *et al.*, 2015; Madrid *et al.*, 2016; Bu *et al.*, 2019; de Simone *et al.*, 2020; Siddiqiui *et al.*, 2020). That said, in the event of an increased rate of SSIs or an outbreak of infections within surgical patients in a hospital, FAW units are one of the potential culprits that should be evaluated in any review.

8.7 Mobile Phones, Tablets and Computers as a Source of Contamination in Operating Rooms

The use of smartphones, tablets and personal computers has become commonplace in healthcare settings, to the extent that many people would be nonplussed if asked not to bring their phones with them into the operating theatre. Smartphones and tablets connected to the internet can be used for information retrieval to facilitate teaching and support patient care, smartphones and tablets with cameras can be used to obtain images necessary for patient records and for teaching purposes, they can be used to access clinical record keeping systems, and they can be used as a method of communication between staff in different areas of the hospital. Although a decade ago many people would not have routinely carried a portable computing device with them into theatre, now it is standard behaviour but without giving due consideration to where else these personal computing devices have travelled and the contamination they may have accrued in the process. Several studies published in recent years confirm significant levels of contamination of smartphones, touch screens and laptop keyboards (Chang *et al.*, 2017; Koscova *et al.*, 2018; Monga *et al.*, 2018; Ide *et al.*, 2019; Qureshi *et al.*, 2020; Qadi *et al.*, 2021). Contamination rates of up to 93% were recorded in one study of mobile phones carried into orthopaedic operating theatres in a human hospital, with contaminants including coagulase-negative staphylococci and *Micrococcus* and *Bacillus* spp. (Qureshi *et al.*, 2020). Another study found a 92% contamination rate, involving coagulase-negative staphylococci, *S. aureus*, bacilli and enteric bacteria (Koscova *et al.*, 2018). In a similar vein, a number of studies have evaluated keyboard contamination on laptops, finding contamination rates of 24–100%, with a range of bacteria isolated including MRSA, vancomycin-resistant enterococci, *Escherichia coli* and *Clostridioides difficile* (Koscova *et al.*, 2018; Ide *et al.*, 2019).

Cleaning mobile phones, tablets and laptop keyboards with simple antibacterial wipes, such as chlorhexidine gluconate wipes, can reduce the bacterial load. Theatre staff, surgeons and anaesthetists should be encouraged to disinfect mobile phones and tablets on a regular basis to reduce the risk of introducing contamination (Koscova *et al.*, 2018). A recent meta-analysis suggested that there may be a link between contamination of items such as mobile phones and patient infection rates, but it is not certain based on current evidence whether this is simple association or true causation (Ide *et al.*, 2019). None the less, if taking a first-principles approach to infection control, decontamination of items such as phones, tablets and laptops is logical as part of an overall infection control policy.

References

Akobeng, A.K. (2005) Understanding randomised controlled trials. *Archives of Disease in Childhood* 90(8), 840–844. DOI: 10.1136/adc.2004.058222.

Al-Benna, S. (2012) Infection control in operating theatres. *Journal of Perioperative Practice* 22(10), 318–322. DOI: 10.1177/175045891602201002.

Albrecht, M., Gauthier, R.L., Belani, K., Litchy, M. and Leaper, D. (2011) Forced-air warming blowers: an evaluation of filtration adequacy and airborne contamination emissions in the operating room. *American Journal of Infection Control* 39(4), 321–328. DOI: 10.1016/j.ajic.2010.06.011.

Almond, S. (2017) Theatre, the ideal design and the nurse's role in maintenance and hygiene. *Veterinary Nursing Journal* 32(7), 188–190. DOI: 10.1080/17415349.2017.1309308.

Alverdy, J.C., Hyman, N. and Gilbert, J. (2021) Re-examining causes of surgical site infections following elective surgery in the era of asepsis. *Lancet Infectious Diseases* 20(3), e38–e43. DOI: 10.1016/S1473-3099(19)30756-X.

Anderson, M.E.C., Foster, B.A. and Weese, J.S. (2013) Observational study of patient and surgeon preoperative preparation in ten companion animal clinics in Ontario, Canada. *BMC Veterinary Research* 9, 194. DOI: 10.1186/1746-6148-9-194.

Andersson, A.E., Bergh, I., Karlsson, J., Eriksson, B.I. and Nilsson, K. (2012) Traffic flow in the operating room: an explorative and descriptive study on air quality during orthopedic trauma implant surgery. *American Journal of Infection Control* 40(8), 750–755. DOI: 10.1016/j.ajic.2011.09.015.

Andrade, N., Schmiedt, C.W., Cornell, K., Radlinsky, M.G., Heidingsfelder, L. *et al.* (2016) Survey of intraoperative bacterial contamination in dogs undergoing elective orthopedic surgery. *Veterinary Surgery* 45(2), 214–222. DOI: 10.1111/vsu.12438.

Baucom, R.B., Phillips, S.E., Ehrenfeld, J.M., Muldoon, R.L., Poulose, B.K. *et al.* (2015) Association of perioperative hypothermia during colectomy with surgical site infection. *JAMA Surgery* 150(6), 570–575. DOI: 10.1001/jamasurg.2015.77.

Beier, R.C., Foley, S.L., Davidson, M.K., White, D.G., McDermott, P.F. *et al.* (2015) Characterization of antibiotic and disinfectant susceptibility profiles among *Pseudomonas aeruginosa* veterinary isolates recovered during 1994-2003. *Journal of Applied Microbiology* 118(2), 326–342. DOI: 10.1111/jam.12707.

Belo, L., Serrano, I., Cunha, E., Carneiro, C., Tavares, L. *et al.* (2018) Skin asepsis protocols as a preventive measure of surgical site infections in dogs: chlorhexidine-alcohol versus povidone-iodine. *BMC Veterinary Research* 14(1), 95. DOI: 10.1186/s12917-018-1368-5.

Berkelman, R.L., Holland, B.W. and Anderson, R.L. (1982) Increased bactericidal activity of dilute preparations of povidone-iodine solutions. *Journal of Clinical Microbiology* 15(4), 635–639. DOI: 10.1128/jcm.15.4.635-639.1982.

Birgand, G., Azevedo, C., Toupet, G., Pissard-Gibollet, R., Grandbastien, B. *et al.* (2014) Attitudes, risk of infection and behaviours in the operating room (the ARIBO Project): a prospective, cross-sectional study. *British Medical Journal Open* 4(1), e004274. DOI: 10.1136/bmjopen-2013-004274.

Birgand, G., Toupet, G., Rukly, S., Antoniotti, G., Deschamps, M.-N. *et al.* (2015) Air contamination for predicting wound contamination in clean surgery: a large multicenter study. *American Journal of Infection Control* 43(5), 516–521. DOI: 10.1016/j.ajic.2015.01.026.

Birgand, G., Haudebourg, T., Grammatico-Guillon, L., Ferrand, L., Moret, L. *et al.* (2019) Improvement in staff behavior during surgical procedures to prevent post-operative complications (ARIBO[2]): study protocol for a cluster randomised trial. *Trials* 20(1), 275. DOI: 10.1186/s13063-019-3370-z.

Bischoff, P., Kubilay, N.Z., Allegranzi, B., Egger, M. and Gastmeier, P. (2017) Effect of laminar airflow ventilation on surgical site infections: a systematic review and meta-analysis. *Lancet Infectious Diseases* 17(5), 553–561. DOI: 10.1016/S1473-3099(17)30059-2.

Boothe, D.M. and Boothe, H.W. (2015) Antimicrobial considerations in the perioperative patient. *Veterinary Clinics of North America – Small Animal Practice* 45(3), 585–608. DOI: 10.1016/j.cvsm.2015.01.006.

Boucher, C., Henton, M.M., Becker, P.J., Kirberger, R.M. and Hartman, M.J. (2018) Comparative efficacy of three antiseptics as surgical skin preparations in dogs. *Veterinary Surgery* 47(6), 792–801. DOI: 10.1111/vsu.12913.

Brown, D.C., Conzemius, M.G., Shofer, F. and Swann, H. (1997) Epidemiologic evaluation of postoperative wound infections in dogs and cats. *Journal of the American Veterinary Medical Association* 210(9), 1302–1306.

Bu, N., Zhao, E., Gao, Y., Zhao, S., Bo, W. *et al.* (2019) Association between perioperative hypothermia and surgical site infection: a meta-analysis. *Medicine* 98(6), e14392. DOI: 10.1097/MD.0000000000014392.

Burger, L. and Fitzpatrick, J. (2009) Prevention of inadvertent perioperative hypothermia. *British Journal of Nursing* 18, 1114–1119. DOI: 10.12968/bjon.2009.18.18.44553.

Chang, C.H., Chen, S.Y., Lu, J.J., Chang, C.J., Chang, Y. *et al.* (2017) Nasal colonization and bacterial contamination of mobile phones carried by medical staff in the operating room. *PloS One* 12(5), e0175811. DOI: 10.1371/journal.pone.0175811.

Charles, D., Heal, C.F., Delpachitra, M., Wohlfahrt, M. and Kimber, D. (2017) Alcoholic versus aqueous chlorhexidine for skin antisepsis: the AVALANCHE trial. *Canadian Medical Association Journal* 189, E1008–E1016. DOI: 10.1503/cmaj.161460.

Chen, S., Chen, J.W., Guo, B. and Xu, C.C. (2020) Preoperative antisepsis with chlorhexidine versus povidone-iodine for the prevention of surgical site infection: a systematic review and meta-analysis. *World Journal of Surgery* 44(5), 1412–1424. DOI: 10.1007/s00268-020-05384-7.

Clayton, K., Vallejo, A.F., Davies, J., Sirvent, S. and Polak, M.E. (2017) Langerhans cells-programmed by the epidermis. *Frontiers in Immunology* 8, 1676. DOI: 10.3389/fimmu.2017.01676.

Dallolio, L., Raggi, A., Sanna, T., Mazzetti, M., Orsi, A. *et al.* (2018) Surveillance of environmental and procedural measures of infection control in the operating theatre setting. *International Journal of Environmental Research and Public Health* 15(1), 46. DOI: 10.3390/ijerph15010046.

Darouiche, R.O., Wall, M.J., Itani, K.M.F., Otterson, M.F. and Webb, A.L. (2010) Chlorhexidine-alcohol versus povidone-iodine for surgical-site antisepsis. *New England Journal of Medicine* 362(1), 18–26. DOI: 10.1056/NEJMoa0810988.

de Oliveira, A.C. and Sarmento Gama, C. (2017) Surgical site infection prevention: an analysis of compliance with good practice in a teaching hospital. *Journal of Infection Prevention* 18(6), 301–306. DOI: 10.1177/1757177417703190.

de Simone, B., Sartelli, M., Coccolini, F., Ball, C.G., Brambillasca, P. *et al.* (2020) Intraoperative surgical site infection control and prevention: a position paper and future addendum to WSES intra-abdominal infections guidelines. *World Journal of Emergency Surgery* 15(1), 10. DOI: 10.1186/s13017-020-0288-4.

Diab-Elschahawi, M., Berger, J., Blacky, A., Kimberger, O., Oguz, R. *et al.* (2011) Impact of different-sized laminar air flow versus no laminar air flow on bacterial counts in the operating room during orthopedic surgery. *American Journal of Infection Control* 39(7), e25–9. DOI: 10.1016/j.ajic.2010.10.035.

Dumville, J.C., McFarlane, E., Edwards, P., Lipp, A., Holmes, A. *et al.* (2015) Preoperative skin antiseptics for preventing surgical wound infections after clean surgery. *Cochrane Database of Systematic Reviews* 2015(4), CD003949. DOI: 10.1002/14651858. CD003949.pub4.

Durani, P. and Leaper, D. (2008) Povidone-iodine: use in hand disinfection, skin preparation and antiseptic irrigation. *International Wound Journal* 5(3), 376–387. DOI: 10.1111/j.1742-481X.2007.00405.x.

Edmiston, C.E. and Leaper, D. (2017) Should preoperative showering or cleansing with chlorhexidine gluconate (CHG) be part of the surgical care bundle to prevent surgical site infection? *Journal of Infection Prevention* 18(6), 311–314. DOI: 10.1177/1757177417714873.

Engesaeter, L.B., Lie, S.A., Espehaug, B., Furnes, O., Vollset, S.E. *et al.* (2003) Antibiotic prophylaxis in total hip arthroplasty: effects of antibiotic prophylaxis systemically and in bone cement on the revision rate of 22,170 primary hip replacements followed 0-14 years in the Norwegian Arthroplasty Register. *Acta Orthopaedica Scandinavica* 74(6), 644–651. DOI: 10.1080/00016470310018135.

Epstein, N.E. (2021) Perspective on ocular toxicity of presurgical skin preparations utilizing chlorhexidine gluconate/hibiclens/chloraprep. *Surgical Neurology International* 12, 335. DOI: 10.25259/SNI_566_2021.

Evans, D. (2003) Hierarchy of evidence: a framework for ranking evidence evaluating healthcare interventions. *Journal of Clinical Nursing* 12(1), 77–84. DOI: 10.1046/j.1365-2702.2003.00662.x.

Gaines, S., Luo, J.N., Gilbert, J., Zaborina, O. and Alverdy, J.C. (2017) Optimum operating room environment for the prevention of surgical site infections. *Surgical Infections* 18(4), 503–507. DOI: 10.1089/sur.2017.020.

Graling, P.R. and Vasaly, F.W. (2013) Effectiveness of 2% CHG cloth bathing for reducing surgical site infections. *Association Perioperative Registered Nurses Journal* 97(5), 547–551. DOI: 10.1016/j.aorn.2013.02.009.

Grönthal, T., Eklund, M., Thomson, K., Piiparinen, H., Sironen, T. *et al.* (2017) Antimicrobial resistance in *Staphylococcus pseudintermedius* and the molecular epidemiology of methicillin-resistant *S. pseudintermedius* in small animals in Finland. *Journal of Antimicrobial Chemotherapy* 72(7), 1021–1030. DOI: 10.1093/jac/dkx086.

Hayes, G., Singh, A., Gibson, T., Moens, N., Oblak, M. *et al.* (2017) Influence of orthopedic reinforced gloves versus double standard gloves on contamination events during small animal orthopedic surgery. *Veterinary Surgery* 46(7), 981–985. DOI: 10.1111/vsu.12688.

Hoffman, P.N., Williams, J., Stacey, A., Bennett, A.M., Ridgway, G.L. *et al.* (2002) Microbiological commissioning and monitoring of operating theatre suites. *Journal of Hospital Infection* 52(1), 1–28. DOI: 10.1053/jhin.2002.1237.

Huang, S.S., Septimus, E., Kleinman, K., Moody, J., Hickok, J. *et al.* (2019) Chlorhexidine versus routine bathing to prevent multidrug-resistant organisms and all-cause bloodstream infections in general medical and surgical units (ABATE Infection trial): a cluster-randomised trial. *Lancet* 393(10177), 1205–1215. DOI: 10.1016/S0140-6736(18)32593-5.

Hu, Q., Zhao, Y., Sun, B., Qi, W. and Shi, P. (2020) Surgical site infection following operative treatment of open fracture: incidence and prognostic risk factors. *International Wound Journal* 17(3), 708–715. DOI: 10.1111/iwj.13330.

Ide, N., Frogner, B.K., LeRouge, C.M., Vigil, P. and Thompson, M. (2019) What's on your keyboard? A systematic review of the contamination of peripheral computer devices in healthcare settings. *BMJ Open* 9(3), e026437. DOI: 10.1136/bmjopen-2018-026437.

Jolivet, S. and Lucet, J.C. (2019) Surgical field and skin preparation. *Orthopaedics & Traumatology, Surgery & Research* 105(1S), S1–S6. DOI: 10.1016/j.otsr.2018.04.033.

Kai, T., Ayagaki, N. and Setoguchi, H. (2019) Influence of the arrangement of surgical light axes on the air environment in operating rooms. *Journal of Healthcare Engineering* 2019, 4861273. DOI: 10.1155/2019/4861273.

Kampf, G. (2016) Acquired resistance to chlorhexidine - is it time to establish an "antiseptic stewardship" initiative? *Journal of Hospital Infection* 94(3), 213–227. DOI: 10.1016/j.jhin.2016.08.018.

Koscova, J., Hurnikova, Z. and Pistl, J. (2018) Degree of bacterial contamination of mobile phone and computer keyboard surfaces and efficacy of disinfection with chlorhexidine digluconate and triclosan to its reduction. *International Journal of Environmental Research and Public Health* 15(10), 2238. DOI: 10.3390/ijerph15102238.

Lidwell, O.M., Lowbury, E.J., Whyte, W., Blowers, R., Stanley, S.J. *et al*. (1982) Effect of ultraclean air in operating rooms on deep sepsis in the joint after total hip or knee replacement: a randomised study. *British Medical Journal* 285(6334), 10–14. DOI: 10.1136/bmj.285.6334.10.

Liu, Z., Liu, H., Yin, H., Rong, R., Cao, G. *et al*. (2021) Prevention of surgical site infection under different ventilation systems in operating room environment. *Frontiers of Environmental Science & Engineering* 15(3), 36. DOI: 10.1007/s11783-020-1327-9.

Lucero, S. and Dryden, M. (2019) Antisepsis, asepsis and skin preparation. *Surgery* 37(1), 45–50. DOI: 10.1016/j.mpsur.2018.11.008.

Lv, Q., Lu, Y., Wang, H., Li, X., Zhang, W. *et al*. (2021) The possible effect of different types of ventilation on reducing operation theatre infections: a meta-analysis. *Annals of the Royal College of Surgeons of England* 103(3), 145–150. DOI: 10.1308/rcsann.2020.7021.

Madrid, E., Urrútia, G., Roqué i Figuls, M., Pardo-Hernandez, H., Campos, J.M. *et al*. (2016) Active body surface warming systems for preventing complications caused by inadvertent perioperative hypothermia in adults. *Cochrane Database of Systematic Reviews* 4(4), CD009016. DOI: 10.1002/14651858. CD009016.pub2.

Makhni, M.C., Jegede, K., Lombardi, J., Whittier, S., Gorroochurn, P. *et al*. (2018) No clear benefit of chlorhexidine use at home before surgical preparation. *Journal of the American Academy of Orthopaedic Surgeons* 26(2), e39–e47. DOI: 10.5435/JAAOS-D-16-00866.

Mayhew, P.D., Freeman, L., Kwan, T. and Brown, D.C. (2012) Comparison of surgical site infection rates in clean and clean-contaminated wounds in dogs and cats after minimally invasive versus open surgery: 179 cases (2007-2008). *Journal of the American Veterinary Medical Association* 240(2), 193–198. DOI: 10.2460/javma.240.2.193.

Melekwe, G.O., Uwagie-Ero, E.A., Zoaka, H.A. and Odigie, E.A. (2018) Comparative clinical effectiveness of preoperative skin antiseptic preparations of chlorhexidine gluconate and povidone iodine for preventing surgical site infections in dogs. *International Journal of Veterinary Science and Medicine* 6(1), 113–116. DOI: 10.1016/j.ijvsm.2018.03.005.

Monga, A., Gupta, B. and Thanveer, K. (2018) Risk of microbial contamination of laptop keyboard in clinical area of dental settings. An *in vitro* study. *Journal of Dental and Medical Sciences* 17, 64–68.

Montiel, V., Pérez-Prieto, D., Perelli, S. and Monllau, J.C. (2021) Fellows and observers are not a problem for infection in the operating rooms of teaching centers. *Tropical Medicine and Infectious Disease* 6(2), 43. DOI: 10.3390/tropicalmed6020043.

Murad, M.H., Asi, N., Alsawas, M. and Alahdab, F. (2016) New evidence pyramid. *Evidence-Based Medicine* 21(4), 125–127. DOI: 10.1136/ebmed-2016-110401.

NICE Guideline Updates Team (2019) *Surgical Infection: Prevention and Treatment. Evidence Review for the Effectiveness of Skin in the Prevention of Surgical Site Infection*. NICE guideline NG125. National Institute for Health and Care Excellence, London.

Nikolić, N., Kienzl, P., Tajpara, P., Vierhapper, M., Matiasek, J. *et al*. (2019) The antiseptic octenidine inhibits langerhans cell activation and modulates cytokine expression upon superficial wounding with tape stripping. *Journal of Immunology Research* 2019, 5143635. DOI: 10.1155/2019/5143635.

Osuna, D.J., DeYoung, D.J. and Walker, R.L. (1990a) Comparison of three skin preparation techniques in the dog part 1: experimental trial. *Veterinary Surgery* 19(1), 14–19. DOI: 10.1111/j.1532-950x.1990.tb01136.x.

Osuna, D.J., DeYoung, D.J. and Walker, R.L. (1990b) Comparison of three skin preparation techniques part 2: clinical trial in 100 dogs. *Veterinary Surgery* 19(1), 20–23. DOI: 10.1111/j.1532-950x.1990.tb01137.x.

Osuna, D.J., DeYoung, D.J. and Walker, R.L. (1992) Comparison of an antimicrobial adhesive drape and povidone-iodine preoperative skin preparation in dogs. *Veterinary Surgery* 21(6), 458–462. DOI: 10.1111/j.1532-950x.1992.tb00081.x.

Pada, S. and Perl, T.M. (2015) Operating room myths: what is the evidence for common practices. *Current Opinion in Infectious Diseases* 28(4), 369–374. DOI: 10.1097/QCO.0000000000000177.

Pelosi, A. (2018) The operating room. In: Johnston, S.A. and Tobias, K.M. (eds) *Veterinary Surgery: Small Animal*, 2nd edn. Elsevier, St Louis, Missouri, pp. 177–192.

Preston Stubbs, W., Bellah, J.R., Vermaas-Hekman, D., Purich, B. and Kubilis, P.S. (1996) Chlorhexidine gluconate versus chloroxylenol for preoperative skin preparation in dogs. *Veterinary Surgery* 25(6), 487–494. DOI: 10.1111/j.1532-950x.1996.tb01448.x.

Qadi, M., Khayyat, R., AlHajhamad, M.A., Naji, Y.I. and Maraqa, B. (2021) Microbes on the mobile phones of healthcare workers in Palestine: identification, characterization, and comparison. *Canadian Journal of Infectious Diseases and Medical Microbiology* 2021, 8845879. DOI: 10.1155/2021/8845879.

Qureshi, N.Q., Mufarrih, S.H., Irfan, S., Rashid, R.H., Zubairi, A.J. *et al.* (2020) Mobile phones in the orthopedic operating room: microbial colonization and antimicrobial resistance. *World Journal of Orthopedics* 11(5), 252–264. DOI: 10.5312/wjo.v11.i5.252.

Reed, M., Kimberger, O., McGovern, P.D. and Albrecht, M.C. (2013) Forced-air warming design: evaluation of intake filtration, internal microbial buildup, and airborne-contamination emissions. *American Association of Nurse Anesthiosology Journal* 81(4), 275–280.

Reichman, D.E. and Greenberg, J.A. (2009) Reducing surgical site infections: a review. *Reviews in Obstetrics & Gynecology* 2(4), 212–221.

Reynolds, H. and Nichols, A. (2019) Which skin preparation technique is most effective to minimise bacterial contamination? *Veterinary Nurse* 10(3), 162–166. DOI: 10.12968/vetn.2019.10.3.162.

Rezk, F., Stenmarker, M., Acosta, S., Johansson, K., Bengnér, M. *et al.* (2021) Healthcare professionals' experiences of being observed regarding hygiene routines: the Hawthorne effect in vascular surgery. *BMC Infectious Diseases* 21(1), 420. DOI: 10.1186/s12879-021-06097-5.

Ritter, M.A., Eitzen, H., French, M.L.V. and Hart, J.B. (1975) The operating room environment as affected by people and the surgical face mask. *Clinical Orthopaedics and Related Research* 111, 147–150. DOI: 10.1097/00003086-197509000-00020.

Roesler, R., Halowell, C.C., Elias, G. and Peters, J. (2018) Chasing zero: our journey. *Association of Perioperative Registered Nurses Journal* 91, 224–235.

Rosewell, L. (2015) Contamination control : part 1 – preventing surgical site infections. *Veterinary Times* 15, 22–24.

Sadrizadeh, S., Tammelin, A., Ekolind, P. and Holmberg, S. (2014) Influence of staff number and internal constellation on surgical site infection in an operating room. *Particuology* 13, 42–51. DOI: 10.1016/j.partic.2013.10.006.

Sadrizadeh, S., Aganovic, A., Bogdan, A., Wang, C., Afshari, A. *et al.* (2021) A systematic review of operating room ventilation. *Journal of Building Engineering* 40, 102693. DOI: 10.1016/j.jobe.2021.102693.

Scaltriti, S., Cencetti, S., Rovesti, S., Marchesi, I., Bargellini, A. *et al.* (2007) Risk factors for particulate and microbial contamination of air in operating theatres. *Journal of Hospital Infection* 66(4), 320–326. DOI: 10.1016/j.jhin.2007.05.019.

Sessler, D.I. (2008) Temperature monitoring and perioperative thermoregulation. *Anesthesiology* 109(2), 318–338. DOI: 10.1097/ALN.0b013e31817f6d76.

Siddiqiui, T., Pal, K.M.I., Shaukat, F., Mubashir, H., Akbar Ali, A. *et al.* (2020) Association between perioperative hypothermia and surgical site infection after elective abdominal surgery: a prospective cohort study. *Cureus* 12(10), e11145. DOI: 10.7759/cureus.11145.

Silberberg-Sinakin, I. and Thorbecke, G.J. (1980) Contact hypersensitivity and langerhans cells. *Journal of Investigative Dermatology* 75(1), 61–67. DOI: 10.1111/1523-1747.ep12521144.

Singh, A., Walker, M., Rousseau, J. and Weese, J.S. (2013) Characterization of the biofilm forming ability of *Staphylococcus pseudintermedius* from dogs. *BMC Veterinary Research* 9, 93. DOI: 10.1186/1746-6148-9-93.

Singh, S. and Blakley, B. (2018) Systematic review of ototoxic pre-surgical antiseptic preparations - what is the evidence? *Journal of Otolaryngology – Head and Neck Surgery* 47(1), 18. DOI: 10.1186/s40463-018-0265-z.

Small, C., Beatty, N. and El Helou, G. (2021) *Staphylococcus pseudintermedius* bacteremia in a lung transplant recipient exposed to domestic pets. *Cureus* 13(5), e14895. DOI: 10.7759/cureus.14895.

Somayaji, R., Priyantha, M.A.R., Rubin, J.E. and Church, D. (2016) Human infections due to *Staphylococcus pseudintermedius*, an emerging zoonosis of canine origin: report of 24 cases. *Diagnostic Microbiology and Infectious Disease* 85(4), 471–476. DOI: 10.1016/j.diagmicrobio.2016.05.008.

Stine, S.L., Odum, S.M. and Mertens, W.D. (2018) Protocol changes to reduce implant-associated infection rate after tibial plateau leveling osteotomy: 703 dogs, 811 TPLO (2006-2014). *Veterinary Surgery* 47(4), 481–489. DOI: 10.1111/vsu.12796.

Stocks, G.W., Self, S.D., Thompson, B., Adame, X.A. and O'Connor, D.P. (2010) Predicting bacterial populations based on airborne particulates: a study performed in nonlaminar flow operating rooms during joint arthroplasty surgery. *American Journal of Infection Control* 38(3), 199–204. DOI: 10.1016/j.ajic.2009.07.006.

Stonecypher, K. (2009) Going around in circles: is this the best practice for preparing the skin? *Critical Care Nursing Quarterly* 32(2), 94–98. DOI: 10.1097/CNQ.0b013e3181a27b86.

Tanner, J. and Melen, K. (2021) Preoperative hair removal to reduce surgical site infection. *Cochrane Database of Systematic Reviews* 8(8), CD004122. DOI: 10.1002/14651858.CD004122.pub5.

Theodorou, C., Simpson, G.S. and Walsh, C.J. (2021) Theatre ventilation. *Annals of the Royal College of Surgeons of England* 103(3), 151–154. DOI: 10.1308/rcsann.2020.7146.

Thomas, L., Maillard, J.Y., Lambert, R.J.W. and Russell, A.D. (2000) Development of resistance to chlorhexidine diacetate in *Pseudomonas aeruginosa* and the effect of a "residual" concentration. *Journal of Hospital Infection* 46(4), 297–303. DOI: 10.1053/jhin.2000.0851.

Troughton, R., Mariano, V., Campbell, A., Hettiaratchy, S., Holmes, A. *et al*. (2019) Understanding determinants of infection control practices in surgery: the role of shared ownership and team hierarchy. *Antimicrobial Resistance and Infection Control* 8, 116. DOI: 10.1186/s13756-019-0565-8.

Webster, J. and Osborne, S. (2015) Preoperative bathing or showering with skin antiseptics to prevent surgical site infection. *Cochrane Database of Systematic Reviews* 2(2), CD004985. DOI: 10.1002/14651858.CD004985.pub5.

Wood, A.M., Moss, C., Keenan, A., Reed, M.R. and Leaper, D.J. (2014) Infection control hazards associated with the use of forced-air warming in operating theatres. *Journal of Hospital Infection* 88(3), 132–140. DOI: 10.1016/j.jhin.2014.07.010.

Xu, H., Wang, Z., Guan, X., Lu, Y., Malone, D.C. *et al*. (2020) Safety of intraoperative hypothermia for patients: meta-analyses of randomized controlled trials and observational studies. *BMC Anesthesiology* 20(1), 202. DOI: 10.1186/s12871-020-01065-z.

9 Monitoring and Prevention of Surgical-Site Infections

DENIS VERWILGHEN[1] AND KELLY L. BOWLT BLACKLOCK[2]*

[1]University of Sydney, Camperdown, NSW 2006, Australia; [2]Royal (Dick) School of Veterinary Studies, University of Edinburgh, Roslin, UK

9.1 Introduction

Despite (and sometimes because of) advances in surgery, surgical-site infections (SSIs) remain a burden of surgery and continue to have a major impact on healthcare costs due to additional treatment, antibiotics, hospital stay and mortality (Ahern *et al.*, 2010). While a 0% SSI rate goal is probably unachievable, the toll that infections are taking on the success rates of surgical procedures remains unacceptably high, and current SSI rates can undoubtedly be reduced further.

Ever since the development of germ theory, it has become clear that 'instead of fighting bacteria in wounds, it is likely better not to introduce them'. In the wake of this statement by Pasteur, surgeons such as Koch, Lister and Halsted developed the principles of antisepsis and later asepsis (Table 9.1), elements that have had an enormous impact on patient survival and surgical success rates. With the waning effectiveness of our antibiotic arsenal, the adoption and adherence to simple and cost-effective methods of aseptic techniques are the key components of SSI prevention.

9.2 What Are SSIs? Definition and Classification

Recognition and surveillance of SSIs are key elements for their treatment and prevention. Proper identification and monitoring is best performed by direct visual inspection of the wound by someone who understands and applies a standardized definition of an SSI (Mannien *et al.*, 2006). In the absence of veterinary-specific definitions, those reported in the US Centers for Disease Control and Prevention

(CDC) documents on SSI definitions (CDC, 2022) and the European CDC *Surveillance of Surgical Site Infections in European Hospitals – HAISSI protocol* (ECDC, 2012) can be used. The definitions below have been adapted from these two documents to be useful in veterinary settings, as some of the standard human criteria are not applicable to veterinary medicine. A group of human and veterinary experts are currently revising these definitions to be most suitable for use in our field via a Delphi consensus process. Updates to these should be available in the coming year in veterinary surgical literature.

9.2.1 Procedural definitions

Surgical procedure

This is defined as a procedure that takes place during an operation in which at least one incision is made through the skin or mucous membrane, or where there is reoperation via an incision that was left open during a previous operative procedure. Surgical procedures can be divided into four categories:

- *Elective surgery.* This is performed by choice and can be scheduled because it does not involve a life-threatening medical emergency.
- *Semi-elective surgery.* This is medically indicated to preserve the patient's life but can be scheduled and does not need to be performed immediately.
- *Urgent surgery.* This is where medical stabilization of the patient is warranted prior to the intervention, which must be performed within 24–48 h to preserve the patient's life.
- *Emergency surgery.* This must be performed without delay to preserve the patient's life.

---

*Corresponding author: Kelly.blacklock@ed.ac.uk

DOI: 10.1079/9781789244977.0009

Table 9.1. Antisepsis versus asepsis.

Antisepsis	Asepsis
The process of destroying germs. Introduced by Lister, the method of antisepsis was meant to fight infection when already present.	Working germ free. Further introduced after the discovery of the germ theory of disease, the method of asepsis focuses on preventing the occurrence of sepsis rather than fighting it. Aseptic technique includes the use of antiseptics to destroy germs.
TREATMENT	PREVENTION

Duration of the anaesthetic procedure

This is the interval in minutes and hours between the time of induction of the patient until full conscious recovery is obtained.

- *General anaesthesia.* This involves the administration of drugs that enter the general circulation and affect the central nervous system to render the patient pain free, amnesic, unconscious and often paralysed with relaxed muscles.
- *Anaesthetic time.* This is the time between induction of the anaesthetic state and the end of the procedure.
- *Preparation time.* This is the time between induction of the anaesthetic state and the start of the surgical procedure. This time includes the time for full preparation of the surgical field and surgical team, including draping.
- *Recovery time.* This is the time between the end of the procedure and the full recovery of consciousness (end of anaesthetic time) of the patient.

Duration of the surgical procedure

This is the interval between the procedure/surgery start time and the procedure/surgery finish time. (Donham *et al.*, 1996):

- *Procedure start time.* This is defined as the time when a procedure is begun (e.g. incision is made for a surgical procedure).
- *Procedure finish time.* This is recorded as the time when all instruments, sharps and sponge counts are completed and verified as correct, all post-operative radiological studies to be done in the operating room are completed, all dressings and drains are secured, and the surgeons have completed all procedural activities on the patient.

9.2.2 Wound definitions

The following types of wounds can be distinguished:

- *Surgical wound.* This is a wound or wounds created by the surgical intervention that were not present on the patient before the procedure.
- *Trauma.* This is a blunt or penetrating injury that occurs prior to the start of the surgical procedure.
- *Wound class.* This is an assessment of the degree of contamination of the surgical wound related to the primary principal procedure being performed at the time of the operation (Table 9.2).
- *Wound contamination and wound closure.* These definitions are given in Tables 9.3 and 9.4, respectively.

9.2.3 Infection definitions

The use of standard and consistent wound infection definitions is critical for proper identification of SSIs, for comparing rates over time and for consistent overall surveillance. Current definitions based on depth of infection and/or the involved structures are reported in Tables 9.5 and 9.6. Additional important definitions include:

- *SSI date of event.* This is the date when the first element used to meet the criteria of an SSI occurs for the first time during the surveillance period.
- *SSI appearance interval.* This is the number of days between the date of the procedure (defined as day 1) and the SSI date of event.

9.3 Epidemiology of SSIs

Epidemiological studies provide important information concerning groups, factors and procedures that are most associated with the risk of SSI. Understanding risk factors can help identify

Table 9.2. Wound class definitions.

Wound class	Definition
Clean	An uninfected operative wound in which no inflammation is encountered and the respiratory, alimentary, genital or uninfected urinary tract is not entered. In addition, clean wounds are primarily closed and, if necessary, drained with closed (active suction) drainage. Operative incisional wounds that follow non-penetrating (blunt) trauma should be included in this category if they meet the criteria.
Clean-contaminated	An operative wound in which the respiratory, alimentary, genital or urinary tracts are entered under controlled conditions and without contamination.
Contaminated	Open, fresh, accidental wounds. In addition, operations with major breaks in sterile technique or gross spillage from the gastrointestinal tract, and incisions in which acute, non-purulent inflammation is encountered, including necrotic tissue without evidence of purulent drainage are included in this category. This includes open surgical wounds returning to the operating room. Examples of major break in sterile technique include, but are not limited to, non-sterile equipment or debris found in the operative field.
Dirty/infected	Traumatic wounds with retained devitalized tissue and those that involve existing clinical infection or perforated viscera. This definition suggests that the organisms causing post-operative infection were present in the operative field before the operation.

Note that placement of any drain at the time of surgery does not change the classification of the wound. Operations performed in high wound classes are not reasons for exclusion of the patient for later meeting criteria for a surgical-site infection (SSI) (e.g. animals that develop an SSI following excision of a purulent process will still be eligible for SSI recording).

Table 9.3. Wound contamination definitions.

Wound contamination	Definition
Wound contamination	The presence of bacteria within a wound without any host reaction.
Wound colonization	The presence of bacteria within a wound that multiply and do not create a host reaction.
Critical wound colonization	Multiplication of bacteria causing a delay in wound healing, usually associated with an exacerbation of pain but still without an overt host reaction.
Wound infection	The deposition and multiplication of bacteria in tissue with an associated host reaction.

Table 9.4. Wound closure definitions.

Closure type	Definition
Primary closure	Closure of the skin during the original procedure regardless of the presence of drains or other devices extruding through the incision. Thus, if any portion of the incision is closed by any means, a designation of primary closure is attributed.
Non-primary closure	Closure other than primary, and includes surgeries where the skin is left completely open during the original procedure. The deep tissue layers may be closed (with skin left open), or deep and superficial layers may both be left completely open. Wounds with non-primary closure may or may not be packed.

individuals who are the most vulnerable and direct any potential interventions, which can significantly reduce infection rates (Ercole *et al.*, 2007). Such systems are in their infancy in veterinary medicine, and large-scale patient recording systems such the National Nosocomial Infection Surveillance (NNIS) or Hospitals in Europe Link for Infections Control through Surveillance (HELICS) systems (available in America and Europe, respectively) are lacking.

9.3.1 The basic SSI risk index

The traditional wound classification system, which stratifies each wound into one of four categories

Denis Verwilghen and Kelly L. Bowlt Blacklock

Table 9.5. Wound infection definitions. Adapted from CDC guidelines (CDC, 2022).

Wound infection	Definition
Superficial incisional infections	Must meet the following criteria: Infection that occurs within 30 days after any operative procedure OR if the infection can be linked to the surgery independent of the time of appearance AND Involves only the skin and the subcutaneous tissues of the incision AND The patient shows signs of *at least one* of the following: • Purulent drainage with or without laboratory confirmation from the superficial incision • Organisms that are identified following an aseptically obtained specimen from the superficial incision or subcutaneous tissues by culture or non-culture-based microbiological testing • A superficial incision that is deliberately opened and culture or non-culture-based testing is not performed AND The patient has *at least one* of the following signs: • Pain or tenderness • Localized swelling • Erythema • Heat Diagnosis of a superficial incisional SSI by the surgeon or attending physician. Comments: The following do not qualify for superficial SSI: • Diagnosis of cellulitis by itself (redness, warmth, swelling) does not meet the criteria for a superficial wound infection • A singular stitch abscess alone confined to the point of suture penetration

Deep incisional infections	Must meet the following criteria:
	Infection that occurs within 30–90 days after any operative procedure OR if the infection can be linked to the surgery independent of the time of appearance
	AND
	Involves only the deep soft tissues of the incision (e.g. fascial and muscular layers)
	AND
	The patient shows signs of *at least one* of the following:
	• Purulent drainage from the deep incision
	• A deep incision that spontaneously dehisces or is deliberately opened or aspirated by the surgeon and organisms are identified following an aseptically obtained specimen from the tissues by culture or non-culture-based microbiological testing AND the patient has *at least one* of the following signs
	  – Fever (>39.2°C/>102.5°F in dogs and cats)
	  – Localized pain or tenderness
	• Diagnosis of an abscess or other evidence of infection involving a deep incision that is detected on gross anatomical or histopathological examination or an imaging test

Continued

Table 9.5. Continued

Wound infection	Definition
Organ space infections	Must meet the following criteria: Infection that occurs within 30 or 90 days after any operative procedure OR if the infection can be linked to the surgery independent of the time of appearance AND Involves any part of the body deeper than the fascial/muscle layers that is opened or manipulated during the operative procedure AND The patient shows signs of *at least one* of the following: • Purulent drainage from a drain that is placed into the organ/space • Organisms that are identified following an aseptically obtained fluid or tissue from the organ/space by culture or non-culture-based microbiological testing • Diagnosis of an abscess or other evidence of infection involving deep incision that is detected on gross anatomical or histopathological examination or an imaging test AND It meets at least one of the criteria for specific organ/space infection listed for specific organs/spaces (Table 9.6)
Infection present at the time of surgery (PATOS)	PATOS denotes that there is documented evidence of infection at the start or during the surgical procedure Fresh traumatic wounds that are contaminated at the time of surgery are not considered PATOS
Multiple layers involved in the infection	The type of SSI reported should reflect the deepest layer involved

based on the expected contamination level of the wound during the procedure (Table 9.2), is widely used but has major limitations (Gaynes, 2000). This system describes the wound but does not consider the intrinsic patient risk. A composite risk index that captures the combined influences of the wound, procedure and patient status is required before meaningful comparisons between SSI rates can be made.

An example of such an index is the NNIS basic SSI risk index. This index is used to assign SSI development risk to surgical patients and is a significantly better predictor of SSI development compared with previously used parameters (Gaynes, 2000). The index is based on three major criteria: (i) procedure duration; (ii) degree of wound contamination; and (iii) American Society of Anesthesiologists (ASA) classification of the patient. The actual SSI risk index is the sum of the scores, as described in Table 9.7. The duration of procedure is a common recurrent denominator linked to infection risk development. This criterion is therefore included as the 75th percentile of duration of the surgery in minutes rounded to the nearest whole number

of hours. Most standardized operative procedures in human medicine have 75th percentile duration values published, although this information is not readily available for veterinary surgery. However, it is reasonable to assume that in a well-organized surgical environment, the majority of clean routine procedures (e.g. ovariohysterectomy, ovariectomy, castration or some orthopaedic procedures such as tibial plateau levelling osteotomy) can be performed by an experienced surgeon within the time frame of 1 h (Fitzpatrick and Solano, 2010; Peeters and Kirpensteijn, 2011).

9.3.2 Infection rates and risk factors

Various studies have reported SSI rates in veterinary surgery, including overall and procedure-specific infection rates. An overview of these rates can be found in Table 9.8. However, most studies reporting SSI rates have some limitations, often due to the lack of correct or clear definitions of SSI, the absence of proper prospective surveillance and small sample size. In retrospective studies, large numbers of infections (particularly those

Denis Verwilghen and Kelly L. Bowlt Blacklock

Table 9.6. Specific organ infection criteria. Adapted from CDC guidelines (CDC, 2022).

Specific organ infection	Criteria
Bone osteomyelitis	The patient has organisms identified from bone by a culture- or non-culture-based microbiological testing method
	The patient has evidence of osteomyelitis on gross anatomic or histopathologic examination
	The patient has *at least two* of the following localized signs:
	• Fever (>39.2°C / >102.5°F in dogs and cats)
	• Swelling
	• Pain or tenderness
	• Heat
	• Drainage
	AND *at least one* of the following:
	• Organisms identified from blood by a culture- or non-culture-based microbiological testing method in a patient with imaging test evidence suggestive of infection (e.g. radiograph, CT scan, MRI, scintigraphy), which if equivocal is supported by clinical correlation (i.e. clinician documentation of antimicrobial treatment for osteomyelitis)
	• Imaging test evidence suggestive of infection (e.g. radiograph, CT scan, MRI, radiolabelled scan), which if equivocal is supported by clinical correlation (i.e. clinician documentation of antimicrobial treatment for osteomyelitis)
Joint or bursa infection	The patient has organisms identified from synovial fluid by a culture- or non-culture-based microbiologic testing method
	The patient has evidence of joint or bursa infection on gross anatomic or histopathologic examination
	The patient has *at least two* of the following signs with no other recognized cause:
	• Swelling
	• Pain or tenderness
	• Heat
	• Evidence of effusion
	• Limitation of motion
	AND *at least one* of the following:
	• Elevated joint fluid white blood cell count and neutrophil
	• Organisms and white blood cells seen on Gram stain of synovial fluid
	Imaging test evidence is suggestive of infection (e.g. radiograph, CT scan, MRI, radiolabelled scan), which if equivocal is supported by clinical correlation (i.e. physician documentation of antimicrobial treatment for synovial infection)

Continued

Table 9.6. Continued

Specific organ infection	Criteria

Implant-associated infections	Any of the other SSI classifications that have shown to include/spread towards the implant OR
	
	Involvement of any orthopaedic or other implant placed during a surgical procedure:
	• Without external superficial, deep or bone-associated signs of infection
	• With clinical or imaging signs suggestive of implant loosening or infection
	• AND *at least one* of the following is documented:
	  – Pathogenic microorganisms identified by culture from deep tissue or implant specimens
	  – Histological presence of microorganisms in deep tissue specimens, confirmed using specific staining techniques
	  – Analysis of histological specimens or cytological examination of peri-prosthetic joint aspirates using one of the three minor criteria as defined by the International Consensus Meeting on Periprosthetic Joint Infection (Zmistowski *et al.*, 2014) demonstrates: (i) ≥2 PMNs per high-power field (×400) in ten consecutive high-power fields (Fink *et al.*, 2013); (ii) ≥23 PMNs in ten consecutive high-power field (field ×20, field of view diameter 0.625 mm) (Morawietz *et al.*, 2009); or (iii) ≥50 CD15⁺ PMNs in a single focal point of one high-power field (CD15 Focus Score) (Kolbel *et al.*, 2015). The value of this criterion has yet to be determined in dogs and cats
	• Increased markers of inflammation, e.g. neutrophil count, C-reactive protein (Lofqvist *et al.*, 2018).

Note that implant-associated infections are caused by microorganisms that grow in biofilms and adhere to the implant surface in a highly hydrated extracellular matrix (Mauffrey *et al.*, 2016). Despite the increasing number of clinical, laboratory and imaging techniques available, the diagnosis of implant infections (in particular peri-prosthetic) may be very difficult and there is no gold standard, although converging evidence can lead to a strong suspicion of infection (Canner *et al.*, 1984; Parvizi *et al.*, 2011; Natoli *et al.*, 2020; Obremskey *et al.*, 2020). Non-culture methods may aid in diagnosing implant-associated infections (see section 9.4). Ultimately, these infections may be hard to identify, as they may produce very similar clinical signs to aseptic mechanical loosening in orthopaedic implants (Parvizi *et al.*, 2011; Cyteval and Bourdon, 2012).
CT, computed tomography; MRI, magnetic resonance imaging; PMN, polymorphonuclear leucocyte; SSI, surgical-site infection.

Table 9.7. Basic SSI risk index calculation factors adapted from European Centre for Disease Prevention and Control definitions, with *T* considered the 75th percentile duration value for a specific procedure.

Calculation	Score = 0 if:	Score = 1 if:
Wound class	Clean Clean-contaminated	Contaminated Dirty
ASA class	ASA-1 ASA 2	ASA-3 ASA-4 ASA-5
Duration of operative procedure, *T*	≤*T*	>*T*
Basic SSI risk index	Sum of scores	

ASA, American Society of Anesthesiologists, SSI, surgical-site infection.

found superficially) may not be reported because they may be treated by veterinarians other than the primary surgeon and/or may not be reported in the medical record at the surgical facility (Sands *et al.*, 1996). Therefore, retrospective studies are likely to be providing an underestimation of true SSI rates by up to 35% (Turk *et al.*, 2015; Garcia Stickney and Thieman Mankin, 2018). The time-consuming and expensive nature of prospective SSI surveillance is a commonly lamented barrier to implementation in veterinary medicine. Recently, a prospective study was presented,

Denis Verwilghen and Kelly L. Bowlt Blacklock

Table 9.8. Reported small animal practice surgical-site infection (SSI) rates, grouped by type of surgery.

Surgical procedure	Sample size (n)	SSI incidence (%)	Reference
All surgical procedures	846	3.0	Turk *et al.* (2015)
	1010	3.0	Eugster *et al.* (2004)
	1574	5.5	Brown *et al.* (1997)
	2063	5.1	Vasseur *et al.* (1988)
Clean-contaminated surgical wounds	239	5.9	Nicholson *et al.* (2002)
Clean surgical wounds	777	4.8	Beal *et al.* (2000)
	863	4.5	Heldmann *et al.* (1999)
	128	0.8	Vasseur *et al.* (1985)
Clean, elective orthopaedic surgical procedures	112	7.1	Whittem *et al.* (1999)
	60	3.3	Holmberg (1985)
Laparoscopy and VATS	179	1.7	Mayhew *et al.* (2012)
TPLO	226	13.3	Nazarali *et al.* (2014)
	208	21.3	Solano *et al.* (2015)
	283	8.8	Etter *et al.* (2013)
	2739	3.8	Savicky *et al.* (2013)
	282	7.4	Gallagher and Mertens (2012)
	476	2.9	Gatineau *et al.* (2011)
	1146	6.6	Fitzpatrick and Solano (2010)
Extracapsular stifle stabilization and TPLO	902	6.1	Frey *et al.* (2010)

TPLO, tibial plateau levelling osteotomy; VATS, video-assisted thoracic surgery.

which compared SSI occurrence as reported by primary-care veterinarians and pet owners. The sensitivity and specificity of owner-reported SSIs was up to 88.9% and 98%, respectively, with active surveillance detecting 36.4% more SSIs than passive surveillance alone. The authors proposed that the questionnaire developed could be used to create a sensitive and specific active surveillance system using client responses with automated distribution, data collection and analysis for SSIs. As a result, personnel time and expense could be greatly reduced, removing barriers to implementation of prospective SSI monitoring (Glenn *et al.*, 2022).

Proper SSI monitoring and establishment of reliable SSI rates requires active, patient-based prospective surveillance using standardized definitions (Table 9.5) (CDC, 2022). In human surgery settings where surveillance programmes are implemented more rigorously, the overall SSI rate is around 5% but is still considered to be an underestimate because of the aforementioned reasons.

Despite their limitations related to the reporting of SSIs, some veterinary studies do provide risk factors related to the occurrence of SSIs (Table 9.9).

9.4 How to Recognize SSIs

9.4.1 Physical examination

Early intervention following identification of an SSI will offer the best chance at resolution. Clinical signs of developing infection include fever that cannot otherwise be explained, increasing post-operative swelling, pain and heat evident at palpation, erythema and persistent wound drainage. In patients undergoing orthopaedic surgeries, the development of post-operative lameness is suggestive of SSI development. All early signs of infection should prompt the surgeon to investigate the wound further. Nevertheless, the key to identifying infection is the ability to recognize the difference between a simple complication of healing, such as a haematoma or seroma, and a surgical wound that has become or is becoming infected. Relying solely

Table 9.9. Reported risk factors associated with small animal surgical procedures.

Risk factor for SSI	Protective factor for SSI	Reference
Hypotension, surgical wound classification and implant	None identified	Turk et al. (2015)
Anaesthesia time	Post-operative administration of antimicrobials	Nazarali et al. (2014)
Use of a non-locking plate in TPLO	Post-operative administration of antimicrobials	Solano et al. (2015)
None identified	Staples instead of suture for skin closure	Etter et al. (2013)
Synthes implant in TPLO	None identified	Savicky et al. (2013)
Hair clipped at surgical site >4 h Surgical time	None identified	Mayhew et al. (2012)
None identified	Post-operative administration of antimicrobials	Gatineau et al. (2011)
TPLO versus extracapsular stifle stabilization	Suture for skin closure Post-operative administration of antimicrobials	Frey et al. (2010)
Increasing body weight Intact male	Post-operative administration of antimicrobials Labrador retriever breed	Fitzpatrick and Solano (2010)
Duration of surgery Increasing number of persons in the operating room Dirty surgical wound classification	Antimicrobial prophylaxis administered	Eugster et al. (2004)
Intact males Concurrent endocrinopathy Duration of surgery Duration of anaesthesia	None identified	Nicholson et al. (2002)
Duration of anaesthesia	None identified	Beal et al. (2000)
Use of propofol for anaesthetic induction	None identified	Heldmann et al. (1999)
Antimicrobial prophylaxis not administered	Antimicrobial prophylaxis administered	Whittem et al. (1999)
Duration of surgery Time of pre-operative clipping	None identified	Brown et al. (1997)
Post-operative rectal temperature Duration of surgery	Antimicrobial prophylaxis administered	Vasseur et al. (1988)

SSI, surgical-site infection; TPLO, tibial plateau levelling osteotomy.

on microbiological results to diagnose infection is unreliable. Most wounds can be colonized with bacteria, but infection occurs when the multiplication and tissue invasion by bacteria (known as virulence) inhibits the ability of the wound to heal (EWMA, 2005). The damage–response framework (Casadevall and Pirofski, 2003) recognizes that microbial pathogenesis is a consequence of the interaction between the host and the microorganism, determined by the extent of damage inflicted by either the microorganism or the host's immune response. In SSIs, ensuing damage will mostly originate from the host immune response to the microbial infection (Casadevall and Pirofski, 2003). Ultimately, infection is a clinical diagnosis based on varied and complex criteria, complicating the process of devising an accurate definition. Consequently, and independent of the definition that is used, a degree of clinical subjectivity will always remain.

9.4.2 Wound evaluation

In human medicine, simple, visual, serial wound inspection is the best method for monitoring the occurrence of SSIs, and is superior to evaluation of

Denis Verwilghen and Kelly L. Bowlt Blacklock

baseline features (e.g. C-reactive protein) (Sanger *et al.*, 2016). Serial evaluation of defined features (wound variables such as wound edge distance, slough/necrosis amount and type, exudate amount and type, granulation/epithelialization score, wound edge colour, wound temperature, wound odour, pain score, haematoma/seroma and wound culture; vital signs such as heart rate, diastolic and systolic blood pressure, and body temperature; and other observations such as the use of a ventilator, antibiotics, nasogastric tube or revision surgery) has been associated with a moderate positive predictive value (0.35) and high negative predictive value (0.93) in ability to predict SSI development 1–5 days before the actual SSI was diagnosed (Sanger *et al.*, 2016). However, this assumes that the attending clinician is familiar with the definitions of an SSI (Mannien *et al.*, 2006), which is not always true. In veterinary medicine, interpretation of what is normal is still extremely variable: in the authors' experience, it is not uncommon for pet owners to indicate that their primary attending veterinarian considered dehiscence and draining in surgical wounds to be a normal phase of surgical wound healing, whereas the authors would consider such changes to be indicative of an SSI and therefore worthy of reporting to the surgical facility.

9.4.3 Markers of SSIs

To guide clinicians in their SSI recognition, human surgeons utilize different markers, which have been tested to allow predictive or differentiating values for septic versus non-septic complications. Parameters such as C-reactive protein and white blood cell counts seem to lack sufficient specificity for this task, but pro-calcitonin (PCT) has shown promise in high-evidence trials (Schuetz *et al.*, 2011). PCT is the prohormone of calcitonin and is produced ubiquitously in response to mediators released during bacterial infections. In humans, PCT shows a clinically favourable kinetic profile because it increases within 6–12 h of stimulation, and circulating levels will halve daily when infection is under control either by antibiotic therapy or the host immune system (Becker *et al.*, 2004). In one study, measuring PCT allowed differentiation of post-operative non-infectious fever from infections occurring after orthopaedic surgeries (Hunziker *et al.*, 2010). PCT measurements have also been shown to be beneficial in monitoring

therapeutic antimicrobial effect in post-operative infections and allowed a reduction in duration of antibiotic treatment without an increase in morbidity and mortality (Schuetz *et al.*, 2011). In cats, elevated PCT (>366 pg ml^{-1}) has been associated with bacterial infection, and in dogs, PCT concentrations are predictive of organ dysfunction and septic shock (Troia *et al.*, 2018; Cho *et al.*, 2021). However, the value of PCT in predicting SSI occurrence or response to treatment has not yet been assessed in small animal clinical practice.

Recently, a novel flexible pH-sensing hydrogel fibre wound dressing was developed for monitoring of wound healing (Tamayol *et al.*, 2016). The skin pH in humans is slightly acidic (pH 4–6), and once the skin barrier is breached by wound fluid, the pH becomes more alkaline (pH 7.4). During the healing processes, the wound pH shifts towards neutral and becomes re-established in the pH 4–6 range upon complete healing. When infected, the local environment will either become very alkaline or acidic (pH 5.4–9.0), and thus continuous pH monitoring of the skin could be beneficial in early detection of superficial SSIs (Dargaville *et al.*, 2013).

9.4.4 Imaging

Ultrasound

Serial ultrasound monitoring of suspect surgical sites may complement visual detection of early signs of wound infection and has been shown to be more reliable than clinical examination alone (O'Rourke *et al.*, 2015). The benefit of ultrasonographic evaluation to detect SSIs in equine ventral midline incisions has long been shown (Wilson *et al.*, 1989), but the technique can be more universally applied to monitor surgical wound healing because it is affordable, easy, portable and non-invasive. Ultrasound examination can prevent an unnecessary procedure or identify occult abscesses that may go on to develop a more severe infection requiring hospitalization (O'Rourke *et al.*, 2015) and has a high negative predictive value in screening for SSI development in high-risk surgical wounds in humans (Barrett *et al.*, 2016). Ultrasonographic features suggestive of wound infection include subcutaneous swelling and oedema, loss of normal tissue architecture around the infected suture line, fistulous tracts, subperiosteal abscesses, fluid pockets around implants, increased tissue echogenicity and/or gas pocketing (either produced by bacteria or because there is wound dehiscence). Ultrasonographic wound evaluation is not without its disadvantages: a competent operator is required and the depth of visualization can be limited. Additionally, interpretation of ultrasonographic changes is made challenging by recent surgery (e.g. a surgical approach will introduce air into the tissues) or where wound healing is complicated but not necessarily infected (e.g. wounds associated with a seroma or hematoma). When performing ultrasonography on surgical wounds, aseptic technique (e.g. a sterile glove over the probe) and the use of alcohol to increase skin contact is preferred over the use of ultrasound gel. Gel may be difficult to completely remove and could itself create a medium for bacterial proliferation, contributing to the establishment of an infection.

Radiography and computed tomography

Early recognition of infections using radiography is difficult because overt bone remodelling needs to occur before radiographic signs appear: approximately 30% of bone resorption is required before it is visible by radiography (Harris and Heaney, 1969; Sutton, 2003; Yochum and Rowe,

2004; Guglielmi *et al.*, 2008). Therefore, even in late stages of infection, radiography has a relatively low sensitivity because the radiographic appearance of the infection will not necessarily be correlated to its severity. In acute infection, the radiographic changes are often limited to non-specific signs such as soft-tissue swelling or separation of tissue planes. In sites where orthopaedic implants have been placed, radiographic changes that are suggestive of infection include radiolucency around the implants and periosteal reaction that cannot be explained by the fracture healing process. Late radiographic signs may include lysis in the cancellous bone and/or the medullary cavity (Fig. 9.1). Serial radiographic evaluation is often needed to confirm the suspicion of infection, although regular monitoring is generally insensitive to evaluate the response to treatment because of the delay in radiographic changes, particularly in bone.

The increasing availability of computed tomography (CT) in veterinary practice will possibly allow earlier and better detection of post-operative infections. CT allows a much higher sensitivity in detecting bone remodelling than radiography and is particularly useful in detecting soft-tissue infections involving gas-producing organisms, and imaging acquisition is rapid (Fig. 9.2) (Altmayer

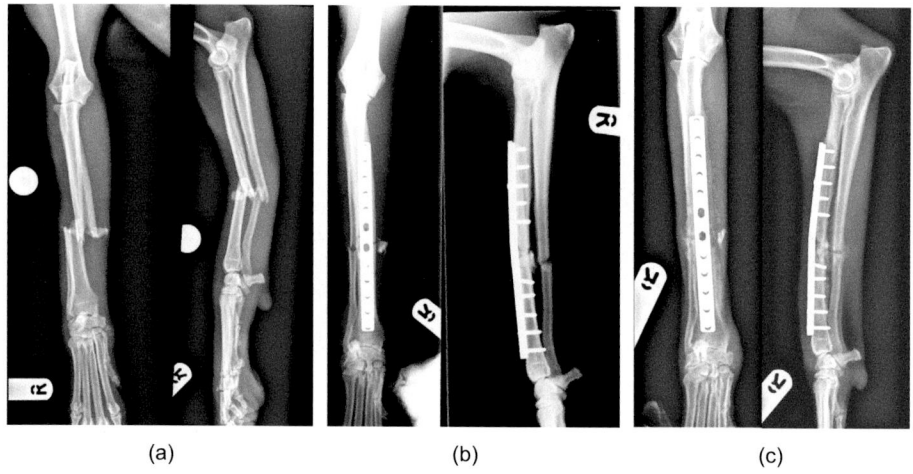

(a)   (b)   (c)

Fig. 9.1. Radiographs of the right forelimb of a 6-year-old lurcher who was hit by a car. (a, b) Craniocaudal and lateral radiograph of the right forelimb before (a) and after (b) surgical repair of the fracture. Surgery comprised placement of a 3.5 mm 12-hole dynamic compression plate with five screws in both the proximal and distal fragments. The fracture gap was packed with cancellous bone chips. (c) Eight weeks after surgery, post-operative radiographs showed a palisading periosteal reaction and delayed union suggestive of a bacterial osteomyelitis. Images courtesy of Tobias Schwarz, University of Edinburgh, Edinburgh, UK.

               Denis Verwilghen and Kelly L. Bowlt Blacklock

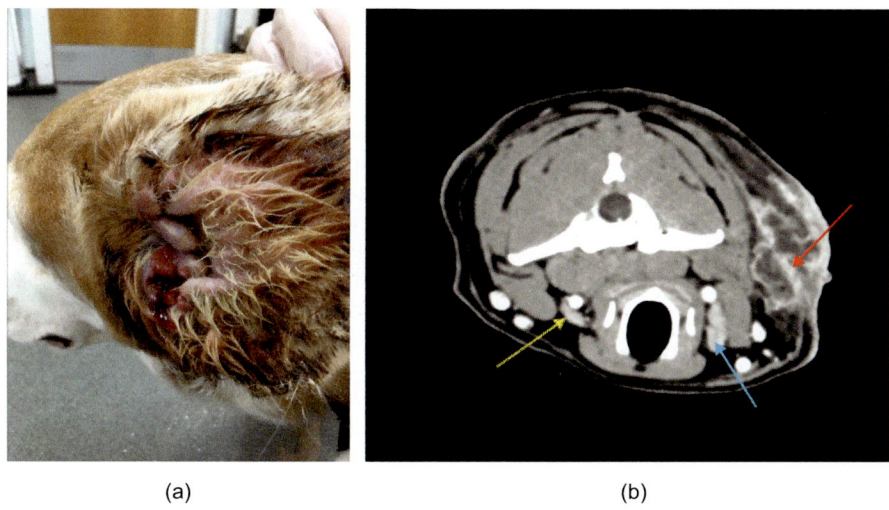

(a)   (b)

Fig. 9.2. (a) Photograph and (b) post-contrast computed tomography (CT) study of the head of a 9-year-old beagle taken 7 months after a left-sided total-ear canal ablation for otitis externa and media. The CT shows left-sided subcutaneous tissues of the caudal aspect of the head and neck (red arrow), measuring approximately 6 cm in length. Multiple rim-enhancing pocket-like lesions have coalesced together and are surrounded by fat stranding. The left medial retropharyngeal lymph node is asymmetrically enlarged (blue arrow) in comparison with the contralateral lymph node (yellow arrow) and is contrast enhancing. These findings are consistent with a left aural abscess with reactive lymphadenomegaly. The abnormal tissue was surgically excised, and histopathology was consistent with a pyogranulomatous inflammatory infiltrate with extensive fibrosis. Bacterial culture did not yield any growth, possibly because the patient was receiving clavulanic acid-amoxicillin prior to admission to the hospital. The patient made an uneventful recovery, and no recurrence of the abscess was detected 1 year after surgery. CT images courtesy of Tobias Schwarz, University of Edinburgh, Edinburgh, UK.

et al., 2020). In human medicine, several small-scale studies have reported that positron emission tomography CT is more accurate than CT alone in diagnosing SSIs following orthopaedic, neurological or sternal surgery (Wang et al., 2016; Lee et al., 2019; Liu et al., 2020). Further studies in small animal surgical patients are required to investigate the accuracy of CT in detecting SSIs.

Scintigraphy

Scintigraphy has also been shown to be valuable in the detection of early orthopaedic infections. For instance technetium 99m-methylene diphosphonate (^{99m}Tc-MDP) three-phase bone scintigraphy provided high predictive values in diagnosing infection in humans following internal fixation of fractures (Yang et al., 2016). The use of so-called 'white blood cell scans' in which white blood cells are tagged with indium-111 is extremely sensitive to the detection of early-onset osteomyelitis but also for detection of so-called hidden soft-tissue infections

(Lewis et al., 2014; Herron and Gossman, 2022). Similar studies in small animal patients are lacking.

Magnetic resonance imaging

In human medicine, magnetic resonance imaging (MRI) is commonly used to identify neurological and musculoskeletal infections because of its superior soft-tissue contrast resolution (Soldatos et al., 2012). MRI findings associated with early SSI include muscle or organ swelling/oedema, which manifests as a high T2-weighted short-tau inversion recovery (T2w/STIR) signal and higher signal on T1w compared with uninvolved structures, as well as contrast enhancement on T1w scans. In more advanced infections, an abscess can be identified, which will demonstrate a high signal on T2w or peripherally enhanced collections of fluid on contrast-enhanced T1w (Altmayer et al., 2020). The accuracy of detecting SSIs using MRI in small animal practice has not been reported.

9.5 Prevention of SSIs

Over the years, it has become apparent that the occurrence of SSI is not related to a single factor, but that a diverse array of pathogen-, patient- and caregiver-related issues influence risk and prevention. As much as the successful outcome of a surgical procedure is not based on the sole responsibility of the surgeon, the entire healthcare team plays a pivotal role in the prevention of SSIs.

9.5.1 Understanding the occurrence of SSIs

The occurrence of SSIs is the result of a complex interplay between multiple factors related to the patient and their environment. Surgical procedures performed in completely sterile environments are impossible. The number of bacteria required for infection to occur will depend on the patient's inherent defence mechanisms against pathogens, the extent and severity of tissue injury, the virulence of the pathogen and the amount of foreign material present (e.g. gross contamination, or implants around which a biofilm may form). Additionally, administration of peri-operative antimicrobials and the intrinsic or acquired antimicrobial resistance of the pathogen must be considered. This theory has been assessed in the veterinary literature. In dogs undergoing clean orthopaedic procedures, bacterial isolates were yielded from 81% of procedures from one or more sources, but the SSI rate was 9% (Andrade *et al.*, 2016). In the same study, bacteria responsible for SSIs did not appear to colonize the patient in the operating room.

The bacterial contamination in a surgical wound can originate from an endogenous or exogenous source. Endogenous sources of contamination include the patient's commensal microbiota at the surgical site or distant body sites (e.g. skin, oropharynx, gastrointestinal tract – linked to surgical wound class). Exogenous sources of contamination are those originating from the surgical team, the environment, and the materials and instruments used. Other risk factors can similarly be divided into endogenous and exogenous. In humans, it has been estimated that approximately half of all identified SSI risk factors are endogenous (e.g. age, systemic disease, history of prior surgery) and many of these are difficult or impossible to modify in the direct pre-operative and peri-operative phase (Uckay *et al.*, 2010). However, many exogenous factors (e.g. change of surgeon during surgery,

visitors during surgery, hair removal methods) can readily be addressed.

Surgical asepsis prevents wound contamination from microorganisms that originate from the patient, the operating room personnel and the environment. The methods and practices that prevent contamination during surgery are defined in part by aseptic surgical technique. Proper SSI prevention measures are not an individual action of the surgeon during the procedure but involve scrupulous preparation of the facilities and environment, surgical site, surgical and anaesthesia team, and surgical equipment. Basic rules are straightforward and simple to implement but unfortunately are not often followed. Every member of a healthcare team, including the surgeon, nurses, assistants, cleaning staff and management group share responsibility for ensuring that aseptic procedures are achieved and are equally responsible for the resulting surgical successes and failures. Adhering to all these practices builds the basis of surgical and operating room team conscience.

The overall aims in the prevention of SSIs are to:

- embrace methods and principles that will reduce the amount of endogenous and exogenous microbiological contamination;
- reduce the pathogenicity of the involved microbes and slow or prevent resistance development (note that SSI prevention methods do not only aim to protect an individual patient from acquiring an infection, they also aim to instigate general measures that eventually protect the surgical population of today and tomorrow);
- increase the host's own defence mechanisms;
- reduce the inflicted tissue trauma; and
- reduce the amount of foreign body material left behind.

Although many of the principles of aseptic technique have found acceptance and evidence validation through their historical merits, although many would have difficulties passing the stringent tests expected in current times. High-level evidence obtained by double-blinded randomized controlled trials is impossible for ethical reasons: for example, it would be unthinkable to compare SSI rates between surgical procedures with or without hand asepsis. Furthermore, the lack of consistent definitions and the use of surrogate outcomes instead of end-point studies have complicated interpretation of findings. Many recommendations are therefore based on theoretical grounds and extrapolation. In

Denis Verwilghen and Kelly L. Bowlt Blacklock

veterinary medicine, evidence for techniques in SSI prevention is even weaker, and extrapolation from human medicine is common. Nevertheless, absence of proof can never be regarded as proof of absence (Smith and Pell, 2003).

9.5.2 SSI preventative measures

Many key aspects of SSI prevention, such as hand hygiene, antimicrobial prophylaxis and surgical-site preparation will be discussed in other chapters. In the sections that follow, we discuss how SSI rates are related to surgical duration, surgeon experience and technique, operating room etiquette, procedural cleanliness and staff compliance with infection-control protocols.

Time

The time taken to complete a procedure is a commonly identified SSI risk factor in human and veterinary studies. Not only is the duration of the surgery itself important, but SSI risk is also related to the overall procedural time from anaesthetic induction to recovery. Longer surgery durations will lead to prolonged exposure of the wound, greater tissue manipulation with more opportunities for pathogens to seed into the wound and increased chance of wound desiccation. Additionally, overall procedure time presumably contributes to the compromise of various host defence mechanisms that are difficult to evaluate specifically. Veterinary literature may not have reported on these facts accurately, yet in human literature the effects of anaesthesia and surgery on the patient's immune status have long been postulated (Walton, 1979). The 'stress' component included in anaesthesia and surgery may play a significant role in the development of SSIs (Walton, 1979). Nevertheless, more recent studies indicate that in generally heathy patients, the effective general anaesthesia component is not considerable; rather, the immune system is mostly influenced by the degree of surgical trauma (Jafarzadeh *et al.*, 2020).

While surgeon experience can be one factor in extending the duration of the surgical procedure, the overall anaesthetic time will be dictated by the entire nursing, surgical and anaesthesia teams. Procedural planning, availability of appropriate instruments and coordination with diagnostic imaging can reduce the overall procedural time (Estrin *et al.*, 2021). In human hospitals, higher SSI rates are associated with longer procedural duration, higher trainee-to-bed ratios, poor communication and higher operative staff turnover (Campbell *et al.*, 2008). In veterinary medicine, several studies have determined that SSI rate increased with procedure time (Nicholson *et al.*, 2002; Eugster *et al.*, 2004; Stetter *et al.*, 2021), and in particular, Pratesi *et al.* (2015) showed an increase in SSIs of 2% with every increasing minute of procedure time. In a pilot study, veterinary undergraduate students observed the team of students performing a surgical and anaesthetic procedure and noted coordination, team responsibility and efficiency. It was reported that better team leadership, equipment preparation, anticipation of needs during the procedure and proactivity in surgical assistance could have reduced the 90 min procedure time by one-third (Denis Verwilghen, personal communication). Improved pre-operative planning and including trained scrub technicians could also significantly reduce intraoperative delays (Estrin *et al.*, 2021).

Surgical experience, technique and operating room etiquette

Many surgeons consider that the most critical factors in prevention of SSIs are sound judgement and proper technique of the surgeon and surgical team, as well as the general patient health (Humphreys, 2009). It is impossible to perform randomized trials on this subjective observation. Adherence to Halsted's principles, maintaining adequate haemostasis while preserving blood supply, gentle handling of the tissues, removal of devitalized tissue, eradication of dead space and appropriate management of the post-operative incision are all gestures and actions that can be learned but for which experience will improve performance and ultimately reduce complications (Aggarwal and Darzi, 2008). This statement is supported by several human studies in which the experience of the surgeon, both in general and for a particular procedure, was associated with lower SSI or wound complication rates (Wurtz *et al.*, 2001). Studies have also reported a higher incidence of wound dehiscence in abdominal procedures when closure was performed by a trainee rather than an attending surgeon (Carlson, 1997; Webster *et al.*, 2003). Similar findings were reported in an equine study in which closure of the abdominal wound by first and second year residents was a significant risk factor for development of SSIs (Torfs *et al.*, 2010).

Considering surgical and anaesthesia time is often reported as a crucial risk factor in complication development, it is easy to relate inexperience with longer surgery. However, in the veterinary study by Torfs *et al.* (2010), surgery and anaesthesia time were not different among level of experience, suggesting that several other factors, such as technique, sound judgement and adherence to aseptic principles contribute to SSI formation to a greater extent with inexperienced surgeons. In the authors' personal experience, increased confidence with procedures grows with an increasing number of years qualified and number of procedures performed, reducing stress and improving decision making. In small animal surgery, no studies have specifically investigated surgeon experience when determining risks for SSI development.

The establishment of proper operating room etiquette receives limited attention in the veterinary community and its importance is likely underestimated. Although probably a surrogate outcome to assess behaviour of the surgical team, noise level in the surgical theatre has been significantly correlated with higher SSI rates in human medicine (Kurmann *et al.*, 2011). Noise leads to a significant decrease in concentration capacity (Kurmann *et al.*, 2011) and to a significant increase in surgical errors (Moorthy *et al.*, 2004). In veterinary surgery, answering questions significantly decreases surgical speed, particularly for less experienced individuals and less experienced male veterinarians and veterinary students (Peterson *et al.*, 2021).

A particularly interesting study by Beldi *et al.* (2009) highlighted how our daily work involves multiple issues that impact outcomes. This prospective investigation involving over 1000 human surgical patients clearly showed that a lapse in discipline by the surgical team was an independent SSI risk factor. Increased movement in theatre, exchange of surgical team members, noise and the presence of visitors in the operating room all independently contributed to an increase in infections rates.

Implementation of checklists into surgical routine has been shown to significantly decrease surgical complications (Haynes *et al.*, 2009), and the authors use a modified World Health Organization Surgical Safety Checklist as standard (freely available online; WHO, 2009), believing that improving theatre discipline may also be able to reduce other surgical-associated patient morbidities in addition to SSIs.

Optimizing surgical cleanliness

Surgical planning is key to success of a procedure. Revising the steps of the surgical procedure and planning the surgical list such that clean procedures precede contaminated/dirty surgeries may be scientifically unsupported strategies but are common sense to reduce SSI risk. For all procedures, operating table setup should be performed with division of instruments from opening to closing of the wound, and instrument boxes should contain duplication of instruments to allow use of new instruments following entry into a contaminated/dirty site. For contaminated and dirty procedures, it is standard practice to have two separate operating tables with different sets of instruments, an extra layer of draping and change of surgical attire once the contaminated part of the procedure is completed.

Various points in the surgical procedure provide opportunities for contamination or mitigation. Proper opening of instruments and the draping procedures reduce initial contamination. Double gloving for draping with discarding the outer pair before the start of the surgery can further reduce contamination risks (Verwilghen, 2018). Preoperative closed gloving is commonly performed in small animal surgery when surgical gowns are worn, because open gloving is associated with increased risk of contamination (Pelosi, 2018). In addition to pre-operative gloving, intraoperative glove changes are recommended any time there is a break in sterility or after potential tumour exposure (Eugster *et al.*, 2004). A recent study demonstrated that the outside of the gown cuff does not seem to represent a major source of contamination during clean procedures in a veterinary population, and therefore intraoperative closed glove exchange does not increase bacterial contamination (Sidhu *et al.*, 2021).

Intraoperative glove exchange may be required after glove perforation, which occurs commonly (in up to 66% of veterinary surgical procedures) (Biermann *et al.*, 2015). As the ability to detect glove perforation during surgery is low (Biermann *et al.*, 2015), double gloving and/or wearing of indicator undergloves may help in reducing and/or identifying perforations in high-risk surgeries. Increased glove contamination and perforation has been shown to occur at around 60 min of procedure time (Ward *et al.*, 2014; Biermann *et al.*, 2015). Changing outer gloves around this time and before handling implants is a potentially useful intervention.

Lack of compliance as a contributor to SSIs

The foremost risk factor for the development of SSI is the behaviour of surgical staff. SSIs are considered the most preventable of all healthcare-associated infections, yet compliance with standard recommendations is often abysmal (Leaper et al., 2014). In human medicine, a systematic review of 96 empirical studies showed a median compliance rate of 40% with hand hygiene guidelines in hospital care (Erasmus et al., 2010). In a survey performed among Canadian human surgeons, 63% did not comply with the current recommended guidelines for patients' pre-operative bathing using chlorhexidine, hair removal techniques, antimicrobial prophylaxis and intraoperative skin preparation (Davis et al., 2008). Shockingly poor adherence to hand hygiene recommendations is also repeatedly noted during observational studies in companion animal clinics. Overall hand hygiene compliance was only 32% in one study, with the lowest compliance seen in the pre-operating room area (20%) and before clean/aseptic procedures (12%) (Schmidt et al., 2021) (discussed in more detail in Chapter 4, this volume). When it comes to pre-surgical hand preparation, despite their own stated beliefs that alcohol hand rubs are superior to aqueous rubs, 66% of respondents to a survey among specialists from the American College of Veterinary Surgeons (ACVS) and European College of Veterinary Surgeons (ECVS) reported that they did not follow these recommendations (Verwilghen et al., 2013). Recommended contact times for surgeon preparation using soap and water are at least 2 min (or up to 7 min in some publications), whereas recommended contact times for alcohol-based hand rubs are 1.5–2 min (or as per the manufacturer's instructions). Despite this, one study showed that contact time during surgeon hand preparation ranged from 7 to 529 s (mean 121 s) for soap and water and from 4 to 123 s (mean 25 s) for alcohol-based hand rubs (Anderson et al., 2013). The same study reported that non-sterile contact with the previously aseptically prepared surgical site occurred in at least 36% of cases (Anderson et al., 2013).

Recommended contact times for pre-operative preparatory solutions for both patients and surgeons are also not universally adhered to. In an observational study, the average patient contact time with soap or alcohol was 75 s (range 10–462 s) and 44 s (range 3–220 s), despite textbooks and manufacturers usually recommending a product-skin contact time of at least 2 min (Anderson et al., 2013). Only 21% of veterinary nurses are reported to be aware of the product concentration and contact time they used while preparing patients (Evans et al., 2009). Depressingly, many similar examples are available in human surgery (Umit et al., 2014), and the most difficult example to understand is probably that of basic hand hygiene, where extremely low compliance is noted.

Use of more extensive hygienic measures than are currently recommended do not seem to have a significant impact on SSIs; however, lack of adherence to the established hospital protocols results in a 3.5-fold increase in the risk for SSI development (Beldi et al., 2009). In human hospital settings where the current SSI rate is around 5%, it is postulated that if full compliance with guidelines and protocols was met, infection rates for clean surgeries would be below 0.5% (Alexander et al., 2011). To minimize anomalies with protocol compliance, the authors' clinics use surgical checklists, regular peer-based observation, and timers to ensure and maintain compliance with current hand hygiene and patient preparation guidelines (Fig. 9.3).

Postponing elective surgeries in case of remote infection or systemic disease

Although randomized trial data are lacking, postponing elective surgeries in patients with remote infections or systemic disease is regarded as high-level evidence by the CDC SSI prevention guidelines (Mangram et al., 1999) and is supported by numerous retrospective reports in human medicine where remote infections were found to be significant risk factors for the development of SSIs (Velasco et al., 1996; Kessler et al., 2012; Pruzansky et al., 2014). The most common sites for remote infections are the gastrointestinal tract and lungs (Uckay et al., 2009). Urinary infections have also been incriminated in increased SSI risk (David and Vrahas, 2000), although the data are less certain (Uckay et al., 2010). Similar studies in veterinary medicine are lacking, although many institutions will evaluate the skin and urinary tract as standard and postpone surgery where an infection is suspected or identified, particularly if the procedure is elective and orthopaedic in nature (Etter et al., 2013).

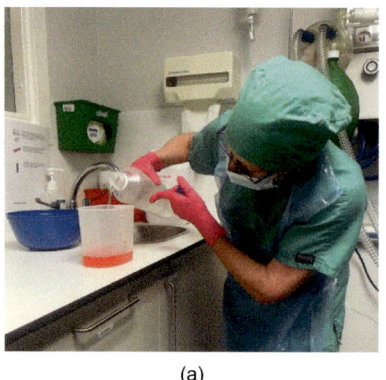 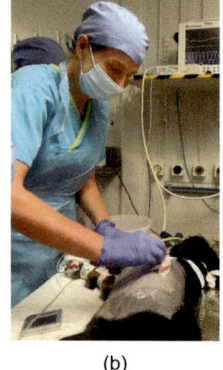 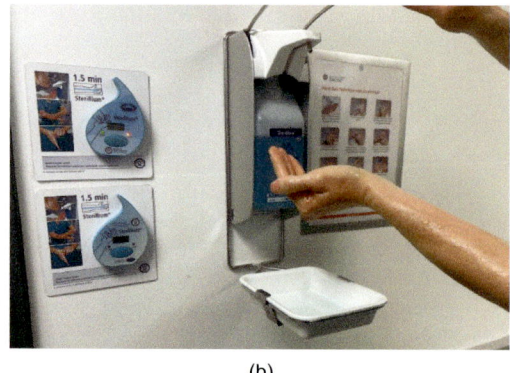

(a) (b) (b)

Fig. 9.3. To minimize anomalies with protocol compliance, accuracy should be ensured by using measuring equipment to make up diluted solutions (a), and peer observation and timers for patient (b) and surgical hand (c) preparation.

The pre-operative systemic inflammatory status of the patient has been correlated with increased risk of SSIs in humans (Mohri *et al.*, 2014; Udofia *et al.*, 2014), as have a number of factors such as obesity, smoking, diabetes, nutritional status of the patient and intake of certain medication (Mangram *et al.*, 1999). Similar findings have been reported in veterinary medicine, and therefore postponing elective surgery in individuals with these conditions is a prudent approach. Routine biochemical and haematological screening of potentially at-risk patients can be considered, with postponement of elective procedures if clinically relevant abnormalities are identified. In a patient affected by concomitant diseases that cannot be controlled before surgical intervention, the benefit of the surgical procedure versus complication risks should be assessed and owners appropriately counselled so that informed consent can be given.

SSI surveillance

Surveillance of SSIs, including appropriate feedback to the surgical team, has long been shown to be an important part of strategies to reduce healthcare-associated infections in general and particularly SSIs (Haley *et al.*, 1985; Gaynes, 2000), and surveillance has now become an essential part of SSI prevention (Anderson *et al.*, 2008). Active surveillance programmes may have an impact on SSI rate decreases, merely by reporting without any other formal form of intervention (Astagneau *et al.*, 2009). Nevertheless, SSI data collection allows calculation of risk-specific infection rates and can

be used by the local hospital and entire healthcare system to set priorities in infection-control programmes, review of protocols and evaluation of the effectiveness of their efforts (Emori *et al.*, 1991). In one of the first large-scale reports from US hospitals published in 1985, it was estimated that 32% of healthcare-associated infections could be avoided by the implementation of a programme (Haley *et al.*, 1985), and a specific surgical wound programme in the same period showed that SSI rates declined from 3.5% to less than 1% after implementation of a surveillance programme (Condon *et al.*, 1983).

Implementation of such programmes requires the use of standardized definitions (see Tables 9.2–9.6), allowing comparisons within and among veterinary healthcare institutions. Putting these strategies into practice is complex, requires engineering changes in behavioural and system aspects (Pittet, 2004; Gould, 2014), and is often frustrating for driving forces behind the programme. However, the efforts have been rewarded with significant reductions in SSI rates, at least in human medicine (Brandt *et al.*, 2006; Rioux *et al.*, 2007).

There are various challenges in identification of SSIs. In humans and veterinary medicine, 20–94% and up to 35% of SSIs are diagnosed following patient discharge from the healthcare facility, respectively (Mannien *et al.*, 2006; Limon *et al.*, 2014; Staszewicz *et al.*, 2014; Turk *et al.*, 2015; Garcia Stickney and Thieman Mankin, 2018). Therefore, a combination of coordinated passive and active surveillance (Table 9.10), along with effective data entry and retrieval, are required for proper SSI surveillance.

Denis Verwilghen and Kelly L. Bowlt Blacklock

Table 9.10. Definitions of passive and active surveillance methods for SSI monitoring.

Passive surveillance	Routine reporting of cases by healthcare providers or non-trained medical personnel; no additional effort is made to identify cases by the surgical facility
Active surveillance	Routine reporting of cases by trained healthcare providers in addition to active contact by infection control team with surgeons and nursing teams in order to identify cases
Active prospective post-discharge surveillance	Active surveillance performed on hospitalized patients and for a period defined by the surgical-site infection (SSI) definition timing, during which monitoring of the development of an SSI is recorded even if the patient has left the healthcare facility

Surveillance period for SSIs

Originally, the CDC classified an SSI as an infection that has developed in a 30–90-day timeframe following a surgical intervention (superficial infections 30 days, deep and organ/space infections up to 90 days) (HICPAC, 2020). A timeframe of 30–90 days may lead to an underestimation of infection rates and in the some documents (ECDC, 2012), an SSI is defined as an infection that occurs up to 1 year after surgery when an implant is used. However, in a small animal prospective active surveillance study in which patients were followed for 1 year, all infections (including those associated with implants) occurred within a 30-day timespan (Turk *et al.*, 2015). In human medicine, limiting post-operative SSI surveillance to 30 days would lead to under-reporting of up to two-thirds of deep incisional and organ space SSIs where implants are used, whereas a 90-day window of surveillance would detect most SSIs across the same procedures (Lankiewicz *et al.*, 2012).

A recent study of over 105,000 human surgical patients assessed the impact of monitoring duration and method on SSI incidence and found that shortening the post-discharge SSI monitoring period from 30 to 21 days (or from 1 year to 90 days for surgeries involving implants) resulted in 6–14% of SSIs being missed (Koek *et al.*, 2015). By contrast, using post-discharge surveillance methods other than the mandatory method resulted in up to 62% of SSIs being missed. These findings led the authors to conclude that international recommendations to limit the maximum post-discharge surveillance duration (for implant surgeries) to 90 days was acceptable, because this approach provides robust insight into trends (Koek *et al.*, 2015).

Overall, the benefits of using more cumbersome long surveillance periods in human settings are not entirely clear, as longer surveillance periods have not resulted in significantly more precise registration of SSI rate. Ultimately, the approach in human medicine is to balance the potential increased case ascertainment associated with a longer follow-up period with the increased resources that would be required (Bryce and Forrester, 2012; Lankiewicz *et al.*, 2012).

In veterinary hospitals, the post-operative monitoring of patients for SSI development is challenging. There is a paucity of active post-discharge surveillance commonly implemented in many national and international human healthcare surveillance systems (ECDC, 2019) or as reported by Turk *et al.* (2015) and Garcia Stickney and Thieman Mankin (2018). Many small animal patients with SSIs are not readmitted to the surgical care facility but rather are treated by primary-care veterinarians who may or may not report the SSI to the surgeon. It is not always possible to establish the time frame for the first occurrence of signs of infection based on discussion with owners, which compromises application of strict SSI definition timeframes. However, any wound infection related to a surgical intervention, independent of the timeframe, should be included in SSI surveillance data, with a clear mention of the timeline of events.

SSI monitoring activities

During the whole 30-day post-operative period, a total of two re-examinations of the patient is recommended. Ideally, these should be planned to occur at the time of suture removal (10–14 days) and at week 4, and performed by the surgeon who performed the procedure. Alternatively, patient and wound examination can be undertaken by another veterinarian or skilled veterinary nurse, or, if previous options are not available, by telemedicine (e.g. telephone consultation based on photos of the wounds obtained at the proposed time points). Reporting should clearly indicate whether the patient was seen by a clinician or whether SSI follow-up was by telephone conversation. In any case, it is important that identification and surveillance of the SSI is performed by a person who is cognisant of SSI definitions (Mannien *et al.*, 2006).

9.6 Conclusion

SSIs are multifactorial in origin and, whereas prevention of SSIs is likely to be the aspect in which we should all invest, realistically achieving 0% infection rates is unlikely to happen. Therefore, attention should also be placed on correct identification and early treatment of SSIs. Furthermore, in terms of prevention, it is not what we already know or do not know that has the largest impact on our infections rates, it is our compliance, or rather our lack of compliance to the application of the basic aseptic principles that effectively results in increased infection rates. In many ways, it is all in our own hands.

Acknowledgements

The authors are grateful to Tobias Schwarz, Dr med. vet., MA, DVR, DipECVDI, DACVR, FRCVS, for his assistance with this chapter.

References

Aggarwal, R. and Darzi, A. (2008) Symposium on surgical simulation for training and certification. *World Journal of Surgery* 32(2), 139–140. DOI: 10.1007/s00268-007-9341-7.

Ahern, B.J., Richardson, D.W., Boston, R.C. and Schaer, T.P. (2010) Orthopedic infections in equine long bone fractures and arthrodeses treated by internal fixation: 192 cases (1990-2006). *Veterinary Surgery* 39(5), 588–593. DOI: 10.1111/j.1532-950X.2010.00705.x.

Alexander, J.W., Solomkin, J.S. and Edwards, M.J. (2011) Updated recommendations for control of surgical site infections. *Annals of Surgery* 253(6), 1082–1093. DOI: 10.1097/SLA.0b013e31821175f8.

Altmayer, S., Verma, N., Dicks, E.A. and Oliveira, A. (2020) Imaging musculoskeletal soft tissue infections. *Seminars in Ultrasound, CT, and MRI* 41(1), 85–98. DOI: 10.1053/j.sult.2019.09.005.

Anderson, D.J., Kaye, K.S., Classen, D., Arias, K.M., Podgorny, K. *et al.* (2008) Strategies to prevent surgical site infections in acute care hospitals. *Infection Control and Hospital Epidemiology* 29 Suppl 1, S51–61. DOI: 10.1086/591064.

Anderson, M.E., Foster, B.A. and Weese, J.S. (2013) Observational study of patient and surgeon preoperative preparation in ten companion animal clinics in Ontario, Canada. *BMC Veterinary Research* 9, 194. DOI: 10.1186/1746-6148-9-194.

Andrade, N., Schmiedt, C.W., Cornell, K., Radlinsky, M.G., Heidingsfelder, L. *et al.* (2016) Survey of intraoperative bacterial contamination in dogs undergoing elective orthopedic surgery. *Veterinary Surgery* 45(2), 214–222. DOI: 10.1111/vsu.12438.

Astagneau, P., L'Hériteau, F., Daniel, F., Parneix, P., Venier, A.-G. *et al.* (2009) Reducing surgical site infection incidence through a network: results from the French ISO-RAISIN surveillance system. *Journal of Hospital Infection* 72(2), 127–134. DOI: 10.1016/j.jhin.2009.03.005.

Barrett, C.D., Celestin, A., Fish, E., Glass, C.C., Eskander, M.F. *et al.* (2016) Surgical wound assessment by sonography in the prediction of surgical wound infections. *Journal of Trauma and Acute Care Surgery* 80(2), 229–236. DOI: 10.1097/TA.0000000000000908.

Beal, M.W., Brown, D.C. and Shofer, F.S. (2000) The effects of perioperative hypothermia and the duration of anesthesia on postoperative wound infection rate in clean wounds: a retrospective study. *Veterinary Surgery* 29(2), 123–127. DOI: 10.1111/j.1532-950x.2000.00123.x.

Becker, K.L., Nylén, E.S., White, J.C., Müller, B. and Snider, R.H. (2004) Clinical review 167: Procalcitonin and the calcitonin gene family of peptides in inflammation, infection, and sepsis: a journey from calcitonin back to its precursors. *Journal of Clinical Endocrinology and Metabolism* 89(4), 1512–1525. DOI: 10.1210/jc.2002-021444.

Beldi, G., Bisch-Knaden, S., Banz, V., Mühlemann, K. and Candinas, D. (2009) Impact of intraoperative behavior on surgical site infections. *The American Journal of Surgery* 198(2), 157–162. DOI: 10.1016/j.amjsurg.2008.09.023.

Biermann, N., Doyle, A., Sanchez, J. and McClure, T. (2015) Observational study on the occurrence of surgical glove perforation and associated risk factors in large animal surgery. *Veterinary Surgery* 44, E41–E73.

Brandt, C., Sohr, D., Behnke, M., Daschner, F., Rüden, H. *et al.* (2006) Reduction of surgical site infection rates associated with active surveillance. *Infection Control and Hospital Epidemiology* 27(12), 1347–1351. DOI: 10.1086/509843.

Brown, D.C., Conzemius, M.G., Shofer, F. and Swann, H. (1997) Epidemiologic evaluation of postoperative wound infections in dogs and cats. *Journal of the American Veterinary Medical Association* 210(9), 1302–1306.

Denis Verwilghen and Kelly L. Bowlt Blacklock

Bryce, E. and Forrester, L. (2012) How long is long enough? Determining the optimal surgical site infection surveillance period. *Infection Control and Hospital Epidemiology* 33(11), 1178–1179. DOI: 10.1086/668037.

Campbell, D.A., Henderson, W.G., Englesbe, M.J., Hall, B.L., O'Reilly, M, *et al*. (2008) Surgical site infection prevention: the importance of operative duration and blood transfusion – results of the first American College of Surgeons – National Surgical Quality Improvement Program Best Practices Initiative. *Journal of the American College of Surgeons* 207(6), 810–820. DOI: 10.1016/j.jamcollsurg.2008.08.018.

Canner, G.C., Steinberg, M.E., Heppenstall, R.B. and Balderston, R. (1984) The infected hip after total hip arthroplasty. *Journal of Bone & Joint Surgery* 66(9), 1393–1399. DOI: 10.2106/00004623-198466090-00012.

Carlson, M.A. (1997) Acute wound failure. *Surgical Clinics of North America* 77(3), 607–636. DOI: 10.1016/s0039-6109(05)70571-5.

Casadevall, A. and Pirofski, L. (2003) The damage-response framework of microbial pathogenesis. *Nature Reviews Microbiology* 1(1), 17–24. DOI: 10.1038/nrmicro732.

CDC (2022) *Surgical Site Infection Event (SSI)*. Centers for Disease Control and Prevention, Atlanta, Georgia. Available at: www.cdc.gov/nhsn/pdfs/pscmanual/9pscssicurrent.pdf (accessed 17 November 2022).

Cho, J.G., Oh, Y.I., Song, K.H. and Seo, K.W. (2021) Evaluation and comparison of serum procalcitonin and heparin-binding protein levels as biomarkers of bacterial infection in cats. *Journal of Feline Medicine and Surgery* 23(4), 370–374. DOI: 10.1177/1098612X20959973.

Condon, R.E., Schulte, W.J., Malangoni, M.A. and Anderson-Teschendorf, M.J. (1983) Effectiveness of a surgical wound surveillance program. *Archives of Surgery* 118(3), 303–307. DOI: 10.1001/archsurg.1983.01390030035006.

Cyteval, C. and Bourdon, A. (2012) Imaging orthopedic implant infections. *Diagnostic and Interventional Imaging* 93(6), 547–557. DOI: 10.1016/j.diii.2012.03.004.

Dargaville, T.R., Farrugia, B.L., Broadbent, J.A., Pace, S., Upton, Z. *et al*. (2013) Sensors and imaging for wound healing: a review. *Biosensors & Bioelectronics* 41, 30–42. DOI: 10.1016/j.bios.2012.09.029.

David, T.S. and Vrahas, M.S. (2000) Perioperative lower urinary tract infections and deep sepsis in patients undergoing total joint arthroplasty. *Journal of the American Academy of Orthopaedic Surgeons* 8(1), 66–74. DOI: 10.5435/00124635-200001000-00007.

Davis, P.J., Spady, D., de Gara, C. and Forgie, S.E. (2008) Practices and attitudes of surgeons toward the prevention of surgical site infections: a provincial survey in Alberta, Canada. *Infection Control and Hospital Epidemiology* 29(12), 1164–1166. DOI: 10.1086/592699.

Donham, R.T., Mazzei, W.J. and Jones, R.L. (1996) Association of anesthesia clincial directors procedure times glossary. *American Journal of Anesthesiology* 23, S1–S12.

ECDC (2012) *Surveillance of Surgical Site Infections In European Hospitals – HAISSI Protocol*. European Centre for Disease Prevention and Control, Stockholm, Sweden. Available at: www.ecdc.europa.eu/sites/default/files/media/en/publications/Publications/120215_TED_SSI_protocol.pdf (accessed 8 January 2023).

ECDC (2019) Healthcare-associated infections: surgical site infections. In: *Annual Epidemiological Report for 2017*. European Centre for Disease Prevention and Control, Stockholm. Available at: www.ecdc.europa.eu/en/publications-data/healthcare-associated-infections-surgical-site-infections-annual-1 (accessed 21 October 2022).

Emori, T.G., Culver, D.H., Horan, T.C., Jarvis, W.R., White, J.W. *et al*. (1991) National nosocomial infections surveillance system (NNIS): description of surveillance methods. *American Journal of Infection Control* 19, 19–35.

Erasmus, V., Daha, T.J., Brug, H., Richardus, J.H., Behrendt, M.D. *et al*. (2010) Systematic review of studies on compliance with hand hygiene guidelines in hospital care. *Infection Control & Hospital Epidemiology* 31, 283–294.

Ercole, F.F., Starling, C.E., Chianca, T.C. and Carneiro, M. (2007) Applicability of the national nosocomial infections surveillance system risk index for the prediction of surgical site infections: a review. *Brazilian Journal of Infectious Diseases* 11, 134–141.

Estrin, A., Rodriguez-Diaz, J.M. and Hayes, G.M. (2021) Real-time analysis of intraoperative delays and variations in intraoperative workflow with level of experience of the primary surgeon in small animal surgery. *Veterinary Surgery* 50, 1600–1608.

Etter, S.W., Ragetly, G.R., Bennett, R.A. and Schaeffer, D.J. (2013) Effect of using triclosan-impregnated suture for incisional closure on surgical site infection and inflammation following tibial plateau leveling osteotomy in dogs. *Journal of the American Veterinary Medical Association* 242, 355–358.

Eugster, S., Schawalder, P., Gaschen, F. and Boerlin, P. (2004) A prospective study of postoperative surgical site infections in dogs and cats. *Veterinary Surgery* 33, 542–550.

Evans, L.K., Knowles, T.G., Werrett, G. and Holt, P.E. (2009) The efficacy of chlorhexidine gluconate in canine skin preparation – practice survey and clinical trials. *Journal of Small Animal Practice* 50, 458–465.

EWMA (2005) *Position Document: Identifying Criteria For Wound Infection*. European Wound Management Association, London. Available at: www.cslr.cz/do

wnload/English_pos_doc_final.pdf (accessed 21 October 2022).

Fink, B., Gebhard, A., Fuerst, M., Berger, I. and Schafer, P. (2013) High diagnostic value of synovial biopsy in periprosthetic joint infection of the hip. *Clinical Orthopaedics and Related Research* 471, 956–964.

Fitzpatrick, N. and Solano, M.A. (2010) Predictive variables for complications after TPLO with stifle inspection by arthrotomy in 1000 consecutive dogs. *Veterinary Surgery* 39, 460–474.

Frey, T.N., Hoelzler, M.G., Scavelli, T.D., Fulcher, R.P. and Bastian, R.P. (2010) Risk factors for surgical site infection-inflammation in dogs undergoing surgery for rupture of the cranial cruciate ligament: 902 cases (2005–2006). *Journal of the American Veterinary Medical Association* 236, 88–94.

Gallagher, A.D. and Mertens, W.D. (2012) Implant removal rate from infection after tibial plateau leveling osteotomy in dogs. *Veterinary Surgery* 41, 705–711.

Garcia Stickney, D.N. and Thieman Mankin, K.M. (2018) The impact of postdischarge surveillance on surgical site infection diagnosis. *Veterinary Surgery* 47, 66–73.

Gatineau, M., Dupuis, J., Plante, J. and Moreau, M. (2011) Retrospective study of 476 tibial plateau levelling osteotomy procedures. Rate of subsequent 'pivot shift', meniscal tear and other complications. *Veterinary and Comparative Orthopaedics and Traumatology* 24, 333–341.

Gaynes, R.P. (2000) Surgical-site infections and the NNIS SSI Risk Index: room for improvement. *Infection Control & Hospital Epidemiology* 21, 184–185.

Glenn, O., Faux, I., Griffin, H. and Blacklock, K. (2022) Accuracy of a client questionnaire at diagnosing surgical site infections in an active surveillance system (abstract). *Veterinary Surgery* 51, O1–O54.

Gould, D. (2014) Infection control practice: interview with 20 nurses reveals themes of rationalising their own behaviour and justifying any deviations from policy. *Evidence-Based Nursing* 18, 59.

Guglielmi, G., Muscarella, S., Leone, A. and Peh, W. (2008) Imaging of metabolic bone diseases. *Radiologic Clinics of North America* 46, 735–754.

Haley, R.W., Culver, D.H., White, J.W., Morgan, W.M., Emori, T.G., Munn, V.P. and Hooton, T.M. (1985) The efficacy of infection surveillance and control programs in preventing nosocomial infections in US hospitals. *American Journal of Epidemiology* 121, 182–205.

Harris, W. and Heaney, R. (1969) Skeletal renewal and metabolic bone disease. *New England Journal of Medicine* 280, 193–202.

Haynes, A.B., Weiser, T.G., Berry, W.R., Lipsitz, S.R., Breizat, A.H. *et al.* (2009) A surgical safety checklist to reduce morbidity and mortality in a global population. *New England Journal of Medicine* 360, 491–499.

Heldmann, E., Brown, D.C. and Shofer, F. (1999) The association of propofol usage with postoperative wound infection rate in clean wounds: a retrospective study. *Veterinary Surgery* 28, 256–259.

Herron, T. and Gossman, W. (2022) *111 Indium White Blood Cell Scan*. StatPearls, Treasure Island, Florida.

HICPAC (2020) *Surgical Site Infection (SSI) Event*. Healthcare Infection Control Practices Advisory Committee, CDC, Atlanta, Georgia.

Holmberg, D.L. (1985) The use of prophylactic penicillin in orthopedic surgery: A clinical trial. *Veterinary Surgery* 14, 160–165. DOI: 10.1111/j.1532-950X.1985.tb00850.x.

Humphreys, H. (2009) Preventing surgical site infection. Where now? *Journal of Hospital Infection* 73, 316–322. DOI: 10.1016/j.jhin.2009.03.028.

Hunziker, S., Hugle, T., Schuchardt, K., Groeschl, I., Schuetz, P. *et al.* (2010) The value of serum procalcitonin level for differentiation of infectious from non-infectious causes of fever after orthopaedic surgery. *Journal of Bone and Joint Surgery* 92, 138–148.

Jafarzadeh, A., Hadavi, M., Hassanshahi, G., Rezaeian, M. and Vazirinejad, R. (2020) General anesthetics on immune system cytokines: a narrative review article. *Anesthesia and Pain Medicine* 10, e103033.

Kessler, B., Sendi, P., Graber, P., Knupp, M., Zwicky, L., Hintermann, B. and Zimmerli, W. (2012) Risk factors for periprosthetic ankle joint infection: a case–control study. *Journal of Bone and Joint Surgery* 94, 1871–1876.

Koek, M.B., Wille, J.C., Isken, M.R., Voss, A. and van Benthem, B.H. (2015) Post-discharge surveillance (PDS) for surgical site infections: a good method is more important than a long duration. *Eurosurveillance* 20, 21042.

Kolbel, B., Wienert, S., Dimitriadis, J., Kendoff, D., Gehrke, T. *et al.* (2015) [CD15 focus score for diagnostics of periprosthetic joint infections: neutrophilic granulocytes quantification mode and the development of morphometric software (CD15 quantifier)]. *Zeitschrift für Rheumatologie* 74, 622–630 (in German).

Kurmann, A., Peter, M., Tschan, F., Muhlemann, K., Candinas, D. and Beldi, G. (2011) Adverse effect of noise in the operating theatre on surgical-site infection. *British Journal of Surgery* 98, 1021–1025.

Lankiewicz, J.D., Yokoe, D.S., Olsen, M.A., Onufrak, F., Fraser, V.J. *et al.* (2012) Beyond 30 days: does limiting the duration of surgical site infection follow-up limit detection? *Infection Control and Hospital Epidemiology* 33, 202–204.

Leaper, D.J., Tanner, J., Kiernan, M., Assadian, O. and Edmiston, C.E. Jr. (2014) Surgical site infection: poor compliance with guidelines and care bundles. *International Wound Journal* 12, 357–362.

Lee, J.W., Yu, S.N., Yoo, I.D., Jeon, M.H., Hong, C.H. *et al.* (2019) Clinical application of dual-phase F-18 sodium-fluoride bone PET/CT for diagnosing surgical site infection following orthopedic surgery. *Medicine (Baltimore)* 98, e14770.

Denis Verwilghen and Kelly L. Bowlt Blacklock

Lewis, S.S., Cox, G.M. and Stout, J.E. (2014) Clinical utility of indium 111-labeled white blood cell scintigraphy for evaluation of suspected infection. *Open Forum Infectious Diseases* 1, ofu089.

Limon, E., Shaw, E., Badia, J.M., Piriz, M., Escofet, R. *et al.* (2014) Post-discharge surgical site infections after uncomplicated elective colorectal surgery: impact and risk factors. The experience of the VINCat Program. *Journal of Hospital Infection* 86, 127–132.

Liu, S., Zhang, J., Yin, H., Pang, L., Wu, B. and Shi, H. (2020) The value of ^{18}F-FDG PET/CT in diagnosing and localising deep sternal wound infection to guide surgical debridement. *International Wound Journal* 17, 1019–1027.

Lofqvist, K., Kjelgaard-Hansen, M. and Nielsen, M.B.M. (2018) Usefulness of C-reactive protein and serum amyloid A in early detection of postoperative infectious complications to tibial plateau leveling osteotomy in dogs. *Acta Veterinaria Scandinavica* 60, 30. DOI: 10.1186/s13028-018-0385-5.

Mangram, A.J., Horan, T.C., Pearson, M.L., Silver, L.C. and Jarvis, W.R. (1999) Guideline for prevention of surgical site infection, 1999. Hospital Infection Control Practices Advisory Committee. *Infection Control & Hospital Epidemiology* 20, 250–278.

Mannien, J., Wille, J.C., Snoeren, R.L. and van den Hof, S. (2006) Impact of postdischarge surveillance on surgical site infection rates for several surgical procedures: results from the nosocomial surveillance network in the Netherlands. *Infection Control & Hospital Epidemiology* 27, 809–816.

Mauffrey, C., Herbert, B., Young, H., Wilson, M.L., Hake, M. *et al.* (2016) The role of biofilm on orthopaedic implants: the "Holy Grail" of post-traumatic infection management? *European Journal of Trauma and Emergency Surgery* 42, 411–416.

Mayhew, P.D., Freeman, L., Kwan, T. and Brown, D.C. (2012) Comparison of surgical site infection rates in clean and clean-contaminated wounds in dogs and cats after minimally invasive versus open surgery: 179 cases (2007–2008). *Journal of the American Veterinary Medical Association* 240, 193–198.

Mohri, Y., Miki, C., Kobayashi, M., Okita, Y., Inoue, M. *et al.* (2014) Correlation between preoperative systemic inflammation and postoperative infection in patients with gastrointestinal cancer: a multicenter study. *Surgery Today* 44, 859–867.

Moorthy, K., Munz, Y., Undre, S. and Darzi, A. (2004) Objective evaluation of the effect of noise on the performance of a complex laparoscopic task. *Surgery* 136, 25–30.

Morawietz, L., Tiddens, O., Mueller, M., Tohtz, S., Gansukh, T. *et al.* (2009) Twenty-three neutrophil granulocytes in 10 high-power fields is the best histopathological threshold to differentiate between aseptic and septic endoprosthesis loosening. *Histopathology* 54, 847–853.

Natoli, R.M., Harro, J. and Shirtliff, M. (2020) Non-culture-based methods to aide in the diagnosis of implant-associated infection after fracture surgery. *Techniques in Orthopaedics* 35, 91–99.

Nazarali, A., Singh, A. and Weese, J.S. (2014) Perioperative administration of antimicrobials during tibial plateau leveling osteotomy. *Veterinary Surgery* 43, 966–971.

Nicholson, M., Beal, M., Shofer, F. and Brown, D.C. (2002) Epidemiologic evaluation of postoperative wound infection in clean-contaminated wounds: a retrospective study of 239 dogs and cats. *Veterinary Surgery* 31, 577–581.

Obremskey, W.T., Metsemakers, W.J., Schlatterer, D.R., Tetsworth, K., Egol, K. *et al.* (2020) Musculoskeletal infection in orthopaedic trauma. Assessment of the 2018 International Consensus Meeting on Musculoskeletal Infection. *Journal of Bone and Joint Surgery-American* 102, e44.

O'Rourke, K., Kibbee, N. and Stubbs, A. (2015) Ultrasound for the evaluation of skin and soft tissue infections. *Missouri Medicine* 112, 202–205.

Parvizi, J., Zmistowski, B., Berbari, E.F., Bauer, T.W., Springer, B.D. *et al.* (2011) New definition for periprosthetic joint infection: from the workgroup of the musculoskeletal infection society. *Clinical Orthopaedics and Related Research* 469, 2992–2994.

Peeters, M.E. and Kirpensteijn, J. (2011) Comparison of surgical variables and short-term postoperative complications in healthy dogs undergoing ovariohysterectomy or ovariectomy. *Journal of the American Veterinary Medical Association* 238, 189–194.

Pelosi, A. (2018) The operating room. In: Johnston, S. and Tobias, K. (eds) *Veterinary Surgery: Small Animal*. Elsevier, St Louis, Missouri, pp. 177–179.

Peterson, J.L., Moore, G.E. and Risselada, M. (2021) Influence of musical preferences and intraoperative questions on suturing speed. *Veterinary Surgery* 50, 1617–1623.

Pittet, D. (2004) The Lowbury lecture: behaviour in infection control. *Journal of Hospital Infection* 58, 1–13.

Pratesi, A., Moores, A.P., Downes, C., Grierson, J. and Maddox, T.W. (2015) Efficacy of postoperative antimicrobial use for clean orthopedic implant surgery in dogs: a prospective randomized study in 100 consecutive cases. *Veterinary Surgery* 44, 653–660.

Pruzansky, J.S., Bronson, M.J., Grelsamer, R.P., Strauss, E. and Moucha, C.S. (2014) Prevalence of modifiable surgical site infection risk factors in hip and knee joint arthroplasty patients at an urban academic hospital. *Journal of Arthroplasty* 29, 272–276.

Rioux, C., Grandbastien, B. and Astagneau, P. (2007) Impact of a six-year control programme on surgical site infections in France: results of the INCISO surveillance. *Journal of Hospital Infection* 66, 217–223.

Sands, K., Vineyard, G. and Platt, R. (1996) Surgical site infections occurring after hospital discharge. *Journal of Infectious Diseases* 173, 963–970.

Sanger, P.C., van Ramshorst, G.H., Mercan, E., Huang, S., Hartzler, A.L. *et al.* (2016) A prognostic model of surgical site infection using daily clinical wound assessment. *Journal of the American College of Surgeons* 223, 259–270.e2.

Savicky, R., Beale, B., Murtaugh, R., Swiderski-Hazlett, J. and Unis, M. (2013) Outcome following removal of TPLO implants with surgical site infection. *Veterinary and Comparative Orthopaedics and Traumatology* 26, 260–265.

Schmidt, J.S., Hartnack, S., Schuller, S., Kuster, S.P. and Willi, B. (2021) Hand hygiene compliance in companion animal clinics and practices in Switzerland: an observational study. *Veterinary Record* 189, e307. DOI: 10.1002/vetr.307.

Schuetz, P., Albrich, W. and Mueller, B. (2011) Procalcitonin for diagnosis of infection and guide to antibiotic decisions: past, present and future. *BMC Medicine* 9, 107. DOI: 10.1186/1741-7015-9-107.

Sidhu, D.S., Gull, T. and Skinner, O.T. (2021) Influence of intraoperative closed glove exchange on glove contamination during clean soft tissue surgeries. *Veterinary Surgery* 50, 1510–1517.

Smith, G.C. and Pell, J.P. (2003) Parachute use to prevent death and major trauma related to gravitational challenge: systematic review of randomised controlled trials. *British Medical Journal* 327, 1459–1461.

Solano, M.A., Danielski, A., Kovach, K., Fitzpatrick, N. and Farrell, M. (2015) Locking plate and screw fixation after tibial plateau leveling osteotomy reduces postoperative infection rate in dogs over 50 kg. *Veterinary Surgery* 44, 59–64.

Soldatos, T., Durand, D.J., Subhawong, T.K., Carrino, J.A. and Chhabra, A. (2012) Magnetic resonance imaging of musculoskeletal infections: systematic diagnostic assessment and key points. *Academic Radiology* 19, 1434–1443.

Staszewicz, W., Eisenring, M.C., Bettschart, V., Harbarth, S. and Troillet, N. (2014) Thirteen years of surgical site infection surveillance in Swiss hospitals. *Journal of Hospital Infection* 88, 40–47.

Stetter, J., Boge, G.S., Grönlund, U. and Bergstrom, A. (2021) Risk factors for surgical site infection associated with clean surgical procedures in dogs. *Research in Veterinary Science* 136, 616–621.

Sutton, D. (2003) *Textbook of Radiology and Imaging*. Churchill Livingstone, London.

Tamayol, A., Akbari, M., Zilberman, Y., Comotto, M., Lesha, E. *et al.* (2016) Flexible pH-sensing hydrogel fibers for epidermal applications. *Advanced Healthcare Materials* 5, 711–719.

Torfs, S., Levet, T., Delesalle, C., Dewulf, J., Vlaminck, L. *et al.* (2010) Risk factors for incisional complications after exploratory celiotomy in horses: do skin staples increase the risk? *Veterinary Surgery* 39, 616–620.

Troia, R., Giunti, M. and Goggs, R. (2018) Plasma procalcitonin concentrations predict organ dysfunction and outcome in dogs with sepsis. *BMC Veterinary Research* 14, 111. DOI: 10.1186/s12917-018-1427-y.

Turk, R., Singh, A. and Weese, J.S. (2015) Prospective surgical site infection surveillance in dogs. *Veterinary Surgery* 44, 2–8.

Uckay, I., Luebbeke, A., Emonet, S., Tovmirzaeva, L., Stern, R. *et al.* (2009) Low incidence of haematogenous seeding to total hip and knee prostheses in patients with remote infections. *Journal of Infection* 59, 337–345.

Uckay, I., Harbarth, S., Peter, R., Lew, D., Hoffmeyer, P. *et al.* (2010) Preventing surgical site infections. *Expert Review of Anti-infective Therapy* 8, 657–670.

Udofia, A.A., Oyetunji, T. and Fossett, D. (2014) 115 Risk factors for laminectomy surgical site infection in a majority minority patient population. *Neurosurgery* 61 (Suppl. 1), 196–197.

Umit, U.M., Sina, M., Ferhat, Y., Yasemin, P., Meltem, K. and Ozdemir, A.A. (2014) Surgeon behavior and knowledge on hand scrub and skin antisepsis in the operating room. *Journal of Surgical Education* 71, 241–245.

Vasseur, P.B., Paul, H.A., Enos, L.R. and Hirsh, D.C. (1985) Infection rates in clean surgical procedures: a comparison of ampicillin prophylaxis vs a placebo. *Journal of the American Veterinary Medical Association* 187, 825–827.

Vasseur, P.B., Levy, J., Dowd, E. and Eliot, J. (1988) Surgical wound infection rates in dogs and cats. Data from a teaching hospital. *Veterinary Surgery* 17, 60–64.

Velasco, E., Thuler, L.C.S., Martins, C.A.D., Dias, L.M.D. and Conalves, V. (1996) Risk factors for infectious complications after abdominal surgery for malignant disease. *American Journal of Infection Control* 24, 1–6.

Verwilghen, D., Findji, S., Weese, J.S., Singh, A., Dupre, G, *et al.* (2013) Evidence based hand hygiene in veterinary surgery: what is holding us back? In: *Annual Symposium of the American College Of Veterinary Surgeons*. San Antonio, Texas.

Verwilghen, D. (2018) The operative risk, the surgical patient, the surgery facility, the operating team. In: Auer, J., Stick, J., Kümmerle, J.M. and Prange, T. (eds) *Equine Surgery*, 5th edn. Elsevier, St Louis, Missouri, pp. 143–183.

Walton, B. (1979) Effects of anaesthesia and surgery on immune status. *British Journal of Anaesthesia* 51, 37–43.

Wang, Y., Cheung, J.P. and Cheung, K.M. (2016) Use of PET/CT in the early diagnosis of implant related wound infection and avoidance of wound debridement. *European Spine Journal* 25 (Suppl. 1), 38–43.

Denis Verwilghen and Kelly L. Bowlt Blacklock

Ward, W.G., Cooper, J.M., Lippert, D., Kablawi, R.O., Neiberg, R.H. and Sherertz, R.J. (2014) Glove and gown effects on intraoperative bacterial contamination. *Annals of Surgery* 259, 591–597.

Webster, C., Neumayer, L., Smout, R., Horn, S., Daley, J., Henderson, W. and Khuri, S. (2003) Prognostic models of abdominal wound dehiscence after laparotomy. *Journal of Surgical Research* 109, 130–137.

Whittem, T.L., Johnson, A.L., Smith, C.W., Schaeffer, D.J., Coolman, B.R. *et al.* (1999) Effect of perioperative prophylactic antimicrobial treatment in dogs undergoing elective orthopedic surgery. *Journal of the American Veterinary Medical Association* 215, 212–216.

WHO (2009) WHO surgical safety checklist. World Health Organization, Geneva, Switzerland. Available at: www.who.int/teams/integrated-health-services/pat ient-safety/research/safe-surgery/tool-and-resources (accessed 25 October 2022).

Wilson, D.A., Badertscher, R.R. 2nd, Boero, M.J., Baker, G.J. and Foreman, J.H. (1989) Ultrasonographic evaluation of the healing of ventral midline abdominal incisions in the horse. *Equine Veterinary Journal* 21(Suppl. 7), 107–110. DOI: 10.1111/j.2042-3306.1989.tb05667.x.

Wurtz, R., Wittrock, B., Lavin, M.A. and Zawacki, A. (2001) Do new surgeons have higher surgical-site infection rates? *Infection Control & Hospital Epidemiology* 22, 375–377.

Yang, F., Yang, Z., Feng, J., Zhang, L., Ma, D. and Yang, J. (2016) Three phase bone scintigraphy with ^{99m}Tc-MDP and serological indices in detecting infection after internal fixation in malunion or nonunion traumatic fractures. *Hellenic Journal of Nuclear Medicine* 19, 130–134.

Yochum, T. and Rowe, L. (2004). *Essentials of Skeletal Radiology*. Lippincott Williams & Wilkins, Baltimore, Maryland.

Zmistowski, B., Della Valle, C., Bauer, T.W., Malizos, K.N., Alavi, A. *et al.* (2014) Diagnosis of periprosthetic joint infection. *Journal of Orthopaedic Research* 32 (Suppl. 1), S98–S107.

10 Treatment of Surgical-Site Infections

Kelly L. Bowlt Blacklock[1*], Owen Glenn[1] and Denis Verwilghen[2]

[1]Royal (Dick) School of Veterinary Studies, University of Edinburgh, Roslin, UK; [2]University of Sydney, Camperdown, NSW 2006, Australia

10.1   Introduction

After one week of hospitalization, a large, grotesque abscess was found at the surgical site on her left groin. At mama's death on May 9, 2012, her left groin, lower left torso and thigh were eaten away. Her underlying flesh and muscle were exposed. It was a brutal death for such a beautiful person.

Franchot Karl, writing about his mother, Gladys Reaves (Karl, 2014)

Infection has forever been the scourge of the surgeon, and rates have historically been of epidemic proportions. The first reliable statistics on operative mortality were published by Malgaigne (1841), which documented a grim average mortality of 60% following limb amputation. The cause of death was recorded as 'hospital diseases': erysipelas, tetanus, pyemia, septicaemia and gangrene. At the time, suppuration and pus formation was considered by most surgeons as a necessary and unavoidable stage of wound healing. The fact that surgeons prided themselves on wearing gowns covered in blood, bodily fluid and dirt from previous operations as a badge of a long and distinguished career probably did much to encourage such 'hospital diseases' (Buicko *et al.*, 2016). The publication of Semmelweis's book, *The Etiology, the Concept and the Prophylaxis of Puerperal Fever*, in 1861 prompted some in the medical world to question whether nosocomial infections were an inevitable consumer of human life following surgery. Inspired by microbiologist Louis Pasteur's germ theory of disease, Joseph Lister's ground-breaking work on surgical asepsis and hand hygiene, while initially ridiculed, led to a decrease in post-operative infections and distinguished him as the 'father of modern surgery'. Over a century after Lister's death, the battles against surgical-site infections (SSIs) are still raging and behind each 'case' is a human or animal patient and their families. In *The Art of War*, Sun Tzu advises that to achieve military success, one must 'know the enemy and know yourself' (Sun Tsu, 2010). So where do we stand now in this war against infection, and what weapons do we have to neutralize our silent enemy?

10.2   Patient Assessment

The best treatment for SSIs is avoiding them in the first place. Most SSIs are caused by contamination of an incision with microorganisms from the patient's own body during surgery, and measures can be taken in the pre-, intra- and post-operative phases of care to reduce the risk of infection (NICE, 2019) (see Section 2 and Chapter 8, this volume). In contrast to the plethora of data regarding preventative strategies, clear guidelines for SSI management are lacking. The post-operative patient should be assessed regularly to allow rapid intervention if infection eventuates. This includes taking the patient's history, physical examination and wound assessment.

10.2.1   Patient history

Typically, SSI symptoms appear within 3–7 days of a surgical procedure. Although we tend to limit ourselves to 30-day monitoring periods, an SSI can express itself at any time following a surgical procedure, whether weeks, months or years later. Patients with a history of endocrinopathies, or who have undergone long or contaminated surgeries, are at increased risk of SSIs (Nicholson *et al.*, 2002).

---

*Corresponding author: Kelly.blacklock@ed.ac.uk

DOI: 10.1079/9781789244977.0010

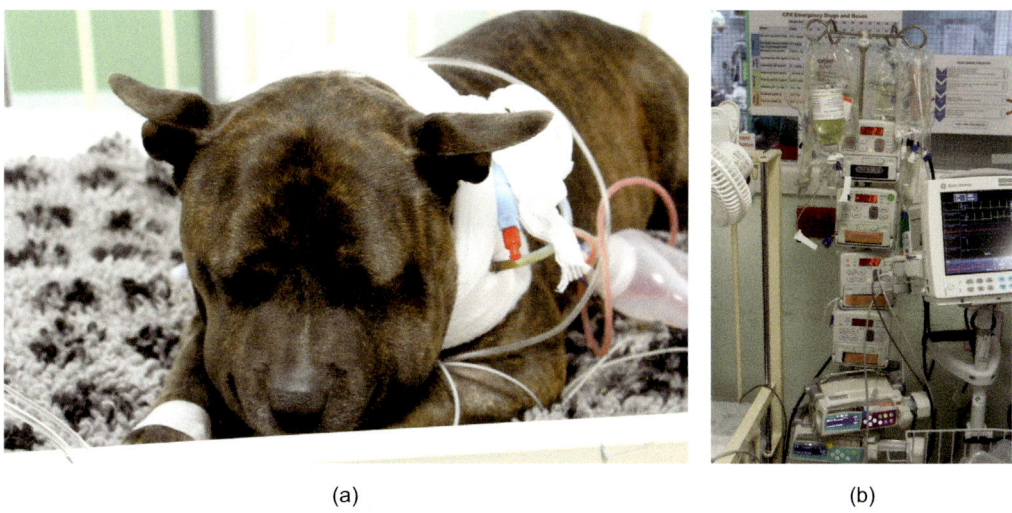

(a)   (b)

Fig. 10.1. (a, b) Wherever possible, patients with sepsis should be referred to a hospital with a dedicated critical care team because of the dynamic nature of their condition, which mandates a bespoke and often complex package of supportive treatment. The patient shown has septic peritonitis and has a feeding tube and abdominal active suction drains in place, as well as several intravenous cannulae to provide numerous intravenous supportive products.

10.2.2 Physical assessment

A full physical examination should be performed to identify comorbidities and to assess the patient for sepsis. Further information pertaining to septic shock can be found in Chapter 19 (this volume), and the clinician is encouraged to contact their local emergency and critical care facility for urgent advice and referral where appropriate (Fig. 10.1).

10.2.3 Wound evaluation

Following surgery, if the incision has been closed, primarily it should be protected by a sterile dressing for 24–48 h (Nelson, 2011). Thereafter, wound coverage may not be beneficial and may hinder the caretaker in monitoring the incision for signs of inflammation/infection (Weese, 2008). The authors use a sterile, liquid skin film adhesive (2-octyl cyanoacrylate) instead of skin sutures/staples, which acts as a physical barrier to bacteria and therefore negates the requirement for a post-operative dressing. In humans, this product has been shown to improve healing rates and reduce SSIs, although similar data in veterinary species are lacking (Towfigh *et al.*, 2008; Wilson, 2008; Rushbrook *et al.*, 2014; Wang *et al.*, 2020).

When evaluating a post-operative wound, dressings should be removed to allow thorough evaluation of the surgical site. Caretakers should wash hands before and after dressing changes and any contact with the surgical site, and should don disposable, non-sterile examination gloves when handling the wound. Interestingly, the duration of hospitalization is associated with a greater risk of infection with multidrug-resistant (MDR) bacteria, and therefore patients should be discharged from the hospital at the earliest safe opportunity (Ogeer-Gyles *et al.*, 2006).

Clinical signs of an SSI include erythema, localized pain, discharge from the wound, persistent pyrexia, wound dehiscence and/or problems with wound healing (Fig. 10.2) (Dellinger, 2015).

Serial photography of the wound is encouraged. In human medicine, the addition of wound photos to clinical notes significantly improves diagnostic accuracy and confidence, and decreases overtreatment: this ultimately decreases costs and improves clinical outcomes (Sanger *et al.*, 2017). In the authors' experience, photographic data allow the wound to be managed more successfully with a team approach and we would encourage practitioners to send photographs of their patients' wounds to a preferred referral hospital who would be delighted to provide advice and assistance. Finally, and importantly, serial photography is a useful reminder of the success achieved to date

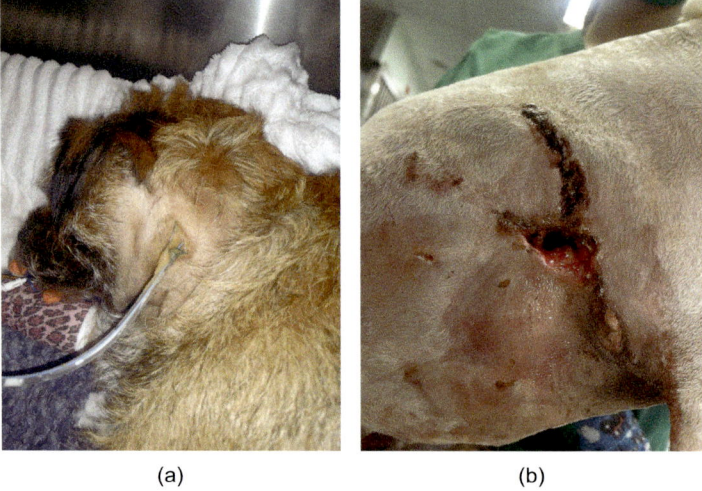

(a)   (b)

Fig. 10.2. (a) Purulent malodorous discharge associated with the stoma of an oesophageal feeding tube in a 5-year-old border terrier, consistent with a surgical-site infection. The infection resolved following removal of the tube, lavage and open-wound management of the site using Manuka honey. No oral antibiotics were administered. (b) Wound dehiscence following a thoracotomy in a 1-year-old cavapoo to treat a penetrating thoracic injury sustained during a dog attack. Bacterial culture of the wound yielded a heavy growth of *Serratia fonticola*, a member of the family *Enterobacteriaceae,* found in a wide array of environments, including drinking water, soil and sewage, and rarely described in human medicine as causing skin and soft-tissue infections following trauma (Aljorayid *et al.*, 2016). The wound resolved after 6 days of negative-pressure wound therapy and was then allowed to heal by second intention. The brown appearance of the surgical site dorsally is secondary to the presence of liquid skin film adhesive, the preferred method of skin closure used by the authors.

when one is lamenting the slow progression of healing.

In human medicine, the incidence of methicillin-resistant *Staphylococcus aureus* (MRSA)-associated SSIs increased from 12% to 23% between 2000 and 2005, and was recorded as 43.7% in 2010 (Young and Khadaroo, 2014). In veterinary medicine, methicillin-resistant *Staphylococcus pseudintermedius* (MRSP) is the most common MDR pathogen (seen in up to 47% of SSIs), followed by MRSA (up to 16% of SSIs) (Turk *et al.*, 2015). Given the prevalence of such resistant bacteria, appropriate barrier nursing protocols should be followed immediately for any patient presenting for any surgical wound-related complication (see Chapter 12, this volume).

10.2.4 Necrotizing fasciitis

Necrotizing fasciitis is a rapidly progressive necrotizing infection of skin, soft tissue and deep fascia. Patients present with rapid fulminant tissue destruction and systemic signs of toxicity. Overall survival rate is up to 47% in a tertiary referral hospital (Buriko *et al.*, 2008). These infections can occur following surgery (at the incision or a distant site), but may also be seen in patients with no known history of surgery or skin trauma.

The clinical features associated with necrotizing fasciitis are illustrated in Table 10.1 and Fig. 10.3. Bacterial culture of affected sites have reportedly yielded a wide spectrum of bacterial species, including Lancefield Group G *Streptococcus* (e.g. *Streptococcus canis*), *Pasteurella multocida*, *Macrococcus caseolyticus*, *Proteus mirabilis*, *Escherichia coli*, *Clostridium* spp. and MRSP (Buriko *et al.*, 2008; Kulendra and Corr, 2008; Mayer and Rubin, 2012; Bowlt *et al.*, 2013; Acheampong *et al.*, 2021). Polymicrobial infections occur in many patients, necessitating broad-spectrum antimicrobial coverage.

Importantly, urgent and extensive operative debridement is recommended to reduce mortality among patients with this condition. It is important that all necrotic tissue is removed, which may require limb amputation or the use of axial pattern flaps to close large defects. In selected patients, a less invasive surgical approach may be taken (e.g.

Table 10.1. Clinical features associated with necrotizing fasciitis. Data from Anaya and Dellinger (2007); Buriko *et al.* (2008); Kulendra and Corr (2008); Weese *et al.* (2009); Bowlt *et al.* (2013); Acheampong *et al.* (2021).

Clinical findings	Imaging	Clinical pathology
Rapid development (within hours) and progression of clinical signs	Subcuticular fluid pockets/ abscesses	Increased white blood cell count (with left shift neutrophilia)
Localized swelling, warmth and erythema progressing to swelling of the site	Enlarged draining lymph nodes	Increased C-reactive protein
Wound/lesion changing from red to purple and then black	Gas in soft tissues	Decreased haemoglobin levels
Blistering necrosis	Asymmetric, contrast-enhancing fascial thickening (CT/MRI)	Metabolic acidosis
Extreme localized pain (disproportionate to the skin changes)		Increased blood lactate levels
Pyrexia		
Tachycardia		
Hypotension		
Collapse/shock/depressed mental status		
Poor response to therapy		

CT, computed tomography; MRI, magnetic resonance imaging.

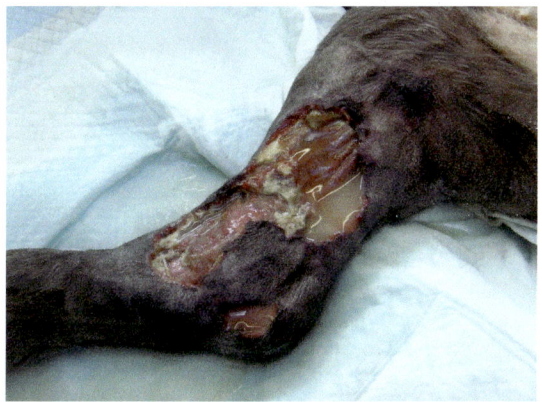

Fig. 10.3. Initial appearance of a wound associated with necrotizing fasciitis in a 2 year old Great Dane who sustained a cat bite in the site only 8 hours previously. Upon presentation, the patient was collapsed, pyrexic and showed extreme pain and bruising in the region of the wound. Over the following 6 hours, she deteriorated despite extensive debridement and intensive care, including generous multi-modal analgesia and cardiovascular support. She died the same day.

less extensive debridement and use of active suction drainage), although in the authors' opinion this is rarely indicated and should be pursued with extreme caution (Csiszer *et al.*, 2010; Bowlt *et al.*, 2013).

10.2.5 Summary

Clinical signs of SSIs typically appear within 3–7 days but can occur at any time following a surgical procedure. A full history and physical examination are essential to rule out comorbidities, especially life-threatening conditions such as sepsis and necrotizing fasciitis. Potential differential diagnoses for SSIs are few but might include other causes of post-operative fever (e.g. urinary tract infection, medications such as opioids in cats (Posner *et al.*, 2010)), pain or post-surgical inflammation without infection.

Emergence of resistant bacteria has reinforced the requirement for antimicrobial stewardship. *S. pseudintermedius* is one of the most commonly cultured bacteria in SSIs, with methicillin-resistant species prevalent. Therefore, bacterial culture of all suspected SSIs is essential to better inform treatment choices. The following section will discuss treatment of patients with SSIs.

10.3 Treatment of SSIs

The thoughtless person playing with penicillin treatment is morally responsible for the death of the man who succumbs to infection with the penicillin-resistant organism.

Sir Alexander Fleming

Clear guidelines for the management of SSIs are lacking, but suggested principles are illustrated

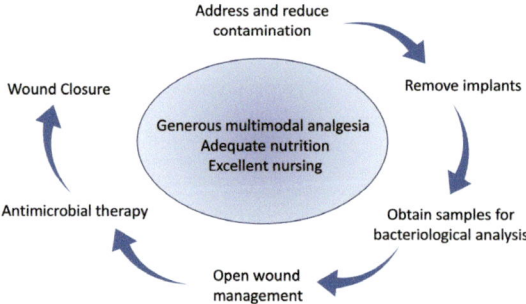

Address and reduce
contamination

Remove implants

Generous multimodal analgesia
Adequate nutrition
Excellent nursing

Wound Closure

Antimicrobial therapy

Obtain samples for
bacteriological analysis

Open wound
management

Fig. 10.4. Suggested treatment protocol for management of surgical-site infections, with generous multi-modal analgesia, adequate nutrition and excellent nursing central to success.

in Fig. 10.4 and further details can be found in the appropriate sections that follow. It is impossible to overemphasize that scrupulous attention must be paid to hand hygiene, cleanliness of the environment and the need for personal protective equipment (Chapters 4, 7 and 6, respectively, this volume).

Infections limited to a mild, superficial, incisional cellulitis without evidence of a wound abscess or deeper extension of infection may be amenable to antibiotic therapy alone (Nelson, 2011). Conversely, not all open wounds require antibiotics; alternative options to facilitate healing should always be explored (Fig. 10.5).

Every surgeon encounters SSIs during their career and the authors would encourage practitioners to contact their local tertiary referral centre for advice at the earliest opportunity: there is nothing more rewarding than helping colleagues to successfully manage their patients' wounds by providing regular bespoke advice, or to accept the responsibility of caring for those patients who need more specialized treatment in a referral environment.

10.3.1 Generous multi-modal analgesia, adequate nutrition and excellent nursing

The provision of tailored and effective multi-modal analgesia for patients with surgical wounds is mandatory. Aside from the negative impact that pain can cause on animal welfare, the surgical stress response and resulting physiological changes can significantly affect bone and wound healing (Huss *et al.*, 2019). While systemic steroid administration can delay wound healing, negligible impact on bone and wound healing is seen when opioids (topical and systemic), local anaesthetics, non-steroidal anti-inflammatories or dissociative agents are administered within authorized dosage regimens (Huss *et al.*, 2019). Alternative analgesics such as tramadol, gabapentin, ketamine and paracetamol also warrant consideration (note: paracetamol cannot be used in cats), and the authors value the

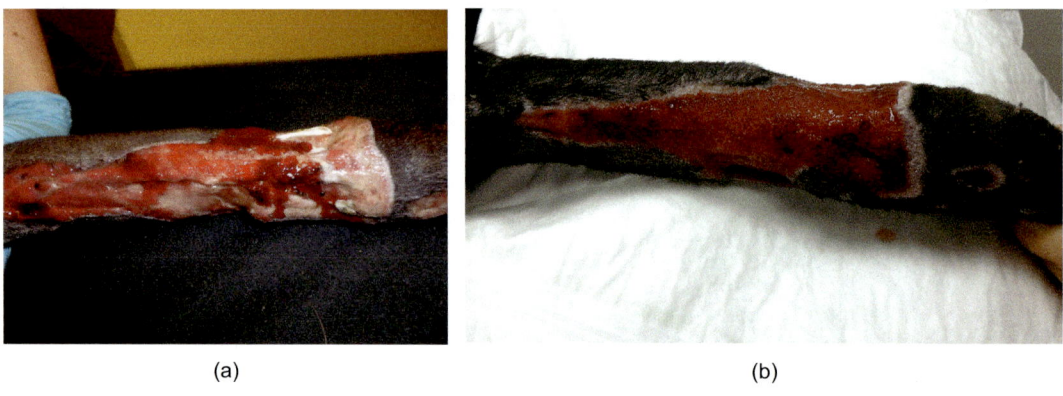

(a)   (b)

Fig. 10.5. (a) A full-thickness skin defect in a 5-year-old cross-breed dog, who presented 3 weeks following a road traffic accident. The wound was lavaged, and bacteriology results yielded a moderate growth of *Staphylococci* spp, that were sensitive to clavulanate-potentiated amoxicillin. A 5-day course of amoxicillin was prescribed. (b) The same wound as in (a), following 10 days of negative-pressure wound therapy. A uniform bed of granulation tissue has formed, which is extremely resistant to infection. Importantly, no further antibiotics are required for this wound. In this patient, a full-thickness skin graft was successfully utilized to close the defect.

regular use of cooling therapy to provide local analgesia.

Like us, most of our sociable companion animals consider food, friends and family to be central to life. It is our role to provide these to our hospitalized patients, and simply spending quality time with them (i.e. when they are not receiving treatment) is hugely beneficial. Every effort should be made to curtail psychological stress while the patient is hospitalized: non-pharmacological options to promote holistic well-being include low-stress handling, pheromone therapy, environmental modifications and sleep promotion (even just turning down the lights in the evening) (Lefman and Prittie, 2019). Using stress scales (https://fearfreepets.com/resources; accessed 25 October 2022) to define stress levels can identify patients for whom additional pharmacological options (e.g. trazodone, benzodiazepines, dexmedetomidine) might be helpful (Lefman and Prittie, 2019).

Eating causes the release of the feel-good chemicals serotonin and dopamine, and patients should be encouraged/assisted to eat as soon as possible. A nursing care plan should allow a resting energy requirement calculation in every inpatient, alongside daily monitoring using a hospitalization sheet. The World Small Animal Veterinary Association (WSAVA) have an excellent nutritional toolkit freely available online (WSAVA, 2022). The presence of a wound causes an increased catabolic state proportional to the severity of the injury, and malnutrition or nutrient deficiency delays healing (Şimşek et al., 2014). Glucose and protein are particularly important during the healing process, and patients should be provided with a high-quality, complete, commercial enteric diet. It may be necessary to place a feeding tube if the patient is unable or unwilling to eat. Some severely hypoproteinaemic, critically ill or septic patients may benefit from additional support (e.g. parenteral nutrition), and advice should be sought from a specialist in emergency and critical care.

Finally, endocrine diseases (e.g. diabetes mellitus, hyperadrenocorticism, hypothyroidism) and uraemia have been implicated in complicating wound healing, and therefore all options to control metabolic disease should be implemented as soon as possible (Lux, 2022).

10.3.2 Addressing and reducing contamination

Once the patient is stabilized, the wound should be opened, debrided and cleaned. Appropriate analgesia, sedation and/or anaesthesia must be provided, and meticulous hand hygiene exercised throughout. Gloves should be worn when handling open wounds. The open wound should be covered with a sterile, water-based lubricant (e.g. K-Y Jelly) to prevent hair entering the wound during clipping. If the fur has regrown around the surgical site (or the original clip was conservative), a large area around the wound should be cleared of fur using clean, well-maintained clippers.

It is imperative that the source of the infection is addressed wherever possible. Necrotic, devitalized and grossly contaminated tissue needs to be removed, and any opportunity for ongoing contamination should be prevented. For example, if the infection is secondary to an enteric wound dehiscence, a resection–anastomosis should be performed and the repair tested for leakage and reinforced (e.g. omentalization, serosal patch) (Fig. 10.6).

Debridement

Wound debridement is an integral element of good wound care and is beneficial because of the presence of devitalized/necrotic tissue within the wound (Gray et al., 2011), which:

- masks or mimic signs of infection;
- provides nutrients for bacteria, particularly anaerobes (e.g. Bacteroides species and Clostridium perfringens) (Urschel, 1999);
- acts as a physical barrier to epithelialization (Kubo et al., 2001);
- prevents the effectiveness of topical preparations (e.g. antimicrobial agents, local anaesthetic); and
- impedes normal matrix formation, angiogenesis, granulation tissue formation and epidermal resurfacing.

Therefore, it is crucial that necrotic tissue is removed as quickly and efficiently as possible to reduce the bioburden and prevent infection (Baranoski and Ayello, 2004), promote wound closure and facilitate wound assessment (Reid and Morison, 1994). Decreasing bioburden also fills the important role of reducing the probability of resistance from

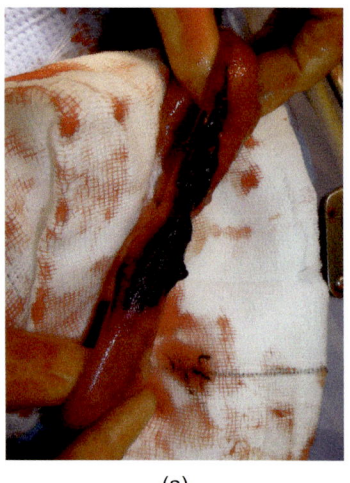 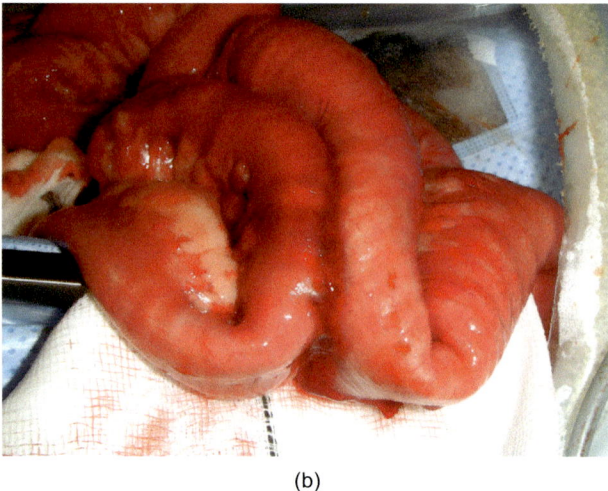

(a)   (b)

Fig. 10.6. (a) Intraoperative photograph of the jejunum in a 3-year-old springer spaniel, 3 days following enterotomy for removal of an intestinal foreign body. Leakage of gastrointestinal contents was apparent from the central portion of the wound, and the enteric wound was blackened along its entire length. (b) The affected length of jejunum was resected, anastomosed and leak tested (Saile *et al.*, 2010; Mullen *et al.*, 2021). A serosal patch was performed and is shown in this image. Thereafter, the abdomen was copiously lavaged and routinely closed. The patient made an uneventful recovery.

antibiotic treatment (Garner *et al.*, 1988; Schiffman *et al.*, 2009; Manna *et al.*, 2021).

There are five main methods of debridement, which are described in Table 10.2. The choice of technique will be based on how quickly debridement is desirable (this will be based on the amount of non-viable tissue present and the anatomical location), availability of skills/products/resources, frequency of care needed and cost implications. Utilizing more than one debridement method will provide consistency in wound bed preparation towards healing.

Wound lavage

Once the source of the infection has been removed or contained, the wound needs to be lavaged to reduce the surface bacterial load and remove any biofilms. Irrigation fluid can splash and spread bacteria to surrounding areas and people, and therefore suitable personal protective equipment is advised (see Chapter 6, this volume), and the patient should be similarly shielded (especially intravenous cannula sites, other open wounds, etc.).

There are three major irrigation variables: delivery method, volume and solution additives. There is a lack of well-designed human and veterinary

trials investigating surgical irrigation practices. Key considerations are discussed below.

SELECTING AN APPROPRIATE IRRIGATION SOLUTION. Normal sterile saline is the favoured irrigation solution because it is isotonic and has the lowest toxicity compared with other solutions. Importantly, the bottle should be discarded after use because bacterial growth can occur in an open container of saline after 24 h. A disadvantage is that saline does not cleanse dirty wounds as effectively as other solutions. Where saline is unavailable, sterile water or tap water could be used, but water toxicity may result when excess volumes are used and microbes (e.g. *Pseudomonas aeruginosa*) can colonize taps (Mena and Gerba, 2009; Fernandez and Griffiths, 2012).

Available alternatives to sterile saline as an irrigation solution are listed in Table 10.3. Commercially available foams, soaps, wipes and solutions with surfactants remove bacteria with less required force due to their surfactant content but can be highly cytotoxic and should be avoided. The use of topical antimicrobial irrigation solutions remains controversial because of resultant cellular toxicity and skin irritation. Worryingly, many bacteria have also developed resistance to antiseptics such that

     Kelly L. Bowlt Blacklock *et al.*

Table 10.2. BEAMS is a mnemonic that is widely used to remember the five types of wound debridement. Data from WoundSource Editors (2018) and Baranoski and Ayello (2004).

Debridement method	Overview	Technique	Advantages	Disadvantages
Biological	Sterile *Lucilia sericata* (green bottle fly) *larvae*.	The sterile maggots are applied to the wound bed with a dressing used to 'confine' the maggots to the wound. Free-range maggots can debride a wound at least twice as fast as those introduced in a biological bag.	Effective, especially in large wounds. Faster than autolytic debridement. Not painful to use. In addition to the larvae ingesting the bacteria and necrotic tissue, they inhibit bacterial growth by releasing ammonia and thereby increasing wound pH, as well as breaking down and preventing biofilm formation.	Maggots may be perceived with distaste. Cannot be used in wounds that communicate with the abdominal or thoracic cavity.
Enzymatic	Exogenous proteolytic, enzymatic liquification of necrotic tissue.	Collagenase digests collagen and necrotic tissue to debride *Clostridium* spp. bacteria.	Not painful to use.	Slow method. Cannot be recommended in heavily contaminated wounds. Antimicrobial agents (including silver-based products) used in conjunction with collagenase can decrease the effectiveness of enzymatic debridement.
Autolytic	Occlusive and semi-occlusive dressings (e.g. hydrogels, hydrocolloids and films).	Most conservative type of debridement, which involves rehydration of necrotic tissue by using a hydrogel or by keeping the wound moist. Endogenous phagocytic cells and proteolytic enzymes then break down necrotic tissue.	Highly selective – only necrotic tissue is affected. Can be used in combination with other debridement techniques. Not painful to use.	Slow method, which increases opportunity for infection, pain and maceration of peri-wound skin. If significant improvement is not seen in 1–2 days, an alternative debridement method should be considered. Requires a functional immune system.

Continued

Table 10.2. Continued

Debridement method	Overview	Technique	Advantages	Disadvantages
Mechanical	Irrigation, hydrotherapy, wet-to-dry dressings, abrasion.	Wet-to-dry dressings are the most commonly used form of mechanical debridement in veterinary medicine. The top layer of the wound bed dries and adheres to an adherent dressing (e.g. gauze), which is then removed, lifting the underlying tissue away with it.	The dressings are cheap.	Non-selective, painful (sedation/anaesthesia required) method. Can damage healthy tissue. Needs regular changing (e.g. up to every 4–6 hours in heavily exudative wounds).
Surgical/ sharp	Using surgical instruments such as scalpel, curette, scissors, rongeur and forceps.	Layered debridement: most common method; necrotic/contaminated material is removed in a piecemeal fashion, removing superficial tissue and progressing to deeper tissues. Tissue is removed down to viable/clean surfaces and the wound is usually subsequently managed as an open wound. En bloc debridement: complete wide local excision of wound, usually followed by primary closure of the resultant clean defect. Less commonly performed in veterinary medicine.	Rapid, effective, selective debridement method that stimulates angiogenesis. En bloc debridement allows primary wound closure, which may reduce the time and cost associated with open-wound management. However, if used inappropriately, wound infection may result.	Adverse effects from debridement (e.g. haemorrhage). Requires general anaesthesia. Requires surgical expertise.

some authors believe an 'antiseptic stewardship' initiative is required (Kampf, 2016). Finding alternative and more natural antiseptic solutions should be explored in the treatment of wound infections (Yagnik *et al.*, 2018, 2021).

Published data are sufficient to support the elimination of antibiotics in wound irrigation (Barnes *et al.*, 2014). The bioactivity of antibiotics against bacteria requires an interval of time for binding to target sites on the pathogen, which is not afforded by irrigation. Indeed, not only do antibiotics in irrigation fluid lack efficacy but their use poses significant threats, including severe anaphylaxis, systemic absorption and toxicity, tissue irritation and development of resistant strains of bacteria (Anglen, 2001; Damm, 2011).

SELECTING A DELIVERY METHOD AND SUFFICIENT PRESSURE. The ideal irrigation technique and pressure required for optimal outcome are still undetermined in the literature. There is no difference in outcome between pulsed- versus continuous-pressure delivery systems. The American College of Surgeons (ACS) defines high pressure as 15–35 psi and low pressure as 1–15 psi: irrigation pressures lower than 4 psi are insufficient to remove surface pathogens and debris, while high-pressure irrigation is more effective in removing bacteria and foreign material but can impair the local immune response, cause tissue damage and propagate bacteria deeper into tissue or bone (Bhandari *et al.*, 1999; Anglen, 2001; di Pasquale *et al.*, 2007). Current evidence recommends that early irrigation using a low-pressure

Table 10.3. Alternatives to sterile saline as an irrigation solution.

Antimicrobial	Mode of action	Use	Bacterial resistance	Reference(s)
Chlorhexidine	Broad-spectrum biocide with fungicidal and concentration-dependent bacteriostatic or bactericidal properties. Destabilizes cell wall and disrupts osmosis of microorganisms.	Diluted to 0.05% for wound irrigation but may induce fibroblast apoptosis and necrosis. Note that a 2% solution is used as a surgical skin preparation on intact skin.	Resistance reported in numerous bacterial species, including *Proteus*, *Pseudomonas*, *Klebsiella*, *Bacillus* and *Shigella* spp., and *Escherichia coli*.	Dance *et al.* (1987); Kampf (2016)
Iodine-based solutions	Broad-spectrum antibacterial activity and action against spores, fungi, yeasts, viruses and protozoa.	1% or 0.1% solution for wound irrigation, but the short residual activity and inactivation by organic matter means that frequent reapplication is necessary. Similar wound infection rates have been reported in human adult and paediatric populations with saline irrigation versus 1% povidone-iodine. More concentrated solutions are cytotoxic to healthy cells and fibroblasts. Discolours skin and can cause local irritation to peri-wound skin.	To date, no acquired bacterial resistance or cross-resistance has been reported for iodine.	Bigliardi *et al.* (2017)
Hypochlorous acid	Oxidative and proteolytic effects. Commercially available as an oxychloride-based topical veterinary biocide solution.	Unlike sodium hypochlorite (NaOCl) and hydrogen peroxide (H_2O_2), hypochlorous acid is non-irritating, non-sensitizing and non-cytotoxic to mammalian cells within its effective antimicrobial concentration range. Topically applied exogenous hypochlorous acid triggers a cascade of events leading to improved wound perfusion and oxygenation, speedier healing and faster restoration of normal tissue architecture with minimal scarring.	To date, no clinical resistance has been reported, but resistance to hypochlorous acid has been reported in a *Salmonella* isolate from a poultry-processing plant.	Mokgatla *et al.* (1998); Mokgatla *et al.* (2002); Wang *et al.* (2011); Eryılmaz and Palabıyık (2013); Gold *et al.* (2020); WHO (2020)

Continued

Table 10.3. Continued

Antimicrobial	Mode of action	Use	Bacterial resistance	Reference(s)
Polyhexamethylene biguanide (PHMB) 0.1%	Available as an irrigation solution and gel. The commercially available product also contains a surfactant (betaine) to lift microbes and debris and suspend them in solution to prevent wound recontamination.	Broad spectrum of activity against bacteria, viruses and fungi. When used following an initial saline lavage, use of PHMB solution reduces inflammatory signs and accelerates wound healing compared with saline irrigation alone.	No evidence of resistance to date.	Bellingeri *et al.* (2016); NICE (2020)
Hydrogen peroxide 3%	The effervescing cleansing action of hydrogen peroxide may act as a chemical debriding agent to help lift debris and necrotic tissue from the wound surface when used at full strength.	*Not recommended as an irrigation solution.* May be cytotoxic to healthy cells and granulating tissue. Ineffective in reducing bacterial counts. May cause embolic events.		Rodeheaver (2001); Lu and Hansen (2017); Peng *et al.* (2020)
Sodium hypochlorite (Dakin's solution)	Bactericidal effect against most organisms commonly found in open wounds.	Cytotoxic to healthy cells and granulating tissues. *Not recommended as an irrigation solution.*		Mangum *et al.* (2018)
Octenidine dihydrochloride	Cationic surfactant active against Gram-positive and -negative bacteria	Irrigation of wounds in dogs has resulted in severe local complications, including significant necrosis and persistent oedematous changes with secondary wound infection. Similar effects are described in humans. *Not recommended as an irrigation solution.*		Hülsemann and Habenicht (2009); Schupp and Holland-Cunz (2009); Franz and Vogelin (2012); Kaiser *et al.* (2015)

Note that the authors prefer sterile saline as an irrigation solution for wound decontamination because it is isotonic and has the lowest toxicity compared with the other solutions listed here. If a wound is particularly contaminated or a multidrug-resistant bacterium is isolated, the authors will use hypochlorous acid for wound irrigation but rarely use other products. Crucially, these solutions are used alongside, rather than in place of, good wound management.

Kelly L. Bowlt Blacklock *et al.*

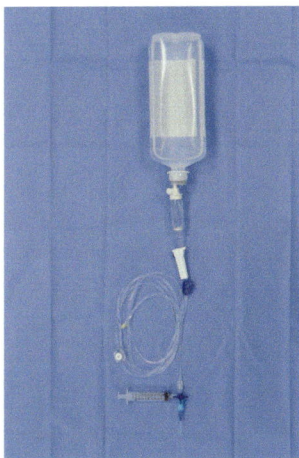

Fig. 10.7. The authors use copious volumes of saline as standard for wound irrigation, delivered via a giving set, three-way tap, needle and piston syringe.

device and saline solution is the best choice in maintaining bacteria clearance for longer than 48 h (Owens *et al.*, 2009). Manually squeezing punctured containers of irrigation fluid is inadequate for pressure irrigation, but needle and syringe-generated pressures of 13 psi (achievable with a 23-gauge needle with a 12 ml piston syringe) are effective in reducing infection (Fig. 10.7) (Longmire *et al.*, 1987; Owens *et al.*, 2009).

DETERMINING A SUFFICIENT VOLUME. Increased irrigation volume improves wound cleansing to a point, but the optimal volume is unknown, and volumes of 50–100 ml cm³ of wound are commonly cited in the literature. The authors determine the necessary irrigation volume according to the wound characteristics and degree of contamination, and recommend that irrigation continues until all visible debris is removed. Performing proper wound irrigation can be tediously time consuming but is a vital part of SSI management.

10.3.3 Removing implants

The presence of a surgical implant presents a unique challenge when treating an SSI. The implant becomes covered in a biofilm, which is a complex structure of the microbiome with bacterial colonies embedded in an extracellular matrix. This biofilm contributes to persistent chronic infections by limiting the effectiveness of host immune responses

and inhibiting development of therapeutic concentrations of antimicrobial drugs at the infection site (Savicky *et al.*, 2013; Sharma *et al.*, 2019). Biofilm must be considered synonymous with antibiotic resistance because of its proficiency in transferring resistance genes between bacterial species, as well as an innate phenotypic tolerance to antibiotics (Bowler *et al.*, 2020).

Biofilms can develop on all indwelling medical implants, including sutures, feeding tubes, drains, catheters, dental implants, orthopaedic implants and cardiovascular devices. Surgical debridement and removal of the implant is recommended in both the human and veterinary literature, and this approach consistently results in a superior outcome (decreased mortality, decreased incidence of chronic infections) compared with antibiotic therapy alone (Donlan, 2001; Fine and Tobias, 2007; Darouiche, 2009; Savicky *et al.*, 2013; Stine *et al.*, 2018). In patients where the implant is essential (e.g. a pacemaker), it is possible to successfully replace the device once the infection is fully resolved (Fine and Tobias, 2007).

In veterinary medicine, the most reported implant-associated infections occur following orthopaedic procedures. The diagnosis of infections associated with orthopaedic implants is based on a combination of clinical signs, laboratory findings and imaging studies. Clinical signs of SSI include lameness, pain on palpation of the surgical site, wound-related complications, sinus tracts/abscesses, soft-tissue swelling or pyrexia. There is no gold standard imaging technique to diagnose implant-associated SSIs: conventional radiography is indispensable, but in human medicine the radiograph is normal in 50% of patients with a confirmed implant-associated SSI. Imaging findings suggestive of post-surgical infection include sequestra, peri-prosthetic lucencies or gas, multifocal zones of osteolysis, implant loosening, sinus tracts, joint effusion and soft-tissue swelling. Additional imaging modalities might be valuable (e.g. computed tomography, magnetic resonance imaging, ultrasonography or, less commonly, bone scintigraphy). To confirm or rule out infection, fine-needle aspiration for cytological and bacteriological analysis of aspirated fluid is the cornerstone of the diagnostic algorithm (Cyteval and Bourdon, 2012). Bacterial analysis is particularly important to inform antibiotic selection, not least because of the high incidence of MDR organisms in implant-associated infections. Culture samples should not

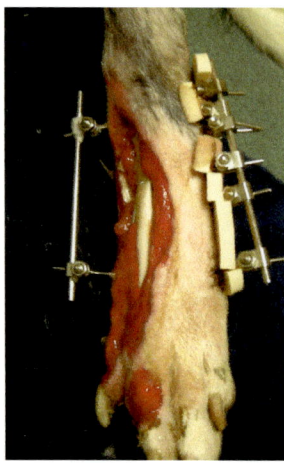

Fig. 10.8. In this canine patient, stabilization of a second and third metatarsal fracture is provided by an external skeletal fixator, allowing open-wound management to proceed unimpeded by implants. Photograph used with permission from Ian Faux, Royal (Dick) School of Veterinary Studies, Roslin, UK.

be collected from grossly contaminated areas, superficial skin or draining tracts but rather from aseptically prepared regions (e.g. at the time of surgery, following wound debridement or during joint lavage) or removed implants, or via fine-needle aspiration of deeper tissues or fluid pockets.

Determining when to remove the implant can be challenging. Fractures can heal in the presence of infection, provided there is adequate stability, but healing will typically be delayed, and ultimately, removal of the implant is necessary to completely resolve the infection (Savicky *et al.*, 2013). Loose implants should be removed or replaced to provide rigid stabilization, and any sequestra identified also needs removing. Alternative options to promote fracture healing can be considered. For example, an external skeletal fixator will allow stabilizing implants to be placed at a site distant to the infection, which will then allow the wound to be managed without the impediment of biofilm-coated implants (Fig. 10.8). If the fracture is not healed (e.g. delayed or non-union), grafting may also be required. In severely affected patients, limb amputation may be indicated.

The largest peer-reviewed publications on implant-associated infection in veterinary medicine are associated with tibial plateau levelling osteotomy (TPLO). Modifications to aseptic surgical protocols can decrease implant-associated infection rates after TPLO, but most infections still involve methicillin-resistant isolates, and implant removal (with or without antibiotics) still provides a superior outcome compared with antibiotic medications without implant removal (Stine *et al.*, 2018). Infection of total hip replacement prosthesis generally requires explantation (Fig. 10.9). However, a case report has described a patient with an MDR peri-prosthetic infection who underwent successful one-stage revision using micro-silver antimicrobial powder and culture-based vancomycin antibiotic-impregnated cement (Ficklin *et al.*, 2016).

In human medicine, CRISPR/CAS9 (clustered regularly interspaced short palindromic repeats/ CRISPR-associated protein 9, a gene editing technique) and photodynamic therapy are proposed as therapeutic approaches to reduce bacterial biofilm infections, but this technology has not yet been trialled in veterinary medicine (Sharma *et al.*, 2019).

10.3.4 Obtaining samples for bacteriological analysis

Following wound debridement and lavage, a bacteriology sample should be collected for aerobic and anaerobic culture using aseptic technique, ideally before antibiotics are provided, into appropriate transport medium and submitted in sealed plastic bags for aerobic and anaerobic bacterial culture (PHE, 2018). This will allow more informed antibiotic stewardship (see Chapters 17 and 19, this volume). In human medicine, Public Health England (PHE) guidance recommends that when using a swab, the superficial areas of the wounds should be cleaned first (e.g. by flushing with sterile saline) and the deepest part of the wound sampled, avoiding the superficial microflora (PHE, 2018).

Samples of pus, if present, are often preferable to swabs and can be aseptically aspirated using a syringe and submitted for analysis in sterile, leak-proof containers (PHE, 2016). If only a minute amount of pus or exudate is available, it is preferable to send a pus/exudate swab in transport medium to minimize the risk of desiccation during transport (PHE, 2016, PHE, 2018). Compliance with local postal, transport and storage regulations is essential.

If a joint infection is suspected, aseptic arthrocentesis can be performed and a semi-quantitative white cell count performed on the synovial fluid to differentiate inflammatory from

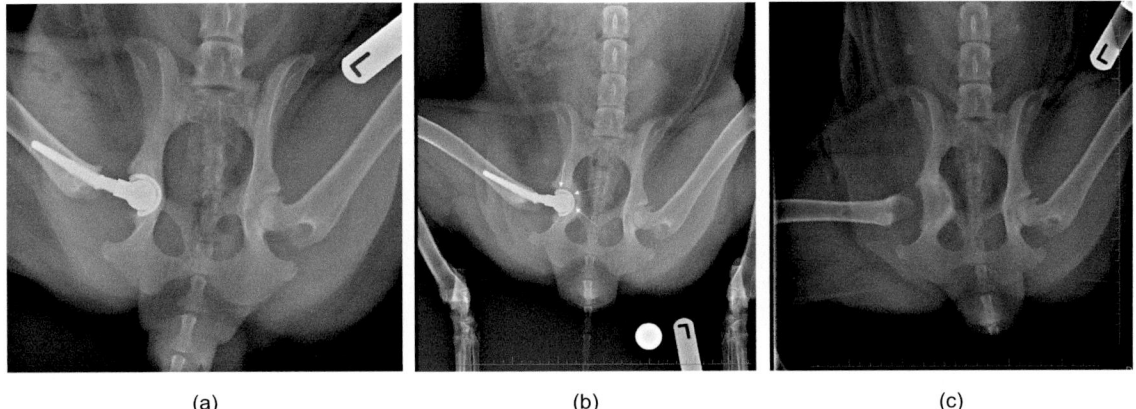

(a)   (b)   (c)

Fig. 10.9. (a) Ventrodorsal radiograph of the pelvis of a 2-year-old Labrador retriever following revision of a right total hip replacement, 3 weeks after the primary surgery. Revision was required for the treatment of a dorsal luxation of the femoral head following a minor traumatic incident. The radiograph shows the placement of a biological fixation (BFX®) prosthetic cup in the right acetabulum and a collared BFX® electron beam melting prosthetic stem in the proximal femur. (b) Ventrodorsal radiographs of the same patient 4 months after total hip replacement. The patient had developed a gradual lameness over the previous few weeks and was perceived to be progressively uncomfortable in the region of the right hip. The radiograph shows the development of pronounced irregular new bone formation around the medial acetabular wall, and a curvilinear radiolucency following the outer shell of the prosthesis (white arrows), which was not appreciable on radiographs taken 4 weeks after revision surgery. Aseptic arthrocentesis yielded a large volume of viscous serosanguinous fluid: cytology was consistent with a severe neutrophilic inflammation and bacterial culture identified a heavy pure growth of penicillin-resistant *Staphylococcus aureus*. (c) The prostheses were surgically explanted, during which the acetabular cup was found to be loose. Four months after explantation, the medial acetabular wall had remodelled and the patient had recovered good function on the right hind limb. Images used with permission from Dylan Clements, Royal (Dick) School of Veterinary Studies, Roslin, UK.

non-inflammatory arthropathies. Additionally, synovial fluid should be submitted for bacterial analysis in enrichment culture because the patient may have already received antibiotics and the number of viable organisms may be very low (PHE, 2021). Specimens should be transported and processed as soon as possible, but if delay is unavoidable, refrigeration of the samples is preferable to storage at ambient temperature (Miller *et al.*, 2018). In human and veterinary medicine, there is no evidence to suggest that assessment of wound infection differs when culture results from swabs or biopsies are available (Haalboom *et al.*, 2019; Stokes *et al.*, 2021).

At some institutions, including that of the authors', point-of-care fluorescence is used to provide information on the presence, location and load of bacteria. This novel, non-contact handheld device has been validated in humans and permits prompt detection and removal of bacterial burden to reduce wound infection and facilitate healing (Andersen *et al.*, 2021; Le *et al.*, 2021; Sandy-Hodgetts *et al.*,

2021). Similar work is ongoing in veterinary medicine, and future peer-reviewed publications will provide more information on which to judge the value of this technology for veterinary applications (Fig. 10.10). Interestingly, mobile thermal imaging has also been used in human medicine to successfully predict an SSI (Fletcher *et al.*, 2021).

Despite the use of optimal techniques, sampling of wounds for bacteriological analysis will never be 100% sensitive and specific. The culture result must be interpreted carefully, with consideration of the body site, common pathogens, sample type and organisms isolated (Weese, 2020). Isolation of multiple organisms should be approached with caution because one or more may be a contaminant. Identification of commensal bacteria of limited virulence (e.g. coagulase-negative staphylococci, enterococci) are typically not clinically relevant. The authors rely much more heavily on the clinical picture to inform treatment options, rather than culture results. When determining whether an isolated

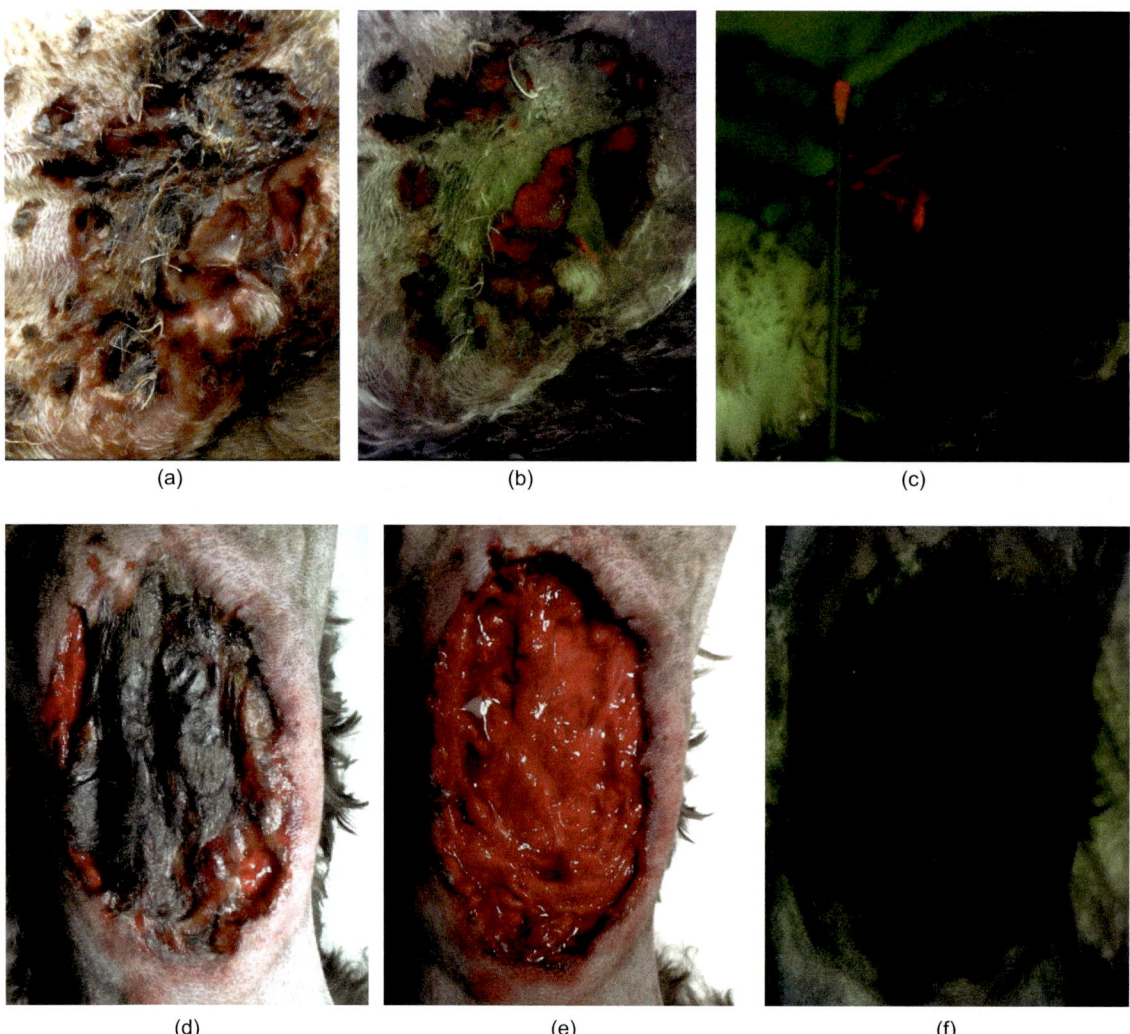

Fig. 10.10. (a) Image taken in white light of a necrotic surgical-site wound on the flank of a canine patient. (b) Fluorescent image of the same wound as in (a), showing the pink blush of the subcutaneous bacterial burden. (c) Fluorescent image of the same wound as in (a) as a direct sample of bacterial colonies is procured. Serial fluorescent imaging following debridement, lavage and open-wound management is helpful to demonstrate decreasing fluorescence associated with decreased bacterial bioburden. (d) Image taken in white light of necrotic tissue associated with a ruptured neck abscess in a spaniel. (e) Image taken in white light of the wound shown in (d) after surgical debridement. (f) Fluorescent image of the wound shown in (d), showing no fluorescence either before or after debridement. Bacterial culture was negative. Open-wound management was instigated, no antibiotics were utilized, and the wound healed completely and uneventfully. Images used with permission from Jon Hall, Wear Referrals, Stockton-on-Tees, UK.

bacterium is clinically important, antimicrobial resistance is irrelevant: resistance and virulence are different. The bacterial species, infection site and degree of bacterial growth, not the susceptibility pattern, should be considered because an MDR bacterium is not more likely to be clinically relevant than a susceptible counterpart (Weese, 2020). Crucially, local laboratories will always welcome a telephone call from the interested clinician who wishes to request assistance with

Kelly L. Bowlt Blacklock *et al.*

the interpretation of recent bacterial culture and susceptibility results.

10.3.5 Open-wound management

Following appropriate debridement and lavage, it is usual for wounds associated with an SSI to be managed as an open wound. Further details on open wound management can be found in Chapter 11 (this volume).

An exception to this rule might include infections associated with the abdominal or thoracic cavity because open-wound management is more challenging in this situation, although not impossible. Referral is strongly recommended in such a scenario. If continued drainage is required from the abdominal cavity, an active suction drain (e.g. Jackson-Pratt) can be placed. There is no place for a passive drain (e.g. Penrose) in this situation. Open peritoneal drainage is possible but rarely indicated, and should only be undertaken at a referral institution because of the intensive nursing requirements and high risk of hypoproteinaemia and nosocomial infections (Staatz *et al.*, 2002). Vacuum-assisted peritoneal drainage has been described but is similarly fraught with difficulties (Cioffi *et al.*, 2012). Intermittent thoracic drainage can be provided via a trocar or small-bore, wire-guided thoracostomy tube, which can also be used to flush the thorax.

10.3.6 Antimicrobial therapy

Not all open wounds require antibiotics. Prophylactic antibiotic use in surgical patients is reviewed comprehensively in Chapter 19 (this volume). If the clinical signs associated with an SSI are severe enough to warrant the provision of antibiotics before culture and sensitivity results are available, a broad-spectrum antibiotic that is appropriate for the likely pathogens should be administered until bacteriology results allow de-escalation (narrowing of the antimicrobial spectrum) (Nelson, 2011). It is imperative that drug doses and intervals are appropriate. In a recent study, samples from most wounds with SSIs yielded growth of MRSP (47.4%) and MRSA (15.8%), with only a minority of SSIs caused by methicillin-susceptible *S. pseudintermedius* (10.5%) or *Enterococcus* (10%), *Klebsiella* (5%), *Pasteurella* (5%) and *Streptococcus* (5%) spp. (Turk *et al.*, 2015).

The impending apocalypse heralded by the increasing incidence of MDR pathogens in veterinary patients is incredibly distressing. Indeed, strains of extensively drug-resistant (XDR) bacteria (non-susceptible to all but two or fewer antimicrobial classes) have been reported (Magiorakos *et al.*, 2012; Detwiler *et al.*, 2013). Importantly, the clinical presentation of MDR pathogens is not dissimilar to that caused by a variety of other MDR and susceptible pathogens, resulting in infections that range from mild/superficial to rapidly fatal (Weese, 2008). The impact of MDR pathogens on patient survival and morbidity have not been investigated thoroughly in small animal practice, but MDR infections are associated with increased mortality and reoperation rates in humans (Jarvis, 1996; Montravers *et al.*, 1996; Wilson, 2003). When MDR infection is identified, infection control precautions and client counselling are important. Clients and veterinary staff should seek up-to-date medical advice from their general practitioner, particularly if they have pre-existing medical conditions.

MRSA

MRSA is a critically important human pathogen and an emerging veterinary and zoonotic (or reverse zoonotic) pathogen. In a recent study, MRSA accounted for nearly 16% of SSIs in dogs following surgery at a veterinary university hospital (Turk *et al.*, 2015). MRSA strains are resistant to all β-lactam antimicrobials (penicillin, cephalosporins and carbapenems) because they possess an altered penicillin-binding protein, but there is often also resistance to other antimicrobial classes (Turk *et al.*, 2015). The use of fluoroquinolones should be avoided wherever possible: not only is their use a significant risk factor for development of MRSA (Weber *et al.*, 2003), but resistance can quickly develop (Morris *et al.*, 2017). Vancomycin is commonly used to treat MRSA infections in humans, which has led to the development of vancomycin-resistant forms (Tenover, 2006). In the authors' opinion, vancomycin should not be used in veterinary species: it is banned in many European countries for veterinary use and poses a genuine ethical dilemma because the promotion of resistance has significant adverse effects on human health.

MRSP

MRSP is currently the most commonly isolated organism in small animal SSIs (up to 47.4%). Like MRSA, MRSP harbours resistance to several other classes of antimicrobials, and susceptibility only to amikacin, rifampicin, vancomycin and linezolid is a widely encountered pattern (Morris *et al.*, 2017). This presents a huge dilemma because of potential drug toxicities and ethical use considerations.

Management of patients with MDR SSIs

Appropriate barrier nursing protocols should be followed immediately for any patient presenting for any surgical wound-related complication (see Chapter 12, this volume). Suggestions for approaches to methicillin-resistant staphylococcal infections of small animals have recently been reported and the interested reader is referred to the clinical consensus guidelines (Morris *et al.*, 2017).

Suggested recommendations for management of MDR SSIs are illustrated in Table 10.4.

SYSTEMATIC ANTIBIOTICS FOR THE MANAGEMENT OF MDR-INFECTED WOUNDS. Sun Tzu's words in *The Art of War* are as relevant today as they were in the 5th century BC: 'The wise warrior avoids the battle.' Wherever possible, we should not engage in providing systemic antibiotics to fuel the MDR bacteria that plague us, irrespective of *in vitro* susceptibility (Barton *et al.*, 2006; Morris *et al.*, 2017; Brown *et al.*, 2021). This is because *in vitro* susceptibility of common antimicrobials may not reflect *in vivo* susceptibility, resistance to common antimicrobials can quickly be induced and further resistance can be induced at other sites where, in the case of staphylococci, carriage of multiple species and multiple genetically unrelated *S. pseudintermedius* strains is common (Lewis and Jorgensen, 2005; Barton *et al.*, 2006; Paul *et al.*, 2012; Brown *et al.*,

Table 10.4. Suggested recommendations for antimicrobial therapy in MDR SSIs. Modified from Morris *et al.* (2017).

Scrupulous hand hygiene and routine cleaning and disinfection protocols are the cornerstone of hospital infection control. Most MDR bacteria are susceptible to commonly used detergents and disinfectants. Appropriate PPE (disposable gown and gloves) should be used.

The pathogenic potential of any isolate should be interpreted in the light of the patient's clinical disease. Antibiotics (especially systemic) are not required for all open wounds.

Minimum reporting by microbiology laboratories should include complete speciation of staphylococci and an antibiogram for all cultured isolates, including commensal species.

Wound cytology is strongly recommended to aid interpretation of the antibiogram results and help target treatment.

In patients with superficial infections, topical antibacterial agents and biocides with proven efficacy against the causal bacteria should be considered in combination with physical management of the wound. Wherever clinically feasible, topical rather than systemic agents should be the sole antibacterial treatment. Discussion with local specialists in soft-tissue surgery, dermatology and microbacteriology is strongly encouraged so that a multi-disciplinary approach can be formulated.

Empirical systemic drug selection is always contraindicated when antimicrobial resistance is suspected based on historical factors (e.g. post-operative or other nosocomial wound and/or recent antibiotic therapy). Antibiotic selection must be based on culture and susceptibility results.

A total restriction-of-use policy should apply to the veterinary use of glycopeptides (vancomycin, teicoplanin and telavancin), linezolid (oxazolidinone), anti-MRSA cephalosporins and potentially new compounds that may be approved in the future for treatment of MDR pathogens in people.

Transmission of methicillin-resistant staphylococci and potentially other MDR bacteria by infected and/or colonized pets to other individuals in the community is known to occur. It is reasonable to restrict animals from contact situations until a clinical response is evident. In the home, this could include social distancing from 'at-risk' individuals and enhanced hygiene measures.

There is currently insufficient evidence to recommend routine screening of clinically normal animals for carriage of methicillin-resistant staphylococci, or for routine decolonization of carrier animals (see Chapter 3, this volume).

Following clinical resolution, passive decolonization in the community by limiting veterinary contact and avoiding antibiotics is recommended.

MDR, multidrug-resistant; MRSA, methicillin-resistant *Staphylococcus aureus*; PPE, personal protective equipment.

Kelly L. Bowlt Blacklock *et al.*

2021). Together, these can lead to treatment failure, induction of XDR bacteria, colonization of MDR bacteria and potentially MDR infections at distant sites.

However, sometimes a battle is unavoidable, and there are situations in which systemic antimicrobials may be warranted, such as where topical treatment is not practical (e.g. septic peritonitis) or where there is evidence of sepsis. If we believe Cicero that 'armed forces abroad are of little value unless there is prudent counsel at home', then the clinician would be well advised to first consult with the microbiology laboratory, who will be supremely placed to guide the selection of an appropriate antimicrobial. Briefly, the antimicrobial must be based on culture and susceptibility results, should be narrow spectrum, and should be administered intravenously initially and at the top of the dosage range to maximize the potential for rapid efficacy and reduced course duration. The patient must be regularly re-evaluated, and repeated culture and susceptibility testing performed to identify further resistance and the earliest time point to stop systemic treatment. Long-acting injectable formulations of antimicrobials should be avoided due to variable tissue concentrations and fixed duration of treatment. In January 2020, the European Medicines Agency (EMA) issued advice on risk categorization of antibiotics for use in animals (EMA, 2020). In this document, four categories of antibiotics were identified:

- *Category A: 'Avoid'*. Antibiotics that are reserved for human treatment only and are not permitted for use in food-producing animals. They may be given to companion animals under exceptional circumstances. Antibiotics in this group include rifamycins, carbapenems and third-generation cephalosporins with β-lactamase inhibitors.
- *Category B: 'Restrict'*. Antibiotics in this category are critically important in human medicine and use in animals should be restricted to mitigate the risk to public health. Antibiotics in this group should be considered for use only when there are no antibiotics in Categories C or D that could be clinically effective, and their use should be based on antimicrobial susceptibility testing. The antibiotics in this group include third- and fourth-generation cephalosporins, quinolones (including fluoroquinolones) and polymyxins.
- *Category C: 'Caution'*. Antibiotics in this category have alternatives in human health but should only be used if there is no alternative lower-risk product available in Category D. Examples include aminoglycosides, first- and second-generation cephalosporins, and macrolides.
- *Category D: 'Prudence'*. Antibiotics in this category should be used as first-line treatments whenever possible, but must be used prudently and only when medically indicated. Examples include tetracyclins, narrow-spectrum penicillins and sulfonamides.

TOPICAL MANAGEMENT OF MDR-INFECTED WOUNDS. Topical management of MDR-infected wounds is preferable. Often, antibiotics that are potentially effective are not available, are toxic or are ethically questionable to use. In such circumstances, the authors believe that lavage, debridement and frequent meticulous dressing changes are often sufficient to resolve the infection without the use of antibiotics, assuming the underlying causes of the infection (e.g. enteric leakage, sequestra, implants) are resolved. Using topical agents may also provide the opportunity to decrease the chance of adverse drug reactions (e.g. gastrointestinal upset) and, more importantly, selection of resistant organisms.

Once the wound has been appropriately lavaged and debrided, additional options for management of MDR-infected wounds without systemic antibiotics are listed briefly below and further details can be found in Chapter 11 (this volume):

- Negative-pressure wound therapy (NPWT), which is the local application of subatmospheric pressure to a wound bed. This reduces oedema and removes exudate, increases wound perfusion, stimulates granulation tissue, increases wound contraction and potentially decreases bacterial contamination. The authors use this technology frequently, with excellent results. Some authors have used NPWT in combination with other products, such as hypertonic salt dressings (Fraccalvieri *et al.*, 2015).
- Manuka honey. This has antibacterial properties attributable to its high osmolarity and acidity (pH 3.6–3.7). It also contains antioxidants and encourages angiogenesis and fibroblast growth through the presence of low levels of hydrogen peroxide (Fig. 10.11).
- Topical antiseptics, such as polyhexamethylene biguanide.

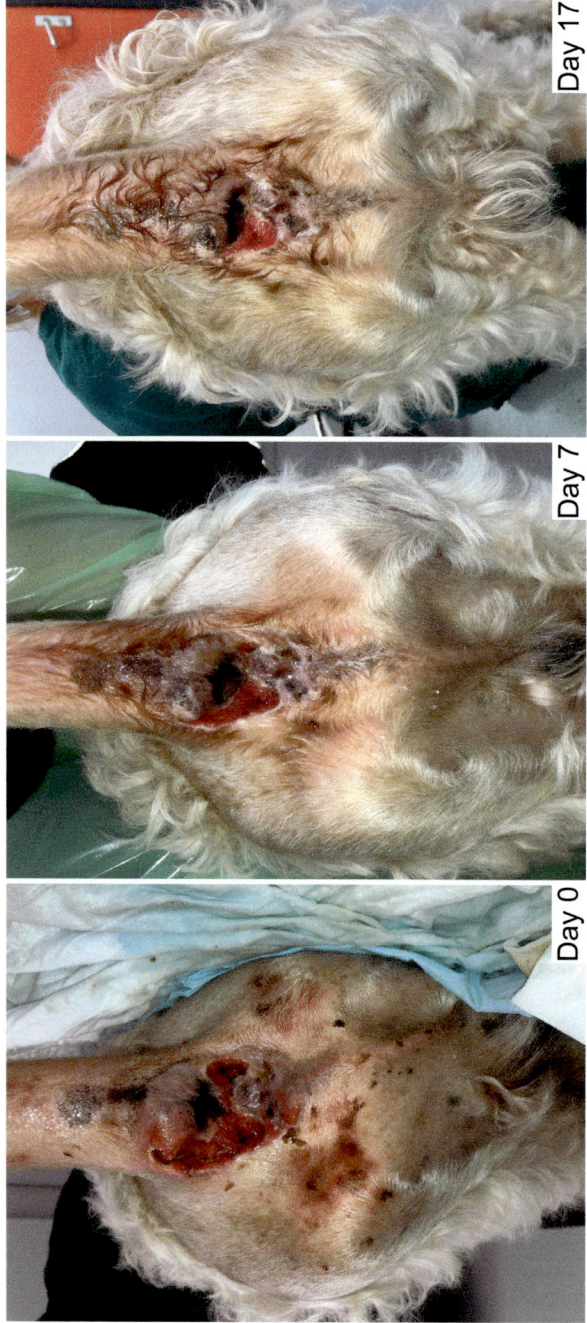

Fig. 10.11. Images of the surgical site of a bilateral anal sacculectomy in a 13-year-old male labradoodle, which has developed an infection 5 days post-operatively. Bacterial culture and sensitivity results from the wound yielded a profuse growth of *Enterococcus faecium* (resistant to penicillins and fluoroquinolones) and *Escherichia coli* (resistant to penicillins, cephalosporins and tetracyclins). The wounds were lavaged with copious quantities of sterile saline and Manuka honey applied three times daily. No antibiotics were provided. The wounds were completely healed by second intention within 1 month of surgery.

Kelly L. Bowlt Blacklock *et al.*

- Nanocrystalline silver. This can be used in combination with NPWT
- Additional novel techniques have been described for open-wound management, including low-level laser therapy and hyperbaric therapy, but limited evidence is available in veterinary patients to date. The authors are particularly excited about recent research into the use of bacteriophages to control MDR-infected wounds in laboratory animals (Fayez *et al.*, 2021), but clinical information is required before this can be added to the hospital armoury against infection.

10.3.7 Wound closure

Once the wound bed is clean and free from necrotic tissue and infection, healing can be completed by:

- primary closure, which is not usually appropriate for wounds considered to be infected;
- delayed primary closure, which is performed 3–5 days after the wound occurs and allows time for elimination of contamination and evidence of ischaemia; closure is performed before a granulation bed forms;
- second intention healing, which is wound healing by contraction and epithelialization; or
- secondary closure, which occurs after the formation of a granulation bed and follows open-wound management for more than 5 days.

Usually, wounds with an SSI are closed via secondary closure or second intention healing. The simplest method of closure is often the most successful.

Second intention healing

Second intention healing is appropriate where the wound is on an extremity and is small, or is in an area surrounded by abundant skin (e.g. flank). Information on how to best support the wound to achieve second intention healing is available in Chapter 11 (this volume).

Secondary closure

Secondary closure allows the wound to close more rapidly than second intention healing and is preferable if vital structures (e.g. tendons, nerves) are exposed, if tissue reconstruction is required for support (e.g. a footpad) or if a scar may limit function (e.g. eyelid, or an extensive wound located over the flexor surface of a joint). An exhaustive description of options for skin closure of the non-infected wound is beyond the scope of this chapter, but the authors refer the interested reader to one of the many beautifully illustrated texts on wound reconstruction (e.g. Williams and Moores, 2009; Pavletic, 2018) and would encourage the practitioner to consult with their local soft-tissue surgery specialist.

If secondary closure is desirable, the granulation bed is surgically excised and the skin closed. Regardless of the technique chosen to achieve apposition of the skin, the single most important consideration is the avoidance of wound tension. Briefly, options for wound closure in this scenario include the following:

- *Local wound reconstructive techniques.* Examples include suturing the wound perpendicular to the lines of skin tension, undermining of surrounding tissues, making a Z- or V-Y-plasty or releasing incisions parallel to the lines of skin tension (take care to consider the local blood supply before doing this). If tension is still too great, wound closure can be facilitated further using tension sutures or skin stretchers.
- *Free skin grafts.* A section of epidermis and dermis is completely removed and transferred to a distant recipient site. The most common type of graft in veterinary medicine is a full-thickness free skin graft.
- *Skin flaps.* Most simple pedicle grafts in dogs and cats are subdermal plexus flaps, which receive blood supply from the subdermal plexus associated with the panniculus muscle or the dermis. Local pedicle grafts (e.g. rotating or advancement flaps) remain the simplest and most practical means of closing wounds where location allows and are suitable for regions such as the trunk or head. They are generally either rotating or advancement flaps. Alternatively, an axial pattern flap can be used, which incorporates a direct cutaneous artery and vein, thereby allowing the graft to be 50% larger than that of subdermal plexus flaps. Axial pattern flaps are particularly useful in distal limbs where neighbouring skin is limited.

Suture selection is important in reducing risk of SSIs. Knotless barbed sutures are available in various sizes and polymers, and contain regular unidirectional or bidirectional barbs that allow tension to be distributed uniformly across the suture length (Goldstein *et al.*, 2014). Elimination of knots achieves a reduction in surgical time and foreign material, and barbed sutures have been used in many human and veterinary studies (Trocchia *et al.*, 2009; Shah *et al.*, 2012; Ehrhart *et al.*, 2013; Spah *et al.*, 2013; Gomes de Lima *et al.*, 2021).

In human medicine, triclosan-coated sutures significantly reduced the risk of SSIs when compared with standard sutures and are therefore recommended in clean and contaminated surgical procedures (Ahmed *et al.*, 2019). In dogs, clinically relevant bacteria isolated from canine wounds (including methicillin-resistant species) adhere more abundantly to uncoated polyglactin 910, and exhibit least adherence to coated monofilament sutures (McCagherty *et al.*, 2020). In the same study, only triclosan-coated materials demonstrated sustained antimicrobial activity (3–29 days) against all tested pathogens, including MDR bacteria. Further studies are required to assess clinical efficacy of triclosan-coated suture materials *in vivo* in veterinary species.

10.4 Conclusion

Despite the most meticulous care and attention, SSIs will haunt every surgeon sooner or later. In these days of impending antibiotic apocalypse, one cannot simply reach for systemic antibiotics. Instead, we must be cleverer, more tactical and one step ahead of our bacterial enemies. To achieve success, we must holistically nurse the whole patient and optimize their well-being so that they can contribute to the fight. We must ambush the infection at its origin, ensuring that the wound is opened, debrided, flushed and appropriately dressed so that there is no opportunity for treatment evasion. Finally, and most importantly, we must liaise with those allies who specialize in microbacteriology and soft-tissue surgery so that the optimal multidisciplinary approach can be formulated, and so that when doubt creeps in, they can provide reassurance that we are all on the same side in this fight.

> Don't depend on the enemy not coming; depend rather on being ready for him.
>
> Tsu (2010).

Acknowledgements

The authors thank the following colleagues for reviewing sections of this chapter pertaining to their areas of expertise: Susan M. Campbell, DipAVN(medical) RVN FHEA CertSAN CertVNECC MBVNA; Efa Llewellyn, BVetMed DACVECC DECVECC FHEA MRCVS; Tim Nuttall, BSc BVSc CertVD PhD CBiol MSB MRCVS; and Gavin Paterson, BSc PhD.

References

Acheampong, O.D., Enyetornye, B., Osei, D. and Pires, I. (2021) Polymicrobial necrotizing fasciitis in a dog: the involvement of *Macrococcus caseolyticus*, *Proteus mirabilis*, and *Escherichia coli*. *Case Reports in Veterinary Medicine* 2021, 1–5. DOI: 10.1155/2021/5544558.

Ahmed, I., Boulton, A.J., Rizvi, S., Carlos, W., Dickenson, E. *et al.* (2019) The use of triclosan-coated sutures to prevent surgical site infections: a systematic review and meta-analysis of the literature. *BMJ Open* 9(9), e029727. DOI: 10.1136/bmjopen-2019-029727.

Aljorayid, A., Viau, R., Castellino, L. and Jump, R.L.P. (2016) Serratia fonticola, pathogen or bystander? A case series and review of the literature. *IDCases* 5, 6–8. DOI: 10.1016/j.idcr.2016.05.003.

Anaya, D.A. and Dellinger, E.P. (2007) Necrotizing soft-tissue infection: diagnosis and management. *Clinical Infectious Diseases* 44(5), 705–710. DOI: 10.1086/511638.

Andersen, C.A., McLeod, K. and Steffan, R. (2021) Diagnosis and treatment of the invasive extension of bacteria (cellulitis) from chronic wounds utilising point-of-care fluorescence imaging. *International Wound Journal* 19(5), 996–1008. DOI: 10.1111/iwj.13696.

Anglen, J.O. (2001) Wound irrigation in musculoskeletal injury. *Journal of the American Academy of Orthopaedic Surgeons* 9(4), 219–226. DOI: 10.5435/00124635-200107000-00001.

Baranoski, S. and Ayello, E.A. (2004) Wound care survey. *Nursing* 34(9), 17. DOI: 10.1097/00152193-200409000-00011.

Barnes, S., Spencer, M., Graham, D. and Johnson, H.B. (2014) Surgical wound irrigation: a call for evidence-based standardization of practice. *American Journal of Infection Control* 42(5), 525–529. DOI: 10.1016/j.ajic.2014.01.012.

Barton, M., Hawks, M., Moore, D., Conly, J., Nicolle, L, *et al.* (2006) Guidelines for the prevention and management of community-associated methicillin-resistant *staphylococcus aureus*: a perspective for Canadian health care practitioners. *Canadian of Infectious Diseases & Medical Microbiology* 17(Suppl. C), 4C–24C.

Bellingeri, A., Falciani, F., Traspedini, P., Moscatelli, A., Russo, A, *et al.* (2016) Effect of a wound cleansing solution on wound bed preparation and inflammation in chronic wounds: a single-blind RCT.

Journal of Wound Care 25(3), 160. DOI: 10.12968/jowc.2016.25.3.160.

Bhandari, M., Schemitsch, E.H., Adili, A., Lachowski, R.J. and Shaughnessy, S.G. (1999) High and low pressure pulsatile lavage of contaminated tibial fractures: an *in vitro* study of bacterial adherence and bone damage. *Journal of Orthopaedic Trauma* 13(8), 526–533. DOI: 10.1097/00005131-199911000-00002.

Bigliardi, P.L., Alsagoff, S.A.L., El-Kafrawi, H.Y., Pyon, J.-K., Wa, C.T.C, *et al.* (2017) Povidone iodine in wound healing: a review of current concepts and practices. *International Journal of Surgery* 44, 260–268. DOI: 10.1016/j.ijsu.2017.06.073.

Bowler, P., Murphy, C. and Wolcott, R. (2020) Biofilm exacerbates antibiotic resistance: Is this a current oversight in antimicrobial stewardship? *Antimicrobial Resistance and Infection Control* 9(1), 162. DOI: 10.1186/s13756-020-00830-6.

Bowlt, K.L., Pivetta, M., Kussy, F., Rossanese, M., Stabile, F. *et al.* (2013) Imaging diagnosis and minimally-invasive management of necrotizing fasciitis in a dog. *Veterinary and Comparative Orthopaedics and Traumatology* 26(4), 323–327. DOI: 10.3415/VCOT-12-08-0100.

Brown, N.M., Goodman, A.L., Horner, C., Jenkins, A. and Brown, E.M. (2021) Treatment of methicillin-resistant Staphylococcus aureus (MRSA): updated guidelines from the UK. *JAC-Antimicrobial Resistance* 3(1). DOI: 10.1093/jacamr/dlaa114.

Buicko, J.L., Lopez, M.A. and Lopez-Viego, M.A. (2016) *From Formalwear and Frocks to Scrubs and Gowns: A Brief History of the Evolution of Operating Room Attire*. American College of Surgeons, Chicago, Illinois. Available at: www.facs.org/media/0ypjk2ki/01_formalwear_and_frocks.pdf (accessed 23 October 2022).

Buriko, Y., Van Winkle, T.J., Drobatz, K.J., Rankin, S.C. and Syring, R.S. (2008) Severe soft tissue infections in dogs: 47 cases (1996-2006). *Journal of Veterinary Emergency and Critical Care* 18(6), 608–618. DOI: 10.1111/j.1476-4431.2008.00370.x.

Cioffi, K.M., Schmiedt, C.W., Cornell, K.K. and Radlinsky, M.G. (2012) Retrospective evaluation of vacuum-assisted peritoneal drainage for the treatment of septic peritonitis in dogs and cats: 8 cases (2003-2010). *Journal of Veterinary Emergency and Critical Care* 22(5), 601–609. DOI: 10.1111/j.1476-4431.2012.00791.x.

Csiszer, A.B., Towle, H.A. and Daly, C.M. (2010) Successful treatment of necrotizing fasciitis in the hind limb of a great dane. *Journal of the American Animal Hospital Association* 46(6), 433–438. DOI: 10.5326/0460433.

Cyteval, C. and Bourdon, A. (2012) Imaging orthopedic implant infections. *Diagnostic and Interventional Imaging* 93(6), 547–557. DOI: 10.1016/j.diii.2012.03.004.

Damm, S. (2011) Intraoperative anaphylaxis associated with bacitracin irrigation. *American Journal of Health-System Pharmacy* 68(4), 323–327. DOI: 10.2146/ajhp090238.

Dance, D.A.B., Pearson, A.D., Seal, D.V. and Lowes, J.A. (1987) A hospital outbreak caused by a chlorhexidine and antibiotic-resistant *Proteus mirabilis*. *Journal of Hospital Infection* 10(1), 10–16. DOI: 10.1016/0195-6701(87)90027-2.

Darouiche, R.O. (2009) Treatment of infections associated with surgical implants. *New England Journal of Medicine* 350(14), 1422–1429. DOI: 10.1056/NEJMra035415.

Dellinger, E.P. (2015) Postoperative wound infections. In: *Clinical Infectious Disease*, 2nd edn. Cambridge University Press, Cambridge, UK, pp. 729–733.

Detwiler, A., Bloom, P., Petersen, A. and Rosser, E.J. (2013) Multi-drug and methicillin resistance of staphylococci from canine patients at a veterinary teaching hospital (2006-2011). *Veterinary Quarterly* 33(2), 60–67. DOI: 10.1080/01652176.2013.799792.

di Pasquale, D.J., Bhandari, M., Tov, A. and Schemitsch, E.H. (2007) The effect of high and low pressure pulsatile lavage on soft tissue and cortical blood flow: a canine segmental humerus fracture model. *Archives of Orthopaedic and Trauma Surgery* 127, 879–884.

Donlan, R.M. (2001) Biofilm formation: a clinically relevant microbiological process. *Clinical Infectious Diseases* 33, 1387–1392.

Ehrhart, N.P., Kaminskaya, K., Miller, J.A. and Zaruby, J.F. (2013) In vivo assessment of absorbable knotless barbed suture for single layer gastrotomy and enterotomy closure. *Veterinary Surgery* 42, 210–216.

EMA (2020) *Categorisation of Antibiotics for Use in Animalsfor Prudent and Responsible Use*. Available at: www.ema.europa.eu/en/documents/report/infographic-categorisation-antibiotics-use-animals-prudent-responsible-use_en.pdf (accessed 23 October 2022).

Eryılmaz, M. and Palabıyık, I.M. (2013) Hypochlorous acid – analytical methods and antimicrobial activity. *Tropical Journal of Pharmaceutical Research* 12, 123–126.

Fayez, M.S., Hakim, T.A., Agwa, M.M., Abdelmoteleb, M., Aly, R.G. *et al.* (2021) Topically applied bacteriophage to control multi-drug resistant *Klebsiella pneumoniae* infected wound in a rat model. *Antibiotics* 10, 1048. DOI: 10.3390/antibiotics10091048.

Fernandez, R. and Griffiths, R. (2012) Water for wound cleansing. *Cochrane Database of Systematic Reviews* 2, CD003861.

Ficklin, M.G., Kowaleski, M.P., Kunkel, K.A.R. and Suber, J.T. (2016) One-stage revision of an infected cementless total hip replacement. *Veterinary and Comparative Orthopaedics and Traumatology* 29, 541–546.

Fine, D.M. and Tobias, A.H. (2007) Cardiovascular device infections in dogs: report of 8 cases and review of the literature. *Journal of Veterinary Internal Medicine* 21, 1265–1271.

Fletcher, R.R., Schneider, G., Bikorimana, L., Rukundo, G., Niyigena, A. *et al.* (2021) The use of mobile thermal imaging and deep learning for prediction of surgical site infection. *Annual International Conference of the IEEE Engineering in Medicine & Biology Society* 2021, 5059–5062.

Fraccalvieri, M., Ruka, E., Morozzo, U., Scalise, A. and Salomone, M. (2015) The combination of a hypertonic saline dressing and negative pressure wound therapy (NPWT) for quick and bloodless debridement of difficult lesions in complicated patients. *Negative Pressure Wound Therapy Journal* 2, 5–7.

Franz, T. and Vogelin, E. (2012) Aseptic tissue necrosis and chronic inflammation after irrigation of penetrating hand wounds using Octenisept®. *Journal of Hand Surgery* 37, 61–64.

Garner, J.S., Jarvis, W.R., Emori, T.G., Horan, T.C. and Hughes, J.M. (1988) CDC definitions for nosocomial infections, 1988. *American Journal of Infection Control* 16, 128–140.

Gold, M.H., Andrieessen, A., Bhatia, A.C., Bitter, P.J., Chilukuri, S. *et al.* (2020) Topical stabilized hypochlorous acid: the future gold standard for wound care and scar management in dermatologic and plastic surgery procedures. *Journal of Cosmetic Dermatology* 19, 270–277.

Goldstein, L.J., Chary, D. and Brennan, S. (2014) Knotless tissue control devices: an asset in plastic surgery. *Plastic Surgical Nursing* 34, 39–42.

Gomes de Lima, H.C., Ribeiro, A.P., de Souza, J.A., Vieira, R.R. and Fernandes, M.F. (2021) Experimental surgery evaluation of barbed suture for celiorrhaphy and subcutaneous closure in bitches with pyometra submitted to ovariohysterectomy. *Acta Cirúrgica Brasileira* 36, e360502.

Gray, D., Acton, C., Chadwick, P., Fumaroa, S., Leaper, D, *et al.* (2011) Consensus guidance for the use of debridement techniques in the UK. *Wounds UK* 7, 77–84.

Haalboom, M., Blokhuis-Arkes, M.H.E., Beuk, R.J., Meerwaldt, R., Klont, R., *et al.* (2019) Culture results from wound biopsy versus wound swab: does it matter for the assessment of wound infection? *Clinical Microbiology and Infection* 25(5), 629. DOI: 10.1016/j.cmi.2018.08.012.

Hülsemann, W. and Habenicht, R. (2009) [Severe side effects after octenisept irrigation of penetrating wounds in children]. *Handchirurgie, Mikrochirurgie, Plastische Chirurgie* 41, 277–282.

Huss, M.K., Felt, S.A. and Pacharinsak, C. (2019) Influence of pain and analgesia on orthopedic and wound-healing models in rats and mice. *Comparative Medicine* 69, 535–545.

Jarvis, W.R. (1996) Selected aspects of the socio-economic impact of nosocomial infections: morbidity, mortality, cost, and prevention. *Infection Control and Hospital Epidemiology* 17, 552–557.

Kaiser, S., Kramer, M. and Thiel, C. (2015) [Severe complications after non-intended usage of octenidine dihydrochloride. A case series with four dogs]. *Tierarztliche Praxis Ausgabe K, Kleintiere/Heimtiere* 43, 291–298.

Kampf, G. (2016) Acquired resistance to chlorhexidine –- is it time to establish an 'antiseptic stewardship' initiative? *Journal of Hospital Infection* 94, 213–227.

Karl, F. (2014) A family's perspective – "The brutality of sepsis will haunt us for the rest of our lives." CDC's Safe Healthcare Blog. 16 September. Available at: https://blogs.cdc.gov/safehealthcare/brutality-of-sepsis-comment-page-4/ (accessed 23 October 2022).

Kubo, M., van de, L., Plantefaber, L.C., Mosesson, M.W., Simon, M. *et al.* (2001) Fibrinogen and fibrin are anti-adhesive for keratinocytes: a mechanism for fibrin eschar slough during wound repair. *Journal of Investigative Dermatology* 117, 1369–1381. DOI: 10.1046/j.0022-202x.2001.01551.x.

Kulendra, E. and Corr, S. (2008) Necrotising fasciitis with sub-periosteal *Streptococcus canis* infection in two puppies. *Veterinary and Comparative Orthopaedics and Traumatology* 21(5), 474–477. DOI: 10.3415/vcot-07-05-0043.

Lefman, S.H. and Prittie, J.E. (2019) Psychogenic stress in hospitalized veterinary patients: causation, implications, and therapies. *Journal of Veterinary Emergency and Critical Care* 29(2), 107–120. DOI: 10.1111/vec.12821.

Le, L., Baer, M., Briggs, P., Bullock, N., Cole, W. *et al.* (2021) Diagnostic accuracy of point-of-care fluorescence imaging for the detection of bacterial burden in wounds: results from the 350-patient fluorescence imaging assessment and guidance trial. *Advances in Wound Care* 10(3), 123–136. DOI: 10.1089/wound.2020.1272.

Lewis, J.S. and Jorgensen, J.H. (2005) Inducible clindamycin resistance in Staphylococci: should clinicians and microbiologists be concerned? *Clinical Infectious Diseases* 40(2), 280–285. DOI: 10.1086/426894.

Longmire, A.W., Broom, L.A. and Burch, J. (1987) Wound infection following high-pressure syringe and needle irrigation. *American Journal of Emergency Medicine* 5(2), 179–181. DOI: 10.1016/0735-6757(87)90121-5.

Lu, M. and Hansen, E.N. (2017) Hydrogen peroxide wound irrigation in orthopaedic surgery. *Journal of Bone and Joint Infection* 2, 3–9.

Lux, C.N. (2022) Wound healing in animals: a review of physiology and clinical evaluation. *Veterinary Dermatology* 33, 91.e27.

Magiorakos, A.-P., Srinivasan, A., Carey, R.B., Carmeli, Y., Falagas, M.E., *et al.* (2012) Multidrug-resistant, extensively drug-resistant and pandrug-resistant

Kelly L. Bowlt Blacklock *et al.*

bacteria: an international expert proposal for interim standard definitions for acquired resistance. *Clinical Microbiology and Infection* 18(3), 268–281. DOI: 10.1111/j.1469-0691.2011.03570.x.

Malgaigne, J. (1841) Etudes statistiques sur tes résultats des grandes opérations dans tes hôpitaux de Paris. *Annales de Médecine Belge et Étrangère* 1841, 241–244.

Mangum, L.C., Franklin, N.A., Garcia, G.R., Akers, K.S., and Wenke, J.C. (2018) Rapid degradation and non-selectivity of Dakin's solution prevents effectiveness in contaminated musculoskeletal wound models. *Injury* 49, 1763–1773.

Manna, B., Nahirniak, P. and Morrison, C.A. (2021) Wound debridement. StatPearls, Treasure Island, Florida. Available at: www.ncbi.nlm.nih.gov/books/NBK507882/ (accessed 23 October 2022).

Mayer, M.N. and Rubin, J.E. (2012) Necrotizing fasciitis caused by methicillin-resistant *Staphylococcus pseudintermedius* at a previously irradiated site in a dog. *Canadian Veterinary Journal* 53, 1207.

McCagherty, J., Yool, D.A., Paterson, G.K., Mitchell, S.R., Woods, S. *et al.* (2020) Investigation of the in vitro antimicrobial activity of triclosan-coated suture material on bacteria commonly isolated from wounds in dogs. *American Journal of Veterinary Research* 81, 84–90.

Mena, K.D. and Gerba, C.P. (2009) Risk assessment of *Pseudomonas aeruginosa* in water. *Reviews of Environmental Contamination and Toxicology* 201, 71–115.

Miller, J.M., Binnicker, M.J., Campbell, S., Carroll, K.C., Chapin, K.C, *et al.* (2018) A guide to utilization of the microbiology laboratory for diagnosis of infectious diseases: 2018 update by the Infectious Diseases Society of America and the American Society for Microbiology. *Clinical Infectious Diseases* 67, e1–e94.

Mokgatla, R.M., Brözel, V.S. and Gouws, P.A. (1998) Isolation of *Salmonella* resistant to hypochlorous acid from a poultry abattoir. *Letters in Applied Microbiology* 27(6), 379–382. DOI: 10.1046/j.1472-765x.1998.00432.x.

Mokgatla, R.M., Gouws, P.A. and Brözel, V.S. (2002) Mechanisms contributing to hypochlorous acid resistance of a *Salmonella* isolate from a poultry-processing plant. *Journal of Applied Microbiology* 92(3), 566–573. DOI: 10.1046/j.1365-2672.2002.01565.x.

Montravers, P., Gauzit, R., Muller, C., Marmuse, J.P., Fichelle, A. *et al.* (1996) Emergence of antibiotic-resistant bacteria in cases of peritonitis after intraabdominal surgery affects the efficacy of empirical antimicrobial therapy. *Clinical Infectious Diseases* 23(3), 486–494. DOI: 10.1093/clinids/23.3.486.

Morris, D.O., Loeffler, A., Davis, M.F., Guardabassi, L. and Weese, J.S. (2017) Recommendations for approaches to meticillin-resistant staphylococcal infections of small animals: diagnosis, therapeutic considerations and preventative measures. *Veterinary Dermatology* 28(3), 304–e69. DOI: 10.1111/vde.12444.

Mullen, K.M., Regier, P.J., Waln, M. and Colee, J. (2021) *Ex vivo* comparison of leak testing of canine jejunal enterotomies: saline infusion versus air insufflation. *Veterinary Surgery* 50(6), 1257–1266. DOI: 10.1111/vsu.13652.

Nelson, L.L. (2011) Surgical site infections in small animal surgery. *Veterinary Clinics of North America: Small Animal Practice* 41, 1041–1056.

NICE (2019) *Surgical Infections: Prevention and Treatment*. NICE Guideline NG125. National Institute for Health and Care Excellence, London. Available at: www.nice.org.uk/guidance/ng125/chapter/Context (accessed 23 October 2022).

NICE (2020) Prontosan for Acute and Chronic Wounds. Medtech Innovation Briefing MIB220. National Institute for Healthand Care Excellence, London. Available at: www.nice.org.uk/advice/mib220 (accessed 14 February 2022).

Nicholson, M., Beal, M., Shofer, F. and Brown, D.C. (2002) Epidemiologic evaluation of postoperative wound infection in clean-contaminated wounds: a retrospective study of 239 dogs and cats. *Veterinary Surgery* 31, 577–581.

Ogeer-Gyles, J., Mathews, K.A., Sears, W., Prescott, J.F., Weese, J.S. *et al.* (2006) Development of antimicrobial drug resistance in rectal *Escherichia coli* isolates from dogs hospitalized in an intensive care unit. *Journal of the American Veterinary Medical Association* 229, 694–699.

Owens, B.B.D., White, D.W. and Wenke, J.C. (2009) Comparison of irrigation solutions and devices in a contaminated musculoskeletal wound survival model. *Journal of Bone and Joint Surgery Series A* 91, 92–98. DOI: 10.2106/JBJS.G.01566.

Paul, N.C., Bärgman, S.C., Moodley, A., Nielsen, S.S. and Guarabassi, L. (2012) *Staphylococcus pseudintermedius* colonization patterns and strain diversity in healthy dogs: a cross-sectional and longitudinal study. *Veterinary Microbiology* 160, 420–427.

Pavletic, M.M. (ed.) (2018) *Atlas of Small Animal Wound Management and Reconstructive Surgery*, 4th edn. Wiley, Hoboken, New Jersey.

Peng, Z., Li, H., Cao, Z., Zhang, W., Li, H. *et al.* (2020) Oxygen embolism after hydrogen peroxide irrigation during hip arthroscopy: a case report. *BMC Musculoskeletal Disorders* 21, 58.

PHE (2016) UK Standards for Microbiology Investigations. Investigation of pus and exudates. PHE publications gateway number: 2016127. Public Health England, London. Available at: www.gov.uk/government/publications/smi-b-14-investigation-of-abscesses-and-deep-seated-wound-infections (accessed 23 October 2022).

PHE (2018) UK Standards for Microbiology Investigations. Investigation of swabs from skin and superficial soft tissue infections. PHE publications gateway number: 2016056. Public Health England, London. Available at: www.gov.uk/government/publications/smi-b-11-investigation-of-skin-superficial-and-non-surgical-wound-swabs (accessed 23 October 2022).

PHE (2021) UK Standards for Microbiology Investigations. Investigation of orthopaedic implant associated infections. PHE publications gateway number: GOV-9410. Public Health England, London. Available at: www.gov.uk/government/publications/smi-b-44-investigation-of-prosthetic-joint-infection-samples (accessed 23 October 2022).

Posner, L.P., Pavuk, A.A., Rokshar, J.L., Carter, J.E. and Levine, J.F. (2010) Effects of opioids and anesthetic drugs on body temperature in cats. *Veterinary Anaesthesia and Analgesia* 37, 35–43.

Reid, J. and Morison, M. (1994) Towards a consensus: classification of pressure sores. *Journal of Wound Care* 3, 157–160.

Rodeheaver, G. (2001) Wound cleansing, wound irrigation, wound disinfection. In: Kraner, D., Rodeheaver, G.T. and Sibbald, R.G. (eds) *Chronic Wound Care: A Clinical Source Book for Healthcare Professionals*, 3rd edn. HM Communications, Wayne, Pennsylvania.

Rushbrook, J.L., White, G., Kidger, L., Marsh, P. and Taggart, T.F. (2014) The antibacterial effect of 2-octyl cyanoacrylate (Dermabond®) skin adhesive. *Journal of Infection Prevention* 15, 236–239.

Saile, K., Boothe, H.W. and Boothe, D.M. (2010) Saline volume necessary to achieve predetermined intraluminal pressures during leak testing of small intestinal biopsy sites in the dog. *Veterinary Surgery* 39, 900–903.

Sandy-Hodgetts, K., Andersen, C.A., Al-Jalodi, O., Serena, L., Teimouri, C. *et al.* (2021) Uncovering the high prevalence of bacterial burden in surgical site wounds with point-of-care fluorescence imaging. *International Wound Journal* 19, 1438–1448.

Sanger, P.C., Simianu, V.V., Gaskill, C.E., Armstrong, C.A., Hartzler, A.L. *et al.* (2017) Diagnosing surgical site infection using wound photography: a scenario-based study. *Journal of the American College of Surgeons* 224, 8–15. DOI: 10.1016/j.jamcollsurg.2016.10.027.

Savicky, R., Simianu, V.V., Gaskill, C.E., Armstrong, C.A.L., Hartzler, A.L. *et al.* (2013) Outcome following removal of TPLO implants with surgical site infection. *Veterinary and Comparative Orthopaedics and Traumatology* 26, 260–265.

Schiffman, J., Golinko, M.S., Yan, A., Flattau, A., Tomic-Canic, M. *et al.* (2009) Operative debridement of pressure ulcers. *World Journal of Surgery* 33, 1396–1402. DOI: 10.1007/s00268-009-0024-4.

Schupp, C.J. and Holland-Cunz, S. (2009) Persistent subcutaneous oedema and aseptic fatty tissue necrosis after using Octenisept®. *European Journal of Pediatric Surgery* 19, 179–183.

Shah, H.N., Nayyar, R., Rajamahanty, S. and Hemal, A.K. (2012) Prospective evaluation of unidirectional barbed suture for various indications in surgeon-controlled robotic reconstructive urologic surgery: Wake Forest University experience. *International Urology and Nephrology* 44, 775–785.

Sharma, D., Misba, L. and Khan, A.U. (2019) Antibiotics versus biofilm: an emerging battleground in microbial communities. *Antimicrobial Resistance & Infection Control* 8, 76.

Şimşek, T., Şimşek, H.U. and Cantürk, N.Z. (2014) Response to trauma and metabolic changes: post-traumatic metabolism. *Turkish Journal of Surgery* 30(3), 153–159. DOI: 10.5152/UCD.2014.2653.

Spah, C.E., Elkins, A.D., Wehrenberg, A., Jaffe, M.H., Baird, D.K., Naughton, J.F. and Payton, M.E. (2013) Evaluation of two novel self-anchoring barbed sutures in a prophylactic laparoscopic gastropexy compared with intracorporeal tied knots. *Veterinary Surgery* 42, 932–942.

Staatz, A.J., Monnet, E. and Seim, H.B. (2002) Open peritoneal drainage versus primary closure for the treatment of septic peritonitis in dogs and cats: 42 cases (1993–1999). *Veterinary Surgery* 31, 174–180.

Stine, S.L., Odum, S.M. and Mertens, W.D. (2018) Protocol changes to reduce implant-associated infection rate after tibial plateau levelling osteotomy: 703 dogs, 811 TPLO (2006–2014). *Veterinary Surgery* 47, 481–489.

Stokes, R.A., Coleman, M.C., Rogovskyy, A.S., Dickerson, V.M. and Mankin, K.M.T. (2021) Comparison of bacteriologic culture results for skin wound swabs and skin wound biopsy specimens. *Journal of the American Veterinary Medical Association* 259, 1416–1421.

Tenover, F.C. (2006) Mechanisms of antimicrobial resistance in bacteria. *American Journal of Infection Control* 34(Suppl. 1), S3–S20. DOI: 10.1016/j.ajic.2006.05.219.

Towfigh, S., Cheadle, W.G., Lowry, S.F., Malangoni, M.A. and Wilson, S.E. (2008) Significant reduction in incidence of wound contamination by skin flora through use of microbial sealant. *Archives of Surgery* 143, 885–891.

Trocchia, A.M., Aho, H.N. and Sobol, G. (2009) A re-exploration of the use of barbed sutures in flexor tendon repairs. *Orthopedics* 32, 731–735.

Tsu, Sun. (2010) *The Art of War*. Capstone Publishing, Chichester, UK.

Turk, R., Singh, A. and Weese, J.S. (2015) Prospective surgical site infection surveillance in dogs. *Veterinary Surgery* 44, 2–8.

Urschel, J.D. (1999) Necrotizing soft tissue infections. *Postgraduate Medical Journal* 75, 645–649.

Wang, L., Belisle, B., Bassiri, M., Xu, P., Debabov, D. *et al.* (2011) Chemical characterization and

Kelly L. Bowlt Blacklock *et al.*

biological properties of NVC-422, a novel, stable N-chlorotaurine analog. *Antimicrobial Agents and Chemotherapy* 55, 2688–2692.

Wang, L.S., Wang, X.-Y., Tu, H.-T., Huang, Y.-F., Qi, X. *et al*. (2020) Octyl-2-cyanoacrylate tissue adhesive without subcuticular suture for wound closure after total hip arthroplasty: a prospective observational study on thirty-two cases with controls for 3 months follow-up. *Journal of Orthopaedic Surgery and Research* 15, 467.

Weber, S.G., Gold, H., Hooper, D.C., Karchmer, A.W. and Carmeli, Y. (2003) Fluoroquinolones and the risk for methicillin-resistant *Staphylococcus aureus* in hospitalized patients. *Emerging Infectious Diseases* 9, 1415–1422.

Weese, J.S. (2008) A review of multidrug resistant surgical site infections. *Veterinary and Comparative Orthopaedics and Traumatology* 21, 1–7.

Weese, J.S. (2020) *Wound Sampling for Culture & Cytology*. Clinician's Brief. Available at: www.cliniciansbrief.com/article/wound-sampling-culture-cytology (accessed 23 October 2022).

WHO (2020) *Hypochlorous Acid (HOCl) for disinfection, antisepsis, and wound care in core categories 15.1, 15.2, and 13*. World Health Organization, Geneva, Switzerland. Available at: https://cdn.who.int/media/docs/default-source/essential-medicines/2021-eml-expert-committee/applications-for-addition-of-new-medicines/a.18_hypochlorous-acid.pdf (accessed 23 October 2022).

Weese, J.S., Poma. R., James, F., Buenviaje, G., Foster, R. and Slavic, D. (2009) *Staphylococcus pseudintermedius* necrotizing fasciitis in a dog. *Canadian Veterinary Journal* 50, 655–656.

Williams, J.M. and Moores, A. (eds) (2009) *BSAVA Manual of Canine and Feline Wound and Reconstruction*. British Small Animal Veterinary Association, Quedgeley, UK.

Wilson, M.A. (2003) Skin and soft-tissue infections: impact of resistant Gram-positive bacteria. *American Journal of Surgery* 186, 35–41.

Wilson, S.E. (2008) Microbial sealing: a new approach to reducing contamination. *Journal of Hospital Infection* 70(Suppl. 2), 11–14. DOI: 10.1016/S0195-6701(08)60018-3.

WoundSource Editors (2018) Wound debridement options: the 5 major methods. WoundSource. Available at: www.woundsource.com/blog/wound-debridement-options-5-major-methods (accessed 23 October 2022).

WSAVA (2022) Nutrition toolkit. WSAVA global nutrition committee. World Small Animal Veterinary Association, Dundas, Ontario. Available at: https://wsava.org/wp-content/uploads/2021/04/WSAVA-Global-Nutrition-Toolkit-English.pdf (accessed 25 October 2022).

Yagnik, D., Serafin, V. and Shah, A.J. (2018) Antimicrobial activity of apple cider vinegar against *Escherichia coli*, *Staphylococcus aureus* and *Candida albicans*; downregulating cytokine and microbial protein expression. *Scientific Reports* 8, 1732. DOI: 10.1038/s41598-017-18618-x.

Yagnik, D., Ward, M. and Shah, A.J. (2021) Antibacterial apple cider vinegar eradicates methicillin resistant *Staphylococcus aureus* and resistant *Escherichia coli*. *Scientific Reports* 11, 1854. DOI: 10.1038/s41598-020-78407-x.

Young, P.Y. and Khadaroo, R.G. (2014) Surgical site infections. *Surgical Clinics of North America* 94, 1245–1264. DOI: 10.1016/j.suc.2014.08.008.

11 Open Wound Management

KELLY L. BOWLT BLACKLOCK*

Royal (Dick) School of Veterinary Studies, University of Edinburgh, Roslin, UK

11.1 Introduction

Open wounds are a common presenting complaint in veterinary practice, and wound management can be challenging but also incredibly rewarding. There is an ever-expanding and sometimes overwhelming array of products, dressings and techniques available that promise to treat all wounds at every stage of the healing journey. Some wounds require extensive initial assistance to prepare them for the road to healing. However, as Ovid said: 'Some wounds are made worse by treatment, as we see: it had been better not to touch them.' Therefore, the clinician should be mindful that novel treatments are not always an improvement on traditional techniques and evidence-based medicine should be practised wherever possible. Wound management is the cornerstone of a soft-tissue surgery specialist's role and the author would encourage practitioners to chat to their local referral institution so that they can gather regular, bespoke advice about how to manage the wound as it evolves. Importantly, this connection will provide the refreshment and reinvigoration that we all need from our colleagues during the vicissitudes of the wound-healing marathon.

The initial management of the wound should include providing generous multi-modal analgesia, addressing contamination, removing implants if necessary and obtaining samples for bacteriological analysis. Further information is provided in Chapter 10 (this volume). This chapter will provide additional information on how to manage the open wound. In the first instance, the practitioner must encourage the wound to form a healthy granulation bed. Once this granulation bed has been achieved, the wound conditions should be optimized to promote wound contraction and epithelialization. This chapter will provide details on dressings that are helpful during each stage of wound healing, and will also offer advice on assessing wound progress. Finally, we will look at how to assess the chronic wound.

11.2 Wound Healing: An Overview

Briefly, wound healing consists of four stages, which occur in a dynamic, overlapping and often simultaneous fashion. It is important to understand these phases, because this knowledge will facilitate the clinician in deciding how to best support the wound:

1. *Inflammation*. The inflammatory phase begins at the time of injury and lasts 3–5 days. It is characterized by increased vascular permeability, chemotaxis and activation of circulatory cells (macrophages, neutrophils, lymphocytes and fibroblasts), and release of cytokines and growth factors. The resultant blood clot and scab facilitate haemostasis, provide a scaffold for migrating cells, and protect the wound from further contamination and fluid loss.
2. *Debridement*. During the debridement phase of healing, neutrophils and monocytes arrive in the wound bed. Neutrophils arrive as soon as 6 h after injury and aim to prevent infection and phagocytose debris and microorganisms. Monocytes arrive later (12 h after injury) and synthesize the growth factors required for the repair and maturation phases of wound healing. After 24–48 h, the monocytes mature into macrophages and secrete collagenase to remove necrotic tissue and phagocytose bacteria.
3. *Repair*. The repair phase begins 3–5 days after injury and comprises fibroblast stimulation, which encourages the fibroblasts to proliferate and migrate into the wound from neighbouring tissue. Initially, the fibroblasts are haphazard in their orientation, but wound tension rapidly encourages

*Kelly.blacklock@ed.ac.uk

© CAB International 2023. *Infection Control in Small Animal Clinical Practice* (eds F. Allerton and K.L. Bowlt Blacklock)
DOI: 10.1079/9781789244977.0011

them to organize themselves such that they are parallel to the wound margin. Angiogenesis is also promoted, resulting in capillary growth into the wound from the surrounding tissue. The result is granulation tissue, which is formed from new capillaries, fibroblasts and fibrous tissue, and is bright red when healthy. Granulation tissue acts as a barrier to infection, a platform for migration of epithelium cells and a source of myofibroblasts (which are essential for wound contraction).

4. *Maturation.* This final phase of wound healing starts around 17–20 days after injury, but can continue for many years. This phase is characterized by collagen deposition and remodelling, which involves the collagen fibres orientating along lines of stress, increasing cross-linking and increasing in thickness. Importantly, only 20% of the final scar strength is achieved in the first 3 weeks (commonly the time of skin suture/staple removal), and the final scar is only 80% of the strength of the original skin.

11.2.1 The ideal wound environment

Maintaining a moist environment is necessary for optimal wound healing: extreme wet or dry conditions can adversely affect healing. Exudate is a combination of vascular fluid and white blood cells, which develops in the wound bed secondary to the increased vascular permeability caused by inflammation. The amount of exudate produced by a wound is related to surface area: the larger the surface area, the greater the likely volume of exudate (Thomas *et al.*, 1996; WUWHS, 2007). Human unspecified granulating wounds produce around 5 g of exudate per 10 cm^2 in 24 h (Lamke *et al.*, 1977), but similar studies in veterinary companion animals are lacking. Some wound types are likely to have high rates of exudate production, including burns or infected wounds. In a healing wound, the volume of exudate generally reduces over time; failure to do so is suggestive of an underlying cause (e.g. infection or ongoing inflammation) which maintains the elevated levels of inflammatory mediators and activated matrix metalloproteinases required for exudate production (WUWHS, 2007). Our role in the management of the open wound is to maximize the positive effects of exudate (e.g. stimulating cell proliferation and facilitating migration; providing water, electrolytes and nutrients for cell metabolism; enabling diffusion of growth and immune factors; assisting autolysis) and minimize the adverse effects (e.g. tissue maceration, saturation of dressings, delayed wound healing, protein loss, discomfort/pain) (WUWHS, 2007).

The following sections will discuss how to support development of a healthy granulation bed and, once this has been achieved, how to support wound contraction and epithelialization.

11.3 Supporting Development of a Healthy Granulation Bed

Granulation tissue is a welcome indicator that a wound is progressing from the inflammatory to the repair/proliferative phase of wound healing. This tissue is a complex of fibroblasts, vascular endothelial cells and macrophages within a matrix of collagen, elastin and fibrin, and is necessary for wound contraction and migration of epithelium. Healthy granulation tissue is recognizable as bright red and cobblestone in appearance (Fig. 11.1a). Importantly, granulation tissue is extremely resistant to infection and antibiotics are not usually indicated at this stage. Changes in the appearance of the granulation tissue (e.g. pale or very dark colour, friable, excessive/proud tissue; Fig. 11.1b) can indicate underlying problems. To encourage formation of healthy granulation tissue, the practitioner may wish to use negative-pressure wound therapy (the author's method of choice), adherent dressings or hydrocolloid gels, with the aim of debriding the tissue and stimulating new vascular growth.

11.3.1 Negative-pressure wound therapy

The most promising recent development in wound management is negative-pressure wound therapy (NPWT), or vacuum-assisted closure. NPWT is well tolerated by patients, is used to optimize the wound bed for surgical closure or second intention healing, and is applicable to a wide variety of canine and feline wounds (Pitt and Stanley, 2014).

NPWT involves local application of negative pressure to a wound bed via an open-cell foam/gauze (Fig. 11.2). Intermittent or continuous suction is applied via a portable suction unit, with wound fluid being evacuated through the tubing into the reservoir canister. Intermittent NPWT more effectively stimulates angiogenesis and granulation tissue compared with continuous NPWT; however, intermittent suction appears to be more painful, and therefore the author uses continuous suction (at –125 mmHg) in clinical patients (Borgquist

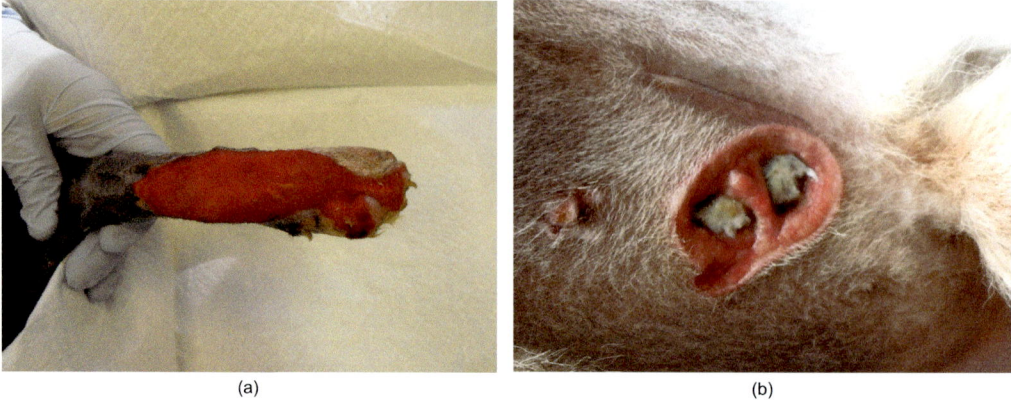

(a)   (b)

Fig. 11.1. (a) Photograph of the distal limb of a cat, showing a healthy bed of granulation tissue. (b) Photograph of an inguinal wound in a dog, showing pale, unhealthy granulation tissue and necrotic tissue, which needs to be debrided to stimulate new ingrowth of blood vessels. Photograph courtesy of Kate Forster.

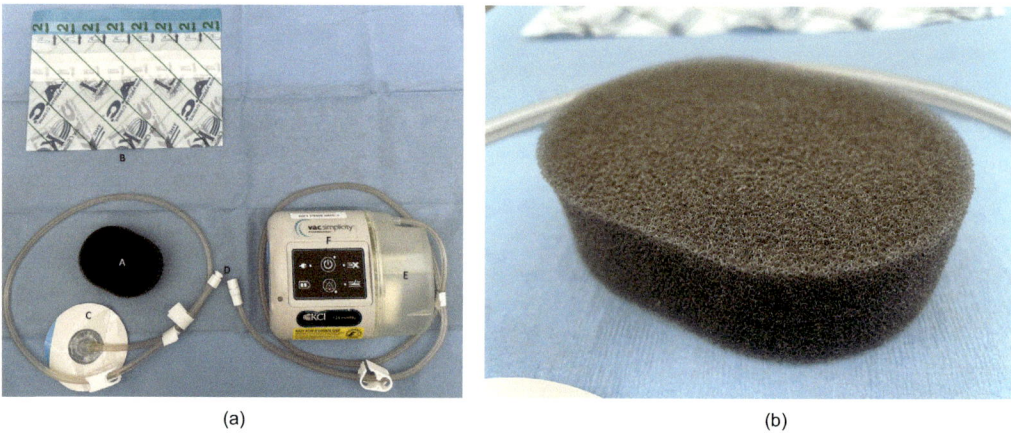

(a)   (b)

Fig. 11.2. Negative-pressure wound therapy involves local application of negative pressure to a wound bed via an open-cell foam/gauze. (a) The foam (A) is covered with an adhesive dressing (B) and a footplate attached (C). The footplate tubing is connected to the tubing from the reservoir cannister (D). The reservoir cannister (E) is disposable and filled with an absorbent material to contain any exudate evacuated from the wound via the tubing. The canister is connected directly to the suction machine (F), which generates the negative pressure in the system. (b) Close-up view of the foam, so that the open cells are visible.

et al., 2010a, b; Timmers *et al.*, 2005). The median duration of NPWT use during wound treatment has been reported as 3 days, with a mean hospitalization of 7.8 days (Pitt and Stanley, 2014). The benefits of NPWT may include:

- reduced oedema and exudate accumulation;
- elimination of strikethrough of bandages because wound fluid is evacuated into the collection canister;

- increased central wound perfusion and vascularization (Chen *et al.*, 2005; Wackenfors *et al.*, 2005; McNulty *et al.*, 2007; Nolff *et al.*, 2018b);
- rapid stimulation of a uniform bed of granulation tissue (Ben-Amotz *et al.*, 2007; Malmsjö *et al.*, 2009; Wilkes *et al.*, 2009; Demaria *et al.*, 2011);
- increased wound fluid partial pressure of oxygen, interleukin-8 and vascular endothelial growth

factor (Labler *et al.*, 2009), and decreased wound matrix metallopeptidase proteinase 9 activity (Nolff *et al.*, 2018a);

- more rapid wound contraction and healing (Owen *et al.*, 2009), with time to healing halved in patients treated with NPWT compared with foam dressings (Nolff *et al.*, 2015); and
- reduced need for bandage changes compared with other dressings used for open-wound management, as NPWT dressings require changing at least every 3 days, compared with every 12–24 h for wet-to-dry dressings; both dressing types require heavy sedation or anaesthesia to permit changing, but the increased duration between changes associated with NPWT permits greater periods of patient recovery and more opportunity for nutritional intact and ambulation (Pitt and Stanley, 2014).

Findings in the literature about the ability of NPWT to reduce wound bacterial contamination are inconsistent (Moües *et al.*, 2004; Weed *et al.*, 2004). However, there is evidence that NPWT-treated wounds show less progression of local infection compared with wounds treated with silver-coated foam dressing (Nolff *et al.*, 2018b). In cats and dogs, NPWT-treated wounds suffered fewer complications and became septic less frequently compared with wounds treated with a polyurethane foam dressing (Nolff *et al.*, 2015, 2017).

NPWT is widely used in many veterinary hospitals to manage a variety of wounds, including traumatic wounds, decubitus ulcers, degloving injuries, distal extremity wounds (Ben-Amotz *et al.*, 2007), thoracic or abdominal wound dehiscence, septic peritonitis (Cioffi *et al.*, 2012), cytotoxic sloughs, burns, perineal wounds, osteomyelitis and traumatic wounds with exposed bone (and even shell; Adkesson *et al.*, 2007), or overexposed orthopaedic implants (Bertran *et al.*, 2013) (Fig. 11.3).

Importantly, prolonged use of NPWT impairs wound contraction and epithelialization (Demaria *et al.*, 2011), and therefore it is important to alter the dressing appropriately once the uniform bed of healthy granulation tissue has been obtained. If the plan is to support the wound to heal by second intention, the author will often select a foam dressing at this stage to maintain an environment conducive to wound contraction and epithelialization.

Complications associated with NPWT are minor. The most common complications include loss of vacuum because of inadequate peri-wound adhesion and mild dermatitis around the wound margin. These are usually readily addressed.

11.3.2 Adherent dressings and hydrogels

Adherent dressings (e.g. wet-to-dry) adhere to the wound bed via proteinaceous exudates penetrating the dressing and drying into the secondary dressing layer. To apply a wet-to-dry dressing, a sterile, open-weave gauze is soaked in saline solution and squeezed by hand to remove as much of the fluid as possible. It is then placed into the wound bed, taking care not to cover the healthy skin beyond the wound edges because this may encourage maceration. The absorbent secondary layer (e.g. Soffban and Knitfix) and finally the tertiary layer (e.g. Vetrap) is applied routinely and the dressing is left in place until dry. Once dried, the contact layer is removed, stripping off the necrotic tissue.

The advantages of wet-to-dry dressing are that only non-viable tissue is removed, and dressing materials are very cheap. However, dressings should be changed every 12–24 h (or more frequently if the exudate is copious) and their removal is painful (therefore heavy sedation or general anaesthesia is required). Importantly, adherent dressings prevent epithelialization and as such are only appropriate in the debridement stage of wound management. Care should be taken that there is no strikethrough of the dressings, which will encourage environmental contamination of the wound.

Some clinicians prefer gentler wound debridement. This can be achieved by using hydrogels (e.g. Intrasite, Granugel), which allow debridement by autolysis and offer increased absorptive capacity. Hydrogels can also be left in place for up to 48 h and can be moulded to the shape of irregular wounds due to their amorphous nature, which is particularly useful in cavities. Once applied, a non-adhesive dressing is required to keep the gel in place. Hydrogels can predispose to excessive granulation tissue and therefore the wound should be closely monitored.

Regardless of the primary layer used in the dressing, the practitioner must ensure that copious padding is applied over bony prominences (e.g. hock, carpus, elbow) and that the pressure exerted by the dressing is uniform along its length so as to minimize the risk of bandage-related complications (e.g. pressure necrosis). Where the location of the wound makes maintaining a dressing *in situ*

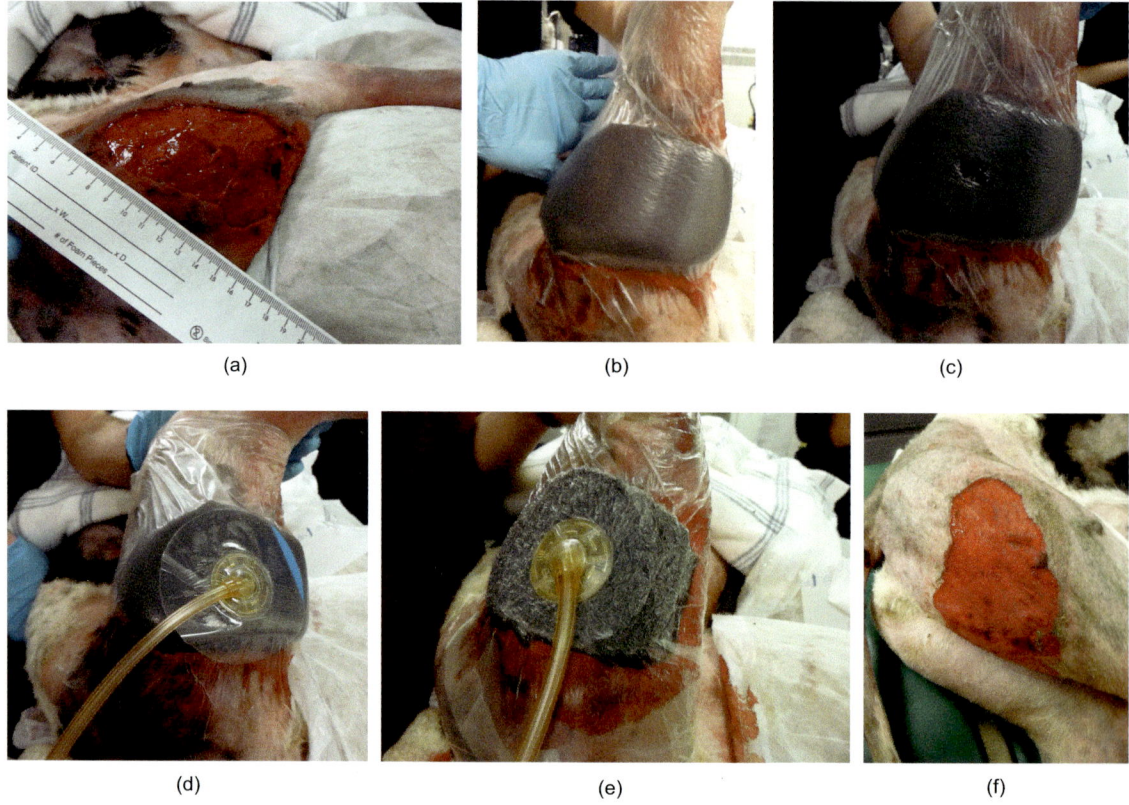

(a)   (b)   (c)

(d)   (e)   (f)

Fig. 11.3. (a) Image of a 12 × 9 cm full-thickness skin wound sustained to the thigh of a greyhound during a dog fight 2 days previously. The injury sustained resulted in significant undermining of the surrounding skin circumferentially around the thigh, and extending from the stifle distally to the mid-lumbar region cranially. (b) An open-pore dressing was cut to the shape of the wound, applied directly to the wound bed, and covered with an adhesive dressing. (c–e) A hole was made in the adhesive dressing (c) to allow the suction footplate to be placed (d) and the negative pressure applied (e). Note how the foam has shrunk in size once the negative pressure is turned on. (f) On day 4, the NPWT was removed: the undermining of the skin had resolved and a uniform bed of healthy granulation tissue was apparent.

challenging, a tie-over dressing might be useful (Fig. 11.4).

11.4 Supporting Wound Contraction and Epithelialization

Once a healthy granulation bed has been achieved, the wound can be supported to heal by second intention or can be closed surgically (e.g. secondary closure using a skin flap or graft). This section will discuss how to achieve wound closure by second intention, with a particular emphasis on dressing choices.

To allow wound contraction and epithelialization over the granulation bed, the dressing should provide the optimal environment for wound healing. It should be:

- moist (but not wet);
- infection and debris free;
- 35–37°C;
- minimally mobile; and
- pH 6 (to prevent bacteria from multiplying).

A daunting array of advanced wound dressings are available that regulate the wound surface by retaining moisture or absorbing exudate, thereby protecting the wound and surrounding tissue. Importantly, the choice of dressing may change as the wound evolves over time.

Kelly L. Bowlt Blacklock

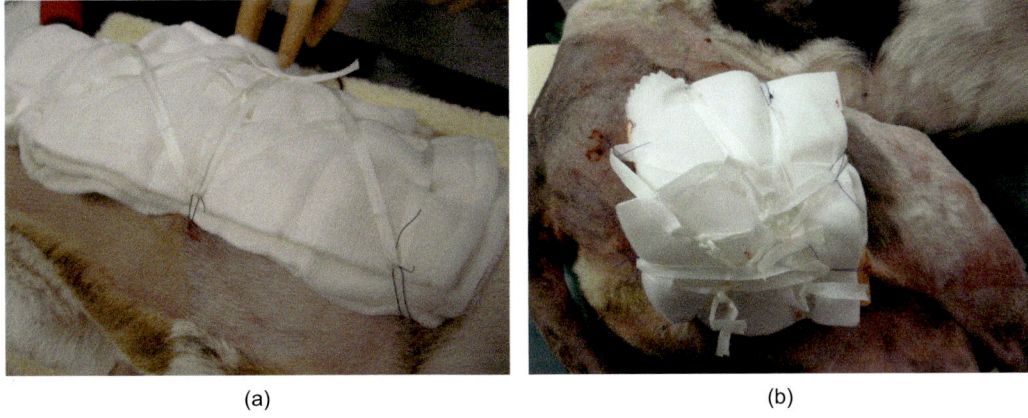

(a)   (b)

Fig. 11.4. (a) A tie-over dressing is useful in regions where maintaining a dressing is challenging (e.g. over the dorsum). Large loops of suture material are placed at regular intervals in the skin neighbouring the wound, and nylon tie is passed through them to secure the underlying dressing in place. (b) After NPWT in the dog shown in Fig. 11.3, a foam dressing was used as a primary layer on the caudal thigh wound, stabilized using a tie-over dressing.

11.4.1   Evidence for dressing types

Dressings are classified as medical devices and therefore the quality of evidence required for their approval is lower than that required for medicines. This is reflected in the small number or poor quality of randomized controlled trials in human medicine, and more so in veterinary medicine. The author has summarized some of the review findings, which may be of interest to the reader in veterinary practice (Table 11.1). Of relevance to this chapter is a further Cochrane review, which aimed to assess the effects of systemic and topical antibiotics, and topical antiseptics for the treatment of surgical wounds healing by secondary intention (Vermeulen *et al.*, 2009). In this review, the authors concluded that there was no robust evidence on the relative effectiveness of any antiseptic/antibiotic/antibacterial preparation evaluated to date for use on surgical wounds healing by secondary intention.

11.4.2   Advanced wound dressings

The National Institute for Health and Care Excellence (NICE) classifies advanced wounds dressings according to their primary component (some dressings comprise several components): hydrogel dressings, hydrocolloid dressings, capillary-acting dressings, foam dressings, odour-absorbent dressings, soft polymer dressings and alginate dressings (BNF, 2022). Importantly, paraffin gauze dressings (e.g. Jelonet) are no longer recommended for

open-wound management, although the author still occasionally uses them following skin grafting procedures. Further details about the more commonly used dressings are presented below, including information about relevant veterinary studies. Some examples of proprietary dressings have also been provided, but other products are also available and further products will certainly come to market in the future.

Hydrogel dressings

Hydrogel dressings (e.g. Intrasite Gel, GranuGel) comprise a water-based, amorphous, cohesive application that is applied to the wound bed and covered with a secondary, non-absorbent dressing. These dressings are used to facilitate autolytic debridement of necrotic wounds and are generally unsuitable for supporting a wound that is progressing towards contraction and epithelialization. Further information is provided in Table 10.2 (Chapter 10, this volume).

Hydrocolloid dressings

Hydrocolloid dressings (e.g. Aquacel, Granuflex, Hydrocoll) consist of carboxymethylated cellulose, pectin and gelatine that forms a non-adherent gel on contact with the wound (Fig. 11.5). The dressing has a flexible, adhesive waterproof backing. In human medicine, hydrocolloid dressings are

Table 11.1. A summary of selected meta-analyses and Cochrane reviews investigating evidence for the use of dressings in wound management in humans. Similar studies in veterinary medicine are lacking, but it is reasonable to assume that results are comparable (as suggested by small veterinary studies).

Study design	Study objectives	Study findings	Limitations	Reference
Meta-analysis	Comparison of silver dressings and control dressings in complete healing of leg wounds and ulcers	No difference in long-term healing between the study groups	All studies considered had quality or bias issues	Carter et al. (2010)
Cochrane review	Comparison of silver- and non-silver-containing dressings on uninfected wound healing	Insufficient evidence to support the use of silver dressings or creams in promoting wound healing or preventing wound infection	Most trials considered were small and of poor quality	Storm-Versloot et al. (2010)
Cochrane review	Assessment of the effects of honey compared with alternative wound dressings and topical treatments on the healing of acute and/or chronic wounds	Honey heals partial thickness burns more quickly than conventional treatment, and infected post-operative wounds more quickly than antiseptics and gauze	Heterogeneous nature of the patient populations and comparators, and low quality of the evidence	Jull et al. (2015)
Cochrane review	Assessment of the effectiveness of dressings and topical agents on surgical wound healing by secondary intention	Foam is best studied as an alternative to gauze and appears to be preferable in terms of pain reduction, patient satisfaction and nursing time	Small, poor-quality trials	Vermeulen et al. (2009)
Cochrane review	Evaluation of the benefits and risks of early versus delayed dressing removal after primary closure of clean and clean-contaminated surgical wounds	The early removal of dressings from clean or clean-contaminated surgical wounds appears to have no detrimental effect on outcomes. Early dressing removal may result in a significantly shorter hospital stay and significantly reduced costs than covering the surgical wound with dressings beyond the first 48 h after surgery	Small, randomized controlled trials	Toon et al. (2015)

helpful for use on clean, uninfected, dry, medium-thickness wounds, whereby they provide a moist environment for wound healing. Care should be taken because the dressings can cause peri-wound maceration or hypergranulation. In the veterinary literature, hydrocolloid dressings have been used to cover first intention healing surgical wounds and were shown to promote organized granulation tissue and decreased inflammatory cells in

the wound bed (Abramo et al., 2008). The use of hydrocolloids in open-wound management is uncommon in veterinary medicine and the evidence is controversial. In a feline model of second intention wound healing, no significant difference in subjective clinical evaluation or planimetry was observed between the hydrocolloid-treated and control wounds (Tsioli et al., 2016, 2018). In these studies, oedema was significantly increased, and

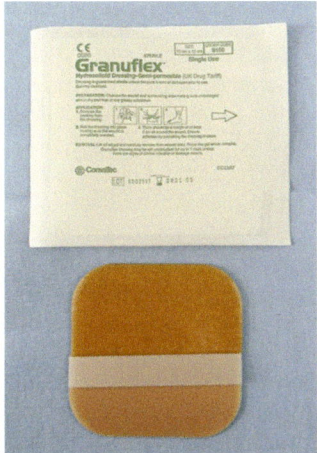

Fig. 11.5. Hydrocolloid dressings consist of carboxymethylated cellulose, pectin and gelatine that form a non-adherent gel on contact with the wound. They are uncommonly used in veterinary medicine.

granulation tissue formation was accelerated in the hydrocolloid-treated wounds.

Capillary-acting dressings

Capillary-acting dressings (e.g. Vacutex) are useful in the management of moderate or heavily exuding wounds. The dressings promote wound debridement and rapid granulation tissue formation by removing exudate, slough and necrotic debris

away from the wound bed. Thereafter, once the wound bed is clean and uniform granulation tissue is apparent, continuation of wound management using this dressing is not optimal. To date, there are no studies assessing the use of capillary-acting dressings in veterinary medicine.

Vapour-permeable films and membranes

Film dressings (e.g. Primapore, Melolin, Leukomed) consist of a sheet of absorbent material between two thin layers of film that contain small pores for the movement of gas and fluid (Fig. 11.6). Movement of fluid into these pores results in the dressing being adherent at these points, and as such, this dressing is unsuitable for open-wound management. Film dressings might be indicated for use on post-operative closed wounds to protect the wound from environmental contamination until a fibrin seal is formed (6–8 h post-surgery). However, the author prefers to use a sterile liquid skin film adhesive (2-octyl cyanoacrylate), which acts as a physical barrier to bacteria and allows the wound to be assessed more easily because it is not obscured by a dressing. There is currently no published research investigating the use of film dressings in small animals.

ACTICOAT is a similar film-like dressing that comprises a nanocrystalline, silver-coated, high-density, polyethylene mesh with a polyester inner core (Fig. 11.7). The dressing releases silver-based

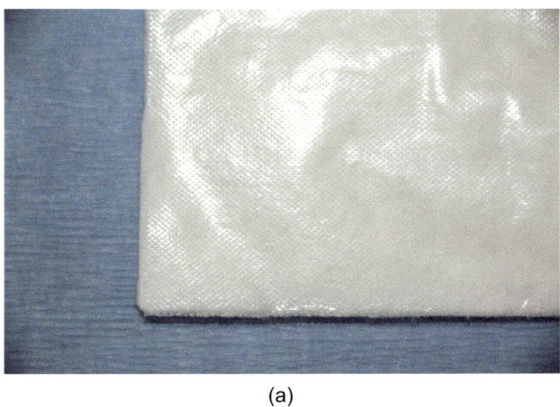

(a)

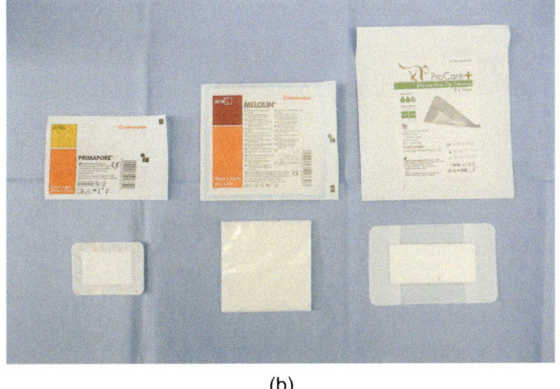

(b)

Fig. 11.6. (a) Close-up image of a film dressing, showing the small pores on the surface through which gas and fluid can move. (b) Film dressings are best reserved for use on post-operative wounds until a fibrin seal is formed, and are available with or without an adhesive backing (e.g. Primapore and Melolin, respectively), or with a silicone contact layer to prevent adhesion to the underlying wound (e.g. ProCare +).

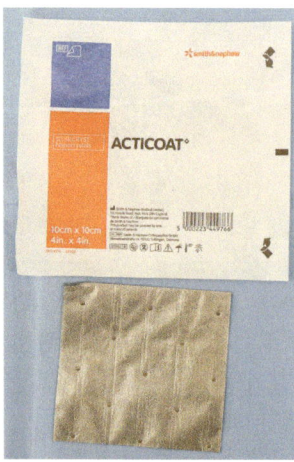

Fig. 11.7. ACTICOAT comprises a nanocrystalline, silver-coated, high-density, polyethylene mesh with a polyester inner core and is effective against a range of multidrug-resistant bacteria.

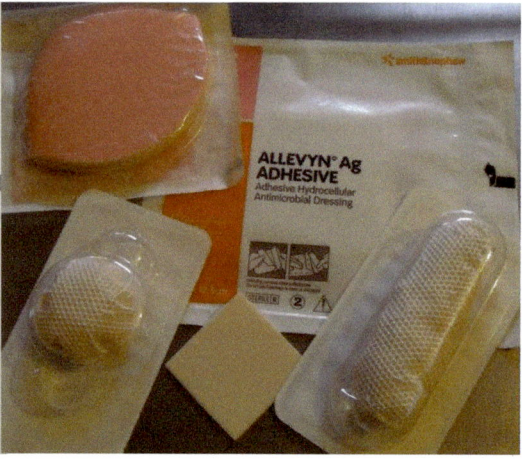

Fig. 11.8. Foam dressings come in a variety of shapes and sizes, including cup shaped (useful over extremities or bony prominences) and pockets (for use in cavities). Products can also be impregnated with silver or polyhexamethylene biguanide.

antimicrobial control, which reportedly lasts for up to 3 days and is effective *in vitro* against multidrug-resistant (MDR) *Pseudomonas* spp., MRSA and vancomycin-resistant *Enterococcus* spp. The author reserves the use of silver film dressings for patients with MDR-infected wounds, sometimes in combination with NPWT, and/or on some full-thickness skin-grafted wounds (Miller *et al.*, 2016).

Foam dressings

Foam dressings (e.g. Kendall Foam, Allevyn, ActivHeal Foam) are hydrophilic dressings made of polyurethane foam, which can be adhesive or non-adhesive and with or without a breathable film backing. The same foam dressings are also available in cup shapes (ideal for elbow wounds) or as pockets for use in cavities (Fig. 11.8). Foam dressings absorb variable amounts of exudate (including extremely large volumes of exudate, up to 1400 g m^2 over 24 h) while maintaining adequate oxygenation.

The non-adhesive nature of foam dressings mean that they are easy to apply, non-painful to remove and easily conform to the affected site. They do not interfere with wound contraction or epithelialization.

In patients with uncomplicated wounds where second intention healing is desirable, the author uses foam dressings once a healthy granulation bed has been achieved and until the wound is completely healed (Fig. 11.9). Foam dressings should be changed at least every 7 days, or when exudate is visible and approaches 1.5 cm from the edge of the dressing, whichever is sooner (Smith+Nephew, 2022). Infected wounds may require dressing changes more frequently. If the dressing becomes saturated, it should be changed more frequently because healthy skin can become macerated if it remains in contact with the wound fluid. Some foam dressings also contain antimicrobial substances, including silver (e.g. Allevyn Ag) and polyhexamethylene biguanide (PHMB, e.g. Kendall AMD). Both products claim to provide sustained antimicrobial properties (including against MDR bacteria) for up to 7 days *in vitro* (Driffield and Woodmansey, 2009), and the addition of silver has shown a reduction in clinical wound infection in human patients (Kotz *et al.*, 2009).

Soft polymer dressings

Soft polymer dressings (e.g. Silflex) are often silicone based, with a non-adherent or gently adherent layer. These dressings are suitable for lightly exudative wounds but can be combined with an overlying absorbent pad (e.g. polyurethane foam film backing such as Advazorb, Eclipse or Allevyn Gentle) for use on heavily exuding wounds (Fig. 11.10). For example, those with an absorbent overlying pad

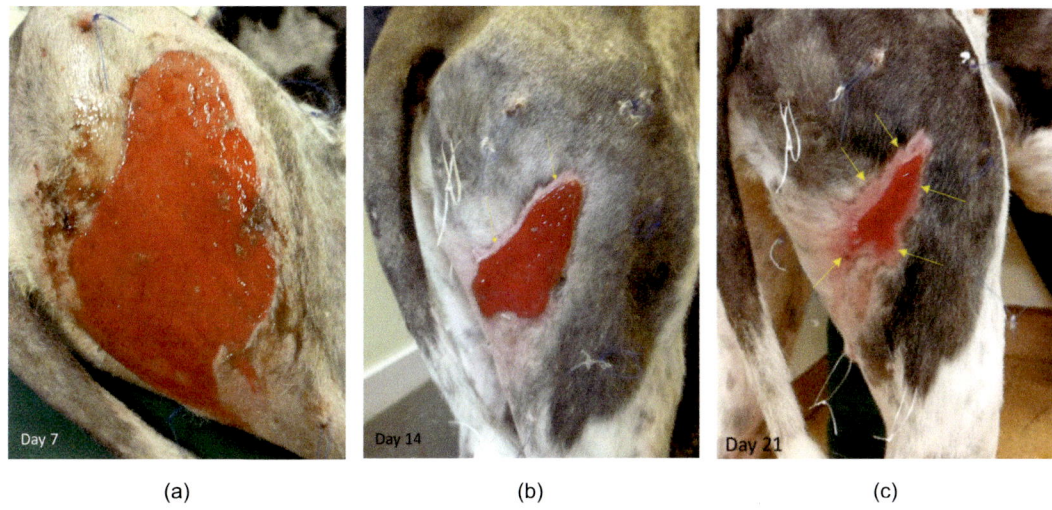

(a)   (b)   (c)

Fig. 11.9. Photographs of the same patient as in Fig. 11.3. A foam dressing was used as a primary layer, supported by a tie-over dressing. The wound pictured on days 7 (a), 14 (b) and 21 (c) shows rapid wound contraction, and epithelialization is evident along the wound edges (yellow arrows). Wound healing was complete by 30 days.

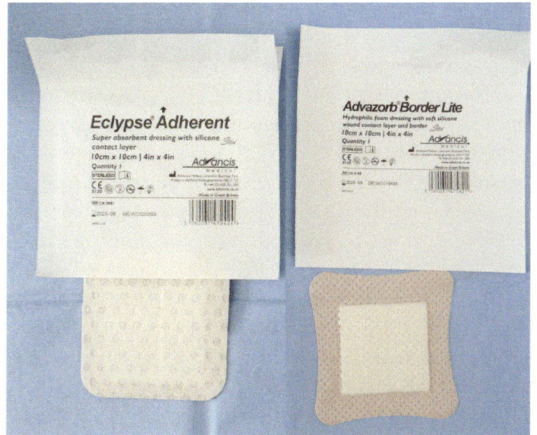

Fig. 11.10. Examples of two dressings with a soft silicone wound contact layer, absorbent layer and film backing. Eclypse has an absorbent layer that forms a gel when in contact with exudate; the absorbent layer in Advazorb is made from polyurethane foam.

can rapidly absorb fluid to a capacity of 600 g m² over 24 h.

Similar to foam dressings, soft polymer dressings can remain in place for up to 7 days but require changing once the dressing becomes saturated with exudate.

Importantly, blood clots can cause the dressing to adhere to the wound bed, and therefore soft polymer dressings are not suitable for bleeding wounds.

Odour-absorbent dressings

Odour-absorbent dressings (e.g. Askina Carbosorb) contain activated charcoal to absorb odour, but are rarely indicated in veterinary medicine. In the author's opinion, wound-related odour is likely to be indicative of an underlying cause (usually infection) and efforts would be more fruitfully directed at addressing the source of the odour.

Alginate dressing

Alginate dressings (e.g. ActivHeal Alginate, Kendall Calcium Alginate, Sorbsan Ribbon) are composed of calcium alginate or calcium sodium alginate, derived from brown seaweed. The woven product is placed into the wound and can absorb large volumes of exudate to form a gel, which is hydrophilic and promotes autolysis, encourages fibroplasias and encourages wound healing. Alginate dressings act as haemostatic agents, but they should not be used where bleeding is heavy and blood clots can cause the dressing to adhere to the wound bed. Alginate dressings are available as sheets or ropes, the latter of which can be layered into deep wounds, cavities and sinuses to absorb exudate and prevent maceration. Alginates can also be impregnated with silver (e.g. ACTICOAT Absorbent).

Miscellaneous

Manuka honey, topical PHMB, low-level laser therapy, hyperbaric therapy and bacteriophages have been briefly discussed in Chapter 10 (this volume).

11.5   Assessment of the Dressing

When regularly assessing the dressing, several factors should be considered, including the following (WUWHS, 2007):

- *Is there leakage of wound fluid?* The dressing should be inspected to ensure that there is no exudate that has penetrated the tertiary layer of the dressing. Strikethrough of the tertiary layer provides a conduit for bacteria to access the wound bed and suggests that the dressing should be changed more frequently (and/or a more absorptive dressing applied).
- *Is there saturation of the secondary dressing layer?* Extensive saturation of the secondary dressing may suggest that more regular dressing changes are indicated.
- *What is the condition of the primary dressing layer?* How much has the dressing adhered to the wound bed and does its removal cause pain to the patient?
- *Has the dressing maintained an appropriate level of wound moisture?* The aim of wound management is to maintain a moist (not wet) wound environment; therefore, if the dressing change frequency is appropriate for the dressing type, small amounts of fluid will be contained within the dressing. However, it will not be saturated.
- *Is the dressing clean?* Have appropriate measures been put in place to avoid patient interference or soiling of the dressing?
- *Is the dressing comfortable?* Are there any sites that are prone to bandage-related injuries, and if so, how can the risk of injury be minimized and/or wounds identified and managed at the earliest opportunity?

11.6   The Chronic Wound

Causes of poor wound healing are described in Table 11.2. When the plan for wound management

Table 11.2. Systemic and local causes of non-healing wounds.

Systemic	Local
Hyper/hypoadrenocorticism	Neoplasia
Exogenous steroid administration	Infection/necrosis
Thyroid disease	Skin edges undermined
Neoplasia	Foreign material present
Anaemia	Continued wound movement
Uraemia	Inappropriate choice of dressing or poor dressing application
Liver disease	Radiation therapy
Chemotherapy	Wound too dry/moist
Malnutrition	Inappropriate wound temperature/ oxygenation

is discussed with the patient's carer(s), it is vital to discuss the potential timescale and costs involved, because unrealistic expectations give the impression that the wound is not progressing, which is frustrating for everyone. Multiple surgeries may be required, and the financial implications (in terms of bandages, time, travel, medications, investigations, etc.) can be substantial. Where the wound looks healthy, often all that is required is more time. The authors initially treat patients with open wounds on an inpatient basis and warn carers that progression to healing can take weeks, if not months.

Ideally, the same clinician should manage the wound wherever possible, and photos should be taken regularly to assess the progress. Anecdotally, traumatic wounds deteriorate rapidly initially as necrotic tissue reveals itself, and then quickly improve as contamination/infection is removed and wound contraction begins. Thereafter, progression is slow because healing relies on epithelialization; carers should be prepared for this slow stage to avoid disappointment.

Where a wound is genuinely non-healing, a thorough physical examination and work-up should be performed to rule out underlying causes. This should include a complete blood count, full serum biochemistry (potentially including assessment for endocrinopathies such as thyroid disease, hyperadrenocorticism, diabetes mellitus) and urinalysis. The author will often also take a bacteriology swab and punch/wedge biopsy of the wound edges to submit for bacterial/fungal culture and histopathology, which is particularly important where the wound is associated with previous tumour removal. Thereafter, the author will often begin the wound healing journey from the beginning, starting with trying to establish a healthy granulation bed using shape excision (e.g. where skin edges are necrotic/undermined), NWPT (preferentially), adherent dressings or hydrogels. Appropriate analgesia is also required. A positive energy balance should be maintained, with adequate feeding and daily weight measurement. Once the granulation bed has been achieved, it is important that the wound remains moist, well oxygenated and warm, and the choice of dressing should provide this environment. The dressing should be reassessed at every bandage change and altered if appropriate. Where the wound is over a region of high mobility (e.g. a joint), the clinician should consider the use of a Robert Jones dressing or splint to immobilize the region and facilitate healing. Alternatively, confinement (e.g. in a kennel) will often aid wound healing.

11.7 Conclusion

The range of dressings available to treat open wounds is vast and often daunting, but understanding the phases of healing will often help in decision making. It is important that those caring for the patient are aware at the onset that the journey may be long, tiring and costly (both financially and emotionally). However, regular wound assessment and flexibility to modify the treatment plan will be helpful. As mentioned at the beginning of this chapter, the author would encourage practitioners to chat to their local referral institution if advice and support are required at any time.

Acknowledgement

The author is grateful for Kate Forster, MA VetMB CertSAS DipECVS MRCVS, for reviewing this chapter.

References

Abramo, F., Argiolas, S., Pisani, G., Vannozzi, I. and Miragliotta, V. (2008) Effect of a hydrocolloid dressing on first intention healing surgical wounds in the dog: a pilot study. *Australian Veterinary Journal* 86(3), 95–99. DOI: 10.1111/j.1751-0813.2007.00243.x.

Adkesson, M.J., Travis, E.K., Weber, M.A., Kirby, J.P. and Junge, R.E. (2007) Vacuum-assisted closure for treatment of a deep shell abscess and osteomyelitis in a tortoise. *Journal of the American Veterinary Medical Association* 231(8), 1249–1254. DOI: 10.2460/javma.231.8.1249.

Ben-Amotz, R., Lanz, O.I., Miller, J.M., Filipowicz, D.E. and King, M.D. (2007) The use of vacuum-assisted closure therapy for the treatment of distal extremity wounds in 15 dogs. *Veterinary Surgery* 36(7), 684–690. DOI: 10.1111/j.1532-950X.2007.00321.x.

Bertran, J., Farrell, M. and Fitzpatrick, N. (2013) Successful wound healing over exposed metal implants using vacuum-assisted wound closure in a dog. *Journal of Small Animal Practice* 54(7), 381–385. DOI: 10.1111/jsap.12055.

BNF (2022) Advanced wound dressings. British National Formulary, National Institute for Health and Care Excellence, London. Available at: https://bnf.nice.org.uk/wound-management/advanced-wound-dressings.html (accessed 25 October 2022).

Borgquist, O., Ingemansson, R. and Malmsjö, M. (2010a) The effect of intermittent and variable negative pressure wound therapy on wound edge microvascular blood flow. *Ostomy Wound Management* 56(3), 60–67.

Borgquist, O., Ingemansson, R. and Malmsjö, M. (2010b) Wound edge microvascular blood flow during negative-pressure wound therapy: examining the effects of pressures from -10 to -175 mmHg. *Plastic and Reconstructive Surgery* 125(2), 502–509. DOI: 10.1097/PRS.0b013e3181c82e1f.

Carter, M.J., Tingley-Kelley, K. and Warriner, R.A. (2010) Silver treatments and silver-impregnated dressings for the healing of leg wounds and ulcers: a systematic review and meta-analysis. *Journal of the American Academy of Dermatology* 63(4), 668–679. DOI: 10.1016/j.jaad.2009.09.007.

Chen, S.Z., Li, J., Li, X.Y. and Xu, L.S. (2005) Effects of vacuum-assisted closure on wound microcirculation: an experimental study. *Asian Journal of Surgery* 28(3), 211–217. DOI: 10.1016/S1015-9584(09)60346-8.

Cioffi, K.M., Schmiedt, C.W., Cornell, K.K. and Radlinsky, M.G. (2012) Retrospective evaluation of vacuum-assisted peritoneal drainage for the treatment of septic peritonitis in dogs and cats: 8 cases (2003-2010). *Journal of Veterinary Emergency and Critical Care* 22(5), 601–609. DOI: 10.1111/j.1476-4431.2012.00791.x.

Demaria, M., Stanley, B.J., Hauptman, J.G., Steficek, B.A., Fritz, M.C. *et al.* (2011) Effects of negative pressure wound therapy on healing of open wounds in dogs. *Veterinary Surgery* 40(6), 658–669. DOI: 10.1111/j.1532-950X.2011.00849.x.

Driffield, K. and Woodmansey, E. (2009) The equivalence of the antimicrobial efficacies of the ALLEVYN ag foam variants against key wound pathogens. Smith & Nephew Research Centre Report Ref: RR-WMP07330-10-03.

Jull, A.B., Cullum, N., Dumville, J.C., Westby, M.J., Deshpande, S. et al. (2015) Honey as a topical treatment for wounds. Cochrane Database of Systematic Reviews 2015(6), CD005083. DOI: 10.1002/14651858.CD005083.pub4.

Kotz, P., Fisher, J., McCluskey, P., Hartwell, S.D. and Dharma, H. (2009) Use of a new silver barrier dressing, ALLEVYN Ag in exuding chronic wounds. International Wound Journal 6(3), 186–194. DOI: 10.1111/j.1742-481X.2009.00608.x.

Labler, L., Rancan, M., Mica, L., Härter, L., Mihic-Probst, D. et al. (2009) Vacuum-assisted closure therapy increases local interleukin-8 and vascular endothelial growth factor levels in traumatic wounds. The Journal of Trauma 66(3), 749–757. DOI: 10.1097/TA.0b013e318171971a.

Lamke, L.O., Nilsson, G.E. and Reithner, H.L. (1977) The evaporative water loss from burns and the water-vapour permeability of grafts and artificial membranes used in the treatment of burns. Burns 3(3), 159–165. DOI: 10.1016/0305-4179(77)90004-3.

Malmsjö, M., Ingemansson, R., Martin, R. and Huddleston, E. (2009) Negative-pressure wound therapy using gauze or open-cell polyurethane foam: similar early effects on pressure transduction and tissue contraction in an experimental porcine wound model. Wound Repair and Regeneration 17(2), 200–205. DOI: 10.1111/j.1524-475X.2009.00461.x.

McNulty, A.K., Schmidt, M., Feeley, T. and Kieswetter, K. (2007) Effects of negative pressure wound therapy on fibroblast viability, chemotactic signaling, and proliferation in a provisional wound (fibrin) matrix. Wound Repair and Regeneration 15(6), 838–846. DOI: 10.1111/j.1524-475X.2007.00287.x.

Miller, A.J., Cashmore, R.G., Marchevsky, A.M., Havlicek, M., Brown, P.M. et al. (2016) Negative pressure wound therapy using a portable single-use device for free skin grafts on the distal extremity in seven dogs. Australian Veterinary Journal 94(9), 309–316. DOI: 10.1111/avj.12474.

Mouës, C.M., Vos, M.C., van den Bemd, G.-J.C.M., Stijnen, T. and Hovius, S.E.R. (2004) Bacterial load in relation to vacuum-assisted closure wound therapy: a prospective randomized trial. Wound Repair and Regeneration 12(1), 11–17. DOI: 10.1111/j.1067-1927.2004.12105.x.

Nolff, M., Albert, R., Wohlsein, P., Baumgärtner, W., Reese, S, et al. (2018b) Histomorphometric evaluation of MMP-9 and CD31 expression during healing under negative pressure wound therapy in dogs. Schweizer Archiv Fur Tierheilkunde 160(9), 525–532. DOI: 10.17236/sat00173.

Nolff, M.C., Fehr, M., Bolling, A., Dening, R., Kramer, S. et al. (2015) Negative pressure wound therapy, silver coated foam dressing and conventional bandages in open wound treatment in dogs. A retrospective comparison of 50 paired cases. Veterinary and Comparative Orthopaedics and Traumatology 28(1), 30–38. DOI: 10.3415/VCOT-14-05-0076.

Nolff, M.C., Fehr, M., Reese, S. and Meyer-Lindenberg, A.E. (2017) Retrospective comparison of negative pressure wound therapy and silver-coated foam dressings in open-wound treatment in cats. Journal of Feline Medicine and Surgery 19(6), 624–630. DOI: 10.1177/1098612X16645141.

Nolff, M.C., Albert, R., Reese, S. and Meyer-Lindenberg, A. (2018a) Comparison of negative pressure wound therapy and silver-coated foam dressings in open wound treatment in dogs: a prospective controlled clinical trial. Veterinary and Comparative Orthopaedics and Traumatology 31(4), 229–238. DOI: 10.1055/s-0038-1639579.

Owen, L.J., Hotston-Moore, A. and Holt, P.E. (2009) Vacuum-assisted wound closure following urine-induced skin and thigh muscle necrosis in a cat. Veterinary and Comparative Orthopaedics and Traumatology 22(5), 417–421. DOI: 10.3415/VCOT-08-12-0123.

Pitt, K.A. and Stanley, B.J. (2014) Negative pressure wound therapy: experience in 45 dogs. Veterinary Surgery 43(4), 380–387. DOI: 10.1111/j.1532-950X.2014.12155.x.

Smith+Nephew (2022) ALLEVYN non-adhesive advanced foam wound dressings. Available at: www.smith-nephew.com/key-products/advanced-wound-management/allevyn/allevyn-non-adhesive/ (accessed 8 January 2023).

Storm-Versloot, M.N., Vos, C.G., Ubbink, D.T. and Vermeulen, H. (2010) Topical silver for preventing wound infection. Cochrane Database of Systematic Reviews 3(3), CD006478. DOI: 10.1002/14651858.CD006478.pub2.

Thomas, S., Fear, M., Humphreys, J., Disley, L. and Waring, M. (1996) The effect of dressings on the production of exudate from venous leg ulcers. Wounds 8, 145–150.

Timmers, M.S., Le Cessie, S., Banwell, P. and Jukema, G.N. (2005) The effects of varying degrees of pressure delivered by negative-pressure wound therapy on skin perfusion. Annals of Plastic Surgery 55(6), 665–671. DOI: 10.1097/01.sap.0000187182.90907.3d.

Toon, C.D., Lusuku, C., Ramamoorthy, R., Davidson, B.R. and Gurusamy, K.S. (2015) Early versus delayed dressing removal after primary closure of clean and clean-contaminated surgical wounds. Cochrane Database of Systematic Reviews 2015(9), CD010259. DOI: 10.1002/14651858.CD010259.pub3.

Tsioli, V., Gouletsou, P.G., Galatos, A.D., Psalla, D., Lymperis, A. *et al.* (2016) Effects of two occlusive, hydrocolloid dressings on healing of full-thickness skin wounds in cats. *Veterinary and Comparative Orthopaedics and Traumatology* 29(4), 298–305. DOI: 10.3415/VCOT-15-04-0058.

Tsioli, V., Gouletsou, P.G., Galatos, A.D., Psalla, D., Lymperis, A. *et al.* (2018) The effect of a hydrocolloid dressing on second intention wound healing in cats. *Journal of the American Animal Hospital Association* 54(3), 125–131. DOI: 10.5326/JAAHA-MS-6604.

Vermeulen, H., Ubbink, D.T., Goossens, A., de Vos, R. and Legemate, D.A. (2009) Dressings and topical agents for surgical wounds healing by secondary intention. *Cochrane Database of Systematic Reviews* 2, CD003554.

Wackenfors, A., Gustafsson, R., Sjögren, J., Algotsson, L., Ingemansson, R. *et al.* (2005) Blood flow responses in the peristernal thoracic wall during vacuum-assisted closure therapy. *Annals of Thoracic Surgery* 79(5), 1724–1730. DOI: 10.1016/j. athoracsur.2004.10.053.

Weed, T., Ratliff, C., Drake, D.B., Fee, T.E. and Mast, B. (2004) Quantifying bacterial bioburden during negative pressure wound therapy: does the wound VAC enhance bacterial clearance? *Annals of Plastic Surgery* 52(3), 276–279. DOI: 10.1097/01.sap. 0000111861.75927.4d.

Wilkes, R., Zhao, Y., Kieswetter, K. and Haridas, B. (2009) Effects of dressing type on 3D tissue microdeformations during negative pressure wound therapy: a computational study. *Journal of Biomechanical Engineering* 131(3), 031012. DOI: 10.1115/1.2947358.

WUWHS (2007) Wound exudate and the role of dressings. A WUWHS Consensus Document. World Union of Wound Healing Societies, Wounds International, London. Available at: www.woundsinternational.com /resources/details/read-more-wound-exudate-and-rol e-dressings-wuwhs-consensus-document (accessed 25 October 2022).

Section 4: Infection Control of the Hospitalized Patient

The hospital environment represents a significant source of infectious disease, and appropriate measures are required to minimize a patient's exposure risk. This section will describe important steps that can be taken when performing invasive procedures (from placement of an intravenous catheter to the care of enteral feeding tubes) and will introduce specific considerations when treating infectious patients in the hospital or those that are at heightened risk from infection due to immunocompromise. To address a situation where disease-prevention measures fail, the final chapter in this section describes the approach to outbreak investigation and management.

This section will cover the following key points:

- Any procedure that penetrates the patient's skin could potentially introduce infectious pathogens into sanctuary sites compromising the body's natural defence mechanisms. Thorough *site preparation, aseptic technique and serial monitoring* of any implanted devices are essential to minimize the risk of healthcare-associated infections.
- Urinary catheters, despite not traversing the patient's skin, still represent a potential conduit for infection to enter and become established within the urinary tract. Catheter care, both during placement and while *in situ*, should follow hygienic principles and facilitate early identification of any catheter-associated infection.
- Hospitalization of patients, suspected or confirmed to have infectious or zoonotic disease, should reflect careful evaluation of the risk posed to other patients and hospital personnel (see Fig. 14.1, Chapter 14, this volume).
- Colour-coding of patients according to their infectious disease categorization (e.g. red for patients deemed to be possibly highly contagious) can provide a readily recognizable visual trigger for staff members.
- Establishing a *dedicated isolation area* is recommended to improve infection control but requires careful consideration in terms of location within the clinic and design to ensure that effective cleaning and decontamination can take place while maintaining excellent patient care and surveillance.
- Investigation of an outbreak of infectious disease requires consideration of the who, what, when, where and why of the problem. Asking (and answering) these individual questions can guide assessment of the seriousness of the problem and identify means to halt its progress and establish underlying reasons for the outbreak.
- Understanding how an infectious disease outbreak arose enables the veterinary team to implement corrective measures and provide recommendations to reduce the likelihood of a future recurrence.

12 Infection Prevention for Invasive Procedures

Lindsey Ashburner, Craig R. Breheny*, Martyna Godniak and Emily Gorman

Royal (Dick) School of Veterinary Studies, University of Edinburgh, Roslin, UK

12.1 Introduction

Healthcare-acquired infections (HAIs) are a major source of morbidity, mortality and expense in both human and veterinary medicine. The World Health Organization (WHO) reports that 7–10% of all hospitalized patients will go on to develop an HAI, and this number increases dramatically when considering intensive care units (Hague *et al.*, 2018). HAIs are not solely a concern for the medical professionals caring for humans but are becoming an emerging problem in the veterinary field. This is especially concerning given the increasing number of treatment options available for our veterinary patients, including a burgeoning number of invasive procedures and a growing number of immunocompromised patients that are being treated. As patients (humans and companion animals) are living longer and coping with multiple comorbidities, with prolonged hospitalization times, the risk for HAIs can only rise.

The aim of this chapter is to summarize some of the commonly performed invasive procedures undertaken in small animals, and to present strategies to minimize the risk of iatrogenic infections.

12.1.1 Procedure site preparation

Aseptic preparation of the sites at which the procedures are performed is described in detail in Chapter 8 (this volume) and is relevant for the techniques discussed in this chapter, with procedure-specific amendments mentioned in each section.

For procedure site preparation, hand hygiene should be performed and examination gloves should be worn. This is discussed in detail in Chapters 4 and 5 (this volume).

12.2 Intravenous Catheters

12.2.1 General considerations

Peripheral venous canulation is one of the most performed procedures in veterinary medicine. While routine, it should not be considered an entirely benign process. Catheters by their nature provide a direct conduit through the barrier of the skin and risk inoculation of bacteria directly into the vasculature.

Peripheral veins have a narrower diameter and slower flow rates, leading to an increased risk of phlebitis after the administration of high-osmolarity medications such as concentrated glucose, potassium chloride and parenteral nutrition. The osmolarity of any fluid administered into a peripheral vein should not exceed 600 mOsm kg^{-1} (Kuwahara *et al.*, 1988). The use of a central venous catheter is advised when concentrated solutions are considered. Similarly, directly caustic medications such as certain chemotherapeutics must be administered with great care to avoid peri-vascular extravasation because this can cause serious injury to the affected limb. Phlebitis will further disrupt the normal protective skin and vascular barriers, and risks secondary infection.

Another point to consider when selecting an appropriate vein is the patient's clinical state and the presence of any underlying pathology. For example, catheterization of the saphenous vein is suboptimal in patients with diarrhoea or urinary incontinence because of the increased risk of gross contamination, which compromises hygiene at the catheter site. In some circumstances, this will be unavoidable, and the clinician could consider

---

*Corresponding author: craig.breheny@ed.ac.uk

modifications of the intravenous (IV) catheter site dressing to incorporate a waterproof surface, or patient management strategies such as placement of a faecal catheter.

A wider IV catheter gauge may be preferred when administering a large volume of fluid. However, if the IV catheter is to be in place for a longer period of time, then use of a smaller bore may reduce the risk of phlebitis (Martinho and Rodrigues, 2008).

12.2.2 IV catheter placement

The patient's limb should be widely clipped to minimize the risk of inadvertent catheter contamination on fur. Substantial feathers to the caudal aspect of the limb should also be clipped to facilitate effective securing of the catheter and avoid contaminating the catheter site.

The site of insertion should then be aseptically prepared (see Chapter 8, this volume). A previous study in human hospitals identified that skin commensals were most frequently cultured from catheter site infections, emphasizing the importance of thorough preparation of the catheter site prior to placement (Malach *et al.*, 2006).

Once the catheter is placed successfully and the stylet has been removed, any blood that escapes should be removed. This is important because blood contamination can act as a nutrition source for local bacteria, promoting growth. For example, blood contamination can be avoided by placing a swab below the catheter before removing the stylet – the swab can then be discarded afterwards.

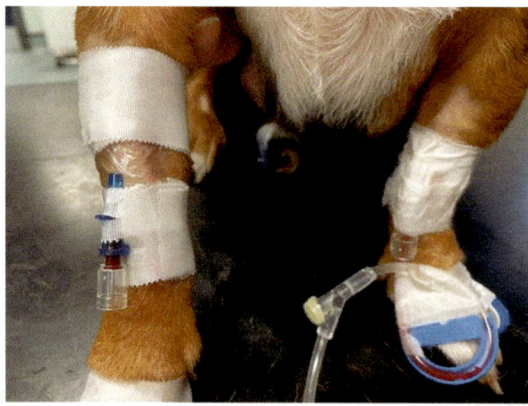

Fig. 12.1. A three-tape method of securing an intravenous catheter.

At the authors' institute, catheters are secured using a three-tape method (Fig. 12.1). A length of Micropore tape is placed distally below the catheter at the point it enters the skin. A second length of Micropore tape is then placed proximally to where the catheter enters the skin. This provides a base layer, after which a final length of waterproof Sleek tape is then applied over both layers and the catheter itself. This allows the Sleek tape to have a fixed grip of the catheter, preventing micromovements and trauma to the vessel, and as it is waterproof, it will also protect the catheter insertion site. The Micropore base layer allows easier dressing removal. A cut swab is then placed below the catheter and secured in place with Micropore tape, preventing upward and downward movement of the catheter. In an unpublished study at the authors' institute, this simpler method was compared with another using a more intensive method of securing with the addition of a sterile translucent film. There was no difference in phlebitis, infection rates or catheter losses between the two groups.

A layer of absorbent dressing is then applied, which will draw moisture into the dressing and away from the IV catheter site. It also provides mechanical protection from the patient interfering with the catheter or inadvertently dislodging it. A final layer of cohesive dressing is then applied.

12.2.3 Monitoring

Once in place, the IV catheter site should be inspected daily, with appropriate hand hygiene performed and examination gloves worn. Inspection should involve removing the bandage material such that the taping around the catheter can be observed directly. The limb should be palpated above and below the dressing for evidence of heat, discomfort or swelling. The development of pyrexia in a previously afebrile patient is an indication that each IV catheter site should be evaluated carefully in addition to the routine daily assessment. The IV catheter should be removed and/or replaced as a precautionary measure. A rapid normalization of the rectal temperature would be expected if the catheter is responsible for this systemic response.

Flushing IV catheters

Sterile 0.9% saline should be used to flush the IV catheter. There is no proven benefit of using heparin to maintain patency, and there is the potential risk of causing harm with dose miscalculations or introduction of infection during preparation of tailored solutions (AACN, 1993; Randolph *et al.*, 1998). The volumes used for flushing catheters should be twice that contained within the catheter itself (INS, 2011). IV catheters should be flushed once every 24 h during the daily catheter assessment. However, if they are not in constant use (e.g. during administration of IV fluid therapy), they may need flushing more frequently to maintain patency. The catheter should be flushed in a pulsatile (push-and-pause) manner, with the area above the catheter site palpated concurrently for evidence of intermittent distension, which confirms that the IV catheter remains in place. Any resistance to flow, limb swelling, discoloration or discomfort upon flushing can be signs of early phlebitis and would warrant removal of the catheter.

Replacing IV catheters

The American Animal Hospital Association (AAHA) recommends replacing the IV fluid tubing every 72 h, which would seem sensible given that this is the component of the system most susceptible to patient interference. Tubing that has been used to administer parenteral nutrition or blood products should be replaced daily if in continual use, and again once the product has been discontinued. A veterinary study identified that bacterial colonization of the IV catheter was significantly more common when the catheter had been used for dextrose infusions or remained in place for 72 h or longer (Sequela and Pages, 2011). The Centers for Disease Control and Prevention (CDC) advise that IV catheters should be replaced every 72–96 h (Tager *et al.*, 1983; Lai, 1998). Despite this, several studies in human medicine have failed to identify a difference in complication rate between catheters that were removed based on clinical assessment compared with those replaced routinely after 72–96 h. These observations support replacing the catheter only where there is a clinical necessity (rather than routinely), which is advantageous to patient welfare and decreases costs. However, routine replacement of IV catheters used for dextrose infusions or blood products would be sensible, despite a lack of supportive evidence at present (Webster *et al.*, 2019).

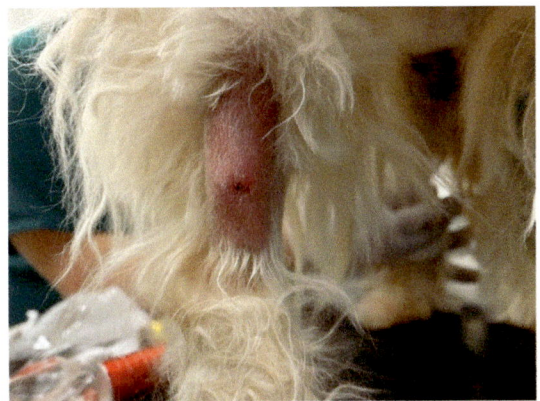

Fig. 12.2. Phlebitis and cellulitis are typically diagnosed based on the appearance of the insertion site and the local tissues, including redness, swelling, pain, damage to overlying skin and discharge from the catheter site.

12.2.4   Evaluating for phlebitis

Phlebitis and cellulitis are typically diagnosed based on the appearance of the insertion site and the local tissues (Fig. 12.2). The hallmarks of inflammation are often identified (see Chapter 11, this volume), and there may also be concurrent discharge from the area. If a definitive diagnosis is sought, a fine-needle aspirate of the region can be performed. Cytological findings suggestive of phlebitis include a predominance of degenerate neutrophils, probably with intracellular bacteria. Gram staining of discharge or aspirated fluid can be used to guide empirical treatment while bacterial culture results are pending.

Bacterial culture of IV catheter tips is not routinely recommended. However, if there is a clinical suspicion of a catheter site infection, then culture of the tip can be helpful. If the catheter has been in place for less than 7 days, the most likely pathogens are skin commensals that are traversing the external surface of the catheter, and rolling the tip surface on an agar plate will be most useful in isolating causative organisms. If the IV catheter has been in place for longer, then colonization of the internal catheter surface is a greater possibility and evaluation of the inner aspect is more useful (Raad *et al.*, 1993). Informing the microbiology laboratory about which samples are submitted and providing a detailed clinical history may help with decision making regarding the optimal plating technique.

If there is active discharging from the catheter site, then obtaining a sample by sterile swab and submitting for culture and sensitivity is recommended. Routine swabbing of an IV catheter site is not recommended.

If the patient is systemically unwell and demonstrating signs that could be compatible with sepsis such as pyrexia, tachycardia and hypotension, then blood cultures could be considered in addition to local sampling. This is discussed in section 12.3.

A recent study demonstrated the clinical utility of ultrasound to detect phlebitis in dogs receiving radiotherapy. Ultrasonographic features consistent with phlebitis included vessel wall thickening, decreased vessel compressibility, filling defects consistent with thrombosis, vessel wall hyperechogenicity and colour flow Doppler alterations (Lodzinska *et al.*, 2019).

12.2.5 Treatment of phlebitis

Once phlebitis is suspected, the catheter should be removed because it is likely to encourage formation of a biofilm, which protects the bacteria from immune defences and therapeutic antibiotics (see Chapter 11, this volume).

In the first instance, local therapy can be attempted if the clinical signs are localized and the patient is systemically well. As most peripheral IV catheters used in general practice are typically in place for less than 7 days, it would be expected that skin commensals are the most likely cause of any infection unless bacterial culture results indicate otherwise. Topical therapies might include warm compresses, appropriate analgesia (e.g. non-steroidal anti-inflammatory medication), or local cleaning with chlorhexidine or hypochlorous acid. If there is evidence of pocketing or abscess formation, then drainage could be attempted.

If the patient is systemically affected, then antimicrobial therapy may be necessary. Amoxicillin-clavulanate or trimethoprim-sulfonamide would be an appropriate empirical choice while bacterial cultures are pending, based on which therapy could be escalated or de-escalated. Any previous antimicrobial history should also be considered, given the risk for resistance to these therapeutics. This information may alter the choice of empirical antimicrobials. Phlebitis can be uncomfortable, and additional analgesic measures should be strongly considered in accordance with the patient's care plan.

12.3 Central Lines

Catheters placed within the jugular veins ('central lines' or 'central venous catheters') confer several additional benefits beyond the provision of IV access. They facilitate repeated sampling without the need for venepuncture, and the wider diameter and faster flow of the jugular vein (compared with a peripheral vein) permits administration of higher osmolarity solutions with a reduced risk of chemical phlebitis.

12.3.1 Central line placement

Many of the considerations and preventative measures for central line placement are similar for IV cannulation, although there are some important differences. The consequences of infections associated with central lines are inherently greater, and patients should be carefully evaluated to ensure they are suitable candidates for such a procedure. For example, the presence of skin disease, particularly if there is evidence of deep pyoderma, would represent a contraindication to placement of a jugular catheter.

In addition to the aseptic site preparation (see Chapter 8, this volume), the use of a fenestrated drape is recommended to further decrease contamination risk. At the authors' institution, a drape with an adhesive skin strip is used to prevent movement of the drape during placement of the central line.

Central lines should be placed by staff who have completed full surgical hand hygiene (see Chapter 5, this volume) and who have donned a surgical cap, mask, sterile gloves and gown (see Chapter 8, this volume), as recommended by the current National Institute for Health and Care Excellence (NICE) guidelines (Newton, 2009).

12.3.2 Monitoring

Central lines should be considered sterile whenever handling is necessary. Needle-free valves should be attached to any port not connected to a fluid pump or infusion. The ports should be cleaned with 70% alcohol wipes and allowed to dry before connecting a syringe or infusion. If total parenteral nutrition (TPN) is being administered via one of the ports, it must be prepared in a sterile manner and, once attached, it is not disconnected until the TPN is discontinued. The TPN mixture makes an excellent bacterial culture medium, and bacterial contamination of the system could be catastrophic.

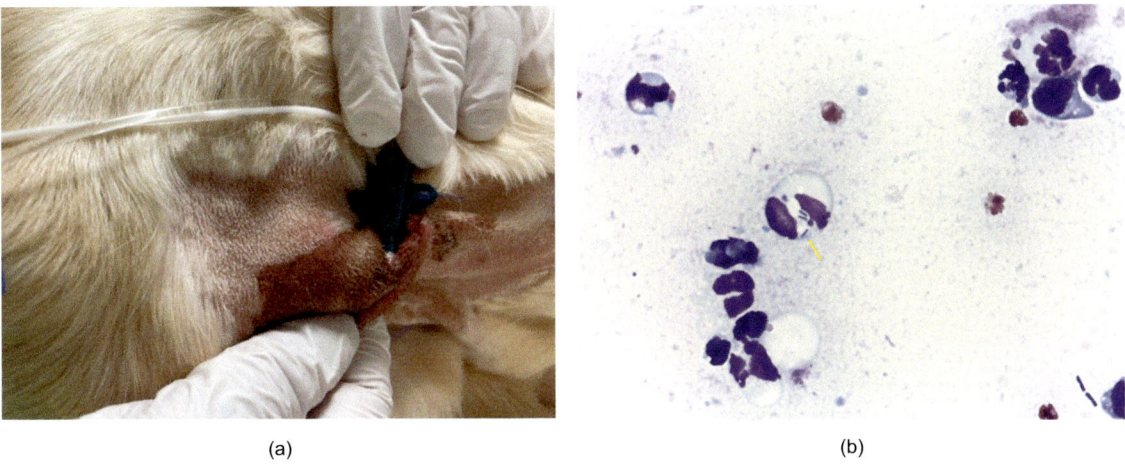

(a)   (b)

Fig. 12.3. (a) Photograph of a central line site with clinical signs of infection, including redness and swelling. (b) Cytological evaluation of a fine-needle aspiration from the site showing degenerate neutrophils and intracellular rods (yellow arrow) contained within a macrophage. Magnification ×100.

As with peripheral IV catheters, the insertion site of the central line should be inspected daily, and the ease of flushing assessed. A sterile translucent dressing can be placed over the insertion site, affording protection from gross contamination while allowing the site to be visualized. Inspection involves visual check of the site where the catheter meets the skin for signs of infection, soiling and for break in the integrity of the dressing. If none of the issues is observed, a clear dressing should be left unchanged for 3-7 days. If any other type of dressing is used, this should be left in place for two days. A pre-defined marker of catheter length/position should be checked to ensure that the catheter has not migrated. Signs of catheter site infection are as for peripheral lines (see section 12.2.2) (Fig. 12.3).

12.3.3 Evaluating for central line-associated phlebitis

The consequences of central line infection are potentially much greater than with a peripheral catheter. An appropriately placed central line should lie in the terminal cranial vena cava, which thereby affords bacteria a direct route to the heart. As such, endocarditis is a possible (albeit infrequent) sequelae to jugular catheter infection.

While any new pyrexia identified in a patient will inevitably raise concerns for a catheter-associated phlebitis, central venous access may still be required for critical patient management. This can lead to difficult decision making because replacement of these devices can be very challenging, although if the site is strongly suspected to be infected then removal is advised.

If there is suspicion of a central catheter-associated infection, two blood samples should be obtained for culture comprising one sample from the catheter and the other from a peripheral vein, taken within 15 min of each other. Ideally, 10 ml of blood is required for human blood culture bottles, which is not always feasible given the range of patient sizes encountered in veterinary medicine (Fig. 12.4). In the authors' experience, we have obtained positive cultures with lesser volumes; however, this probably depends on the degree of the circulating bacteraemia. If a multi-lumen catheter has been placed, a sample should be taken from each port. As with peripheral IV catheters, central catheter tips can also be submitted for bacteria culture.

Ultrasonography of the catheter insertion site can also be useful. Imaging will allow the identification of cellulitis and fluid pockets, and facilitate targeted aspirates if there are pocketed areas of infection that have not breached the skin surface.

12.3.4 Treatment of central line-associated phlebitis

If a catheter-associated bloodstream infection is strongly suspected, then empirical treatment may be necessary.

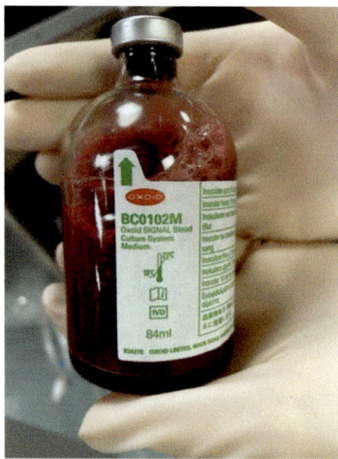

Fig. 12.4. If there is suspicion of a central catheter-associated infection, blood samples should be collected into a blood culture bottle for bacterial culture. This information will inform antibiotic selection.

As with peripheral IV catheter infections, skin commensals are the most likely cause of central venous catheter infections. As previously identified (Sequela and Pages, 2011), the most commonly encountered peripheral catheter-associated pathogens are *Staphylococcus*, *Klebsiella*, *Enterococcus* and *Pseudomonas* spp. and *Escherichia coli*.

Broad-spectrum systemic empirical antibiotic therapy is necessary for patients with central line-associated phlebitis, pending bacterial culture and susceptibility results. Parenterally administered antibiotics should be administered, with amoxicillin-clavulanate being an appropriate empirical choice. However, a history of previous antibiotic administration and the severity of the infection should be considered when deciding on the most appropriate approach for the individual patient. If the culture of the catheter tip or blood (from either peripheral veins or the central catheter ports) yields bacterial growth, then antibiotic choice should be adapted or de-escalated in line with the susceptibility profile of the isolated organism.

12.4 Oesophageal, Gastric and Jejunal Feeding Tubes

Feeding tube placement is a commonly utilized procedure to facilitate medication and address the nutritional needs of hospitalized patients. Oesophageal, gastric and jejunal feeding tubes all bypass the oral and nasal cavities, which allows placement of a larger-gauge tube (compared with nasogastric feeding tubes) and administration of a variety of liquid foods.

With the tube traversing the skin into the gastrointestinal tract, it is simultaneously exposing the stoma site to both skin and gastrointestinal commensals. In previous studies, the infection rate of the oesophageal feeding tube stoma site was 12.8–17.2% in cats and 13.7% in dogs (Breheny *et al.*, 2019; Nathanson *et al.*, 2019).

The use of glucocorticoids may increase the risk of HAIs associated with feeding tubes. In one study, cats with oesophageal feeding tubes who received glucocorticoids or chemotherapeutics had an increased risk (odds ratio 3.91) of developing a stoma site infection compared with those not receiving such medications (Breheny *et al.*, 2019). In dogs who had gastrostomy tubes placed, individuals receiving glucocorticoids were more than twice as likely to experience major complications (43%) than the control group (18%) (Aguiar *et al.*, 2016). In the latter study, a stoma site infection was encountered in 17% of dogs with a gastrostomy tube, with isolated bacteria including *Enterococcus*, *Klebsiella* and *Streptococcus* spp. and *E. coli*. This infection rate compares favourably with that reported in human medicine (30%) (McClave and Neff, 2006).

12.4.1 Feeding tube placement

Surgical-site asepsis and surgeon preparation are as above for central venous catheter placement (see Chapter 5, this volume).

Once the tube is in place, an adhesive, absorptive dressing is cut to shape by cutting a 'Y' from one side. This allows the dressing to conform around the tube and cover the stoma site. An alternative approach, used at the authors' institution, is the use of BIOPATCH (Ethicon, Johnson and Johnson), which is a disc-shaped dressing with a central hole and slit along one radius, allowing the BIOPATCH to wrap around the tube. The dressing is made from polyurethane foam impregnated with chlorhexidine gluconate, allowing wicking of any exudate from the insertion site surface and a sustained release of disinfectant to the local environment. A meta-analysis of BIOPATCH use at IV cannula and epidural catheter sites has shown that they are effective at reducing infections (Ho and Litton, 2006). An additional benefit of the patches is that they can

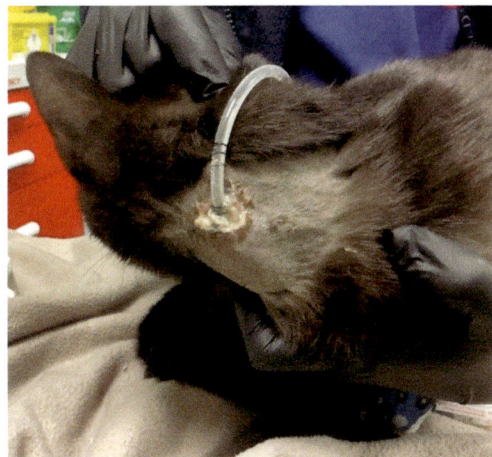

Fig. 12.5. Photograph of an infection at the stoma site of an oesophageal feeding tube in a cat. There is a significant amount of purulent discharge from the site and necrosis of the surrounding skin. This tube requires removal and submission for bacterial culture and sensitivity. The local site should be appropriately cleaned and managed as an open wound (see Chapter 11, this volume).

be left in place for 7 days at a time, increasing the ease of patient management for owners in the home environment.

Following placement of an adhesive dressing over the stoma, a further substantial dressing is also required to secure the tube and minimize opportunity for patient interference. Micromovements of the tube are likely to aggravate the local tissues with resultant inflammation and disruption of local skin barriers. A padding-based dressing can be placed, followed by an elasticated dressing to prevent movement of the tube. Alternatively, a customized outer dressing (e.g. Kitty Collar) can be used in cats and smaller dogs. If a gastrostomy or jejunostomy tube is placed, then these patients require a suitably sized Elizabethan collar and protective shirt or body stocking.

12.4.2 Monitoring

When handling the site, appropriate hand hygiene should be performed and examination gloves worn (see Chapters 4 and 5, this volume). The feeding tube stoma site should be redressed daily, evaluating where the tube enters the skin for signs of inflammation and/or infection (Fig. 12.5). It

is not uncommon for there to be some discharge from the stoma site, although its presence increases the odds of developing infection (Breheny *et al.*, 2019).

The site should also be palpated for heat or evidence of discomfort. If there is discomfort on use of the tube, this immediately warrants further investigation of the tube position and assessment of local tissues.

12.4.3 Evaluating for feeding tube-associated infection

If there is any discharge from the stoma site, a sample should be obtained in a sterile manner and evaluated cytologically for the presence of degenerate neutrophils and intracellular bacteria. A portion of the tube tip should also be retained for bacterial culture and susceptibility if cytology findings are supportive of an infection.

The patient should also be monitored during use of the tube, particularly when volumes of feed are increased to full energy requirements. If the food is administered too rapidly, there is an increased risk of reflux through the stoma site, potentially seeding bacteria within the cervical fascial layers or into the abdomen, depending on the tube type used.

Within the cervical region, pocketing of infection and abscess development are encountered intermittently. This can cause signs of systemic illness, including pyrexia. Performing a focused ultrasonographic examination of the region can be useful to identify abscesses or cellulitis, which can be aspirated for cytological analysis and bacterial culture.

With the use of gastric and jejunal tubes, the risk of leakage into the abdominal cavity, rather than the subcutaneous tissue, is a very real possibility. In the initial days following tube placement, the patient should be evaluated for signs of peritonitis (e.g. monitoring rectal temperature, respiratory rate and abdominal comfort). Frequent abdominal ultrasonography to assess for free abdominal fluid is also sensible to detect leakage at the earliest opportunity. If there is any doubt over tube placement or migration, confirmatory contrast studies should be performed using a water-soluble contrast agent (i.e. not barium, which has a synergistically deleterious effect in patients with septic peritonitis) (Ko and Mann, 2014).

12.4.4 Treatment of feeding tube-associated infection

In the face of a confirmed oesophageal stoma site infection, or when there is a strong suspicion, the oesophagostomy tube should be removed wherever possible. The tube itself can harbour bacteria, allowing the formation of a biofilm, which can act as a nidus for recrudescence of infection. There is also the possibility of selecting for resistant strains should antibiotics be used while the tube is *in situ*.

From veterinary studies, the most commonly isolated bacteria from stoma site infections include *Enterococcus*, *Staphylococcus*, *Streptococcus* and *Pasteurella* spp. and *E. coli*, (Breheny *et al.*, 2019; Nathanson *et al.*, 2019). This is to be expected because these isolates represent either skin-surface or gastrointestinal commensals.

As with all the invasive devices mentioned so far, the ideal remedy for stoma site infection is removal of the tube. In relation to gastrostomy or jejunostomy tubes, this is possible if two criteria are met: (i) the tube has been in place for at least 10 (ideally 14) days to ensure that a secure stoma has formed; and (ii) the tube is no longer required.

As infections associated with feeding tubes tend to be localized rather than systemic, topical treatment in conjunction with tube removal will often lead to resolution without the need for systemic antimicrobial therapy. Topical therapy such as hypochlorous acid is an effective antibacterial that does not interfere with wound healing. Additionally, if an abscess is present or forming, then draining or lancing the abscess and flushing copiously may allow healing and resolution of the infection (see Chapter 11, this volume).

If there is evidence of extensive cellulitis, pyrexia or signs of illness outside the local area, then systemic antibiotics are indicated, with empirical decisions made following cytology and Gram staining while a representative culture sample is pending. If the infection is severe, unresponsive to management or risks deeper penetration into the abdominal cavity, then surgical debridement of the area and reversal of the stoma are necessary.

Patients that have a feeding tube in place are often relatively unwell and may be receiving antibiotic therapy as part of their treatment plan. This is important to consider: if an infection were to develop in a patient who was already receiving antibiotics, there may be increased risk of isolating a multidrug-resistant pathogen. Appropriate personal protective equipment should be used when handling these patients, and the patient should be nursed in an isolation unit (if clinical stability allows) until bacterial culture results return.

12.5 Urinary Catheters

12.5.1 Indications for urinary catheterization

Urinary catheters are employed in the management of patients with a variety of underlying conditions. However, they can also be associated with nosocomial infections and their use could lead to increased surgical risk (Chandler and Middlecote, 2011). One-time or intermittent urethral catheterization can be used to perform contrast radiographic procedures or to relieve an obstruction.

Even a one-time urethral catheterization can introduce bacteria into the lower urinary tract and the sample can be contaminated by bacteria and red blood cells (Smarick, 2015). Indwelling urinary catheters are left in place for variable lengths of time to allow for continuous urine collection and are indicated where urine retention or replacement of the catheter would be detrimental to the patient, such as in a systemically ill cat with urethral obstruction or urethral trauma, or for the monitoring of acute kidney injury.

Recumbency or urinary incontinence in themselves are not justifiable indications for urinary catheterization; however, if urine scalding, skin damage or urine contamination of wounds is occurring and other management methods have proven ineffective, the use of an indwelling urinary catheter can be considered. These recommendations are aimed at avoiding complications such as catheter-associated urinary tract infections (UTIs).

Consideration should be given as to whether a urinary catheter is truly necessary in patients at a higher risk of infection or the development of multidrug resistance. Patients that would be included in these categories include those with diarrhoea, immunosuppression or diabetes mellitus and/or those receiving antimicrobial medications.

12.5.2 Urinary catheter placement

Prior to starting the procedure, all the necessary equipment should be assembled (Box 12.1).

Patient preparation includes clipping the hair from the preputial or vulvar area, incorporating an area at least 3–5 cm from the catheter insertion

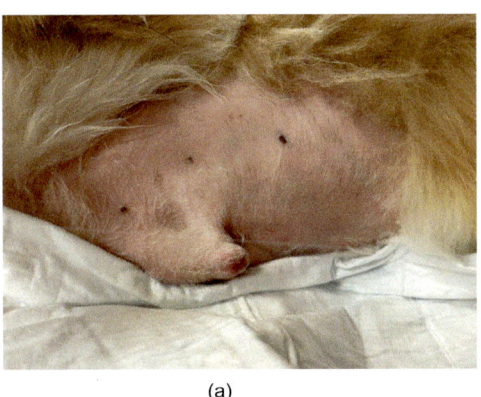
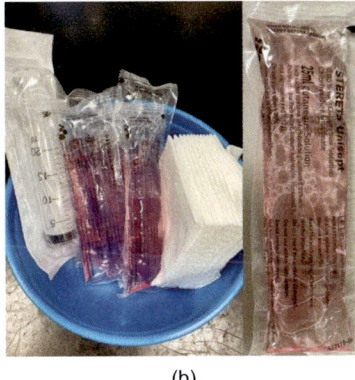
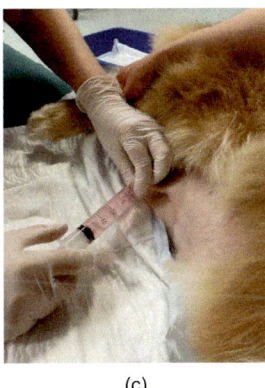

(a)   (b)   (c)

Fig. 12.6. Patient preparation for placement of a urinary catheter in a male dog. (a) The fur around the prepuce is widely clipped to incorporate a 3–5 cm area around the catheter insertion site. (b) Using 0.05% chlorhexidine. (c) The prepuce is flushed with 2–10 ml, dependant on patient size.

site (Fig. 12.6). Hand hygiene should be performed before donning examination gloves and preparing the area with 0.05% chlorhexidine solution. The prepuce or vestibule should be flushed with 2–10 ml of 0.05% chlorhexidine solution, with the volume used dependent on patient size.

A recent study in humans looked at the preventative effect of urethral cleaning versus disinfection for catheter-associated UTIs and found that chlorhexidine was the most effective, followed by clean water, soap and water, and dilute iodine (Cao *et al.*, 2018).

In male dogs and cats, the penis should be extruded and cleaned of any gross exudate with 0.05% chlorhexidine-soaked gauze swabs. No alcohol should be used around the penis or vulva to avoid irritation. An aseptic technique should be maintained when placing the catheter (see Chapter 5, this volume): sterile barrier drapes should be used for the work area, hand hygiene should be performed and sterile gloves donned. The end of

the urinary catheter should be lubricated before placement using a sterile, water-based lubricant. The plastic, sterile packaging in which the catheter arrives can be cut with a blade or sterile scissors to allow easier manipulation of the catheter in an aseptic manner. This involves cutting the sealed end from the packaging, then cutting the last inch of the packaging to provide a tab with which to handle the catheter.

If the catheter is to remain indwelling, it should immediately be connected to a closed collection system after placement and an Elizabethan collar placed to prevent patient interference. If a commercial collection system is not available, a drainage system can be created using an empty IV fluid bag and sterile IV fluid administration set. The bag used should not have been stored longer than 7 days since its original use, should be capped with a sterile device and should not have contained dextrose (Smarick, 2015). An open system or intermittent draining directly from the catheter should be avoided to prevent external contamination, which dramatically increases the risk of developing a UTI.

12.5.3 Management of indwelling urinary catheters

Before handling the urinary catheter or collection system, hand hygiene should always be performed and examination gloves worn. The prepuce or vestibule should be flushed every 4hrs with 0.05% chlorhexidine solution which can be warmed to aid patient comfort. The outside of the collection system, including all connections should also be visually evaluated and wiped with either 0.05% chlorhexidine solution or 70% isopropyl alcohol swabs. This can be performed more frequently, or the collection system replaced, if the system becomes visibly soiled. The urinary collection bag should be emptied every 4 h from the evacuation port and urine production quantified.

To empty the collection bag, the port should be cleaned with 0.05% chlorhexidine before and after emptying. Every effort should be made not to break the closed collection system; however, if the system is thought to be contaminated, a UTI is suspected, or the system is no longer functional, aseptic replacement is warranted. The collection bag should always be positioned below the patient to allow the urine to flow by gravity, preventing retrograde flow of urine from the collection bag back into the patient, which may allow bacterial contamination (Fig. 12.7). The system clamp should be closed when the patient is moved or walked and immediately reopened once below the patient again.

The patient's bladder should be regularly palpated or checked using ultrasound to ensure adequate drainage. There is an increased risk of blockage in patients passing large amounts of debris in their urine, and urinary catheter obstruction should be suspected if urine production is below that expected. If catheter obstruction is a possibility, the catheter should be slightly repositioned and the collection system checked for kinks. When there is a possibility of occlusions, 0.9% sterile saline solution can be used to flush the catheter. Aseptic technique should be used, and the flush directly attached to the urinary catheter rather than the collection system because bacteria may have colonized the collection system (Ackerman, 2016).

12.5.4 Evaluating for urinary catheter-associated infection

The placement of a urinary catheter disrupts the body's natural defences against infection, as well as bypassing the natural sphincters and normograde urine flow. Bacteria can be introduced directly into the bladder at the time of catheterization, and urinary catheter placement can traumatize and

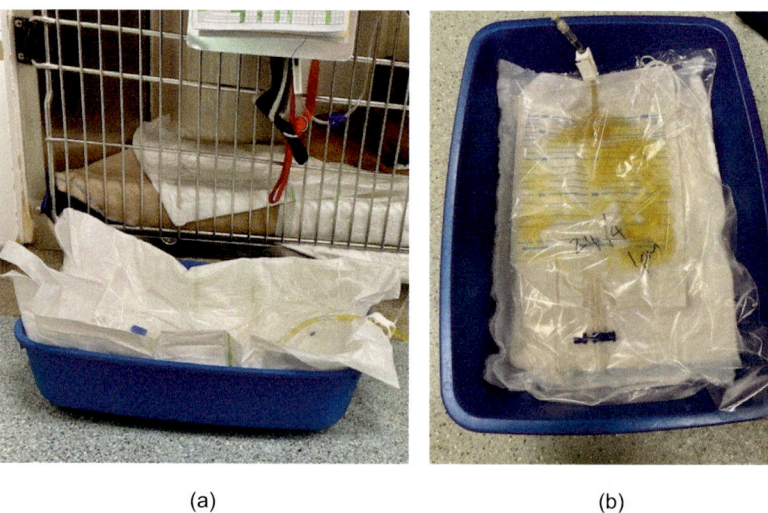

(a)   (b)

Fig. 12.7. The urinary collection bag should be positioned below the level of the patient (a) and off the floor in a clean container (b).

erode the protective glycosaminoglycan layer and mucosal lining of the bladder (Ackerman, 2016). Catheters can also harbour bacteria in their narrow lumens and along their rough, irregular surfaces, promoting bacterial adhesion and colonization (O'Neill and Labato, 2015). Although bacteria are often found in the urine of catheterized animals, it is important to distinguish between subclinical bacteriuria and infection.

The clinician and nurse should be mindful that a catheterized patient is unlikely to display the usual constellation of clinical signs expected with a lower UTI because the urinary catheter will remove the bladder distension required to stimulate voiding and may mask clinical signs of stranguria. If there are gross abnormalities of the urine, such as increased cloudiness or haemorrhage, this is not necessarily a cause for alarm because such changes can be a consequence of having an indwelling urinary catheter, but further investigations would be prudent.

However, if clinical signs such as pyrexia or a novel leucocytosis are seen, further investigations are warranted, and a urine culture should be prioritized. Current recommendations for suspected UTIs in catheterized animals are: (i) to remove the urinary catheter; (ii) to obtain a cystocentesis sample for cytological analysis and bacterial culture; and (iii) to place a new urinary catheter and collection system if it is still required for clinical reasons (Fig. 12.8) (Weese et al., 2019). If cystocentesis is not possible, urine samples can be collected from a newly placed catheter system once the first 5 ml of urine has been discarded. Samples obtained from the collection system for the purposes of bacterial culture should be interpreted with caution due to the potential for the presence of bacteria within the collection system, which may not be reflective of what is occurring within the patient (Loveday et al., 2014).

Studies of dogs with indwelling urinary catheters show bacteriuria in 10–48% of patients. The likelihood of developing bacteriuria increases by 20% with each year of age, by 27% for each day the catheter remains in place and by 454% with antibiotic use (Bubenik et al., 2007). Importantly, bacteriuria is not predictive of a UTI, and risk of UTI development has shown to be minimal if the catheter is left in place for fewer than 3 days, especially if steps are taken to perform aseptic placement and the catheters are managed appropriately (Smarick, 2015). However, it is not recommended to replace the urinary catheter at set time points because this increases the risk of trauma and the opportunities for introducing bacteria. Despite placement of urinary catheters being common in cats to relieve and treat urethral obstruction, few studies have examined the incidence of infection that may develop as a result.

Prophylactic antibiotics should not be administered to patients with indwelling urinary catheters: their use has not been shown to prevent infection but instead increases the risk of HAIs. Antibiotics should only be administered to patients with documented infections, with associated clinical signs such as lower urinary tract signs, pyrexia, systemic clinical signs or evidence of pyelonephritis. If a true infection (rather than subclinical bacteriuria) is suspected, then where possible the urinary catheter should be removed in order to deprive bacteria of the protective biofilm on the catheter surface (Weese et al., 2019). If a true UTI is identified once the catheter has been removed, it should be treated as a sporadic UTI (Weese et al., 2019). The most encountered isolates in dogs with UTIs are E. coli, Enterococcus and Staphylococcus spp. (Wong et al., 2015). The susceptibility patterns can vary, and therefore bacterial culture is recommended to best inform antibiotic selection. If empirical treatment is necessary, a low-tier antibiotic such as amoxicillin should be used to minimize the risk of developing resistance. Repeat urine cultures may be necessary to evaluate for bacterial resistance as treatment progresses.

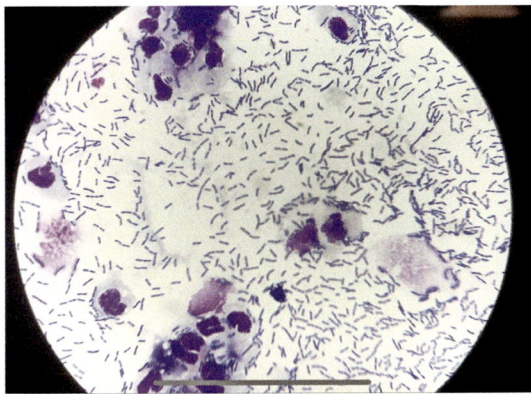

Fig. 12.8. Microscope image of Diffquik-stained urine sediment demonstrating numerous rods and intracellular bacteria. Magnification ×100.

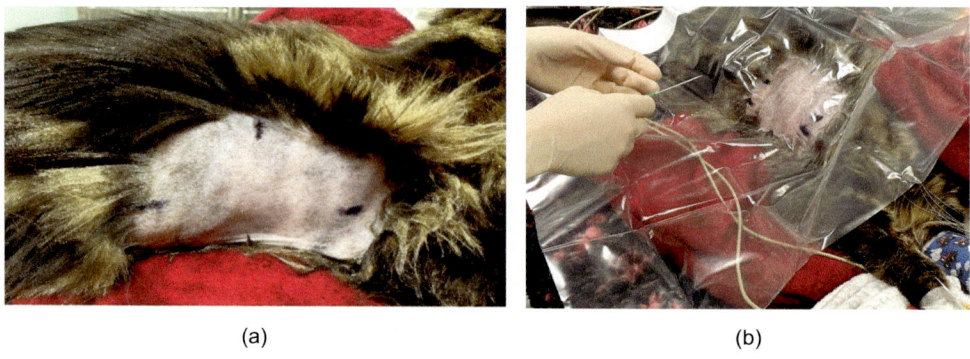

(a)   (b)

Fig. 12.9. (a) The clipped hemithorax of a cat prior to placement of a thoracostomy tube. (b) A sterile dressing has been placed over the insertion site.

Box 12.2. Equipment requirement for placement of a thoracostomy tube.

- Sterile surgical gloves
- Sterile drapes
- Surgical kit
- No. 10 or 15 surgical blade
- Appropriately sized thoracostomy tube
- Lidocaine 2%
- Christmas tree adapter

- Three-way tap
- Needle-free valve
- Appropriately sized syringes for aspiration (5–50 ml)
- Suture material (monofilament)
- Dressing materials

12.6 Thoracostomy Tubes

12.6.1 Indications for thoracostomy tubes

Thoracostomy tubes, also referred to as chest tubes or thoracic drains, are used to remove fluid and/or air from the pleural space to relieve lung retraction and restore pleural subatmospheric pressure (Sigrist, 2015). Pneumothoraces and pleural effusions can be managed initially via thoracocentesis, which can be repeated several times. However, if more than three episodes of needle thoracocentesis are required in a 12–24 h period, if ongoing air leakage or fluid production is expected (e.g. chylothorax), if lavage as well as drainage is required (e.g. pyothorax) or if the patient has just undergone thoracic surgery, then the placement of a thoracostomy tube should be considered (Lynch and Campos, 2019).

12.6.2 Thoracostomy tube placement

Thoracostomy tubes can be placed under sedation or general anaesthesia to allow controlled placement and avoid contamination. The lateral aspect of the selected hemithorax should be clipped using clean, sharp clippers from behind the scapula to the last rib (Fig. 12.9). Aseptic preparation should be undertaken as described previously (see Chapter 8, this volume).

Equipment required for placement of a thoracostomy tube is shown in Box 12.2. The selected thoracostomy tube should then be placed under strict aseptic conditions with surgical scrubbing and sterile gloves donned (Fig. 12.9). The placement procedure is beyond the scope of this chapter. Once the thoracostomy tube has been successfully placed, the area should be cleaned of any blood and a sterile dressing placed over the insertion site. Ideally, this should be a clear dressing so that the insertion site can be visually examined daily (Fig. 12.9).

If a thoracostomy tube has been placed during a life-threatening emergency and sterility may have been compromised, the degree of potential contamination should be considered, and where this is significant, placement of a new tube in a controlled manner might be prudent once the patient is clinically stable.

12.6.3 Management of thoracostomy tubes

Care of thoracostomy tubes

Following placement of the thoracostomy tube, a stocking vest or pet T-shirt should be applied to cover the drain and prevent premature removal. An Elizabethan collar should also be placed to avoid patient interference. Patients with thoracostomy tubes in place require 24 h monitoring with regular respiratory rate and effort checks due to the risk of developing a pneumothorax, either as consequence of placement or secondary to tube obstruction (Savino *et al.*, 2011).

Strict aseptic care is required when dealing with thoracostomy tubes. Hands should be cleaned prior to handling and sterile gloves should be worn (see Chapter 5, this volume). Bandages or dressings need to be checked and changed daily (or more frequently if they slip or become soiled). Daily checks of the insertion site are required to monitor for signs of infection or inflammation. Sutures should be inspected to ensure the drain is still being held securely in place, that the tube does not have any kinks and that it has not migrated.

Evacuation of the thoracic cavity using a thoracostomy tube

Drainage of the thoracic cavity via the thoracostomy tube is achieved using either intermittent or continuous drainage depending on the nature of the pleural space disease and equipment available (Sigrist, 2015).

Intermittent manual syringe aspiration every 1–6 h is sufficient in many patients and allows adequate drainage and maintenance of negative pressure. Following hand hygiene and donning of sterile gloves, the needle-free valve should be wiped clean using a 70% alcohol swab for 30 s and then allowed to dry prior to attaching the syringe. Single-use disinfectant caps that contain a foam impregnated with 70% isopropyl alcohol can also be used, avoiding the need to manually disinfect the needle-free valves (Fig. 12.10). These caps are left in place while the drain is not in use and replaced after each drainage process.

If a large volume of air or fluid is being removed, a three-way tap and Luer lock syringe should be used to avoid multiple removals and reattachments of the syringe to the drain. Care should be taken not to apply too much pressure when aspirating the thoracostomy tube because excessive negative

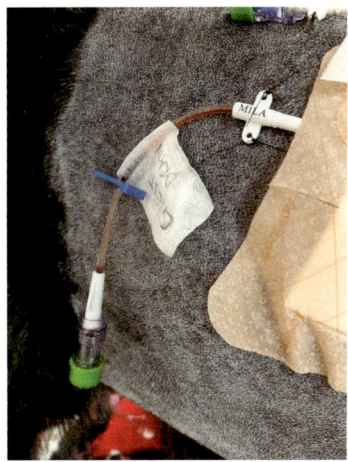

Fig. 12.10. A thoracostomy tube in a dog, with a disposable cap containing 70% alcohol on the inner surface to protect and maintain the sterility of the Luer access valve.

pressure can lead to lung trauma, surgical-site disruption, and occlusion of the tube by mediastinal or pleural tissue. Approximately 5–10 ml of vacuum in a syringe equates to the difference between the pleural pressure and the interalveolar pressure (Sigrist, 2015). As such, no more than 5 ml of negative pressure should be applied to the tube to avoid iatrogenic damage.

The volume and characteristics of all fluid and air should be documented after each aspiration. In cases of continuous air leaks or severe fluid accumulation, continuous active suction may be necessary. This method allows sustained lung expansion and better healing of leaks by pleural adhesion. Various devices such as the Pleur-evac or Thopaz are commercially available and provide a suction pressure of 10–20 cmH$_2$O (Fig. 12.11). These devices can be disconnected from the patient for short periods of time if required. Aseptic technique should be followed when handling the tubes and all ends sealed with a sterile bung when not in use.

Some patients, such as those diagnosed with a pyothorax, may benefit from intermittent flushing or lavage of the chest via the thoracostomy tube. There is little evidence available detailing the best method to perform this and it appears to be based largely on clinician preference and the individual patient. The authors' experience involves instilling 5–10 ml kg^{-1} of warmed sterile 0.9% saline into the pleural space via the thoracostomy tube, allowing

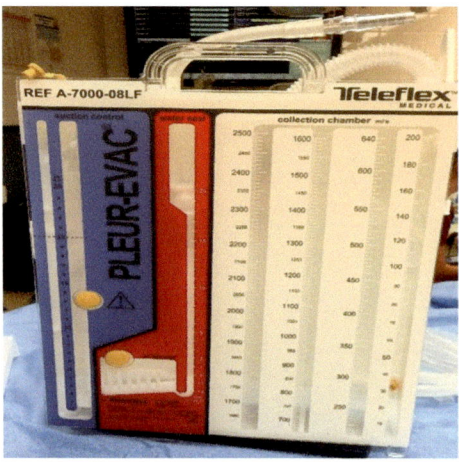

Fig. 12.11. A commercially available unit for continuous active suction of the thoracic cavity via a thoracostomy tube.

the fluid to dwell for 20–30 min, and then draining the chest. This process is performed under strict aseptic conditions: hand hygiene is performed, sterile gloves are donned and the needle-free valves are wiped clean using alcohol wipes before any syringes are attached. If possible, two thoracostomy tubes should be placed: one used to instil and the other to remove the lavage fluid. Two syringes should be used for this process, a 'clean' syringe to instil the saline and a second 'dirty' syringe to remove the exudate.

Generous multi-modal analgesia (including local anaesthetic via the thoracostomy tube) should be provided to all patients while a thoracostomy tube is in place.

12.6.4 Evaluating for thoracostomy tube-associated infection

There appears to be little evidence of infection risks associated with thoracostomy tube placement. In human medicine, skin infections, pyothorax and even necrotizing infections have been known to occur at the insertion site (Kwiatt *et al.*, 2014). By acting as a foreign body, the thoracostomy tube may provide a route for infectious exposure between the insertion site, the chest wall and the pleural space. The tube insertion site should be checked daily for any signs of local infection such as erythema, swelling or discharge.

Point-of-care ultrasound to evaluate the pleural space and fluid characteristics can be helpful. An increase in fluid volume or alteration in appearance (e.g. an increase in fluid echogenicity) would be an indication for further investigation. Needle thoracocentesis should then be performed, if safe to do so, to obtain a sample for analysis without the potential contamination encountered if sample collection were to occur via the thoracostomy tubes.

If there is a change in the appearance of the fluid being removed from the thoracostomy tube, it should be examined for signs of bacterial infection. If a pyothorax was the reason for tube placement, cytological changes in bacterial populations could be an indication for repeating culture. A newly documented pyrexia or changes in the patient's blood results (e.g. development of a leucocytosis or left shift) could also be indicative of infection. In humans, pyothorax after thoracostomy tube placement has a reported incidence of 1–25%, with the presence of a pleural effusion prior to tube placement carrying a higher risk of infection (Chan *et al.*, 1997).

Prophylactic antibiotic use prior to thoracostomy tube placement is controversial and such use should be considered on an individual basis. In patients with pyothorax, antimicrobial therapy should be given based on the expected bacterial organisms involved and subsequently guided by culture and susceptibility. Obligate anaerobes are isolated from 60% of dogs and 89% of cats with positive cultures in a pyothorax, and suitable antibiotic choices could include potentiated amoxicillin or metronidazole (Wray and Hill, 2008), or a fluoroquinolone with clindamycin (Lappin *et al.*, 2017). In human medicine, it is recommended that prophylactic antibiotics should be given to all patients with penetrating chest trauma to reduce the incidence of chest infections. However, in patients with blunt trauma, antibiotic use should be considered on a case-by-case basis (Ayoub *et al.*, 2014).

12.6.5 Thoracostomy tube removal

An eventual consideration that arises following successful patient treatment is timing of thoracostomy tube removal. The presence of tubes alone will result in inflammation and the development of effusion, even in the absence of a disease process. In a study of thoracostomy tube placement in 8 healthy dogs they caused continued fluid production, 3 subsequently developed pyothorax (caused by *Staphylococcus*

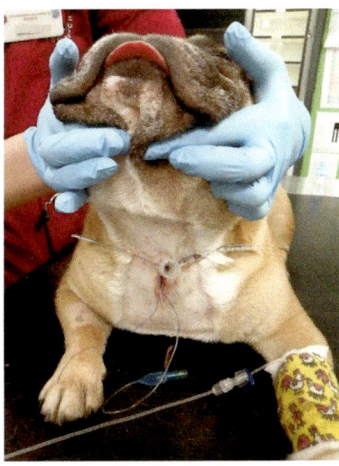

Fig. 12.12. Home-made temporary tracheostomy tube in a French bulldog.

pseudintermedius and *Streptococcus equi*) (Hung *et al.*, 2016). This confirms that thoracostomy tubes are not benign and should be removed as early as clinically possible. Typically, it is advised that thoracostomy tubes should be removed when the volume of fluid produced is below 2 ml kg^{-1} day^{-1} (Sigrist, 2015). However, a recent study reported that thoracostomy tubes were removed with a fluid production range of 16.8 ml kg^{-1} day^{-1} (mean 2.2 ml kg^{-1} day^{-1}); the underlying disease process and presence of pre-operative effusion, but *not* the volume produced from the tube at the time of discharge, was related to the risk of effusion recurrence (Racette *et al.*, 2022).

12.7   Tracheostomy Tubes

Temporary tracheostomy tubes (TTTs) can be life-saving in patients with upper airway obstruction, and can either be placed electively, when the risk of obstruction is known and instituted prophylactically, or emergently (Fig. 12.12).

12.7.1   Indications for a TTT: routine versus emergent

Placement of a TTT requires general anaesthesia, with orotracheal intubation (if possible) to facilitate oxygenation during the procedure.

Routine placement allows for a controlled environment, aseptic technique and provision of a secure airway. Emergent placement involves a

higher risk to the patient, as some of these requirements may not be achievable.

The ventral cervical neck should be clipped widely from the angle of the mandibles to the manubrium and laterally to beyond the jugular veins (Mann and Flanders, 2012). Aseptic preparation of the area prior to placement is required and sterile technique should be used throughout the procedure (see Chapter 8, this volume). A drape should be used, when possible, to minimize contamination. Patients undergoing general anaesthesia who are at risk of requiring emergent TT placement on recovery may have the insertion site clipped pre-emptively to speed up the process.

12.7.2   Management of TTTs

Where possible, patients with a TTT should be placed in an environment where they are constantly breathing humidified oxygen in order to protect the respiratory mucosa, which is integral in combatting inhaled pathogens. If this is not possible, humidification of the airway should be carried out intermittently, with nebulization being the most effective method for patients who are breathing spontaneously. Nebulization should be performed every 4–6 h for 10–15 min using sterile 0.9% saline. If the nebulizer does not provide oxygen, and the patient is particularly sensitive to handling, oxygen can be delivered by attaching the nebulization chamber directly on to an oxygen source tubing.

12.7.3   Tracheostomy tube (TT) maintenance supply station

A station should be set up, ready for use at all times, which contains the necessary equipment for maintenance and replacement of the TTT (Box 12.3). The imminent dangers of tube obstruction or dislodgement are life threatening and should be addressed immediately.

12.7.4   Routine maintenance

Routine maintenance should be carried out every 2–4 h depending on the patient's individual requirements as follows:

● Place the patient in an easy-to-access area with one person carrying out the tube care and another restraining the patient's head/providing flow by oxygen.

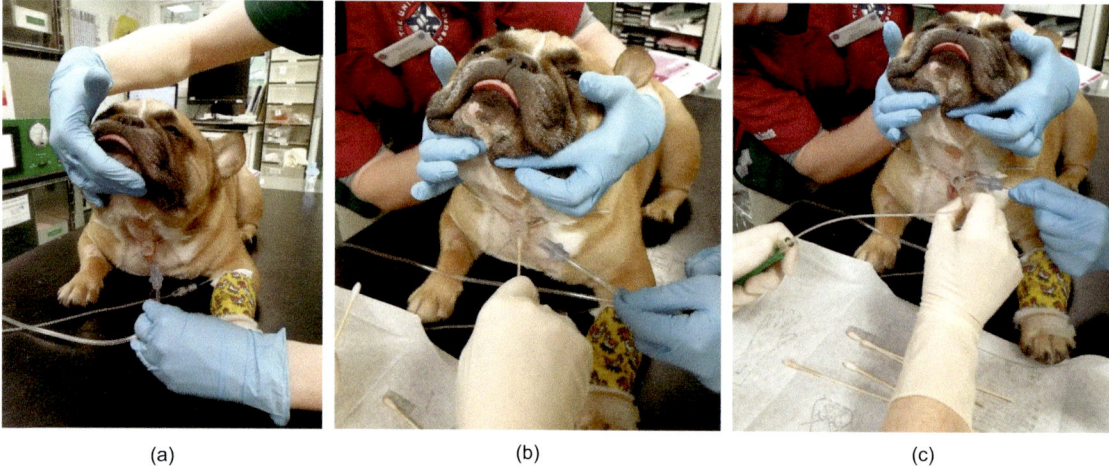

Fig. 12.13. (a) Pre-oxygenation of the lungs prior to TTT suctioning. (b) Aseptic cleaning of the TTT inner lumen prior to suctioning. (c) Sterile suctioning of the TTT lumen.

- Perform hand hygiene.
- Open all of the sterile supplies and fill the bowl with sterile saline aseptically.
- Perform hand hygiene and don sterile gloves.
- An assistant should hold the patient's head up and provide flow by oxygen throughout the procedure, ensuring pre-oxygenation for a few minutes prior to suctioning (Fig. 12.13a) (Savino *et al.*, 2011).
- Using saline-dipped sterile cotton buds, clean the inner lumen of the tube connector, removing any gross, visible secretions (Fig. 12.13b).
- Once the tube connector is clean and the patient adequately pre-oxygenated, insert the suction catheter into the TTT and advance to a few centimetres beyond the distal tip of the tube. Suction should not be applied during advancement of the suction catheter to avoid traumatizing any tissues. Care should be taken to avoid contamination of the suction tubing during this time.
- Gently withdraw the suction catheter using a circular motion to encompass the entire lumen, while intermittently suctioning (Fig. 12.13c). Only moderate suction should be used, (80–120 mmHg) to avoid suction-based trauma to the mucosa.

- The suction catheter should be in place for no more than 10-15 s.
- Once removed, clean the outside of the suction catheter with a sterile saline-soaked swab, then suck up some saline to remove any debris from the inside of the catheter tip.
- During suction catheter cleaning, the assistant should monitor the patient closely for any signs of distress, continue providing flow by oxygen and ensuring complete recovery before a second pass of the suction catheter.
- Check the patient's respiratory pattern and listen at the tube opening for continued noise before resuctioning.
- If deemed necessary, repeat the process two to four times depending on the volume of secretions present and how well the patient is tolerating it.
- Perform hand hygiene.

Alternatively, if the patient is showing no clinical signs to indicate the need for suctioning (e.g. dyspnoea, noisy breathing, coughing/gurgling, increased respiratory rate/effort), suctioning the tube should only be carried out at most every 4 h if deemed necessary, as suctioning can be very stressful for the patient. It can also cause iatrogenic damage of the tracheal mucosa and risks inoculating bacteria into the airways if performed too frequently.

If the patient starts coughing during the procedure, it is probably due to advancement of the catheter too far distally causing irritation to the mucosa of the trachea or bronchi.

The use of sterile supplies and aseptic technique during maintenance is vital to prevent bacteria being introduced iatrogenically into the lower airways.

After suctioning

After the patient has recovered from suctioning:

- Clean around the outer rim of the tube connector with sterile saline-soaked swabs.
- Clean the skin around the stoma site with sterile saline-soaked swabs and pat the area dry. Take care not to touch the tissues within the incision to avoid introducing a nosocomial secondary bacterial infection to the area. A moderate amount of discharge from the surgical incision is to be expected in the first few days.
- Check the umbilical tape or ties securing the TTT behind the patient's neck (Fig. 12.14) to ensure the TTT has not become dislodged during the cleaning process. These tapes can be tightened if necessary.

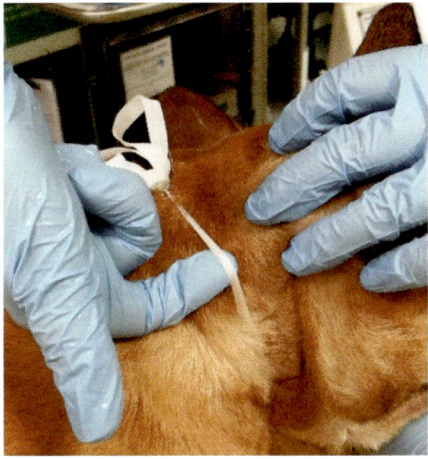

Fig. 12.14. Correct placement of the TTT securement tapes. They should be tight enough to minimize the chance of tube dislodgement but comfortable for the patient with no obstruction to breathing.

- Frequent evaluation of these tapes for gross contamination should be performed, and soiled tapes/ties removed, as these could be a nidus for infection.

As soon as routine maintenance is complete, any supplies used from the station should be replaced immediately as they may be required urgently if the patient were to obstruct again.

The TTT should be replaced every 24 h with a new sterile tube (Fudge, 2009). If the tube is even partially occluded by secretions, the resultant narrowing of the available airway can cause an increased respiratory workload for the patient leading to increased stress, hyperthermia, hypoxia and potential respiratory fatigue. The secretions can also allow bacteria to proliferate and increase the risk of biofilm formation.

The stoma site should also be evaluated daily for signs of infection.

Vaseline, or other types of barrier cream, may be used on the skin around the stoma and surgical incision site to prevent any maceration or excoriation of the tissues. This can occur if the site is producing a lot of secretions and should be decided on a case-by-case basis.

12.7.5 Evaluation for pneumonia

Patients with a TTT in place have circumvented the normal anatomy, which, in healthy animals,

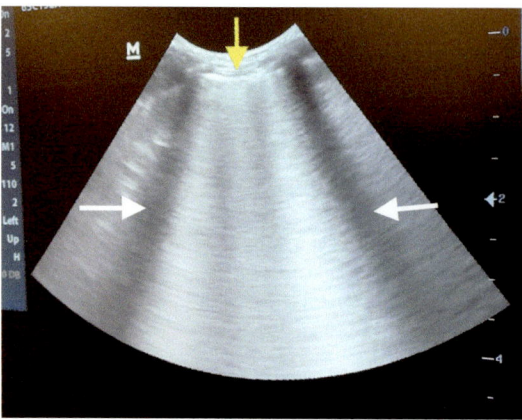

Fig. 12.15. This is a still image acquired by point-of-care ultrasound (POCUS). The black areas extending throughout the image represent the ribs and their associated acoustic shadow. Within the intercostal space are the lung fields, the hyperechoic lines radiating from the level of the muscle downward, almost like rays shining down, termed B-lines. They indicated a gas–fluid interface and can be seen with oedema, haemorrhage or purulent material as encountered in pneumonia.

acts to prevent bacterial inhalation. The first line of defence is provided by the nasal turbinates, which filter, warm and humidify the inspired air. Secondly, the glottis helps prevent foreign material from being aspirated. Patients with a TTT have bypassed these normal protective elements, increasing the risk of nosocomial pneumonia. Clinical signs to evaluate for pneumonia include coughing, pyrexia, tachypnoea, dyspnoea and increased frequency of TTT obstruction. If there is a clinical suspicion of pneumonia, diagnostic imaging is warranted, including thoracic radiographs or computed tomography, and/or identification of B-lines on point-of-care ultrasound in the cranioventral lung fields (Fig. 12.15). Bronchoalveolar lavage or a transtracheal lavage could be performed to obtain samples to submit for cytological evaluation and bacterial culture and sensitivity testing. Gram staining can aid with empirical antibiotic choices, if required.

12.8 Conclusion

With the increasing advantages that medical advances can afford our patients, there is also the potential for increased harm when infection occurs

as a consequence of our interventions. One of the key aspects and areas where we can prevent this is by ensuring a robust approach to aseptic technique during initial placement of medical equipment such as catheters and tubes, and also throughout their time in place.

Another aspect is the diligent monitoring of procedure sites for early indicators of site infection and taking a proactive approach towards obtaining samples and submitting these for culture early in the disease process, while also considering the relative benefits of local or systemic treatment in each case.

The final area to be consistently questioning is whether these interventions continue to be needed daily, and at what point does their use have a greater negative impact than the positive ones they initially presented.

References

AACN (American Association of Critical-Care Nurses) (1993) Evaluation of the effects of heparinized and nonheparinized flush solutions on the patency of arterial pressure monitoring lines: the AACN thunder project. *American Journal of Critical Care* 2(1), 3–15.

Ackerman, N. (2016) Managing indwelling urinary catheters. *Clinicians Brief* 14, 23–26.

Aguiar, J., Chang, Y.M. and Garden, O.A. (2016) Complications of percutaneous endoscopic gastrostomy in dogs and cats receiving corticosteroid treatment. *Journal of Veterinary Internal Medicine* 30(4), 1008–1013. DOI: 10.1111/jvim.13969.

Ayoub, F., Quirke, M. and Frith, D. (2014) Use of prophylactic antibiotic in preventing complications for blunt and penetrating chest trauma requiring chest drain insertion: a systematic review and meta-analysis. *Trauma Surgery & Acute Care Open* 4, e000246.

Breheny, C.R., Boag, A., Le Gal, A., Hōim, S.-E., Cantatore, M. *et al.* (2019) Esophageal feeding tube placement and the associated complications in 248 cats. *Journal of Veterinary Internal Medicine* 33(3), 1306–1314. DOI: 10.1111/jvim.15496.

Bubenik, L.J., Hosgood, G.L., Waldron, D.R. and Snow, L.A. (2007) Frequency of urinary tract infection in catheterized dogs and comparison of bacterial culture and susceptibility testing results for catheterized and noncatheterized dogs with urinary tract infections. *Journal of the American Veterinary Medical Association* 231(6), 893–899. DOI: 10.2460/javma.231.6.893.

Cao, Y., Gong, Z., Shan, J. and Gao, Y. (2018) Comparison of the preventive effect of urethral cleaning versus disinfection for catheter-associated urinary tract infections in adults: a network meta-analysis. *International Journal of Infectious Diseases* 76, 102–108. DOI: 10.1016/j. ijid.2018.09.008.

Chan, L., Reilly, K.M., Henderson, C., Kahn, F. and Salluzzo, R.F. (1997) Complication rates of tube thoracostomy. *American Journal of Emergency Medicine* 15(4), 368–370. DOI: 10.1016/s0735-6757(97)90127-3.

Chandler, S. and Middlecote, L. (2011) Principles of general nursing. In: Cooper, B., Muullineaux, E. and Turner, L. (eds) *BSAVA Textbook of Veterinary Nursing*, 5th edn. BSAVA Publications, Gloucester, UK, pp. 409–441.

Fudge, M. (2009) Tracheostomy. In: Silverstein, D.C. and Hopper, K. (eds) *Small Animal Critical Care Medicine*. Saunders, Elsevier, pp. 75–77.

Hague, M., Sartelli, M., McKimm, J. and Abu Bakar, M. (2018) Health care-associated infections - an overview. *Infection and Drug Resistance* 11, 2321–2333. DOI: 10.2147/IDR.S177247.

Ho, K.M. and Litton, E. (2006) Use of chlorhexidine-impregnated dressing to prevent vascular and epidural catheter colonization and infection: a meta-analysis. *Journal of Antimicrobial Chemotherapy* 58(2), 281–287. DOI: 10.1093/jac/dkl234.

Hung, G.C., Gaunt, M.C., Rubin, J.E., Starrak, G.S. and Sakals, S.A. (2016) Quantification and characterization of pleural fluid in healthy dogs with thoracostomy tubes. *American Journal of Veterinary Research* 77(12), 1387–1391. DOI: 10.2460/ajvr.77.12.1387.

INS (Infusion Nurses Society) (2011) Infusion nursing standards of practice. *Journal of Infusion Nursing* 34(Suppl.), S1–S110.

Ko, J.J. and Mann, F.A.T. (2014) Barium peritonitis in small animals. *Journal of Veterinary Medical Science* 76(5), 621–628. DOI: 10.1292/jvms.13-0220.

Kuwahara, T., Asanami, S. and Kubo, S. (1988) Experimental infusion phlebitis: tolerance of peripheral venous endothelial cell. *Nutrition* 14, 496–501.

Kwiatt, M., Tarbox, A., Seamon, M.J., Swaroop, M., Cipolla, J. *et al.* (2014) Thoracostomy tubes: a comprehensive review of complications and related topics. *International Journal of Critical Illness and Injury Science* 4(2), 143–155. DOI: 10.4103/2229-5151.134182.

Lai, K.K. (1998) Safety of prolonging peripheral cannula and i.v. tubing use from 72 hours to 96 hours. *American Journal of Infection Control* 26(1), 66–70. DOI: 10.1016/s0196-6553(98)70063-x.

Lappin, M.R., Blondeau, J., Boothe, D., Breitschwerdt, E.B., Guardabassi, L, *et al.* (2017) Antimicrobial use-guidelines for treatment of respiratory tract disease in dogs and cats:Antimicrobial Guidelines Working Group of the International Society for Companion Animal Infectious Diseases. *Journal of Veterinary Internal Medicine* 31(2), 279–294. DOI: 10.1111/jvim.14627.

Lodzinska, J., Leigh, H., Parys, M. and Liuti, T. (2019) Vascular ultrasonographic findings in canine patients with clinically diagnosed phlebitis. *Veterinary Radiology & Ultrasound* 60(6), 745–752. DOI: 10.1111/vru.12805.

Loveday, H.P., Wilson, J.A., Pratt, R.J., Golsorkhi, M., Tingle, A. *et al.* (2014) epic3: national evidence-based guidelines for preventing healthcare-associated infections in NHS hospitals in England. *Journal of Hospital Infection* 86(Suppl 1), S1–70. DOI: 10.1016/S0195-6701(13)60012-2.

Lynch, A. and Campos, S. (2019) Thoracostomy tube placement. In: Drobatz, K.J., Hopper, K., Rozanski, E. and Silverstein, D.C. (eds) *Textbook of Small Animal Emergency Medicine*. Wiley, Hoboken, New Jersey, pp. 1199–1201.

Malach, T., Jerassy, Z., Rudensky, B., Schlesinger, Y., Broide, E. *et al.* (2006) Prospective surveillance of phlebitis associated with peripheral intravenous catheters. *American Journal of Infection Control* 34(5), 308–312. DOI: 10.1016/j.ajic.2005.10.002.

Mann, F.A. and Flanders, M.M. (2012) Temporary tracheostomy. In: Burkitt Creedon, J.M. and Davis, H. (eds) *Advanced Monitoring and Procedures for Small Animal Emergency and Critical Care*. Wiley, Chichester, UK, pp. 306–317. DOI: 10.1002/9781118997246.

Martinho, R.F.S. and Rodrigues, A.B. (2008) Occurrence of phlebitis in patients on intravenous amiodarione. *Einstein* 6, 459–462.

McClave, S.A. and Neff, R.L. (2006) Care and long-term maintenance of percutaneous endoscopic gastrostomy tubes. *Journal of Parenteral and Enteral Nutrition* 30, S27–38. DOI: 10.1177/01486071060300S1S27.

Nathanson, O., McGonigle, K., Michel, K., Stefanovski, D. and Clarke, D. (2019) Esophagostomy tube complications in dogs and cats: retrospective review of 225 cases. *Journal of Veterinary Internal Medicine* 33(5), 2014–2019. DOI: 10.1111/jvim.15563.

Newton, J. (2009) Central venous cannulation – transforming training and safety. London: National Institute for Health and Care Excellence. Available at: www. nice.org.uk/sharedlearning/central-venous-cannulation-transforming-training-and-safety (accessed 25 October 2022).

O'Neill, K.E. and Labato, M.A. (2015) Urinary catheters & infection. *Clinician's Brief*, November 2015. Available at: www.cliniciansbrief.com/article/urinary-catheters-infection (accessed 27 October 2022).

Raad, I., Costerton, W., Sabharwal, U., Sacilowski, M., Anaissie, E. *et al.* (1993) Ultrastructural analysis of indwelling vascular catheters: a quantitative relationship between luminal colonization and duration of placement. *Journal of Infectious Diseases* 168(2), 400–407. DOI: 10.1093/infdis/168.2.400.

Racette, M.A., Sharkey, L.C., Rendahl, A.K., Heinrich, D.A. and Chow, R.S. (2022) Retrospective evaluation of fluid production at the time of thoracostomy tube removal following elective and emergency surgery in dogs (2010-2017): 185 cases. *Journal of Veterinary Emergency and Critical Care* 32(1), 58–67. DOI: 10.1111/vec.13138.

Randolph, A.G., Cook, D.J., Gonzales, C.A. and Andrew, M. (1998) Benefit of heparin in peripheral venous and arterial catheters: systematic review and meta-analysis of randomised controlled trials. *British Medical Journal* 316(7136), 969–975. DOI: 10.1136/bmj.316.7136.969.

Savino, E., Petrollini, E.A. and Hughes, D. (2011) Nursing care of the critical patient. In: King, L.K. and Boag, A. (eds) *BSAVA Manual of Canine and Feline Emergency and Critical Care*, 2nd edn. BSAVA, Quedgeley, UK, pp. 372–382.

Sequela, J. and Pages, J.O. (2011) Bacterial and fungal colonisation of peripheral intravenous catheters in dogs and cats. *Journal of Small Animal Practice* 52(10), 531–535. DOI: 10.1111/j.1748-5827.2011.01101.x.

Sigrist, N.E. (2015) Thoracostomy tube placement and drainage. In: Silverstein, D.C. and Hopper, K. (eds) *Small Animal Critical Care Medicine*, 2nd edn. Elsevier, pp. 1032–1035.

Smarick, S. (2015) Urinary catheterisation. In: Silverstein, D.C. and Hopper, K. (eds) *Small Animal Critical Care Medicine*, 2nd edn. Elsevier, pp. 1069–1072.

Tager, I.B., Ginsberg, M.B., Ellis, S.E., Walsh, N.E., Dupont, I. *et al.* (1983) An epidemiologic study of the risks associated with peripheral intravenous catheters. *American Journal of Epidemiology* 118(6), 839–851. DOI: 10.1093/oxfordjournals.aje.a113702.

Webster, J., Osborne, S., Rickard, C.M. and Marsh, N. (2019) Clinically-indicated replacement versus routine replacement of peripheral venous catheters. *Cochrane Database of Systematic Reviews* 1(1), CD007798. DOI: 10.1002/14651858.CD007798.pub5.

Weese, J.S., Blondeau, J.M., Boothe, D., Breitschwerdt, E.B., Guardabassi, L. *et al.* (2019) Antimicrobial use guidelines for treatment of urinary tract disease in dogs and cats: antimicrobial guidelines working group of the International Society for Companion Animal Infectious Diseases. *Veterinary Medicine International* 2011, 263768.

Wong, C., Epstein, S.E. and Westropp, J.L. (2015) Antimicrobial susceptibility patterns in urinary tract infections in dogs (2010-2013). *Journal of Veterinary Internal Medicine* 29(4), 1045–1052. DOI: 10.1111/jvim.13571.

Wray, J.D. and Hill, N. (2008) Pyothorax. In: *British Small Animal Veterinary Congress 2008*. Available at: www.vin.com/apputil/content/defaultadv1.aspx?pId=11254&id=3862995 (accessed 25 October 2022).

13 Management of the Infectious Patient

ELEANOR HASKEY[1]* AND TOM REILLY[2]

[1]The Royal Veterinary College, Hawkshead Lane, Brookmans Park, Hatfield, UK; [2]Willows Veterinary Centre and Referral Service, Highlands Road, Shirley, Solihull, UK

13.1 Introduction

Infection control strategies are a critical step in preventing the spread of diseases that may increase patient morbidity and mortality. They also protect staff and the public from zoonoses. Healthcare-associated infections can lead to prolonged hospital stays, increased antimicrobial resistance and increased use of antimicrobials, all of which have financial implications for the pet owner. Veterinary clinics have professional, moral and legal requirements to reduce the risks to hospitalized patients and to provide a safe work environment for the veterinary team (Weese, 2004). Therefore, infection control and prevention (ICP) should be taken seriously, and it is fundamental that the veterinary team adhere to local policies and processes to optimize quality of care as well as patient and personnel safety. Evidence-based veterinary research is currently limited, and many recommendations are therefore extrapolated from human healthcare. Understanding disease transmission is vital to prevent contamination or infection – it is important to understand where the risks are.

The 'one style fits all' infectious disease policy is no longer appropriate in modern veterinary practice. There is a need for more evidence-based polices to demonstrate the most effective approaches to barrier nursing, vaccination protocols and client education. Currently, there is limited evidence to measure the benefits of ICP plans in veterinary practice (Stull et al., 2018). However there is evidence from other healthcare fields (WHO, 2019). For this reason, it is generally accepted that veterinary clinics should have a written ICP plan similar to those used in paraprofessions. The ICP plan should be available as a quick reference guide for the whole team to access and should be reviewed and updated annually.

The ICP plan must be tailored to the individual clinic, giving consideration to the patients treated and the procedures undertaken. There are several published veterinary guidelines including:

- *Guidelines for Veterinary Personal Biosecurity* published by the Australian Veterinary Association (AVA, 2017);
- *Infection Control, Prevention, and Biosecurity Guidelines* published by the American Animal Hospital Association (AAHA) (Stull et al., 2018); and
- *Infection Prevention and Control Best Practices for Small Animal Veterinary Clinics* published by the Canadian Committee on Antibiotic Resistance (2008).

These guidelines include step-by-step instructions for creating an ICP plan in the clinic (Fig. 13.1). They document recommendations on establishing a coordinator, developing evidence-based standard operating procedures (SOPs) for specific tasks, identifying areas for improvement, staff training and education, implementing surveillance and maintaining compliance. They detail specific information about personal protective actions and equipment, environmental infection control, employee health, disinfectants and sterilants.

When a potentially infectious or confirmed infectious patient presents to the clinic, the veterinary team needs to respond quickly and efficiently according to the clinic ICP plan in order to minimize the risk of harm to other patients or personnel. Compliance with ICP plans relies on effective training and education of the team, financial investment from the practice management, appropriate

---

*Corresponding author: ehaskey@rvc.ac.uk

© CAB International 2023. *Infection Control in Small Animal Clinical Practice* (eds F. Allerton and K.L. Bowlt Blacklock)
DOI: 10.1079/9781789244977.0013

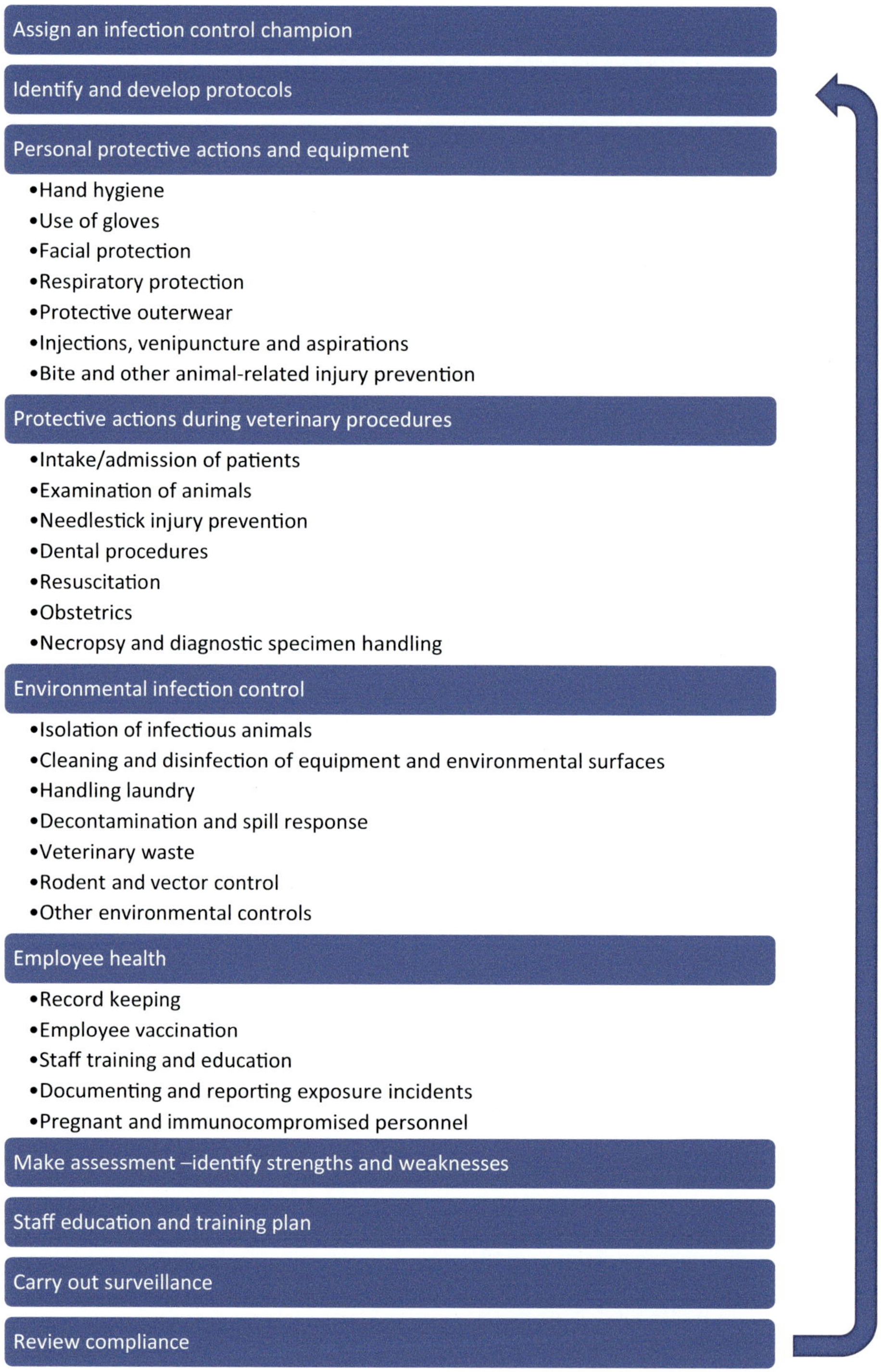

Assign an infection control champion

Identify and develop protocols

Personal protective actions and equipment
- Hand hygiene
- Use of gloves
- Facial protection
- Respiratory protection
- Protective outerwear
- Injections, venipuncture and aspirations
- Bite and other animal-related injury prevention

Protective actions during veterinary procedures
- Intake/admission of patients
- Examination of animals
- Needlestick injury prevention
- Dental procedures
- Resuscitation
- Obstetrics
- Necropsy and diagnostic specimen handling

Environmental infection control
- Isolation of infectious animals
- Cleaning and disinfection of equipment and environmental surfaces
- Handling laundry
- Decontamination and spill response
- Veterinary waste
- Rodent and vector control
- Other environmental controls

Employee health
- Record keeping
- Employee vaccination
- Staff training and education
- Documenting and reporting exposure incidents
- Pregnant and immunocompromised personnel

Make assessment –identify strengths and weaknesses

Staff education and training plan

Carry out surveillance

Review compliance

Fig. 13.1. Step-by-step instructions for creating an infection control and prevention plan.

Eleanor Haskey and Tom Reilly

workload, and access to appropriate equipment and materials. Compliance also involves a cultural shift within the clinic – it can take time to change habits, and reinforcement with further training and follow-up is very beneficial.

13.2 Principles of Isolation

The principles of isolation of patients considered potentially infectious date back to the late 1800s when the emphasis was on separating patients into 'infectious disease hospitals' (Weese, 2004). By the 1970s, the Centers for Disease Control and Prevention (CDC) recommended that patients were isolated dependent on their condition: strict isolation, contact isolation, or enteric, wound/skin or blood precautions. In later years, more recent CDC guidelines have put the emphasis on the hospital ICP committee's decision making and developing protocols specific to the hospital. In veterinary medicine, the Royal College of Veterinary Surgeons Practice Standards Scheme is an accreditation initiative to promote high standards of veterinary care in clinics (RCVS, 2015). The core standards recommend that clinics 'must provide designated accommodation for the isolation of infectious and zoonotic cases or have a written policy for dealing with such cases that is known to all members of the team'. Clinics are encouraged to be proactive by nominating an infection control champion who takes an active lead in developing the ICP plan for the clinic.

There are five guiding principles in the hierarchy of control that the veterinary team need to consider in their ICP plan when dealing with infectious patients (Gibbins and MacMahon, 2015):

1. Elimination: eliminating the risk.
2. Substitution: reducing the risk with a safer alternative.
3. Engineering controls: building features into the clinic to facilitate infection control measures.
4. Administrative controls: implementing protocols, staff training and supervision.
5. Personal protective equipment: as an adjunct to other principles to help contain the infectious agent.

Isolating a patient must be considered when a patient poses a risk to other patients or personnel. Isolation facilities vary across clinics, and the method of isolation will depend on factors such as patient stability, staffing, cost implications, virulence of the infection and route of transmission. Many large clinics have dedicated isolation facilities, but smaller clinics may not, and so provisions need to be made as to how to offer a safe place to hospitalize the patient. Upon initial patient assessment or triage, the stability of the patient needs to be ascertained as well as an assessment of the risk that patient carries. Based on the stability of the patient, there are a number of options, including management as an outpatient versus immediate hospitalization. The greatest challenge arises when the patient presents with a high level of risk in an unstable condition and needs hospitalization and intensive treatment for a number of days.

A simple flow chart can aid in the decision-making process for where it is safest to manage the patient (Fig. 13.2).

13.3 Identifying Infectious Patients

Identifying infectious patients can sometimes be challenging, as some will be asymptomatic carriers of an animal pathogen (e.g. feline herpes virus) or harbouring microorganisms that are pathogenic to humans (e.g. leptospirosis). In human medicine, patient management systems can be programmed with algorithms to help identify high-risk patients at the time of triage or when clinical parameters are logged on the patient record. As many veterinary clinics do not operate paperless systems, there should be an emphasis on screening patients. Checklists have been associated with improved outcomes, reduced rates of death and complications in hospital settings (Haynes *et al.*, 2009). Checklists could be implemented to help identify and screen infectious patients at the time of admission to the clinic (e.g. AAHA phone triage list accessible at: www.aaha. org/globalassets/02-guidelines/infection-control/ aahaphonetriagechecklist.pdf; accessed 27 October 2022). Other factors that should be considered at this time include age, concurrent ill health, pregnancy, immunosuppression and reduced defence mechanisms (e.g. skin disease), as these factors may increase susceptibility to becoming infected.

13.4 Zoonotic Diseases

A zoonotic disease is a disease that is transmissible from animals to humans. Zoonotic pathogens may be viral, parasitic or bacterial in nature and can be transmitted via direct or indirect contact depending on the disease. Some examples of zoonotic diseases are shown in Table 13.1.

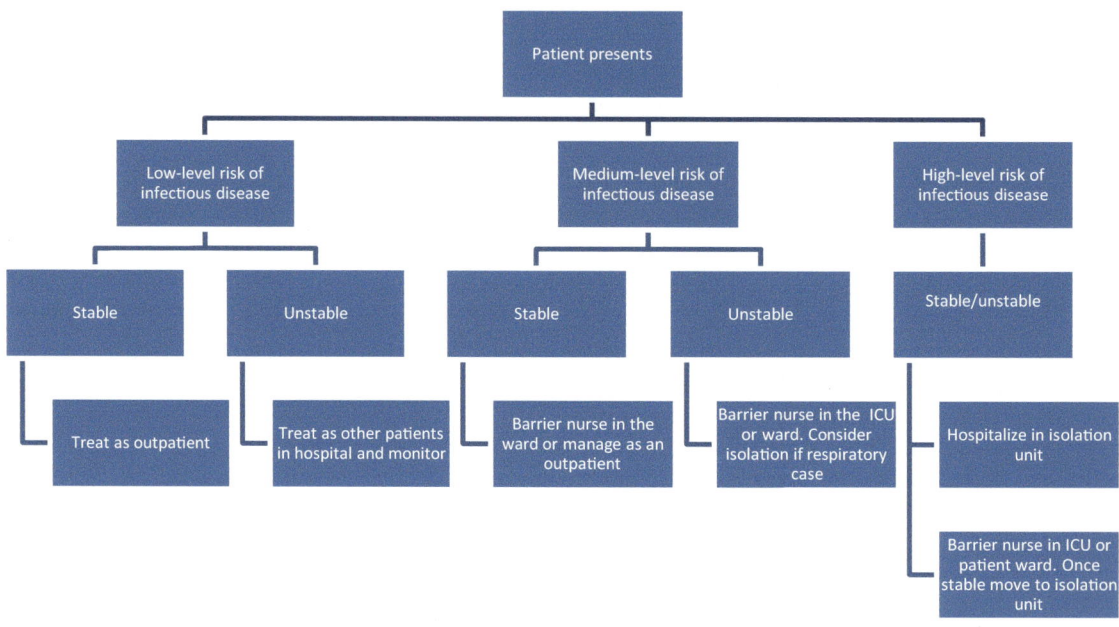

Fig. 13.2. Flowchart for hospitalization considerations of infectious patients. ICU, intensive care unit.

Table 13.1. Examples of zoonotic diseases.

Zoonosis	Agent	Clinical symptoms (dogs/cats)	Transmission	Human symptoms
Brucellosis	*Brucella canis*, *Brucella suis*	Late-term abortions	Direct contact or via aerosol transmission; semen and vaginal discharge	Flu-like symptoms of fever, malaise, fatigue and headache
Campylobacter	*Campylobacter jejuni*	Diarrhoea, anorexia, intermittent vomiting	Faeces	Abdominal pain, diarrhoea
Leptospirosis	*Leptospira icterohaemorrhagiae*, *Leptospira canicola*	Primarily affects the liver or kidneys, with patients not uncommonly presenting in renal or hepatic failure; can affect the nervous, respiratory, cardiovascular, reproductive or ophthalmic systems	Direct or indirect contact with infected urine	Fever, headache, chills, muscle ache, vomiting, jaundice, diarrhoea
Rabies	Rabies virus, family Rhabdoviridae	Behavioural changes, hypersalivation, fever	Saliva/animal bites	Death, fever, hydrophobia, seizures
Salmonellosis	*Salmonella* spp.	Diarrhoea, anorexia, vomiting and malaise	Faeces, raw meat exposure	Diarrhoea, abdominal pain, fever

238

Eleanor Haskey and Tom Reilly

There are special precautions for dogs that carry an increased risk of brucellosis in light of the potentially serious zoonotic implications associated with exposure to dogs infected with *Brucella canis* and the increasing importation of animals (into the UK) from countries where infections levels remain higher (e.g. Eastern Europe), so additional measures are warranted.

Clinicians are encouraged to consult up-to-date guidance from their local authorities in relation to:

- recommended screening protocols for animals imported from 'at-risk' countries;
- the use of appropriate personal protective equipment (PPE) whenever handling suspected or confirmed cases;
- critical information to communicate to veterinary diagnostic laboratories whenever submitting samples from animals with undetermined infection status (e.g. relevant travel history); and
- management of inadvertent exposure of staff (e.g. where the patient's infection status is only identified after handling/performance of diagnostic tests or therapeutic interventions).

13.5   Infectious Diseases

Infectious diseases are diseases that can be transmitted directly or indirectly from one animal to another. Infectious diseases can come in the form of viruses, bacteria, parasites or fungi. Some examples of infectious diseases are shown in Table 13.2.

13.6   Admission and Hospitalization

Establishing SOPs for the admission, hospitalization and discharge of infectious patients ensures that all members of staff are aware of the expectations and requirements needed to effectively and safely care for patients with infectious diseases. SOPs have been demonstrated to work best and gain better staff compliance when they are evidence based and tailored to the specific disease rather than a generic infectious disease SOP. Infection control SOPs play a critical role in preventing the spread of potentially deadly diseases among our patients. Understanding the source of infection, host susceptibility and methods of transmission will empower veterinary staff with the knowledge required to effectively manage and hospitalize the infectious patient.

Establishing a practice-wide infection control strategy that is understood by staff members can lower the risk of disease exposure and can aid in the prevention of healthcare-associated infections. Assigning a biosecurity status to each patient admitted to the hospital taking into account signalment, clinical history, physical findings and diagnostic findings can be used to determine where the patient should be hospitalized and under what

Table 13.2. Examples of infectious diseases.

Disease	Agent	Clinical symptoms	Transmission
Canine parvovirus	Canine parvovirus, family Parvoviridae	Death, anorexia, vomiting, haemorrhagic diarrhoea, depression	Direct contact with faecal matter
Canine distemper	Canine distemper virus, genus Morbillivirus	Pyrexia, hyperkeratosis of the pads, nasal discharge, diarrhoea, cough	Aerosol or ingestion
Bordetella (kennel cough)	*Bordetella bronchiseptica*	Hacking cough, nasal discharge, ocular discharge	Direct or indirect contact with aerosol droplets
Feline immunodeficiency virus	Feline immunodeficiency virus, family Retroviridae	Pyrexia, weight loss, lymphadenopathy	Saliva via bite wounds
Feline leukaemia virus	Feline leukaemia virus, family Retroviridae	Diarrhoea, anorexia, vomiting, malaise	From mother to kittens via placenta or milk; or from saliva via bites
Feline upper respiratory tract disease	Feline calicivirus, family Caliciviridae, and feline herpesvirus, family Herpesviridae	Sneezing, nasal discharge, ocular discharge, loss of appetite	Direct or indirect contact with aerosol respiratory tract droplets and nasal discharge

conditions (O'Dwyer, 2013). This holistic outlook and individual tailoring of the biosecurity status ensures that all aspects are considered before the patient arrives at a ward, minimalizing the risk of spreading disease. All patients admitted to the practice should have their infection control status assessed and then should be assigned a biosecurity status that is clear for all staff to understand and access.

13.7 Selecting Biosecurity Tiers

Four biosecurity levels are recognized:

- *Tier 1.* These patients are at high risk of acquiring an infection due to poor or compromised immune status but do not currently actually have any known infection. These patients include neonates, unvaccinated juveniles, chemotherapy patients, burn patients, immunosuppressed patients and long-term, critically ill patients. These patients can be hospitalized in general wards but should be protected from other patients to prevent them from being exposed to infections in the hospital environment. PPE should be worn when handling tier 1 patients including gloves and aprons. Hand hygiene is paramount, and direct contact between other patients must be avoided. Unnecessary handling of patients should be avoided. Consideration should be given to the type of patients housed near or around these patients.
- *Tier 2.* These patients have no history, clinical findings or laboratory results that provide evidence of contagious disease. These patients will be the bulk of patients admitted to the hospital for elective surgery, work-ups, trauma cases, etc. They require normal hospitalization and can be housed anywhere within the hospital.
- *Tier 3.* These patients either have, or are thought to have, a contagious disease or infection that can be considered mildly or moderately contagious to other patients or staff members. If there is any indication that a contagious disease is present, then patients should be graded as tier 3 patients until proven otherwise. Once a contagious disease has been ruled out, the patient can be downgraded to a tier 2 patient. These patients can be hospitalized in general ward areas provided the patients are barrier nursed, appropriate PPE is worn and, where necessary, a perimeter is marked on the floor to prevent

urine or faecal contamination. There should be consideration of any tier 1 patients within the ward that any tier 3 patients are housed in.
- *Tier 4.* These patients are known or suspected to have a highly contagious disease. Tier 4 patients should be housed within the isolation unit without movement through any wards and with minimal movement around the hospital. The patient should either be carried or trolleyed around the practice and not walked. Examination tables, consult rooms and, if required, sections of reception should be cleaned and disinfected. These patients should remain isolated until discharged.

After the patient's biosecurity status has been assigned, careful consideration should be given as to which kennel the patient should be housed in, and a ground-floor kennel should be used to prevent the spreading of the pathogens through faecal matter or vomitus leaking into other kennels. Transportation of any infectious patient through the hospital should be kept to a minimum. When necessary, the patient should be transported using a stretcher or trolley to prevent direct contact with the floor. The types of disinfectants used should be researched to ensure they are capable of destroying the desired pathogen, and the correct dilution rates should be establish and the same disinfectant used to clean the unit as well as the footbaths. Hand hygiene has been proven to be one of the most important aspects of controlling the spread of infection within the veterinary practice, but has also been found to be one of the least compliant areas (see Chapter 5, this volume). Effective hand hygiene will prevent the translocation of pathogens between staff, patients and the hospital and will decrease the risk of exposure and prevent infection (Anderson, 2015).

Owner visitation of infectious patients can prove to be a controversial topic; most of the literature indicates that client interaction with the hospitalized patient could lead to greater risk of cross-contamination both within the hospital and in the greater environment. However, the lack of contact and loss of familiar comforts, such as the owner and home environments, inherent to the isolation of patients, can lead to stress. By providing familiar comforts, this stress may be reduced. Any owner visitation must ensure the owner is compliant with the practice's infection control policy. Depending on the pathogen and predicted survival of the patient, it is often difficult to prevent owner visitation through fear their pet may not survive and the need to make informed decisions regarding their pet's care.

Barrier nursing is an important infection control consideration to ensure that further spread of pathogens is prevented. Infectious patients should be housed in an isolation ward equipped with foot baths, PPE, and separate monitoring and cleaning equipment. All PPE should be disposable and is required to fully cover any area that may come into contact with the patient or its environment. PPE should also be water resistant to prevent strikethrough, which may contaminate clothing underneath. Designated staff members should be assigned to the isolation unit to prevent any cross-contamination that may occur and to ensure consistency of patient care. Nursing staff working in the isolation unit should have minimum contact with patients housed in the general wards to ensure that no staff members become vectors for the disease by transporting it outside the isolation facility. Signage hung on the patient's kennel allows all staff members to quickly identify the need to barrier nurse the patient and leads to greater compliance. Identification of the suspected or known pathogen will also aid staff in understanding what PPE is required. The need to isolate the infectious patient is often unavoidable, for the safety of staff and other patients in the hospital.

13.7.1 Risk assessments

All members of the veterinary team should be actively engaged with the practice's biosecurity policy to help identify potentially high-risk patients. The practice biosecurity policy should include risk assessments that help protect practice staff, visitors and clients. Groups that are deemed as at risk include infants, pregnant team members and immunocompromised people.

Infants and young children

Any children visiting the practice should be closely supervised, and contact with infectious or suspected infectious patients should be avoided at all times.

Pregnant team members

Pregnant team members are more susceptible to certain zoonotic diseases, with some pathogens potentially posing a health risk to the unborn child. Regular risk assessments with line managers should be undertaken to ensure that the status of the expectant mother is fully understood so that risks can be reduced. Expectant mothers should avoid contact with confirmed or potentially zoonotic patients. Correctly identifying and labelling patients as zoonotic is vital to help protect pregnant staff and reduce the risk to them.

Immunocompromised people

Staff members should inform line managers if they have an immunocompromised status so that appropriate measures can be instigated to protect them from zoonotic diseases present within the hospital. Any immunocompromised staff members should avoid contact with patients with suspected or confirmed zoonotic diseases.

Ensuring an accurate patient history is taken before the patient arrives for the appointment can help prevent the spread or introduction of pathogens into the practice. Several studies have demonstrated the relationship between decreases in hospital-acquired infections and educating the team on infection control principles. Asking simple questions while scheduling the appointment can help identify any high-risk patients. Some questions to consider include:

- patient age: rapid identification of juvenile and geriatric patients;
- vaccination status;
- any high levels of mixing with other animals, such as boarding kennels, catteries or day care;
- any travel abroad;
- salient clinical signs that may increase the risk of disease transmission (e.g. diarrhoea, vomiting, coughing or sneezing); and
- medications that could affect the immune system such as chemotherapy drugs or steroids.

If an infectious disease is suspected prior to the consultation appointment, the patient should not be invited into the practice and the client should be advised to wait outside. Each practice should have an SOP to handle infectious patients that should determine the route by which these patients should be admitted into the practice, where the consultation and examination will take place, and where best to house these patients.

On some occasions, patients may only be identified as possibly infectious when they are already within the practice, such as during the consultation appointment or in some circumstances after they have been hospitalized. In this event, the practice protocol should be followed as soon as the possible infectious patient is identified. All team members, areas, other patients and surfaces that have come in contact with the patient should be established. These areas should immediately be disinfected.

13.7.2 PPE

PPE should be used as part of the infection control strategy and not as a lone preventative measure. The function of PPE is to reduce contamination of clothing and skin in an effort to reduce the transmission of pathogens. It is important that PPE is used correctly and that the user understands the purpose of wearing the PPE and how it protects against transmitting the pathogen so transmission can be actively monitored (see Chapter 8, this volume, for more details).

Gloves

PPE is no replacement for effective hand washing, and hand hygiene is still required before and after glove usage. Glove wearing has been noted as a barrier to hand hygiene in human healthcare settings and can give a false belief that hand washing is less important if gloves are worn. Sterile gloves should be considered when the primary concern is contaminating the patient with microbes, such as treating clean wounds. Non-sterile gloves can be used in any situation where the risk of contaminating hands is deemed to be increased and should be worn to protect the user from exposure as well as protecting other patients from cross-contamination. Gloves should be checked for defects or tears before and after wear, and hands should be washed before donning and after doffing to minimize the risk of contamination through barrier failure while using gloves (see Chapter 6, this volume, for more details).

Face mask

Disposable single-use facemasks should be considered for use in any situation where an individual may be at risk of splash or droplet transmission. Wound lavage and dental procedures should only be undertaken while wearing masks to shield the user. When dealing with patients with suspected zoonotic pathogens (especially patients with

potential mycobacterial disease), N95 masks or respirators should be worn, as standard disposable single-use facemasks will not provide sufficient protection.

Clothing

Disposable single-use aprons and gowns should be worn if contamination of clothing from the patient could put practice staff or other patients at risk. Clothing can become contaminated with microbes from patient excretions, aerosol droplets or fluid discharge. Disposable aprons and gowns should be impermeable to avoid microbial strikethrough. Disposable PPE should not be reused even when treating the same patient, and sufficient care should be taken when removing PPE so as not to accidently contaminate the user's clothing or skin.

Some veterinary clinics and human hospitals work using a colour-coded system to help with identification of infectious patients in the clinic: red for highly contagious patients, yellow for suspected infectious or those at risk of infection (e.g. immunosuppressed), and green for those that are not infectious or at risk of infection. Such systems are easy to implement and act as a visual trigger for the veterinary team working with the patient (Weese, 2004).

13.8 Clinics with Isolation Facilities

Many larger hospitals will have a separate isolation ward area in which they can hospitalize infectious cases. In an ideal world, isolation areas should consist of an anteroom where staff can don PPE and wash their hands before entering the ward area/isolation room. The ward area/isolation room should be designed and equipped to function as a self-sufficient unit. It should separate infectious cases and allow for routine procedures to be performed, such as dressing changes. The aim is to have minimal movement of personnel and equipment between the isolation area and main hospital.

The ideal properties of an isolation area are discussed below.

13.8.1 Purpose-built ward area

The isolation area should be built with consideration to infection control including the location within the clinic and the interior design of the area to ensure that effective cleaning and decontamination can take place. If a new clinic is being designed or renovations are taking place, careful discussion and consideration should be made with regard to infection control from the start of the project. Rao (2004) published a checklist of features that should be included in isolation rooms such as a hand-washing basin, a door with door closer and a sealed room with independent exhaust. The International Healthcare Facility Guidelines (2017) recommend there should be an anteroom attached to the isolation room, which allows transfer of equipment, controls entry and exit of contaminated air from the isolation room, and acts as a controlled area where personnel can don PPE before entry to the isolation room. Consideration should also be given to the items within the unit such as kennels, examination table, oxygen supply, sink for hand washing and sink for washing equipment. Items should be made from non-porous, easy-to-clean materials so the room can be decontaminated effectively between patients (AVA, 2017).

13.8.2   Clear signage and documentation

The isolation ward area should be clearly identifiable to the team, and the patient details including the identity of any likely infectious agent(s) should be visible to personnel at the entry point of the ward. There should be information about the level of risk and the safety precautions that are required when handling the patient. In some hospitals, individual patient risk assessments may be carried out, which staff should read and sign before entering the isolation area and coming into contact with the patient. It is also recommended to have a log system so that the personnel who come into contact with the patient are traceable. Access should be limited to essential personnel only to minimize unnecessary traffic and exposure.

13.8.3   Separate medical equipment and consumables

Only essential medical equipment such as drip pumps should come into contact with the patient. Any medical equipment that could be contaminated should be disinfected after use according to the manufacturer's guidelines (CDC, 2007). Some equipment may be able to be sterilized (e.g. with ethylene oxide or by cold sterilization) after use to prevent patient-to-patient spread of pathogens. In some human settings, single-use medical equipment such as surgical kits or bronchoscopes are being used to minimize spread of pathogens. Non- essential equipment such as computers should be located outside the isolation area to prevent contamination with infectious agents. Single-use consumables (e.g. needles and syringes) should be disposed of in a sharps bin or in clinical waste after use and should not be resterilized. The Canadian Committee on Antibiotic Resistance published guidelines on infection prevention in 2008. They found that there is little to no objective information on how to disinfect or resterilize consumables and how often this can be done without compromising the integrity of the item, so disposable items should be used where possible. The room should be stocked with anticipated supplies for the following 24 h so that excess stock and clutter is kept to a minimum within the isolation area.

13.8.4   Separate husbandry items

Disposable cardboard bowls and litter trays can be used for patients in the isolation unit. If non-disposable bowls and trays are used, these can be decontaminated by dishwashing on a hot wash or soaking in a dilute bleach solution (one part bleach to nine parts water). Any other items such as chew toys or feed toys can either be machine washed on a hot wash or discarded. Many larger clinics have a colour-coded system for bedding. For example, the authors' clinic uses red bedding for infectious cases – this acts as an immediate visual reminder that the patient and also the bedding is potentially infectious. Bedding and other fabric items such as toys should always be handled with gloves. Soiled bedding should be contained within the isolation unit before being taken to be washed separately. It can be placed into vinegar beds prior to placing them in the washing machine to avoid spread of pathogens. Fabric items should be washed with detergent and hot water at 70°C for 25 min (WHO, 2014b) and either machine dried or hung out in direct sunlight to dry.

13.8.5   PPE

When dealing with an infectious patient it is necessary to wear PPE as an additional protective layer to minimize the risk. In most veterinary clinics, the veterinary team wear protective outerwear such as scrub tops/consultation tops or laboratory coats, which should be removed before donning PPE in the anteroom, prior to entering the isolation room and coming into contact with the patient. PPE usually consists of non-sterile, long-sleeved gowns or full body overalls, shoe covers and gloves. If the patient has a zoonotic disease or there is a concern regarding transmission via aerosols/droplets, then the addition of masks, respirators and/or eye protection may be necessary. It is important that staff are trained in the correct way to don and doff PPE in order to prevent contamination of themselves or the surrounding environment. The AAHA (Stull *et al.*, 2018) and World Health Organization (WHO, 2014a) have published protocols for entering and exiting an isolation unit:

- Before entering the isolation area, remove practice outerwear (e.g. laboratory coat) and any equipment (e.g. stethoscope, scissors, thermometer, watch, cell phone) and leave outside the isolation unit/anteroom.
- Gather any necessary supplies and medications before putting on PPE.
- Perform hand hygiene and then put on shoe covers, gown and gloves before entering the isolation room.
- Attend to the patient in isolation as needed. *Do not* bring treatment sheets, pens or electronic devices such as laptops, cell phones or tablets into the isolation room.
- Clean and disinfect any equipment used while caring for the patient.
- Before leaving the isolation room, remove PPE. Clean and disinfect non-disposable PPE (e.g. eye protection). Place used disposable PPE in the waste container lined with a biohazard bag in the isolation room. *Do not save disposable PPE for reuse.* Avoid contact with external portions of the door when exiting the isolation room.
- Perform hand hygiene and then disinfect any surfaces (e.g. doorknobs) that may have accidentally been contaminated when the room was exited. Make any needed chart entries. Wash hands again before leaving the anteroom.

13.8.6 Dedicated cleaning supplies and cleaning protocols

There should be a written policy to include daily cleaning and upkeep of the area and also how to decontaminate the area when the infectious patient has been discharged. Daily cleaning to maintain cleanliness levels includes cleaning the direct patient environment (kennel area), horizontal surfaces, high-touch areas (e.g. door handles) and sinks, and mopping the floor. Damp cleaning can help to reduce the generation of aerosols (WHO, 2014b). Decontamination of the area involves a more thorough clean in which all surfaces and items are wiped down, any consumables that have potentially been contaminated are disposed of and equipment is disinfected. After the area has been decontaminated, the room is shut down and left clean and empty ready for admission of the next infectious patient. The veterinary clinic should choose a disinfectant that works against the common pathogens that they see in their patient population. The manufacturer's instructions should be followed regarding correct dilution rates and contact times to maximize the effectiveness of the disinfectant. The isolation area should have separate cleaning equipment (e.g. bucket, mops), which are cleaned and dried after use (WHO, 2014b). Aerosol disinfection can be considered as part of the cleaning protocol after infectious respiratory cases. Personnel engaged in cleaning should be trained in safe practices and should be provided with the necessary safety equipment according to the product's safety data sheet (AVA, 2017). There have been a number of studies to evaluate the effectiveness of aerosolized disinfectants, steam cleaning and disinfection with UVC light (Andersen *et al.*, 2006). Although many of these methods help to reduce bacterial contamination, further research into the cost versus benefit and efficacy of such methods is needed and so disinfection via correct manual cleaning is still considered superior (Boyce, 2016).

13.8.7 Hand hygiene

Hand hygiene was recognized as the cornerstone of modern infection prevention in the 1890s and even today is considered the most important action in reducing the transmission of microorganisms between patients, healthcare workers and the environment (Liang *et al.*, 2014). The WHO has published extensive guidelines on hand hygiene in healthcare (WHO, 2009). Hand washing is considered necessary for hands that are soiled with organic matter, whereas alcohol-based gels/foams are recommended for routine hand care. Hand rubs involve less time than hand washing and are often more accessible, leading to increased adherence to their use. Hand sanitizers should be located at the entry and exit points of the isolation area in addition to inside the unit. All personnel interacting with the patient should abide by the five key moments of hand hygiene (WHO, 2009). With hand hygiene seen to be at the forefront of infection control policies, many clinics are now following the NHS policy of 'bare below the elbow' in an attempt to reduce the spread of infections. 'Bare below the elbow' is defined as the hands and arms up to the elbow/mid-forearm being exposed and free from clothing, jewellery, watches, false nails and nail varnish. However, it is important to note that not all infectious agents are inactivated or killed by hand sanitizers, and effective barrier nursing is imperative.

13.8.8 Separate ventilation and drainage

Air from the clinic and isolation area should not mix, so negative-pressure ventilation is recommended to reduce airborne pathogens (Stull *et al.*, 2018). It is recommended that there should be 6–12 air changes h^{-1}, and air should be vented outside (Rao, 2004; CDC, 2007). Air filters can be incorporated into these systems to trap large particles such as hair. High-efficiency particulate air (HEPA) filters are superior but are expensive and require regular replacement. This means that they are often not suitable for many clinics. For rooms that do not have negative ventilation, a window can be left ajar to encourage passive ventilation and some air change; however, this poses a safety/security risk.

13.8.9 Waste-disposal protocol

Veterinary waste is a potential source of infectious or zoonotic pathogens. Therefore, the following principles should be considered to reduce the risk of transmission (AVA, 2017):

- segregating clinical or hazardous waste;
- using an appropriate colour-coded system;
- wearing PPE when handling waste;
- performing appropriate hand hygiene and wearing appropriate PPE when handling waste; and
- storing waste safely away from the general public and vermin.

Waste should be disposed of inside the isolation area. Double bagging is not necessary unless the outside of the bag has been contaminated (WHO,

2014b). The veterinary clinic should have a clear policy outlining the correct disposal of clinical waste and cadavers in line with their local authorities and governing bodies.

13.8.10 Direct access to outside

It is recommended that isolated infectious canine patients should not be walked outside in public areas used by other animals. An ideal isolation unit would incorporate an outdoor exercise area, so isolated patients have the opportunity to urinate and defaecate outside. Separate runs would be required for each animal, which are disinfected between uses. If clinics do not have a separate exercise area, then isolated patients could be carried or trolleyed outside to a separate area, away from where other patients exercise. This solution is not ideal, as it requires movement of the patient through the clinic and therefore increases the risk of spreading the infectious pathogens. Alternatively, the patient could be given a period of supervised free roaming within the isolation area and the opportunity to toilet outside their kennel on the floor if they are the only patient housed in the unit. If the patient needs to be moved out of the isolation area for procedures that cannot take place in the unit (e.g. radiographs), this should be scheduled at the end of the day when there is minimal movement of other patients and staff. Transportation of infectious patients through the hospital should be kept to a minimum, and when necessary the patient should be transported using a stretcher or trolley to prevent direct contact with the floor. PPE should be worn and any area cleaned and disinfected once used.

13.8.11 Nursing care

The clinic should have clear SOPs for the management of any indwelling medical devices. Intravenous catheter care in infectious patients is important to prevent the access of bacteria into the venous system or surrounding tissues. Catheter sites should be observed for signs of infection at the site including inflammation, cellulitis and phlebitis. If left unnoticed or untreated, this can progress to bacteraemia, septicaemia and potential organ failure. Patients with diarrhoea need more vigilance to ensure this does not contaminate the catheter site. Attention to treatment scheduling should be made so treatment times can be grouped together, resulting in fewer trips in and out of the isolation unit and allowing time for patient rest without interruption. Other staffing considerations include the allocation of patients to nurses; for example, a nurse who is caring for an infectious cat flu patient should not nurse other feline patients during that shift to minimize the risk of cross-contamination.

13.9   Clinics Without Isolation Facilities

Depending on the infectious agent, there are a number of options available that can be considered to help with management of the patient:

- A consult room can be set up with a collapsible kennel and turned into a temporary isolation area. As many of the considerations discussed above for an isolation unit as possible should be implemented, including minimal access, PPE, cleaning protocols and disposal of waste.
- The patient could be hospitalized and barrier nursed in a ward area with the opposite species; for example, a feline patient with cat flu could be housed in the canine ward as the risk of cross-species infection is very low. Stress reducing measures should be implemented if this option is chosen as patients will be in a mixed ward area. Clear signage, separate equipment for the patient and separate waste should all be implemented.
- In line with the CDC (2007) guidelines for isolation precautions, patients with the confirmed same infectious pathogen can be housed together in the same area and barrier nursed (e.g. a litter of puppies with parvovirus). Strict barrier nursing must be implemented and patients should be kept in separate kennels. The use of additional collapsible kennels may help to keep patients segregated.
- The patient can be referred to a facility where isolation within a unit is possible. This is suggested for confirmed infectious cases that carry a high risk to other patients in the hospital such as distemper or kennel cough.
- The patient is barrier nursed in the regular ward area. This option is often considered when patients are deemed unstable and there is concern surrounding the level of observation they require and this not being possible if they are in the isolation unit. Strict barrier nursing must be implemented to reduce the risk of spreading the infectious pathogen to other inpatients.

- Careful consideration should be given to where the infectious patient should be hospitalized. A ground-floor kennel should be used to prevent the spread of pathogens through faecal matter or vomitus leaking into other kennels.

13.10   Other Considerations

13.10.1   Adverse effects of isolation

Depending on clinic setups, workload and local policies, there is often a tendency to spend less direct nursing time with the patient. This can lead to compromised patient observations and care. Abad *et al.* (2010) conducted a systematic review of the adverse effects experienced by human patients hospitalized in isolation facilities. They concluded that isolating patients can lead to reduced care provider and patient contact along with negative psychological and safety effects on the patient. Direct patient care was either less frequent or shorter in isolated patients compared with non-isolated patients. Patient safety was also affected with examples of fewer patient clinical records, more incomplete recordings of clinical parameters and fewer nursing notes in the isolated patient group. Patients reported a negative impact on their mood, including feelings of depression, anxiety, fear and hostility. Hewson (2014) also reported similar altered behaviour in animals hospitalized in the clinic. She suggested a number of environmental factors that can be implemented to help reduce stress in the hospitalized patient. Cats like to have an area such as a cardboard box that they can either hide in or perch on. Toys or food games can act as distractions for young canine patients. Pheromones in the form of plug-ins or sprays can be used if a single species is hospitalized in the isolation area. There is evidence in human and veterinary medicine that patients can benefit from listening to music while hospitalized, so having a radio playing during the daytime can be considered (Herron and Shreyer, 2014). It is important to try and maintain a circadian rhythm, so lights off at night time and an uninterrupted period for sleep should be factored into the care plan. The lack of contact and loss of familiar comforts such as the owner and home environments demonstrated that the isolation of patients can lead to stress. By providing familiar comforts, this stress may be reduced. In essence, careful consideration must be given to the selection of patients to isolate and how best to manage these patients so that high-quality care can be delivered.

13.10.2 Maximizing observations in isolated patients

A concern many veterinary professionals have about isolating patients is the reduced visual observation of the patient as part of the treatment plan. There are a number of solutions that can be implemented to try and increase visual observation including the use of a webcam system, which display the video to a screen outside the isolation area, the use of a baby monitor to hear and visualize the patient, or the use of telemetry monitoring so that vital parameters such as ECG, non-invasive blood pressure and temperature are displayed on a screen outside the isolation area. In new purpose-built clinics, having isolation facilities with glass walls may mean that there is opportunity for extra observation of these patients without having to enter the unit.

13.10.3 Owner visits to isolated or barrier-nursed patients

Owner visitation for infectious patients is a controversial topic. Most literature indicates that client interaction with the hospitalized patient could lead to greater risk of cross-contamination both within the hospital and in the wider environment, and also carries a risk to the pet owner. The CDC published recommendations for people visiting relatives with COVID-19 in the hospital within their published COVID-19 guidelines (CDC, 2020). They recommended one visitor per patient at any one time, education of visitors on the potential risks and making it compulsory to wear PPE during the visit. The use of gowns, gloves and masks by visitors to veterinary hospitals has not been addressed in the literature; however, pet owners are likely to have more direct contact with their patient than perhaps when visiting a human in hospital. It is considered sensible to employ PPE for owners visiting and to minimize direct contact for patients with zoonotic disease potential. If pet owners come to visit hospitalized infectious patients, they should not come into contact with other patients in order to minimize transmission of pathogens.

13.10.4 Personal items

Consideration should be given to wearing and handling personal items. Many hospitals operate a 'bare below the elbow' policy to reduce the transmission of pathogens and also to increase adherence to hand hygiene. Pagers or mobile phones are likely to become contaminated when being used for communication or as a calculator on the clinic floor. Disinfection of such items is rarely carried out, and these devices can act as a vector for pathogen transmission in the veterinary clinic and outside environment. Staff should be discouraged from using phones in the clinical setting, but if necessary, then a culture of good hand hygiene should be instilled to reduce contamination to devices (Weese, 2004). Another item that is regularly used in the clinic and likely to become contaminated is a stethoscope. It has been documented that 69% of stethoscopes in a human healthcare setting were contaminated and most of the isolated organisms were potential nosocomial pathogens (Weese, 2004). A dedicated stethoscope should be used for infectious patients (WHO, 2014b), and personal stethoscopes should be disinfected between each use/patient with 70% alcohol (Bernard et al., 1999).

13.10.5 Audits

Clinical audits allow staff compliance to be investigated, as well as highlighting the importance of infection control. Online practice auditing facilities are currently provided free of charge by the Bella Moss foundation and, although geared more towards a background of methicillin-resistant Staphylococcus aureus and methicillin-resistant Staphylococcus pseudintermedius, they provide a useful framework to work from.

13.11 Conclusion

The importance of having a tailored ICP plan cannot be overemphasized. Successful management of the infectious patient is a team effort, which relies on early identification of 'at-risk' patients, adherence to local policies or SOPs, and clear communication. Isolation and barrier nursing precautions along with simple measures such as hand hygiene and the use of checklists have been proven to have a profound effect on reducing the spread of pathogens. A robust ICP plan and an engaged team will lead to a safer environment for both patients and personnel.

References

Abad, C., Fearday, A. and Safdar, N. (2010) Adverse effects of isolation in hospitalised patients: a systematic review. *Journal of Hospital Infection* 76, 97–102.

Andersen, B., Bånrud, H., Bøe, E., Bjordal, O. and Drangsholt, F. (2006) Comparison of UV C light and chemicals for disinfection of surfaces in hospital isolation units. *Infection Control and Hospital Epidemiology* 27, 729–734.

Anderson, M.E.C. (2015) Contact precautions and hand hygiene in veterinary clinics. *Veterinary Clinics: Small Animal Practice* 45, 343–360.

AVA (2017) *Guidelines for Veterinary Personal Biosecurity*, 3rd edn. Australian Veterinary Association, Sydney, Australia. Available at: www.ava.com.au/library-resources/other-resources/veterinary-personal-biosecurity/ (accessed 26 October 2022 (accessed 26 October 2022).

Bernard, L., Kereveur, A., Durand, D., Gonot, J., Goldstein, F. *et al.* (1999) Bacterial contamination of hospital physicians' stethoscopes. *Infection Control and Hospital Epidemiology* 20, 626–628.

Boyce, J.M. (2016) Modern technologies for improving cleaning and disinfection of environmental surfaces in hospitals. *Antimicrobial Resistance and Infection Control* 5, 10. DOI: 10.1186/s13756-016-0111-x.

Canadian Committee on Antibiotic Resistance (2008) In: *Infection Prevention and Control Best Practices for Small Animal Veterinary Clinics*. Canadian Committee on Antibiotic Resistance, Guelph, Ontario. Available at: www.wormsandgermsblog.com/files/2008/04/CCAR-Guidelines-Final2.pdf (accessed 26 October 2022).

CDC (2007) *2007 Guideline for Isolation Precautions: Preventing Transmission of Infectious Agents in Healthcare Settings*. Centres for Disease Control and Prevention, Atlanta, Georgia. Available at: www.cdc.gov/infectioncontrol/pdf/guidelines/isolation-guidelines-H.pdf (accessed 9 January 2023).

CDC (2020) Operational considerations for containing COVID-19 in non-US healthcare settings. Atlanta, Georgia: Centres for Disease Control and Prevention. Available at: www.cdc.gov/coronavirus/2019-ncov/hcp/non-us-settings/hcf-visitors.html (accessed 9 January 2023).

Gibbins, J.D. and MacMahon, K. (2015) Workplace safety and health for the veterinary health care team. *Veterinary Clinics of North America: Small Animal Practice* 45(2), 409–426. DOI: 10.1016/j.cvsm.2014.11.006.

Haynes, A.B., Weiser, T.G., Berry, W.R., Lipsitz, S.R., Breizat, A.-H.S. *et al.* (2009) A surgical safety checklist to reduce morbidity and mortality in a global population. *New England Journal of Medicine* 360, 491–499.

Herron, M.E. and Shreyer, T. (2014) The pet-friendly veterinary practice: a guide for practitioners. *Veterinary Clinics of North America: Small Animal Practice* 44, 451–481.

Hewson, C. (2014) Evidence-based approaches to reducing in-patient stress – Part 3: how to reduce in-patient stress. *Veterinary Nursing Journal* 29, 234–236.

International Healthcare Facility Guidelines (2017) Isolation rooms. Available at: www.healthfacilityguidelines.com/ViewPDF/ViewIndexPDF/iHFG_part_d_isolation_rooms (accessed 26 October 2022).

Liang, S.Y., Riethman, M. and Fox, J. (2014) Infection prevention in the emergency department. *Annals of Emergency Medicine* 64, 299–313.

O'Dwyer, L. (2013) How to implement an infection control strategy. *Veterinary Nurse* 4, 558–564.

Rao, S.K.M. (2004) Designing hospital for better infection control: an experience. *Medical Journal Armed Forces India* 60, 63–66.

RCVS (2015) Practice standards scheme. Royal College of Veterinary Surgeons, London. Available at: www.rcvs.org.uk/setting-standards/practice-standards-scheme/ (accessed 26 October 2022).

Stull, J.W., Bjorvik, E., Bub, J., Dvorak, G. and Petersen, C. (2018) 2018 AAHA infection control, prevention, and biosecurity guidelines. *Journal of American Animal Hospital Association* 54, 297–326.

Weese, J. (2004) Barrier precautions, isolation protocols and personal hygiene in veterinary hospitals. *Veterinary Clinics of North America Equine Practice* 20, 543–559.

WHO (2009) WHO guidelines on hand hygiene in health care. World Health Organization, Geneva, Switzerland. Available at: http://whqlibdoc.who.int/publications/2009/9789241597906_eng.pdf (accessed 26 October 2022).

WHO (2014a) *Infection Prevention and Control of Epidemic- and Pandemic-Prone Acute Respiratory Infections in Health Care. Annex E, Isolation Rooms or Areas*. World Health Organization, Geneva, Switzerland. Available at: www.ncbi.nlm.nih.gov/books/NBK214341/ (accessed 26 October 2022).

WHO (2014b) *Infection Prevention and Control of Epidemic- and Pandemic-Prone Acute Respiratory Infections in Health Care. Annex B, Isolation Precautions*. World Health Organization, Geneva, Switzerland. Available at: www.ncbi.nlm.nih.gov/books/NBK214342/ (accessed 26 October 2022).

WHO (2019) *Minimum Requirements for Infection Prevention and Control Programmes*. World Health Organization, Geneva, Switzerland. Available at: www.who.int/publications/i/item/9789241516945 (accessed 26 October 2022).

Eleanor Haskey and Tom Reilly

14 Investigation and Management of Outbreaks

Brandy A. Burgess*

College of Veterinary Medicine, University of Georgia, Athens, Georgia, USA

14.1 Introduction

Disease outbreaks have been recognized throughout history, and for centuries, we have been investigating these epidemics to discover their origins. A classic example of an outbreak investigation was that conducted by John Snow (1813–1858) during the 1854 cholera epidemic in London (Snow, 1855). It is notable that this was long before the germ theory was the prevailing scientific philosophy underpinning the occurrence of infectious disease (which did not gain widespread acceptance until the 1860s with Pasteur, Lister and Koch), and yet, by meticulously orienting disease by person, place and time, Snow was able to deduce its source as the Broad Street public water pump. This investigation exemplifies the power of observation and systematic data collection, and illustrates the central tenet of epidemiology – that disease does not occur randomly.

As we begin to discuss outbreak investigation, it is important to ensure that we are working from common definitions. Broadly, disease may be described as endemic or epidemic in a given locale or population, or it may be described as a pandemic if it encompasses a larger region such as a country. By definition, *endemic disease* is the normal or expected level of disease that occurs with predictable regularity, while *epidemic disease* is the clustering of disease in space and time in excess of normal expectations (Fig. 14.1). Note that it may be normal for the level of endemic disease to fluctuate over time, for example as seen with seasonal flu, and that an *outbreak* is generally considered to be more localized than an epidemic (although we often use these terms interchangeably).

So, when does the occurrence of disease become an outbreak? The challenge here is that there is no set number of individuals who need to be affected to be deemed an 'outbreak.' It is a relative term that will vary from situation to situation. One thing is certain: irrespective of size of the outbreak, the investigation should use a systematic approach to identify contributing factors with the ultimate goal of control and prevention.

14.2 Outbreak Investigation

Generally, the objectives of an outbreak investigation include defining the problem, halting progress of disease, determining the reason for the outbreak, implementing corrective measures and providing recommendations to reduce the likelihood of recurrence (Martin *et al.*, 1987). In practice, it is helpful to iteratively work through the five Ws and an H – who, what, when, where, why and how – to achieve these objectives.

14.2.1 What and how much: defining the problem

First things first – determine if, in fact, there is a problem. A practitioner may be called at any time during a perceived disease event. Each time, they should ask whether disease is occurring (or has occurred) in excess of what would be expected for this region, in this type of a population, managed in this way. For example, the prevalence of canine respiratory disease expected in a rescue shelter would differ from that expected in a breeding facility or in a veterinary hospital because facility management and animal populations are likely to differ.

Next, make sure everyone has a clear understanding of what is being counted. This begins by creating a working definition of the problem, which

*Brandy.Burgess@uga.edu

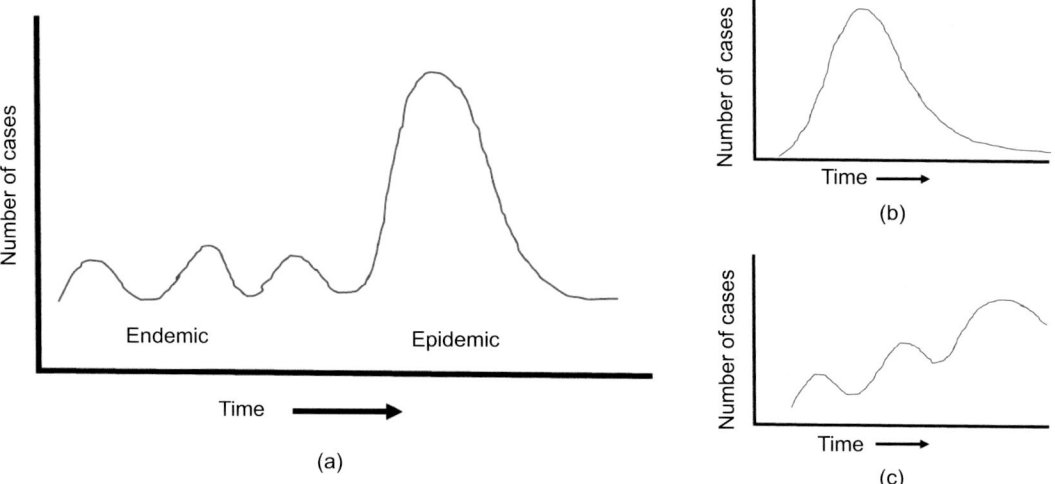

Fig. 14.1. Common disease patterns. (a) Distribution of cases over time, illustrating endemic versus epidemic disease. (b) A point-source epidemic. (c) A propagating epidemic.

may include clinical signs as well as the presumptive diagnosis. For example, in an outbreak of canine influenza virus in December 2017, the working definition was dogs with upper respiratory signs that were linked to dogs that had been shipped from South Korea (Weese *et al.*, 2019). This working definition should be refined throughout the investigation, and any presumptive diagnoses should be confirmed. In the case of the canine respiratory disease outbreak, it was determined to be canine influenza virus (H3N2) (Weese *et al.*, 2019). This working definition will ultimately be refined into the case definition used when analysing factors that may be contributing to the outbreak (i.e. when making comparisons between groups).

14.2.2 Who, where and when: orienting the problem

Now you can begin to orient the problem by animal, place and time – the who, where and when – refining the working definition into a case definition, placing cases on a facility map and creating an epidemic curve.

The who: defining a case and a non-case

A case definition is crucial to an investigation, demarcating a case (affected) from a non-case (unaffected), and should include animals with the primary disease of concern while excluding healthy animals and those with other unrelated conditions. This allows focused data collection and is necessary to calculate rates of disease when cases and non-cases are cross-classified by potential exposures or risk factors for the development of disease.

The where and when: defining the pattern of disease in space and time

Remember the adage 'a picture is worth a thousand words?' Never is this truer than in outbreak investigation. Mapping cases on a facility diagram and charting them over time can give the investigator critical insights into potential sources and important factors.

Obtain a facility layout or draw the layout, highlighting housing locations and animal and human movement. Pay particular attention to the date of disease onset in different areas of the facility, as well as how each area is used. For example, an outbreak investigation of diarrhoeal disease and death among puppies at a greyhound breeding facility used a facility diagram to show the spatial orientation of important management areas and guided investigators in their investigation (Morley *et al.*, 2006), while in an outbreak of neurological disease at an equine boarding facility, investigators showed the progression of disease spread on a facility map, which informed mitigation and containment efforts

Brandy A. Burgess

(Burgess *et al.*, 2012). Once you have a facility map, confirm locations during a site visit to ensure a complete understanding of the layout and spread of disease within the facility.

Create an epidemic curve depicting the distribution of disease over time. This curve is a pictorial representation charting case count along the vertical axis and time along the horizontal access. These curves can often give insights into the mode of transmission and ultimately the source. For example, a point-source epidemic results from a common source of exposure over a short period of time for all affected individuals. Graphically, this results in an epidemic curve with a steep upslope and a more gradual downslope (Fig. 14.1). Alternatively, with a propagated epidemic, a diseased animal will be the source of infection for a subsequent animal, so on and so forth. This results in an epidemic curve with multiple peaks over time, each a bit higher than the previous depicted as a more gradual upslope. Eventually, the epidemic will wane as the number of susceptible individuals declines or as a result of mitigation efforts (Fig. 14.1).

14.2.3 Why and how: identifying key determinants

Disease does not occur randomly in populations. In other words, there are factors (also referred to as 'exposures') that may contribute to the development of disease or to its prevention. As the investigation progresses, it is useful to think through the epidemiological triad to ensure factors related to the agent, the host and the environment are being considered and that relevant data are being collected. Note that these classifications of factors are not exclusive and you may find that a single factor may have an effect on the agent, host and/or environment.

- *The agent.* In general, the agent can be biological, chemical or physical. Furthermore, when considering biological agents, infectivity, virulence and pathogenicity may be important characteristics contributing to morbidity and mortality among those affected. While outbreak investigations tend towards biological agents, do not discount chemical or physical agents that may present as point-source epidemics. For example, an outbreak associated with poor water quality may at first appear to be due to an infectious agent, as highlighted in a reported outbreak of

death and diarrhoea in a horse herd (Burgess *et al.*, 2010). Additionally, when considering biological agents, insect vectors and reservoirs may play important roles in transmission and/ or in maintaining the agent in the environment.

- *The host.* Important features of the host that may contribute to susceptibility include intrinsic factors, such as age, sex, breed, immune status, general health status and behaviour, and extrinsic factors, such as population structure and dynamics, as well as facility management. This is in no way an exhaustive list. The clinician should recognize that many different elements may affect immunity, general health and behaviour, and that population structure and facility management may change over time.

- *The environment.* Environmental factors are generally thought of as external factors that can be categorized as abiotic (physical or non-living) or biotic (living) factors. Abiotic factors may include such things as air, soil and water, the climate, the materials used in the built environment, and the structure of the facilities and their use. Biotic factors refer to the flora and fauna contributing to the larger ecosystem, including other animals in or near the facility, wildlife and insect vectors that may be important in the chain of transmission or in an agent's life cycle.

Once data are collected and collated, the investigator can begin to analyse it, comparing attack rates between animals exposed to a factor of interest with those not exposed. These calculations may be done at any time to gain an understanding of the scope and impact of the outbreak as it is occurring.

- *Collating the data.* Early on, investigators need to determine standard data that will be collected for all members of the susceptible population, if possible, or at least a representative sample, and a database should be created. Data should include basic demographic information, housing location, animal group (e.g. litter, room or kennel), and other factors that may be of interest. Animals in the population at risk should be cross-classified regarding factors of concern and disease status. This will make it easier to create an attack rate table.

- *Calculating attack rates.* The attack rate is an incidence rate that is commonly used in outbreak investigations to quantify the proportion of the at-risk population that is disease positive. The attack rate equals the number

Table 14.1. An attack rate table for workplace-related exposures of Q fever in an animal refuge and veterinary clinic. Data from Malo *et al.* (2018).

Factor or exposure	Exposed			Unexposed			Risk ratio (AR_{exp}/AR_{unexp})
	Cases	Total	AR (%)	Cases	Total	AR (%)	
Visit to cat impound	7	31	22.6%	0	9	0.0%	NA
Direct contact with cats or kittens	7	28	25.0%	0	3	0.0%	NA
Handling cats or kittens at birth, or present during birthing events	4	13	30.8%	3	18	16.7%	1.8
Providing or assisting with euthanasia of cats or kittens	4	9	44.4%	3	22	13.6%	3.3
Disposal of deceased cats or kittens	5	11	45.5%	2	20	10.0%	4.5
Cleaning of cat impound, cages or changing litter	3	12	25.0%	4	19	21.1%	1.2

AR, attack rate (number of cases/number at risk at the beginning of the outbreak); NA, not applicable.

of cases divided by the number at risk at the beginning of the outbreak. An attack rate table can be developed from the database, listing risk factors vertically and exposed and unexposed horizontally (Table 14.1). Attack rates can then be calculated and compared either directly, if a representative cross-section of the population at risk is included, or by calculating a ratio if the data are non-representative.

The attack rate table allows investigators to gain perspective on the likely source and contributing factors in the outbreak, and gives direction to control measures should attack rates be determined in real time. For example, in a 2018 outbreak investigation of Q fever in people at an animal refuge and veterinary clinic in Australia, investigators reported close contact with parturient products from infected cats as the likely cause (Malo *et al.*, 2018). Indeed, risk ratios suggested individuals assisting with euthanasia and disposal in this outbreak to be at greatest risk (Table 14.1) (Malo *et al.*, 2018). Knowing this would allow additional personal protective equipment (PPE) to be worn to protect personnel and to encourage strict adherence to its use, as well as employing rigorous cleaning and disinfection protocols. Attack rate tables should be included in the final summary report provided to stakeholders.

14.3 Outbreak Management

A primary goal in outbreak management is to limit spread to unaffected animals, areas within a facility, facilities and/or regions. Thus, it is critical to gain perspective on the likely cause whether it is physical, chemical or biological. If the presumptive diagnosis is an infectious agent, then measures should be taken to disrupt the chain of transmission. Recall that the chain of transmission includes a source of agent, portal of exit, mechanism of transmission, portal of entry and a susceptible host. Significant effort is typically focused on the mechanism of transmission – broadly classified as contact (direct or indirect), airborne (aerosol or droplet formation) or vector-borne – with efforts intended to disrupt one or more of these transmission routes.

Common objectives in outbreak management include reducing contact between infectious and susceptible animals (e.g. separation, quarantine, animal movement controls, avoid mixing and common-use equipment), to reduce the number of susceptible animals (e.g. vaccination, close the population) and to decrease the amount of infectious agent (e.g. by cleaning and disinfection). In real-time outbreak management, it can be useful to consider five key areas – access, people, animals, environment and movement – to achieve these objectives.

14.3.1 Access

Anything animals mutually share or contact can transmit disease (e.g. people, feed/water bowls, tools, walkways, fences, exercise areas). With this in mind, it is critical to have rules and guidelines in place to limit contact with people and other animals including wildlife, as well as maintaining

Brandy A. Burgess

separation between exposed and non-exposed individuals. Facilities should limit access to personnel and visitors to those who are necessary. Note that it is prudent to have contingency planning in place to facilitate end-of-life decision making with owners.

14.3.2 People

People can carry pathogens from affected to unaffected and/or susceptible individuals on their equipment, clothing and hands. As such, it is important not only to limit the necessary individuals who need to access the affected facility and/or animals, but also that defined rules and protocols are in place to decrease the likelihood of transmission. Availability of required PPE and hand hygiene supplies is key in this effort, as this has been identified as a barrier to compliance in small animal veterinary practice (Anderson and Weese, 2016).

14.3.3 Animals

There are often many animal species and risk groups in animal facilities. Depending on the suspected or confirmed agent associated with an outbreak, multiple species could be affected, requiring a more extensive investigation and expansive mitigation efforts. While the general animal population is considered to be 'healthy', by design, many animals coming into a veterinary hospital will be compromised in some way (e.g. severe illness, immunosuppression, pregnancy, neonate), are there seeking specialized therapy that may increase susceptibility (e.g. chemotherapy) or need critical care, which predisposes to the development of a healthcare-associated infection (Ruple-Czerniak et al., 2013).

14.3.4 Environment

Microorganisms can remain on surfaces and equipment and in soil, faeces, wood and water for long periods of time. Weather and temperature can also affect a microorganism's ability to multiply and/or survive outside of the host. Therefore, it is important to consider materials used in facility construction – cleanable surfaces are a must for cleaning and disinfection to be effective. Porous materials should be sealed and cracks should be repaired. Outdoor exercise areas can be particularly challenging as you cannot disinfect dirt. Remember, the solution to pollution is dilution; thus, removal of faeces and breaking up and distribution of material that cannot be removed are key in this effort.

14.3.5 Movement

An early management strategy in the course of an outbreak is to stop animal movement. This is particularly important if you believe you are dealing with a reportable disease (in the USA, this can be at the State or Federal level) or if the agent is potentially zoonotic. Once the appropriate authorities have been contacted and a plan is put in place, lifting of movement restrictions can be considered. Limiting animal movement also applies to moving animals within the facility. In general, animals housed in a group should be maintained in those groups. The situation may warrant separation of groups into exposed, infected and non-exposed, although this will depend on the situation and capacity of the facility. During an outbreak, human movement should also be managed with policies in place to restrict personnel movement from outbreak housing areas into general housing areas without taking appropriate precautions (e.g. PPE, shower-out).

14.4 Outbreak Communication

Do not underestimate the power of communication, or the lack thereof. In general, transparent communications should occur during the outbreak (i.e. real-time communication), as well as after the investigation is complete in an investigative summary report.

14.4.1 Real-time communication

While proactive communication of risk-related information is generally good practice, outbreaks can adversely impact the organization's 'brand' and may present legal liability (practice managers/owners should contact their legal counsel for advice). That being said, it is critical that real-time communication be clear and actionable and based on the best available evidence at that time. Controlling the message ensures alignment of perceived and actual risk among personnel and clients, potentially reducing negative information and facilitating a more rapid return to 'normal'. In the context of a veterinary hospital, consider clients' confidence in that organization and a return to a 'normal' case load after the outbreak is fully mitigated.

14.4.2 Investigation summary report

An important component to any outbreak investigation is reporting the investigative process and its findings back to stakeholders. This report should include an explanation of the processes used in the investigation, interpretation of test results and an analysis of factors determined to contribute to the outbreak. Additionally, it should present prevention strategies to reduce the likelihood for recurrence and, if the outbreak is still ongoing, should provide refinement of the current mitigation efforts and outbreak management plan.

14.5 Conclusion

Outbreak investigation is not really about the diagnosis per se but rather about discovering the origin. While some outbreaks may progress slowly, affecting only a few animals in a single facility or small region, others may progress very rapidly, affecting many animals and facilities in a wide geographical region.

As the first line of defence, veterinary practitioners should have a plan in place to systematically compile information (the five Ws and an H) to determine whether an epidemic is actually occurring and to identify important factors in its propagation and prevention. They should be ready to manage disease in individual animals as well as the population (movement control, contact control, hygiene), and to seek expert advice from colleagues and the appropriate authorities as warranted.

Upon recognition of an outbreak, treatment of affected animals should be initiated as soon as possible (symptomatically until a presumptive diagnosis can be established), and generic control measures should be put in place (e.g. movement restriction and PPE) for containment. As the outbreak progresses and data are collected and analysed, investigators will develop a much clearer understanding of the scope of the problem and be able to implement agent-specific treatment and prevention strategies, as well as more refined mitigation efforts.

Note that outbreak investigation and management is in no way a linear process. Rather, it is a circular, iterative process that builds on the evidence as it is discovered. Just like John Snow in the 1854 London cholera epidemic, a little shoe-leather epidemiology (i.e. field epidemiology) can go a long way to prevent additional morbidity and mortality in the present and future.

References

Anderson, M.E.C. and Weese, J.S. (2016) Self-reported hand hygiene perceptions and barriers among companion animal veterinary clinic personnel in Ontario, Canada. *Canadian Veterinary Journal* 57(3), 282–288.

Burgess, B.A., Lohmann, K.L. and Blakley, B.R. (2010) Excessive sulfate and poor water quality as a cause of sudden deaths and an outbreak of diarrhea in horses. *Canadian Veterinary Journal* 51(3), 277–282.

Burgess, B.A., Tokateloff, N., Manning, S., Lohmann, K., Lunn, D.P. *et al.* (2012) Nasal shedding of equine herpesvirus-1 from horses in an outbreak of equine herpes myeloencephalopathy in Western Canada. *Journal of Veterinary Internal Medicine* 26(2), 384–392. DOI: 10.1111/j.1939-1676.2012.00885.x.

Malo, J.A., Colbran, C., Young, M., Vasant, B., Jarvinen, K. *et al.* (2018) An outbreak of Q fever associated with parturient cat exposure at an animal refuge and veterinary clinic in southeast Queensland. *Australian and New Zealand Journal of Public Health* 42(5), 451–455. DOI: 10.1111/1753-6405.12784.

Martin, S.W., Meek, A.H. and Willeberg, P. (1987) *Veterinary Epidemiology – Principles and Methods.* Ames, Iowa, Iowa State University.

Morley, P.S., Strohmeyer, R.A., Tankson, J.D., Hyatt, D.R., Dargatz, D.A. *et al.* (2006) Evaluation of the association between feeding raw meat and *Salmonella enterica* infections at a Greyhound breeding facility. *Journal of the American Veterinary Medical Association* 228(10), 1524–1532. DOI: 10.2460/javma.228.10.1524.

Ruple-Czerniak, A., Aceto, H.W., Bender, J.B., Paradis, M.R., Shaw, S.P. *et al.* (2013) Using syndromic surveillance to estimate baseline rates for healthcare-associated infections in critical care units of small animal referral hospitals. *Journal of Veterinary Internal Medicine* 27(6), 1392–1399. DOI: 10.1111/jvim.12190.

Snow, J. (1855) *On the Mode of Communication of Cholera.* John Burchill, London.

Weese, J.S., Anderson, M.E.C., Berhane, Y., Doyle, K.F., Leutenegger, C. *et al.* (2019) Emergence and Containment of Canine Influenza Virus A(H3N2), Ontario, Canada, 2017-2018. *Emerging Infectious Diseases* 25(10), 1810–1816. DOI: 10.3201/eid2510.190196.

Brandy A. Burgess

Section 5: Antibiotic Use

The discovery of antibiotics heralded a phenomenal advancement in the management of infectious disease and has saved countless lives and reduced morbidity over the last 90 or more years. For future generations to be able to continue to benefit from these life-saving medications, there is a pressing need to adopt measures to preserve their efficacy. Antibiotic use is a primary driver of antibiotic resistance due to the application of selection pressure for resistant strains. As a direct consequence, all prescribers must ensure that antibiotics are used appropriately and that all unnecessary use is avoided. This section offers recommendations on when to use and, possibly more importantly, when not to use antibiotics. Understanding how antibiotics work, how to recognize when they are needed and how to monitor their impact will contribute to optimal antibiotic stewardship benefitting both our patients and wider society.

The following key points are covered:

- Antibiotics kill bacteria or impair their growth by targeting structural defensive barriers (e.g. the cell wall), bacterial protein or nucleic acid synthesis, or by disrupting critical biochemical pathways.
- Bacteria resist the effects of antibiotics by modifying the antibiotic (leading to its inactivation), modifying the antibiotic target site or reducing the concentration of the antibiotic at its target (by preventing its access or by purposefully expelling it from the cell via efflux pumps).
- Antimicrobial resistance (AMR) is recognized as a serious threat to human (and animal) health and is already responsible for millions of deaths globally each year.

- Antibiotic stewardship initiatives have been developed to encourage veterinary practitioners to follow rational stewardship principles that will help conserve the efficacy of antibiotics in the future.
- Certain antibiotics (e.g. fluoroquinolones and third-generation cephalosporins such as cefovecin) have been classified as *highest-priority critically important antibiotics* and should be reserved as much as possible for human use. They should only be used in companion animals when other (lower-tier) antibiotics would not be effective.
- The use of antibiotics to prevent a possible infection developing, antibiotic prophylaxis, is warranted in some immunosuppressed patients as a protective measure and can reduce the likelihood of surgical-site infections when used prior to and during surgical interventions.
- Antibiotic prophylaxis is not a substitute for surgical asepsis, and most clean or clean-contaminated procedures do not require any antibiotics to be administered.
- Multiple resources and antibiotic-use guidelines have been created by groups working across Europe to support antibiotic decision making for veterinarians. Frequent reference to these documents will help veterinarians play their role in the war against AMR.
- A non-prescription form can facilitate client communication and ensure that owners share in the conversation regarding withholding antibiotics wherever appropriate.
- Monitoring trends in antibiotic use will help identify areas that can be improved and evaluate the success of stewardship interventions.

15 Management of the Immunosuppressed Patient

JOCELYN BISSON*

Royal (Dick) School of Veterinary Studies, University of Edinburgh, Roslin, UK

15.1 Introduction

Veterinary patients may become immunosuppressed for a variety of reasons. Primary immunosuppressive disorders are rare, but secondary immunodeficiency is common, occurring in numerous disease processes, including diabetes mellitus and hyperadrenocorticism. Drug-induced immunosuppression is also increasingly common as more and more patients are treated for neoplastic and immune-mediated diseases.

There are several factors to consider when contemplating antimicrobial treatment options for the immunosuppressed patient. This chapter focuses primarily on antimicrobial treatment for immunosuppression during cancer chemotherapy, as this is where the largest evidence base can be found. However, it also considers antimicrobial use with other immunosuppressive drugs and naturally occurring immunosuppression.

15.2 Immunosuppression Following Cancer Chemotherapy

Neutropenia is the primary dose-limiting toxicity for the majority of chemotherapeutic agents in both humans and veterinary patients, and the risk of infection with increasing neutropenia is well documented (Boudreaux, 2014; Bisson *et al.*, 2018). Although most chemotherapy agents cause a generalized bone marrow suppression, neutrophils are the cell line most frequently depleted as they have a short half-life and require regular replenishment from bone marrow precursors (Boudreaux, 2014). However, patients receiving maximum tolerated dose cancer chemotherapy also experience depletion of circulating lymphocytes, indicating

that both innate and adaptive immunosuppression occurs in these patients (Rasmussen *et al.*, 2017). In addition to immunosuppression associated with chemotherapy, cancer patients may also experience immunomodulation due to surgical procedures, pain and opioid administration (Perry and Douglas, 2019).

Typically, the reference range for absolute neutrophil count (ANC) in dogs and humans is between 2×10^9 and 7×10^9 cells l^{-1}, although this varies among laboratories. Studies in humans in the 1960s identified an increased risk of infection when ANC fell below 2×10^9 cells l^{-1}, with patients with counts less than 0.5×10^9 cells l^{-1} considered to be high risk (Bodey *et al.*, 1966). Most human oncology guidelines and studies now focus on an ANC of less than 0.5×10^9 cells l^{-1} (Phillips *et al.*, 2012). The Veterinary Cooperative Oncology Group – Common Terminology Criteria for Adverse Events (VCOG-CTCAE) classifies any ANC below 0.5×10^9 cells l^{-1} as grade 4, severe neutropenia (Table 15.1) (LeBlanc *et al.*, 2021). In many veterinary guidelines and hospitals, a VCOG-CTCAE grade 3 neutropenia (less than 1×10^9 cells l^{-1}) is considered clinically concerning (Thamm and Vail, 2007; Vail, 2009; Boudreaux, 2014).

For most chemotherapeutic agents used in veterinary medicine, the time to development of the ANC nadir is approximately 7 days, although this varies from patient to patient (Boudreaux, 2014; Britton *et al.*, 2014). Prolonged neutrophil nadirs as late as 3 weeks after chemotherapy administration have been documented for chemotherapy agents such as lomustine and carboplatin (Page *et al.*, 1993; Moore *et al.*, 1999).

In humans, the prevalence of neutropenia at less than 1×10^9 cells l^{-1} varies widely from around 10%

*Jocelyn.bisson@ed.ac.uk

Table 15.1. Veterinary Cooperative Oncology Group – Common Terminology Criteria for Adverse Events grades of neutropenia.

Grade	Absolute neutrophil count ($\times 10^9$ l^{-1})
1	≥1.50
2	1.00–1.49
3	0.50–0.99
4	<0.50

to more than 40%, depending on the chemotherapy protocol used and specific patient risk factors (Jolis *et al.*, 2013; Teillant *et al.*, 2015). The prevalence of neutropenia in dogs is generally considered to be lower than this but varies widely among studies and depends on the chemotherapy protocol used (Garrett *et al.*, 2002; MacDonald *et al.*, 2005; Chretin *et al.*, 2007). A recent retrospective study in dogs receiving various chemotherapy agents for a variety of tumour types found that grade 3 or 4 neutropenia occurred after 15.3% of chemotherapy administrations (Bisson *et al.*, 2020).

In oncology patients, we tend to consider two main categories of neutropenia: neutropenia where the patient is clinically unwell (generally referred to as febrile neutropenia (FN)) and neutropenia where the patient has no clinical signs (generally referred to as asymptomatic neutropenia). Neutropenic patients that are unwell require a very different level of intervention compared with those where the neutropenia is clinically silent (Fig. 15.1).

15.2.1 Febrile neutropenia

Definition and frequency

Neutropenic patients are unable to mount a typical inflammatory response to infection and therefore any infection may progress rapidly to bacteraemia and overwhelming bacterial sepsis (Morgan *et al.*, 2021). This lack of typical inflammatory response may also mean that neutropenic patients do not present with the classical clinical signs of infection (Rodriguez *et al.*, 1973). The initial harbinger of infection is typically fever, although dogs and cats may also have accompanying vague clinical signs such as decreased appetite, lethargy, vomiting and diarrhoea (Pierro *et al.*, 2017; Bisson *et al.*, 2020). It is therefore extremely important to treat any patient with fever and concurrent neutropenia (i.e. FN) as

having the potential to develop fatal sepsis and provide aggressive emergency therapy (Fig. 15.2).

The definition of FN varies widely among studies. In humans, definitions of FN include temperature of more than 38–38.5°C accompanied by a neutropenia of less than 0.5$\times 10^9$ cells l^{-1} or less than 1.0$\times 10^9$ cells l^{-1}, and expected to fall to less than 0.5$\times 10^9$ cells l^{-1} within 48 h (Morgan *et al.*, 2021). The National Institute for Health and Care Excellence (NICE) guidelines advise considering any ANC of 0.5$\times 10^9$ cells l^{-1} or less and a fever greater than 38°C as FN (Phillips *et al.*, 2012). However, a 2017 audit found that only 64% of UK hospitals were using the NICE definition (Morgan and Phillips, 2018).

Veterinary studies tend to use a more conservative definition of FN including any ANC of less than 2.5 $\times 10^9$ cells l^{-1} in conjunction with a rectal temperature greater than 39.2°C (Britton *et al.*, 2014; Bisson *et al.*, 2020).

Importantly, not all neutropenic patients with infection will present with fever. This is probably due to a lack of pyrogenic cytokine release in severely immunosuppressed patients (Boudreaux, 2014). A study assessing the outcome of FN in dogs found that there was an increased probability of death in patients with lower temperatures at admission, most likely due to an inadequate immune response (Britton *et al.*, 2014). Another study found no significant difference in the incidence of bacteraemia or bacteriuria between clinically unwell but afebrile dogs and febrile neutropenic dogs (Shaffer *et al.*, 2016). It is therefore important to treat any clinically unwell neutropenic patient aggressively, regardless of their body temperature at admission. The NICE guidelines also recommend that human patients without fever but with other signs or symptoms consistent with sepsis be treated in the same way as FN patients (Phillips *et al.*, 2012).

Human chemotherapy protocols are classified as high, intermediate or low risk for inducing FN, with high-risk protocols defined as those inducing FN in more than 20% of patients (Lyman *et al.*, 2014). The majority of human FN patients are hospitalized, with hospital mortality rates of around 8% (Weycker *et al.*, 2014). The risk of FN appears to be lower in veterinary patients, with most studies reporting rates of less than 10% (Garrett *et al.*, 2002; Vail, 2009). A recent study reported only four episodes of FN out of 586 chemotherapy administrations in 181 dogs; however, this study only assessed FN occurring after the predicted

Jocelyn Bisson

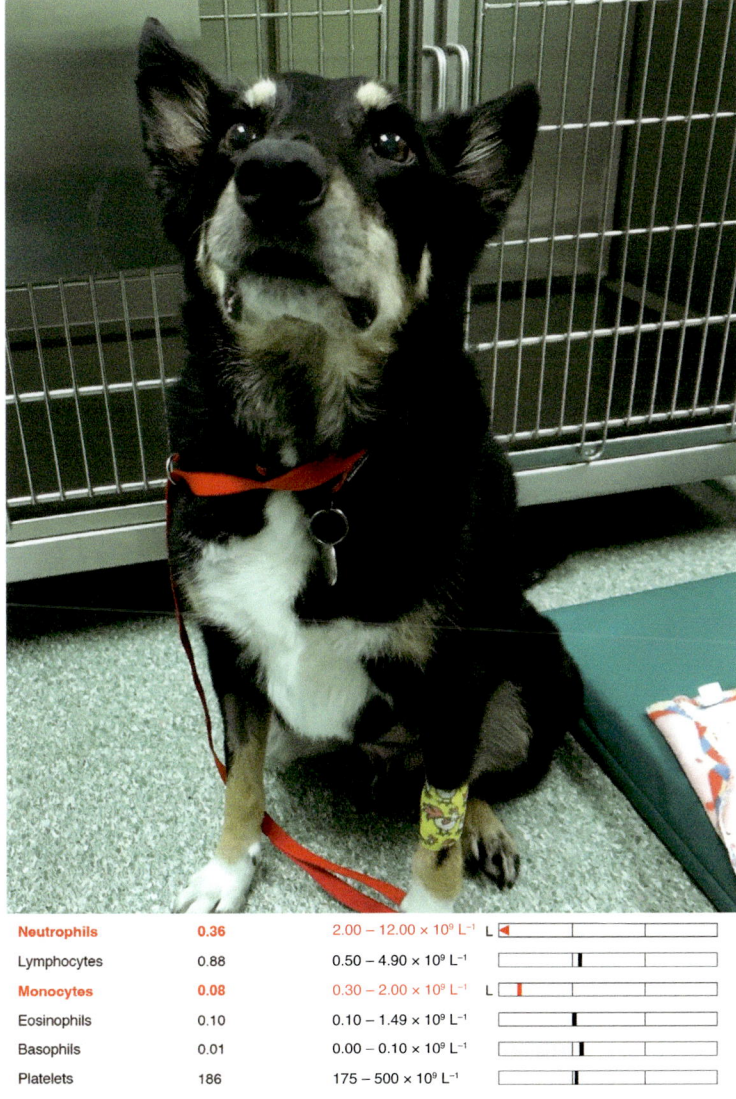

Neutrophils	**0.36**	2.00 – 12.00 × 10⁹ L⁻¹	
Lymphocytes	0.88	0.50 – 4.90 × 10⁹ L⁻¹	
Monocytes	**0.08**	0.30 – 2.00 × 10⁹ L⁻¹	
Eosinophils	0.10	0.10 – 1.49 × 10⁹ L⁻¹	
Basophils	0.01	0.00 – 0.10 × 10⁹ L⁻¹	
Platelets	186	175 – 500 × 10⁹ L⁻¹	

Fig. 15.1. A clinically well lymphoma patient with a VCOG-CTAE (Veterinary Cooperative Oncology Group – Common Terminology Criteria for Adverse Events) grade 4 neutropenia 1 week after lomustine chemotherapy. Parameters in red are below laboratory reference range. Reference ranges are also indicated by the bars and boxes to the right of the numerical values. Bars within the central box demonstrate a value within reference range, while the bar and arrowhead in the left boxes demonstrate a value below or well below the reference range.

neutrophil nadir (Bisson *et al.*, 2020). Higher rates of FN are reported with more intensive veterinary chemotherapy protocols (Northrup *et al.*, 2002). Mortality rates among hospitalized canine patients are similar to human rates at around 8% (Britton *et al.*, 2014).

Origin of infection

In most FN patients, the source of infection is from their own gastrointestinal (GI) tract. Chemotherapy-induced damage to the physical defence barrier of the GI mucosa leads to increased intestinal permeability and bacterial translocation (Britton *et al.*,

---

Management of the Immunosuppressed Patient

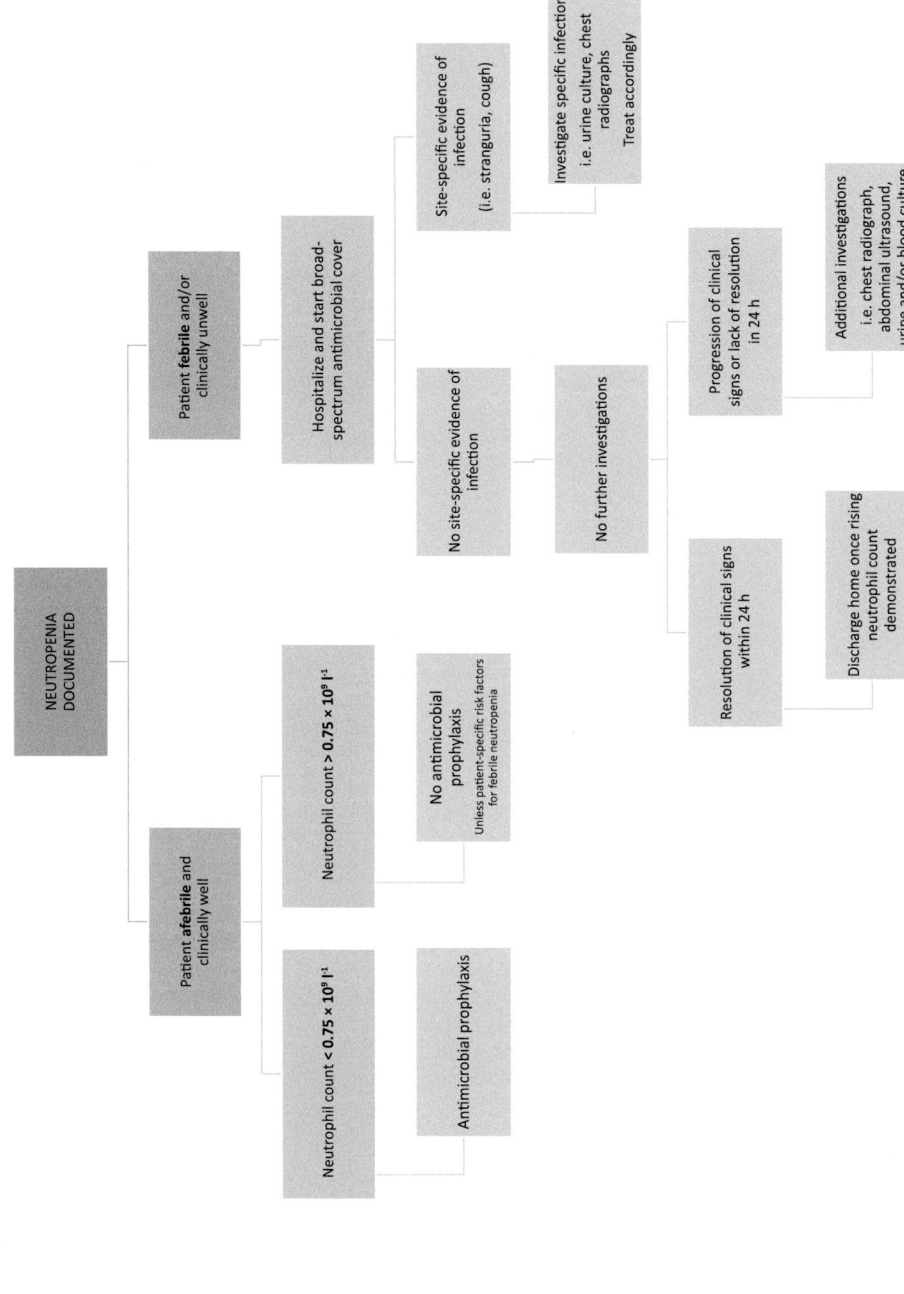

Fig. 15.2. Algorithm for neutropenia management in veterinary cancer chemotherapy patients.

Jocelyn Bisson

2014). However, other sources or sites of infection, such as the urinary or respiratory tract or skin, are also possible. Human guidelines recommend that at least two sets of blood cultures are performed at the time of hospital admission from two separate venepuncture sites (Freifeld *et al.*, 2011; Phillips *et al.*, 2012; Rapoport *et al.*, 2021). However, in a large study of children with FN, 59% had no documented clinical or microbiological evidence of infection (Morgan *et al.*, 2021). This indicates that searching for the underlying bacterial infection can ultimately be unrewarding, even with relatively advanced techniques such as multiple blood cultures. Human guidelines therefore do not recommend additional investigations, such as urine culture or chest radiographs, unless there are specific clinical signs that indicate a localized infection (Freifeld *et al.*, 2011; Phillips *et al.*, 2012).

This also holds true for veterinary patients. In a study of FN in dogs, an infectious focus was only identified in 25.7% (18/70) of dogs: nine dogs had radiographic evidence of pneumonia, five had urinary tract infection, three had active skin infections and one had confirmed bacteraemia on blood culture (Britton *et al.*, 2014). Blood culture was only performed in two patients in this study and was negative in the second patient tested (Britton *et al.*, 2014). A study in 55 neutropenic dogs found that the overall incidence of bacteraemia detected on blood culture was 12.5% and bacteriuria was 7.5% (Shaffer *et al.*, 2016). Of the blood cultures that were positive, six out of seven were Gram-positive organisms (similar to rates reported in human literature) and three out of seven demonstrated evidence of antimicrobial resistance (Kuderer *et al.*, 2006; Shaffer *et al.*, 2016). While blood culture is considered the gold standard in management of people with potential sepsis, it can be challenging and costly to perform in veterinary patients. Given the low level of detection of bacteraemia on blood culture in FN patients and the fact that the vast majority of veterinary patients will respond to empirical therapy, routine blood culture in these patients does not appear to be justified as a first-line investigation (Vail, 2009; Shaffer *et al.*, 2016). Some centres have attempted to use urine culture as a proxy for bacteraemia; however, the sensitivity of urine to reflect concordant bacteraemia is only 30% and cannot be used as a substitute or screen for blood culture (Barash *et al.*, 2018).

Rapid polymerase chain reaction (PCR)-based diagnostic technologies that detect small amounts of specific bacterial DNA in patients' whole-blood samples are becoming increasingly available in human medicine and, in theory, can help with rapid bacterial identification and treatment (Buss *et al.*, 2018; Morgan *et al.*, 2021). However, their clinical and cost effectiveness are still debatable, and there are few studies exploring their use in a FN setting. Therefore, they are yet to be widely recommended (Stevenson *et al.*, 2016).

In patients displaying any specific clinical signs of infection, such as productive cough or stranguria, localized testing such as chest radiographs or urine culture is indicated. Additionally, if patients do not respond clinically to empirical antimicrobials within 12–24 h, then additional testing for any resistant or site-specific infections should be considered, including abdominal ultrasound, echocardiography and blood culture from two sites. Adding an additional antimicrobial to broaden the spectrum can also be considered at this time point while awaiting culture results (Boudreaux, 2014). It is important to consider that many of the clinical signs displayed by affected patients, including lethargy and pyrexia, may actually be associated with tumour progression rather than the neutropenia itself, and therefore careful reanalysis of the tumour burden is indicated in patients that do not improve rapidly.

Treatment

FN patients are at risk of very rapid deterioration and it is not indicated to wait for culture results before proceeding with empirical therapy (Boudreaux, 2014). Indeed, human guidelines recommend antimicrobial administration within 1 h of hospital admission, with an association between longer time to antibiotic administration and impaired safety noted in a recent systematic review (Phillips *et al.*, 2012; Koenig *et al.*, 2020). The concept of this 'golden hour' is widely recommended in the management of sepsis in people and should be considered a reasonable target to aim for in the management of veterinary FN cases, particularly as these patients are likely to present later to the hospital than human patients would.

ANTIMICROBIAL CHOICE. Empirical veterinary treatment recommendations vary among studies and institutions. Overall, the recommendation is to hospitalize FN patients and provide empirical, broad-spectrum, intravenous (IV) antimicrobial coverage. Typical antimicrobial combinations recommended in dogs include marbofloxacin (2 mg kg⁻¹ IV every 24 h) and metronidazole (15 mg kg⁻¹ IV every 12 h), a penicillin-like drug such as ampicillin (22 mg/kg IV every 8 h) and amikacin (10 mg kg⁻¹ IV every 24 h) with careful monitoring of renal function, or a first-generation cephalosporin such as cefazolin (20 mg g⁻¹ IV every 8 h) and enrofloxacin (5–10 mg kg⁻¹ IV every 24 h) (Thamm and Vail, 2007; Vail, 2009; Bisson et al., 2020). Similar combinations of antimicrobials are also reported in cats (Pierro et al., 2017). Significantly, human oncology guidelines are now advising against this level of extensive antimicrobial cover, recommending monotherapy alone (e.g. a fluoroquinolone or a broad-spectrum β-lactam antibiotic with a β-lactamase inhibitor, i.e. amoxicillin-clavulanic acid) and no additional antimicrobial cover unless there is a patient-specific indication such as a documented resistant infection (Freifeld et al., 2011; Phillips et al., 2012). This is due to extensive evidence from a meta-analysis that additional antimicrobials do not improve survival and are associated with higher levels of morbidity and adverse events (Paul et al., 2013). Successful monotherapy approaches with IV penicillin-like drugs alone have been documented in four cats, with FN resolving in all treated cats (Pierro et al., 2017). This approach warrants further consideration in veterinary medicine; however, a sufficient evidence base is lacking, and further comparative clinical studies are required before a definitive recommendation can be made. Any veterinary FN patient receiving monotherapy alone should be closely monitored for deterioration or lack of response to therapy in case additional antimicrobial cover is required.

Care must be taken when administering enrofloxacin to cats due to the risk of retinal degeneration; the manufacturer's guidelines should be closely adhered to and dose reduction may need to be considered in geriatric cats or those with renal impairment (Wiebe and Hamilton, 2002). Fluoroquinolones are also extremely important for human medicine (discussed in section 15.2.2); while their use may be considered justified in this setting due to the life-threatening nature of FN, careful antimicrobial stewardship is encouraged. The pharmacokinetics and pharmacodynamics of the chosen antimicrobial should also be carefully considered. It is vital to use the antimicrobial at an appropriately high dose in order to try to avoid the development of antimicrobial resistance (Onufrak et al., 2016).

HOSPITALIZATION. There is increasing evidence in human oncology that FN episodes are heterogeneous, and the risk of significant infection and complications varies between patients (Rapoport et al., 2021). Human guidelines now recommend a risk-stratified approach to FN management with intensive management for high-risk patients but more relaxed and even outpatient management strategies for those considered low risk. One of the most commonly used risk stratification tools is the Multinational Association for Supportive Care in Cancer (MASSC) index. This index found that FN patients were more likely to have septic complications if they presented with conditions such as hypotension, respiratory failure, altered mental status, arrhythmias or renal failure (Rapoport et al., 2021). Analysis of several human randomized controlled trials has found that oral antimicrobials were as effective in preventing mortality as IV antimicrobials in FN patients considered to be low risk on the MASCC index (Vidal et al., 2013). A meta-analysis also found that oral treatment is an acceptable alternative to IV antimicrobials in FN patients who are haemodynamically stable and do not have organ failure, acute leukaemia, pneumonia, infection of a central line or a severe soft-tissue infection (Vidal et al., 2013). Biomarkers to predict infection or severity of illness have been explored, particularly in paediatric FN patients (Morgan et al., 2021). The most commonly implicated markers include procalcitonin, C-reactive protein, and interleukin (IL)-6 and IL-8; however, a lack of good-quality evidence, alongside high costs and limited availability, mean that very few risk stratification strategies to date have incorporated biomarker use (Morgan et al., 2021).

In agreement with human risk stratification studies, a study in 70 dogs hospitalized for FN found that tachycardia on admission, decreasing neutrophil count after admission and documented infection (pneumonia or urinary tract infection) were all associated with a prolonged hospital stay (Britton et al., 2014). Additionally, hypotension and granulocyte colony-stimulating factor (GCSF) use were significantly associated with death in hospital, although the result for GCSF was suspected to be due to bias (Britton et al., 2014). Patients presenting with FN and any of these risk factors should be carefully monitored and the prognosis considered to be more guarded. Oral treatment at home for low-risk FN patients would potentially have considerable advantages for veterinary patients,

Jocelyn Bisson

including reduced exposure to nosocomial infections and maintenance of better quality of life (the ultimate goal in veterinary chemotherapy patients) (Vidal *et al.*, 2013; Walther *et al.*, 2017). However, human guidelines also consider social factors when determining appropriate management for FN patients, and patients that live far from the hospital would not be treated as outpatients (Phillips *et al.*, 2012; Morgan *et al.*, 2021). Many veterinary oncology patients live several hours away from specialist out-of-hours care and the vague clinical signs of progressive FN may be hard for owners to detect. With these factors in mind and the lack of veterinary evidence to support outpatient FN management at present, the majority of veterinary oncologists continue to manage affected individuals as inpatients initially.

TREATMENT DURATION. There is increasing debate over the length of hospitalization and antimicrobial course required in FN patients. The majority of veterinary patients respond rapidly to therapy, and neutrophil counts typically rise quickly after the nadir. Most animals are clinically well and afebrile within 12–24 h (Vail, 2009; Boudreaux, 2014; Bisson *et al.*, 2020). Current veterinary publications recommend discharge from hospital once the patient is clinically well and afebrile and their neutrophil count has risen (in most cases to greater than 1×10^9 cells l^{-1}). These texts also recommend continuation of oral antimicrobials at home (typically for 3–7 additional days) (Vail, 2009; Boudreaux, 2014). However, such recommendations are not evidence based, and there are increasing data to show that long antimicrobial courses may not be required in FN patients.

In human oncology, there are generally two possible approaches to antimicrobial course length: (i) a 'short course', where antimicrobials are discontinued as soon as a patient is afebrile and/or clinically well; or (ii) a 'long course', where antimicrobials are continued until neutropenia has resolved. A trial in the 1970s demonstrated an increased risk of death in patients with a short course of antimicrobials compared with a long course, and this understandably led to caution. The recent standard has been to continue antimicrobials until the patient is afebrile, free of documented infection and has a neutrophil count greater than 0.5×10^9 cells l^{-1} (Pizzo *et al.*, 1979; Morgan *et al.*, 2021). Additional studies on shorter antimicrobial cover duration are limited and those available contain marked heterogeneity between patients with regard to risk status, type of malignancy and treatment. However, a recent human systematic review found no significant difference in rates of mortality or clinical failures between short and long antimicrobial courses in patients with FN (Stern *et al.*, 2019).

Increasingly in human infection control, the dogma of 'completing the course' of antimicrobials is being challenged. There is limited evidence that discontinuing antimicrobials early encourages antimicrobial resistance but increasing evidence that treating with antimicrobials for longer than necessary actually builds resistance (Llewelyn *et al.*, 2017). A systematic review and multi-centre study in human patients (including some who were immunocompromised due to cancer chemotherapy) found that those receiving 7-day courses of antimicrobials for hospital-acquired pneumonia or *Enterobacteriaceae* bacteraemia had the same clinical outcomes as those receiving longer (10–15-day) courses (Pugh *et al.*, 2015; Chotiprasitsakul *et al.*, 2018). Importantly, the same studies also documented lower numbers of multidrug-resistant infections among patients receiving shorter antimicrobial courses (Pugh *et al.*, 2015; Chotiprasitsakul *et al.*, 2018).

For the majority of veterinary patients, the neutrophil count will recover within a few days of the nadir compared with human patients where neutropenia may last weeks (Ettinger *et al.*, 2017). While further studies are needed in veterinary patients, withdrawal of antimicrobials as soon as clinical signs have resolved and the neutrophil count has demonstrated signs of recovery appears to be a far more reasonable approach than prescribing empirical 5- or 7-day courses of antimicrobials after an FN episode.

15.2.2 Asymptomatic neutropenia

Evidence for antimicrobial prophylaxis

The lack of evidence on antimicrobial use in FN patients is nothing when compared with the lack of evidence on prophylactic antimicrobial use in neutropenic patients that are clinically well. Debate on the best course of action in these patients still rages in both the veterinary and human oncology fields.

It is relatively standard practice in veterinary institutions to perform a routine complete blood count (CBC) in patients at the predicted time of their neutrophil nadir following chemotherapy (although the exact frequency and timing of these CBCs is empirical and varies among institutions). Antimicrobial prophylaxis is often implemented in asymptomatic patients that are demonstrated to be neutropenic on this CBC to try to prevent them from developing FN. However, there is limited evidence as to whether antimicrobial prophylaxis actually benefits these patients, and what level of neutropenia requires prophylaxis.

There is increasing evidence from human randomized controlled trials and meta-analyses that the use of prophylactic fluoroquinolones (most commonly levofloxacin) reduces fever, microbiologically documented infections and hospitalization in neutropenic patients when compared with placebo (Drayson *et al.*, 2019; Owattanapanich and Chayakulkeeree, 2019). Some studies and meta-analyses have also found a difference in mortality between the two groups, but this is not a consistent finding, with many studies underpowered to detect a difference in mortality (Gafter-Gvili *et al.*, 2005, Gafter-Gvili *et al.*, 2012; Lo and Cullen, 2006; Owattanapanich and Chayakulkeeree, 2019).

Veterinary evidence for antimicrobial prophylaxis in dogs receiving chemotherapy is far more limited. However, a double-blinded, placebo-controlled trial assessed prophylactic trimethoprim-sulfonamide (TMPS) administration versus placebo during doxorubicin chemotherapy in dogs with lymphoma and osteosarcoma. Dogs that received TMPS had significantly lower rates of GI toxicity, suspected infections and hospitalization compared with placebo controls (Chretin *et al.*, 2007). However, in a study evaluating hospital stays in dogs with FN, 22% had been receiving various prophylactic antimicrobials and still went on to develop FN; these patients also had the same length of hospitalization and survival as patients with FN who had not received prophylaxis (Britton *et al.*, 2014). This finding demonstrates that antimicrobial prophylaxis may not prevent FN or improve FN outcomes in a significant subset of patients. This finding is corroborated by a recent study where in two of the four episodes of FN recorded the dogs were already receiving TMPS (Britton *et al.*, 2014; Bisson *et al.*, 2020).

Any reduction in toxicity and hospitalization rates is certainly very important to consider, especially in veterinary chemotherapy patients where most protocols are palliative, and it is important that adverse effects should be kept to an absolute minimum. It is tempting to consider prescribing prophylactic antimicrobials for all patients on chemotherapy. However, there are key disadvantages to this blanket approach.

Evidence against antimicrobial prophylaxis

Of great concern is the influence of antimicrobial prophylaxis on the development of antimicrobial resistance. Reports of resistant bacterial isolates from cancer chemotherapy patients receiving antimicrobial prophylaxis are widespread. A literature review from the USA reported resistance to standard prophylactic antimicrobials in 26.8% of the pathogens causing infections after chemotherapy (Teillant *et al.*, 2015). In addition, several human hospitals have reported increases in fluoroquinolone-resistant organisms cultured among commensals from the bowel and throat of patients receiving fluoroquinolone prophylaxis (Gustafsson *et al.*, 2003; Timmers *et al.*, 2004). Fluoroquinolone prophylaxis has also been suggested to increase the risk of intestinal translocation of extended-spectrum β-lactamase producing *Enterobacteriaceae* leading to bacteraemia (Timmers *et al.*, 2004). One study recorded fluoroquinolone resistance rates of more than 50% in *Escherichia coli* bloodstream isolates in cancer patients receiving fluoroquinolone prophylaxis (Kern *et al.*, 2005).

Equivalent veterinary studies in chemotherapy patients are not available. However, prior antimicrobial use is a risk factor for the isolation of resistant *Staphylococcus pseudintermedius* from the skin and ear in dogs (Zur *et al.*, 2016). In addition, a case–control study involving 150 veterinary practices found that an increased number of prior antimicrobial courses was associated with development of methicillin-resistant *Staphylococcus aureus* (Magalhães *et al.*, 2010).

As global antimicrobial resistance rates continue to rise and few new antimicrobials are approved, veterinary antimicrobial stewardship is vital. The American Veterinary Medical Association (AVMA) urges vets to 'commit to stewardship' and to consider alternatives to antimicrobial drugs in bacterial disease prevention, while the PROTECT ME guidelines of the British Small Animal Veterinary Association (BSAVA) encourage vets to reduce prophylactic antimicrobial use (BSAVA/SAMSoc, 2018; AVMA, 2022).

In addition to the concerns for antimicrobial resistance, prophylactic antimicrobials may also have detrimental effects on patients' microbiomes.

Jocelyn Bisson

Systemically administered antimicrobials impact the composition and function of the GI microbiome, which in turn may increase GI colonization by pathogenic, multidrug-resistant bacterial species (Galloway-Peña *et al.*, 2017). Concerningly, there is also increasing evidence that disruption of the microbiome may actually reduce the efficacy of certain chemotherapy agents. The GI microbiome appears to be essential for functions such as non-pathogenic bacterial translocation and subsequent activation of T-cells, induction of reactive oxygen species and modulation of the tumour microenvironment, all of which may influence the response to chemotherapy (Galloway-Peña *et al.*, 2017). Studies in mouse models of melanoma, sarcoma and colon carcinoma have revealed reduced tumour necrosis after platinum chemotherapy and failure of response to CTLA-4 blockade immunotherapy in mice pre-treated with antimicrobials (Viaud *et al.*, 2013; Vétizou *et al.*, 2015). In addition, antimicrobials with a Gram-positive spectrum reduced the efficacy of cyclophosphamide when administered to mice with lymphoma (Iida *et al.*, 2013; Viaud *et al.*, 2013; Vétizou *et al.*, 2015). A study in human patients receiving cyclophosphamide for leukaemia also found that those receiving antimicrobials with a Gram-positive spectrum (more likely to disrupt the microbiome) had significantly reduced progression-free and overall survival times compared with those receiving primarily Gram-negative-spectrum antimicrobials or no antimicrobials at all (Pflug *et al.*, 2016).

Disruptions to the microbiome may also cause other detrimental effects to patient health, such as alterations in metabolites, cytokine profiles and inflammatory responses. Human oncologists describe a 'catch-22' situation where mucosal injury and neutropenia induced by chemotherapy necessitate prophylactic antimicrobials, but their use induces microbial dysbiosis leading to potential complications such as pulmonary disease, reduced responses to chemotherapy, inflammatory colitis, and *Clostridioides difficile* and resistant infections (Galloway-Peña *et al.*, 2017).

There are several studies indicating that prophylactic antimicrobials may have similar effects in disrupting microbial diversity in dogs. One study reported that the administration of the macrolide antimicrobial tylosin altered the GI microbial composition for prolonged periods, with changes continuing for over 28 days after completion of the antimicrobial course (Suchodolski *et al.*, 2009).

Another study demonstrated that oral administration of metronidazole markedly decreased bacterial diversity in the gut microbiome, with an increase in potentially pathogenic bacteria such as *Enterococcaceae*, *Enterobacteriaceae* and *Streptococcus* spp. (Igarashi *et al.*, 2014).

Appropriate cut-offs for initiating antimicrobial prophylaxis

For some neutropenic patients receiving chemotherapy, prophylactic antimicrobials can markedly reduce morbidity. However, there are also significant disadvantages to their use, and it is therefore important that they are reserved for those patients that truly benefit. The level of neutropenia that truly increases the risk of bacterial infection and 'requires' prophylaxis remains poorly defined in both human and veterinary patients. Most modern veterinary texts recommend prophylactic antimicrobials for any ANC less than 1.0×10^9 cells l^{-1} (Vail, 2009; Ettinger *et al.*, 2017; Gustafson and Bailey, 2019; Vail *et al.*, 2019). A survey of veterinarians with an interest in oncology found that 4% used an ANC cut-off of less than 0.5×10^9 cells l^{-1}, 58% used a cut-off of less than 1.0×10^9 cells l^{-1} and 29% used a cut-off of less than 1.5×10^9 cells l^{-1} (Regan *et al.*, 2013). This differs considerably from human guidelines where an ANC cut-off of less than 0.5×10^9 cells l^{-1} is routinely recommended in the UK and is as low as less than 0.1×10^9 cells l^{-1} for some patients in the USA (Phillips *et al.*, 2012; Flowers *et al.*, 2013). A recent veterinary study found that an ANC cut-off of less than 0.75×10^9 cells l^{-1} was very well tolerated in the 181 dogs studied, and there was no significant difference in the incidence of post-nadir FN or non-haematological toxicity between dogs receiving prophylactic antimicrobials and neutropenic dogs above the cut-off (neutrophil counts $0.75–3.6 \times 10^9$ cells l^{-1}) who did not receive prophylactic antimicrobials (Bisson *et al.*, 2020).

As with FN treatment, there is a suggestion that a patient's requirement for prophylactic antimicrobials can be stratified according to certain risk factors for the development of FN. In human oncology, patient factors such as acute leukaemia, stem-cell transplants, high-dose chemotherapy protocols and the first cycle of chemotherapy predispose patients to development of FN (Rapoport *et al.*, 2021). Similar risk factors have been recorded in dogs, including lower body weight, lymphoma, doxorubicin or vincristine administration, and dogs that are homozygous for the ABCB1-1Δ mutation (Box 15.1, Fig. 15.3) (Sorenmo *et al.*, 2010; Bisson *et al.*, 2018).

Cats have been found to be at higher risk of FN after lomustine or vinca alkaloid administration (Box 15.1) (Pierro *et al.*, 2017). The fact that most vets implement the same ANC cut-off for prophylaxis regardless of patient-specific risk factors has tended to form part of the argument for using higher cut-offs. However, in a study assessing an ANC cut-off of less than 0.75×10^9 cells l^{-1}, there was no significant difference in the incidence of non-haematological toxicity or post-nadir FN between patients with different weights or tumour types, or receiving different chemotherapy agents or chemotherapy dose numbers (Bisson *et al.*, 2020). This is despite the finding that lower neutrophil counts were significantly associated with lomustine

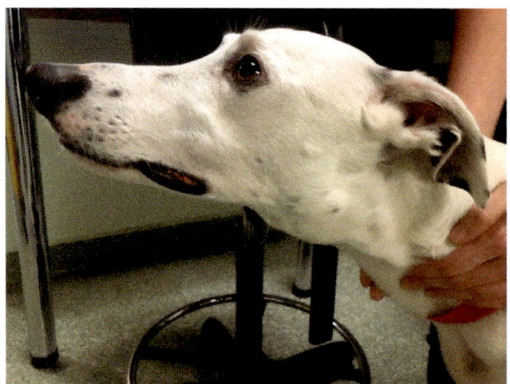

Fig. 15.3. A patient with high-grade multi-centric lymphoma prior to chemotherapy. Note the enlarged submandibular lymph nodes. Although the risk of developing febrile neutropenia is low, there is a higher risk for patients with lymphoma and those receiving vincristine or doxorubicin.

administration and earlier doses of chemotherapy (consistent with the first or second cycle). These findings suggest that even when taking into account some of the previously recognized risk factors for FN, this cut-off is well tolerated. However, it is important to note that vincristine administrations were not assessed in this study, and there were no dogs with the ABCB1-1Δ mutation (Bisson *et al.*, 2020). Attention to these risk factors is therefore warranted when considering antimicrobial prophylaxis for patients (Fig. 15.2). Genetic testing is also recommended for dogs of breeds with a known risk of the ABCB1-1Δ mutation (e.g. collies and herding breeds) prior to initiation of treatment with drugs transported by the P-glycoprotein pump that the gene encodes (including vincristine and doxorubicin) (Mealey *et al.*, 2008).

It is important to note that the numbers of animals developing FN after standard veterinary cancer chemotherapy protocols are very low and the risk of serious complications of this FN even lower. However, the development of mild to moderate asymptomatic neutropenia is relatively common. Using an ANC cut-off of less than 1.5×10^9 cells l^{-1} would increase antimicrobial prescriptions by more than 50% compared with the cut-off of less than 0.75×10^9 cells l^{-1} assessed in a recent study, and these prescriptions appeared to be unnecessary (Bisson *et al.*, 2020). As well as the risks of antimicrobial resistance and disruption of the microbiome, frequent antimicrobial prescription during chemotherapy can create significant additional financial pressure for owners, as well as the stress of administering medication to patients at home.

It could be argued that the ANC cut-off of less than 0.75×10^9 cells l^{-1} assessed by Bisson *et al.* (2020) was too conservative and could be lowered further to match human guidelines. However, there

Jocelyn Bisson

is currently no evidence to support this opinion, and caution is advised for several reasons. The exact timing of the neutrophil nadir is heterogeneous in dogs: as CBC is typically measured only once after chemotherapy administration, its timing may not represent the 'true' neutrophil nadir, with the ANC potentially continuing to drop thereafter. In addition, clinical signs of FN may be harder to detect in veterinary patients than in humans, and pet owners may be more likely to discontinue chemotherapy treatment if any adverse effects occur. Future studies are needed to investigate the tolerability of lower ANC cut-offs and the possible benefit of stratifying ANC cut-offs according to individual risk factors for developing FN.

Appropriate antimicrobials for prophylactic use

Most human guidelines recommend fluoroquinolones for antimicrobial prophylaxis in neutropenic patients. Fluoroquinolones are favoured as they have a broad spectrum but relatively little anaerobic action, which helps to spare the GI flora. TMPS has similar broad-spectrum and anaerobe-sparing qualities but has been found to cause more adverse effects in humans including myelosuppression and *C. difficile* colitis (Bisson *et al*., 2018). However, there were no significant differences in mortality, febrile episodes or bacteraemia between fluoroquinolones and TMPS in a meta-analysis (Gafter-Gvili *et al*., 2012).

Fluoroquinolones are notorious for driving the evolution of resistant bacteria, and NICE guidelines recommend that cancer centres in which patients are receiving fluoroquinolones for antimicrobial prophylaxis should closely monitor rates of antimicrobial resistance (Phillips *et al*., 2012). One human literature review and modelling study in the USA suggested that for a 30% reduction in antimicrobial efficacy, there would be 683 additional deaths per year in patients receiving chemotherapy for haematological malignancies (Teillant *et al*., 2015). This demonstrates the importance of such antimicrobials in human oncology and the real human cost of increasing rates of resistance. Fluoroquinolones are listed by the World Health Organization (WHO) as critically important for human medicine and should be safeguarded; any prophylactic use in veterinary medicine is therefore strongly discouraged (Bisson *et al*., 2018).

TMPS has been associated with a number of adverse effects in dogs including blood dyscrasias, keratoconjunctivitis sicca, hypothyroidism, hyperkalaemia, cholestasis, acute hepatic necrosis and skin disease (Trepanier, 2004). This association decreased their popularity as a viable clinical choice in the past. However, these effects are reasonably rare, and no adverse effects attributable to TMPS have been reported in the two main veterinary studies assessing antimicrobial prophylaxis in veterinary chemotherapy patients (Chretin *et al*., 2007; Bisson *et al*., 2020). TMPS is therefore considered the most appropriate antimicrobial for prophylactic use in these patients. For individual cases where TMPS is contraindicated, such as patients with a known intolerance or risk factor (e.g. those with existing keratoconjunctivitis sicca), an alternative antimicrobial such as a penicillin-like drug or (after very careful consideration) a fluoroquinolone may be used. However, penicillin-like drugs are not considered an ideal initial choice due to their increased anaerobic activity and negative effect on the GI microbiome when compared with TMPS.

The length of prophylactic antimicrobial course required is very poorly studied. Typically, neutropenia will resolve rapidly after the neutrophil nadir, usually within 24–48 h. However, CBC results obtained on one day is very much a 'snapshot in time' and does not indicate whether the patient's ANC is rising or falling (Boudreaux, 2014). Therefore, veterinary texts typically recommend a 3–7-day course of prophylactic antimicrobials following documentation of the neutropenia (Bisson *et al*., 2018). Based on the discussion of course length above, it would appear prudent to opt for the shortest course possible, ideally with repetition of another CBC after 2–3 days, and discontinuation of antimicrobials as soon as the ANC is above the cut-off value.

Alternative strategies for reducing infection

As discussed above, for most FN patients the source of infection is from their own GI tract. Historically, upon documentation of neutropenia, many human protocols have recommended the initiation of a 'neutropenic diet' due to the risk of certain uncooked foods, particularly fresh fruits and vegetables, containing *E. coli*, *Pseudomonas aeruginosa* and other Gram-negative bacilli (Gardner *et al*., 2008). Generally, neutropenic diets advise cooking of all food and limiting raw ingredients; however, there is poor evidence that these diets actually help to prevent infections or reduce mortality (Carr and Halliday, 2015). Recently, there has been increasing concern over the risk of bacterial pathogens affecting dogs fed raw meat-based diets; a recent study revealed a significant increase in the excretion of zoonotic and resistant bacteria in the faeces of dogs fed raw meat-based diets compared with those fed dry kibble (Runesvärd et al., 2020). While no studies exist to guide recommendations on raw feeding in dogs on chemotherapy, it would appear prudent to advise against raw feeding in these patients given the increased risk of GI colonization by pathogenic bacteria and presumed subsequent risk of translocation and bacteraemia.

Additionally, there is no evidence for the use of other infection-control measures in neutropenic veterinary chemotherapy patients. However, well-known infection control measures such as reverse barrier nursing of hospitalized patients to avoid transfer of nosocomial infections and strict aseptic technique when placing IV cannulas or performing other procedures is strongly recommended. As discussed above, clinically well patients should be cared for at home to reduce the risk of nosocomial infections.

Occasionally, human oncologists will also utilize GCSF in an attempt to combat severe neutropenia. GCSF is a haematopoietic growth factor that promotes the proliferation and maturation of neutrophil precursors in the bone marrow, thus increasing the neutrophil count (Xu et al., 2000). There are several synthetic, injectable versions available such as filgrastim and pegfilgrastim. In human patients, prophylactic administration of these drugs has been shown to reduce the duration of grade 3 or 4 neutropenia (ANC less than 1×10^9 cells l^{-1}) and decrease the incidence of FN (Jolis et al., 2013). However, their use in human oncology remains controversial, with several studies unable to demonstrate a reduction in mortality for patients receiving GCSF (Skoetz et al., 2015). US and UK guidelines recommend against offering GCSF for most patients unless they are undergoing a high-risk chemotherapy protocol (such protocols are not used in veterinary patients) (Phillips et al., 2012; Flowers et al., 2013).

There is very limited evidence on the use of GCSF in dogs. Both canine recombinant and human GCSF products are extremely expensive and have limited availability (Bisson et al., 2018). The use of human GCSF products in dogs carries a risk of cross-species antibody production, which has been reported to neutralize not only the human GCSF but also the endogenous canine GCSF, leading to an even more severe neutropenia (Yamamoto et al., 2011). One study in six healthy research beagles found that canine GCSF accelerated the recovery from neutropenia following cyclophosphamide treatment; however, it is difficult to apply this finding to all canine patients. In a study of 70 dogs hospitalized for FN, GCSF use was significantly associated with death in hospital; although this was suspected to be related to bias, it is a potentially concerning finding (Britton et al., 2014). It is therefore not possible to recommend the use of GCSF in veterinary patients, except in cases of very severe neutropenia that is expected to be prolonged, or if a known chemotherapy overdose has occurred (Bisson et al., 2018).

Counterintuitively, there are numerous studies where dogs experiencing neutropenia during chemotherapy protocols had improved disease outcomes; this is probably due to more appropriate dosing and complies with the maximum tolerated dose concept of chemotherapy administration (Gustafson and Bailey, 2019). Despite this, any patient with neutropenia requiring antimicrobial prophylaxis (and certainly any incidence of FN) should be considered an unacceptable haematological toxicity, and reduction of any subsequent dose of chemotherapy would be advised. Specific guidelines for dose reductions are not available, and clinicians will empirically reduce the dose by between 10% and 25% following severe haematological toxicity (Gustafson and Bailey, 2019).

For neutropenia that does not result in the patient being clinically unwell or requiring antimicrobial prophylaxis, chemotherapy dose reduction may not be required. However, if this neutropenia causes the subsequent chemotherapy dose to be delayed, then a dose reduction is advised to prevent further dose delays. A study in 64 dogs receiving CHOP (cyclophosphamide, doxorubicin, vincristine and prednisolone) chemotherapy for lymphoma found that chemotherapy administered for any ANC of more than 1.5×10^9 cells l^{-1} did not result in any increased toxicity compared with other ANC cut-offs (Fournier et al., 2018). Therefore, no chemotherapy dose reductions should be required for any ANC of more than 1.5×10^9 cells l^{-1} unless the patient is clinically unwell or has other chemotherapy adverse effects such as GI effects.

Jocelyn Bisson

15.3 Other Immunosuppressive Medications

In addition to cancer chemotherapy, numerous other immunosuppressive medications are widely used in veterinary practice, primarily to treat immune-mediated and inflammatory disease or to prevent organ rejection following renal transplantation in cats (Ettinger *et al.*, 2017). Although secondary infections have been reported following treatment with a wide variety of immunosuppressive agents including glucocorticoids, azathioprine, mycophenolate mofetil and leflunomide, infections after cyclosporine are prominently reported in the literature (Archer *et al.*, 2014). In one study, dogs receiving cyclosporine treatment for immune-mediated disease were 7.1 times more likely to develop an opportunistic invasive fungal infection compared with dogs receiving other immunosuppressive medications (McAtee *et al.*, 2017). In 95 dogs receiving cyclosporine at immunosuppressive dosages, the prevalence of secondary bacterial infection was 17%, with infections occurring most frequently in the GI, urinary and respiratory systems and often at more than one body site (High and Olivry, 2020). Interestingly cyclosporine has not been associated with myelosuppression and neutropenia but rather exerts its potent immunosuppressive function via T-cell suppression (Archer *et al.*, 2014). Cyclosporine forms a complex with cyclophilin A, an abundant immunophilin in T-cells, leading to blocked T-cell activation (Narayanan *et al.*, 2020).

The management of infections secondary to immunosuppressive agents depends on the severity of the infection and of the underlying disease. For severe infections it would typically involve stopping or reducing the dose of the immunosuppressive agent and providing appropriate antimicrobials based on culture and susceptibility testing and the site of infection (Archer *et al.*, 2014). For patients where the dose of the immunosuppressive cannot be reduced due to the underlying immune-mediated disease, the prognosis is more guarded. However, some successes have been reported in fungal disease by reducing the cyclosporine dose and increasing the glucocorticoid dose to compensate (McAtee *et al.*, 2017). A recent study revealed that T-cell expression of IL-2 and interferon-γ in healthy dogs starts to return to pre-cyclosporine treatment values within 24 h of cessation of the drug; however, it may take several days for consistent cytokine expression, an important consideration when treating severe or

life-threatening infectious complications in these patients (Narayanan *et al.*, 2020).

No veterinary guidelines on antimicrobial prophylaxis for patients on immunosuppressive therapy are available. Gleaning relevant information from the human literature is also challenging, as there is marked heterogeneity in the immunosuppressive medications used and conditions treated and a lack of standardized human medical guidelines. In general, antimicrobial prophylaxis in humans is reserved for those patients on high-dose immunosuppressive agents with additional risk factors such as old age or coexisting pulmonary disease (Malpica *et al.*, 2019). These patients may be offered TMPS as prophylaxis for *Pneumocystis jirovecii* pneumonia (Malpica *et al.*, 2019). TMPS has also been found to reduce the incidence of major infection in patients receiving immunosuppressives for systemic lupus erythematosus but is still not widely recommended in the majority of patients (Ganu *et al.*, 2021).

An important consideration in human patients on immunosuppressants is the recrudescence of viral diseases such as hepatitis B, and screening and vaccination are often performed prior to starting the immunosuppressive (Malpica *et al.*, 2019). Consideration of concurrent conditions prior to implementing immunosuppression is also important in veterinary patients, with possible complicating factors including but not limited to: feline caliciviruses and herpesviruses, *Toxoplasma gondii*, surgical implants such as pacemakers or urinary stents, or the presence of severe osteoarthritis, laryngeal paralysis or megaoesophagus (Ettinger *et al.*, 2017). Many immune-mediated conditions present with severe disease, leaving the clinician little choice but to start rapid immunosuppression. However, for patients with underlying conditions, careful consideration of their management plan including the dose and route of administration of the immunosuppressive agent and any additional monitoring that may be required is recommended (Ettinger *et al.*, 2017). Correct dosing regimens can be challenging to refine; for instance, a cyclosporine dosing protocol has not been established in the dog, and even individual dogs with the same blood cyclosporine concentration may vary in immune response (Riggs *et al.*, 2013). However, a quantitative reverse transcription PCR-based assay has now emerged allowing monitoring of cyclosporine action at a molecular level in order to achieve acceptable immunosuppressive effects while minimizing the risk of secondary infections (Riggs *et al.*, 2013). Owners should be counselled on careful monitoring for any evidence of fever or other signs of secondary infection. Human guidelines emphasize the importance of patient counselling, and human patients are advised to minimize infection via careful hand hygiene and food preparation (Malpica *et al.*, 2019). These precautions also apply to veterinary patients with reverse barrier nursing during hospitalization, and consideration of avoiding raw diets (as discussed above) is recommended.

15.4 Naturally Occurring Immunosuppression

In addition to drug-induced immunosuppression, 'naturally occurring' immunodeficiency is also reported. Primary immunodeficiency is rare in dogs and cats but includes numerous congenital disorders that affect innate or adaptive immunity such as Pelger–Huët syndrome and canine cyclical haematopoiesis. Unfortunately, due to their rarity, data on infection control in affected patients are extremely limited (DeBey, 2010).

Secondary immunodeficiency is far more common in dogs and cats, and can occur for multiple reasons including endocrinopathy (in particular hyperadrenocorticism and diabetes mellitus), barrier damage (burns, urinary catheters, IV cannulas) and myelodysplastic disorders (Ettinger *et al.*, 2017). The best evidence for the management of infections due to secondary immunodeficiency is found in relation to the management of urinary tract infections, and the International Society for Companion Animal Infectious Diseases (ISCAID) has produced extensive guidelines (Weese *et al.*, 2019). Taking the example of diabetes mellitus and urinary tract infections in cats, such infections are common in diabetic patients and occur regardless of the diabetic control status (Bailiff *et al.*, 2006). Routine screening of diabetic cats for bacteriuria has previously been recommended; however, this practice is becoming increasingly controversial as there is no evidence to demonstrate a beneficial effect of antimicrobial treatment in subclinical, culture-positive cats (Dorsch *et al.*, 2019). In addition, there is no evidence for the use of prophylactic antimicrobials in these patients (Weese *et al.*, 2019). Overall, any infection resulting from secondary immunodeficiency is typically best addressed by treating the underlying cause of the immunodeficiency, such as removing the urinary catheter or improved control of the endocrinopathy (Ettinger *et al.*, 2017). To treat clinical infections more effectively, the clinician needs to recognize the key features of primary or secondary immunodeficiency in patients, including recurrent or chronic infections, opportunistic infection with normally harmless or commensal organisms, an adverse response to modified live vaccines or ill-thrift in neonates. However, there is little evidence for further intervention such as screening for subclinical infection or providing prophylactic antimicrobials to at-risk patients (Ettinger *et al.*, 2017; Dorsch *et al.*, 2019).

15.5 Conclusion

There is limited evidence available to guide veterinary clinicians when prescribing antimicrobials for immunosuppressed patients. However, a few key points are clear. Immunosuppressed patients that are unwell with clinical signs of neutropenic sepsis require rapid intervention and broad-spectrum antimicrobial cover. Conversely, clinically well, immunosuppressed patients require careful consideration before prophylactic antimicrobials are prescribed; any benefits of antimicrobial use must be balanced with the risks of generating antimicrobial resistance and the effects on the patient's microbiome.

References

Archer, T.M., Boothe, D.M., Langston, V.C., Fellman, C.L., Lunsford, K.V. *et al.* (2014) Oral cyclosporine treatment in dogs: a review of the literature. *Journal of Veterinary Internal Medicine* 28(1), 1–20. DOI: 10.1111/jvim.12265.

AVMA (2022) Antimicrobial stewardship definition and core principles. American Veterinary Medical Association, Schaumburg, Illinois. Available at: www.avma.org/resources-tools/avma-policies/antimicrobial-stewardship-definition-and-core-principles (accessed 28 October 2022).

Bailiff, N.L., Nelson, R.W., Feldman, E.C., Westropp, J.L., Ling, G.V. *et al.* (2006) Frequency and risk factors for urinary tract infection in cats with diabetes mellitus. *Journal of Veterinary Internal Medicine* 20(4), 850–855. DOI: 10.1892/0891-6640(2006)20[850:farffu]2.0.co;2.

Barash, N.R., Birkenheuer, A.J., Vaden, S.L. and Jacob, M.E. (2018) Agreement between parallel canine blood and urine cultures: is urine culture the poor man's blood culture? *Journal of Clinical Microbiology* 56(9), e00506-18. DOI: 10.1128/JCM.00506-18.

Bisson, J.L., Argyle, D.J. and Argyle, S.A. (2018) Antibiotic prophylaxis in veterinary cancer chemotherapy: a review and recommendations. *Veterinary and Comparative Oncology* 16(3), 301–310. DOI: 10.1111/vco.12406.

Bisson, J.L., Fournier, Q., Johnston, E., Handel, I. and Bavcar, S. (2020) Evaluation of a 0.75×10^9/L absolute neutrophil count cut-off for antimicrobial prophylaxis in canine cancer chemotherapy patients. *Veterinary and Comparative Oncology* 18(3), 258–268. DOI: 10.1111/vco.12544.

Bodey, G.P., Buckley, M., Sathe, Y.S. and Freireich, E.J. (1966) Quantitative relationships between circulating leukocytes and infection in patients with acute leukemia. *Annals of Internal Medicine* 64(2), 328–340. DOI: 10.7326/0003-4819-64-2-328.

Boudreaux, B. (2014) Antimicrobial use in the veterinary cancer patient. *Veterinary Clinics of North America. Small Animal Practice* 44(5), 883–891. DOI: 10.1016/j.cvsm.2014.05.004.

Britton, B.M., Kelleher, M.E., Gregor, T.P. and Sorenmo, K.U. (2014) Evaluation of factors associated with prolonged hospital stay and outcome of febrile neutropenic patients receiving chemotherapy: 70 cases (1997-2010). *Veterinary and Comparative Oncology* 12(4), 266–276. DOI: 10.1111/vco.12001.

BSAVA/SAMSoc (2018) PROTECT ME. British Small Animal Veterinary Association/Small Animal Medicine Society, Quedgeley, UK. Available at: www.bsava.com/Resources/Veterinary-resources/PROTECT-ME/ (accessed 28 October 2022).

Buss, B.A., Baures, T.J., Yoo, M., Hanson, K.E., Alexander, D.P. et al. (2018) Impact of a multiplex pcr assay for bloodstream infections with and without antimicrobial stewardship intervention at a cancer hospital. *Open Forum Infectious Diseases* 5, ofy258. DOI: 10.1093/ofid/ofy258.

Carr, S.E. and Halliday, V. (2015) Investigating the use of the neutropenic diet: a survey of U.K. dietitians. *Journal of Human Nutrition and Dietetics* 28(5), 510–515. DOI: 10.1111/jhn.12266.

Chotiprasitsakul, D., Han, J.H., Cosgrove, S.E., Harris, A.D., Lautenbach, E. et al. (2018) Comparing the outcomes of adults with Enterobacteriaceae bacteremia receiving short-course versus prolonged-course antibiotic therapy in a multicenter, propensity score-matched cohort. *Clinical Infectious Diseases* 66(2), 172–177. DOI: 10.1093/cid/cix767.

Chretin, J.D., Rassnick, K.M., Shaw, N.A., Hahn, K.A., Ogilvie, G.K. et al. (2007) Prophylactic trimethoprim-sulfadiazine during chemotherapy in dogs with lymphoma and osteosarcoma: a double-blind, placebo-controlled study. *Journal of Veterinary Internal Medicine* 21(1), 141–148. DOI: 10.1892/0891-6640(2007)21[141:ptdcid]2.0.co;2.

DeBey, M.C. (2010) Primary immunodeficiencies of dogs and cats. *Veterinary Clinics of North America: Small Animal Practice* 40(3), 425–438. DOI: 10.1016/j.cvsm.2010.01.001.

Dorsch, R., Teichmann-Knorrn, S. and Sjetne Lund, H. (2019) Urinary tract infection and subclinical bacteriuria in cats: a clinical update. *Journal of Feline Medicine and Surgery* 21(11), 1023–1038. DOI: 10.1177/1098612X19880435.

Drayson, M.T., Bowcock, S., Planche, T., Iqbal, G., Pratt, G., et al. (2019) Levofloxacin prophylaxis in patients with newly diagnosed myeloma (TEAMM): a multicentre, double-blind, placebo-controlled, randomised, phase 3 trial. *Lancet Oncology* 20(12), 1760–1772. DOI: 10.1016/S1470-2045(19)30506-6.

Ettinger, S.J., Feldman, E.C. and Côté, E. (2017) *Textbook of Veterinary Internal Medicine: Diseases of the Dog and the Cat*, 8th edn. Elsevier, St Louis, Missouri.

Flowers, C.R., Seidenfeld, J., Bow, E.J., Karten, C., Gleason, C. et al. (2013) Antimicrobial prophylaxis and outpatient management of fever and neutropenia in adults treated for malignancy: American Society of Clinical Oncology clinical practice guideline. *Journal of Clinical Oncology* 31(6), 794–810. DOI: 10.1200/JCO.2012.45.8661.

Fournier, Q., Serra, J.C., Handel, I. and Lawrence, J. (2018) Impact of pretreatment neutrophil count on chemotherapy administration and toxicity in dogs with lymphoma treated with CHOP chemotherapy. *Journal of Veterinary Internal Medicine* 32(1), 384–393. DOI: 10.1111/jvim.14895.

Freifeld, A.G., Bow, E.J., Sepkowitz, K.A., Boeckh, M.J., Ito, J.I, et al. (2011) Clinical practice guideline for the use of antimicrobial agents in neutropenic patients with cancer: 2010 update by the Infectious Diseases Society of America. *Clinical Infectious Diseases* 52(4), e56–93. DOI: 10.1093/cid/cir073.

Gafter-Gvili, A., Fraser, A., Paul, M. and Leibovici, L. (2005) Meta-analysis: antibiotic prophylaxis reduces mortality in neutropenic patients. *Annals of Internal Medicine* 142(12 Pt 1), 979–995. DOI: 10.7326/0003-4819-142-12_part_1-200506210-00008.

Gafter-Gvili, A., Fraser, A., Paul, M., Vidal, L., Lawrie, T.A, et al. (2012) Antibiotic prophylaxis for bacterial infections in afebrile neutropenic patients following chemotherapy. *Cochrane Database of Systematic Reviews* 1(1), CD004386. DOI: 10.1002/14651858.CD004386.pub3.

Galloway-Peña, J.R., Jenq, R.R. and Shelburne, S.A. (2017) Can consideration of the microbiome improve antimicrobial utilization and treatment outcomes in the oncology patient? *Clinical Cancer Research* 23(13), 3263–3268. DOI: 10.1158/1078-0432.CCR-16-3173.

Ganu, S.A., Mathew, A.J., Nadaraj, A., Jeyaseelan, L. and Danda, D. (2021) Cotrimoxazole prophylaxis prevents major infective episodes in patients with systemic lupus erythematosus on immunosuppressants: a non-concurrent cohort study. *Lupus* 30(6), 893–900. DOI: 10.1177/0961203321995238.

Gardner, A., Mattiuzzi, G., Faderl, S., Borthakur, G., Garcia-Manero, G. *et al.* (2008) Randomized comparison of cooked and noncooked diets in patients undergoing remission induction therapy for acute myeloid leukemia. *Journal of Clinical Oncology* 26(35), 5684–5688. DOI: 10.1200/JCO.2008.16.4681.

Garrett, L.D., Thamm, D.H., Chun, R., Dudley, R. and Vail, D.M. (2002) Evaluation of a 6-month chemotherapy protocol with no maintenance therapy for dogs with lymphoma. *Journal of Veterinary Internal Medicine* 16(6), 704–709. DOI: 10.1892/0891-6640(2002)016<0704:eoacpw>2.3.co;2.

Gustafson, D.L. and Bailey, D.B. (2019) Cancer chemotherapy. In: Vail, D.M., Thamm, D.H. and Liptak, J.M. (eds) *Withrow and MacEwen's Small Animal Clinical Oncology*, 6th edn. Elsevier, Philadelphia, Pennsylvania, pp. 182–208.

Gustafsson, I., Sjölund, M., Torell, E., Johannesson, M., Engstrand, L, *et al.* (2003) Bacteria with increased mutation frequency and antibiotic resistance are enriched in the commensal flora of patients with high antibiotic usage. *Journal of Antimicrobial Chemotherapy* 52(4), 645–650. DOI: 10.1093/jac/dkg427.

High, E.J. and Olivry, T. (2020) The prevalence of bacterial infections during cyclosporine therapy in dogs: a critically appraised topic. *Canadian Veterinary Journal* 61, 1283–1289.

Igarashi, H., Maeda, S., Ohno, K., Horigome, A., Odamaki, T. *et al.* (2014) Effect of oral administration of metronidazole or prednisolone on fecal microbiota in dogs. *PloS One* 9(9), e107909. DOI: 10.1371/journal.pone.0107909.

Iida, N., Dzutsev, A., Stewart, C.A., Smith, L., Bouladoux, N. *et al.* (2013) Commensal bacteria control cancer response to therapy by modulating the tumor microenvironment. *Science* 342(6161), 967–970. DOI: 10.1126/science.1240527.

Jolis, L., Carabantes, F., Pernas, S., Cantos, B., López, A. *et al.* (2013) Incidence of chemotherapy-induced neutropenia and current practice of prophylaxis with granulocyte colony-stimulating factors in cancer patients in Spain: a prospective, observational study. *European Journal of Cancer Care* 22(4), 513–521. DOI: 10.1111/ecc.12057.

Kern, W.V., Klose, K., Jellen-Ritter, A.S., Oethinger, M., Bohnert, J, *et al.* (2005) Fluoroquinolone resistance of *Escherichia coli* at a cancer center: epidemiologic evolution and effects of discontinuing prophylactic fluoroquinolone use in neutropenic patients with leukemia. *European Journal of Clinical Microbiology & Infectious Diseases* 24(2), 111–118. DOI: 10.1007/s10096-005-1278-x.

Koenig, C., Schneider, C., Morgan, J.E., Ammann, R.A., Sung, L. *et al.* (2020) Association of time to antibiotics and clinical outcomes in patients with fever and neutropenia during chemotherapy for cancer: a systematic review. *Supportive Care in Cancer* 28(3), 1369–1383. DOI: 10.1007/s00520-019-04961-4.

Kuderer, N.M., Dale, D.C., Crawford, J., Cosler, L.E. and Lyman, G.H. (2006) Mortality, morbidity, and cost associated with febrile neutropenia in adult cancer patients. *Cancer* 106(10), 2258–2266. DOI: 10.1002/cncr.21847.

LeBlanc, A.K., Atherton, M., Bentley, R.T., Boudreau, C.E., Burton, J.H, *et al.* (2021) Veterinary Cooperative Oncology Group – Common Terminology Criteria for Adverse Events (VCOG-CTCAE v2) following investigational therapy in dogs and cats. *Veterinary and Comparative Oncology* 19(2), 311–352. DOI: 10.1111/vco.12677.

Llewelyn, M.J., Fitzpatrick, J.M., Darwin, E., SarahTonkin, C., Gorton, C, *et al.* (2017) The antibiotic course has had its day. *British Medical Journal* 358, j3418. DOI: 10.1136/bmj.j3418.

Lo, N. and Cullen, M. (2006) Antibiotic prophylaxis in chemotherapy-induced neutropenia: time to reconsider. *Hematological Oncology* 24(3), 120–125. DOI: 10.1002/hon.783.

Lyman, G.H., Abella, E. and Pettengell, R. (2014) Risk factors for febrile neutropenia among patients with cancer receiving chemotherapy: a systematic review. *Critical Reviews in Oncology/Hematology* 90(3), 190–199. DOI: 10.1016/j.critrevonc.2013.12.006.

MacDonald, V.S., Thamm, D.H., Kurzman, I.D., Turek, M.M. and Vail, D.M. (2005) Does L-asparaginase influence efficacy or toxicity when added to a standard CHOP protocol for dogs with lymphoma? *Journal of Veterinary Internal Medicine* 19(5), 732–736. DOI: 10.1892/0891-6640(2005)19[732:dlieot]2.0.co;2.

Magalhães, R.J., Loeffler, A., Lindsay, J., Rich, M., Roberts, L, *et al.* (2010) Risk factors for methicillin-resistant staphylococcus aureus (MRSA) infection in dogs and cats: a case–control study. *Veterinary Research* 41, 55.

Malpica, L., van Duin, D. and Moll, S. (2019) Preventing infectious complications when treating non-malignant immune-mediated hematologic disorders. *American Journal of Hematology* 94(12), 1396–1412. DOI: 10.1002/ajh.25642.

McAtee, B.B., Cummings, K.J., Cook, A.K., Lidbury, J.A., Heseltine, J.C. *et al.* (2017) Opportunistic invasive cutaneous fungal infections associated with administration of cyclosporine to dogs with immune-mediated disease. *Journal of Veterinary Internal Medicine* 31(6), 1724–1729. DOI: 10.1111/jvim.14824.

Mealey, K.L., Fidel, J., Gay, J.M., Impellizeri, J.A., Clifford, C.A. *et al.* (2008) ABCB1-1Delta polymorphism can predict hematologic toxicity in dogs treated with vincristine. *Journal of Veterinary Internal Medicine* 22(4), 996–1000. DOI: 10.1111/j.1939-1676.2008.0122.x.

Moore, A.S., London, C.A., Wood, C.A., Williams, L.E., Cotter, S.M. *et al.* (1999) Lomustine (CCNU) for the treatment of resistant lymphoma in dogs. *Journal of*

Veterinary Internal Medicine 13(5), 395–398. DOI: 10.1892/0891-6640(1999)013<0395:lfttor>2.3.co;2.

Morgan, J.E. and Phillips, B. (2018) Winter 2017 Children's Cancer and Leukaemia Group febrile neutropenia audit. *Archives of Disease in Childhood* 103(12), 1187. DOI: 10.1136/archdischild-2018-315249.

Morgan, J.E., Phillips, B., Haeusler, G.M. and Chisholm, J.C. (2021) Optimising antimicrobial selection and duration in the treatment of febrile neutropenia in children. *Infection and Drug Resistance* 14, 1283–1293. DOI: 10.2147/IDR.S238567.

Narayanan, L., Mulligan, C., Durso, L., Thames, B., Thomason, J. *et al.* (2020) Recovery of T-cell function in healthy dogs following cessation of oral cyclosporine administration. *Veterinary Medicine and Science* 6(3), 277–282. DOI: 10.1002/vms3.230.

Northrup, N.C., Rassnick, K.M., Snyder, L.A., Stone, M.S., Kristal, O. *et al.* (2002) Neutropenia associated with vincristine and L-asparaginase induction chemotherapy for canine lymphoma. *Journal of Veterinary Internal Medicine* 16(5), 570–575. DOI: 10.1892/0891-6640(2002)016<0570:nawval>2.3.co;2.

Onufrak, N.J., Forrest, A. and Gonzalez, D. (2016) Pharmacokinetic and pharmacodynamic principles of anti-infective dosing. *Clinical Therapeutics* 38(9), 1930–1947. DOI: 10.1016/j.clinthera.2016.06.015.

Owattanapanich, W. and Chayakulkeeree, M. (2019) Efficacy of levofloxacin as an antibacterial prophylaxis for acute leukemia patients receiving intensive chemotherapy: a systematic review and meta-analysis. *Hematology* 24(1), 362–368. DOI: 10.1080/16078454.2019.1589706.

Page, R.L., McEntee, M.C., George, S.L., Williams, P.L., Heidner, G.L. *et al.* (1993) Pharmacokinetic and phase I evaluation of carboplatin in dogs. *Journal of Veterinary Internal Medicine* 7(4), 235–240. DOI: 10.1111/j.1939-1676.1993.tb01013.x.

Paul, M., Dickstein, Y., Schlesinger, A., Grozinsky-Glasberg, S., Soares-Weiser, K, *et al.* (2013) Beta-lactam versus beta-lactam-aminoglycoside combination therapy in cancer patients with neutropenia. *Cochrane Database of Systematic Reviews* 2013(6), CD003038. DOI: 10.1002/14651858.CD003038.pub2.

Perry, J.A. and Douglas, H. (2019) Immunomodulatory effects of surgery, pain, and opioids in cancer patients. *Veterinary Clinics of North America: Small Animal Practice* 49(6), 981–991. DOI: 10.1016/j.cvsm.2019.07.008.

Pflug, N., Kluth, S., Vehreschild, J.J., Bahlo, J., Tacke, D. *et al.* (2016) Efficacy of antineoplastic treatment is associated with the use of antibiotics that modulate intestinal microbiota. *Oncoimmunology* 5(6), e1150399. DOI: 10.1080/2162402X.2016.1150399.

Phillips, R., Hancock, B., Graham, J., Bromham, N., Jin, H, *et al.* (2012) Prevention and management of neutropenic sepsis in patients with cancer: summary of NICE guidance. *British Medical Journal* 345, e5368. DOI: 10.1136/bmj.e5368.

Pierro, J., Krick, E., Flory, A., Regan, R., DeRegis, C. *et al.* (2017) Febrile neutropenia in cats treated with chemotherapy. *Veterinary and Comparative Oncology* 15(2), 550–556. DOI: 10.1111/vco.12198.

Pizzo, P.A., Robichaud, K.J., Gill, F.A., Witebsky, F.G., Levine, A.S, *et al.* (1979) Duration of empiric antibiotic therapy in granulocytopenic patients with cancer. *American Journal of Medicine* 67(2), 194–200. DOI: 10.1016/0002-9343(79)90390-5.

Pugh, R., Grant, C., Cooke, R.P.D. and Dempsey, G. (2015) Short-course versus prolonged-course antibiotic therapy for hospital-acquired pneumonia in critically ill adults. *Cochrane Database of Systematic Reviews* 2015(8), CD007577. DOI: 10.1002/14651858.CD007577.pub3.

Rapoport, B.L., Cooksley, T., Johnson, D.B., Anderson, R. and Shannon, V.R. (2021) Treatment of infections in cancer patients: an update from the neutropenia, infection and myelosuppression study group of the Multinational Association for Supportive Care in Cancer (MASCC). *Expert Review of Clinical Pharmacology* 14(3), 295–313. DOI: 10.1080/17512433.2021.1884067.

Rasmussen, R.M., Kurzman, I.D., Biller, B.J., Guth, A. and Vail, D.M. (2017) Phase I lead-in and subsequent randomized trial assessing safety and modulation of regulatory T cell numbers following a maximally tolerated dose doxorubicin and metronomic dose cyclophosphamide combination chemotherapy protocol in tumour-bearing dogs. *Veterinary and Comparative Oncology* 15(2), 421–430. DOI: 10.1111/vco.12179.

Regan, R.C., Kaplan, M.S.W. and Bailey, D.B. (2013) Diagnostic evaluation and treatment recommendations for dogs with substage-a high-grade multicentric lymphoma: results of a survey of veterinarians. *Veterinary and Comparative Oncology* 11(4), 287–295. DOI: 10.1111/j.1476-5829.2012.00318.x.

Riggs, C., Archer, T., Fellman, C., Figueiredo, A.S., Follows, J. *et al.* (2013) Analytical validation of a quantitative reverse transcriptase polymerase chain reaction assay for evaluation of T-cell targeted immunosuppressive therapy in the dog. *Veterinary Immunology and Immunopathology* 156(3–4), 229–234. DOI: 10.1016/j.vetimm.2013.09.019.

Rodriguez, V., Burgess, M. and Bodey, G.P. (1973) Management of fever of unknown origin in patients with neoplasms and neutropenia. *Cancer* 32(4), 1007–1012. DOI: 10.1002/1097-0142(197310)32:4<1007::aid-cncr2820320437>3.0.co;2-m.

Runesvärd, E., Wikström, C., Fernström, L.-L. and Hansson, I. (2020) Presence of pathogenic bacteria in faeces from dogs fed raw meat-based diets or dry kibble. *Veterinary Record* 187(9), e71. DOI: 10.1136/vr.105644.

Shaffer, K., Bach, J. and Chun, R. (2016) Prospective study evaluating the incidence of bacteraemia and bacteriuria in afebrile and febrile neutropaenic dogs undergoing chemotherapy. *Veterinary Medicine and Science* 2(4), 281–294. DOI: 10.1002/vms3.49.

Skoetz, N., Bohlius, J., Engert, A., Monsef, I., Blank, O. *et al.* (2015) Prophylactic antibiotics or G(M)-CSF for the prevention of infections and improvement of survival in cancer patients receiving myelotoxic chemotherapy. *Cochrane Database of Systematic Reviews* 2015(12), CD007107. DOI: 10.1002/14651858. CD007107.pub3.

Sorenmo, K.U., Harwood, L.P., King, L.G. and Drobatz, K.J. (2010) Case-control study to evaluate risk factors for the development of sepsis (neutropenia and fever) in dogs receiving chemotherapy. *Journal of the American Veterinary Medical Association* 236(6), 650–656. DOI: 10.2460/javma.236.6.650.

Stern, A., Carrara, E., Bitterman, R., Yahav, D., Leibovici, L, *et al.* (2019) Early discontinuation of antibiotics for febrile neutropenia versus continuation until neutropenia resolution in people with cancer. *Cochrane Database of Systematic Reviews* 1(1), CD012184. DOI: 10.1002/14651858.CD012184.pub2.

Stevenson, M., Pandor, A., Martyn-St James, M., Rafia, R., Uttley, L, *et al.* (2016) Sepsis: the lightcycler septifast test MGRADE®, sepsitest™ and IRIDICA BAC BSI assay for rapidly identifying bloodstream bacteria and fungi - a systematic review and economic evaluation. *Health Technology Assessment* 20, 1–246.

Suchodolski, J.S., Dowd, S.E., Westermarck, E., Steiner, J.M., Wolcott, R.D. *et al.* (2009) The effect of the macrolide antibiotic tylosin on microbial diversity in the canine small intestine as demonstrated by massive parallel 16S rRNA gene sequencing. *BMC Microbiology* 9, 210. DOI: 10.1186/1471-2180-9-210.

Teillant, A., Gandra, S., Barter, D., Morgan, D.J. and Laxminarayan, R. (2015) Potential burden of antibiotic resistance on surgery and cancer chemotherapy antibiotic prophylaxis in the USA: a literature review and modelling study. *Lancet Infectious Diseases* 15(12), 1429–1437. DOI: 10.1016/S1473-3099(15)00270-4.

Thamm, D.H. and Vail, D.M. (2007) Aftershocks of cancer chemotherapy: managing adverse effects. *Journal of the American Animal Hospital Association* 43(1), 1–7. DOI: 10.5326/0430001.

Timmers, G.J., Dijstelbloem, Y., Simoons-Smit, A.M., van Winkelhoff, A.J., Touw, D.J. *et al.* (2004) Pharmacokinetics and effects on bowel and throat microflora of oral levofloxacin as antibacterial prophylaxis in neutropenic patients with haematological malignancies. *Bone Marrow Transplantation* 33(8), 847–853. DOI: 10.1038/sj.bmt.1704431.

Trepanier, L.A. (2004) Idiosyncratic toxicity associated with potentiated sulfonamides in the dog. *Journal of Veterinary Pharmacology and Therapeutics* 27(3), 129–138. DOI: 10.1111/j.1365-2885.2004.00576.x.

Vail, D.M. (2009) Supporting the veterinary cancer patient on chemotherapy: neutropenia and gastrointestinal toxicity. *Topics in Companion Animal Medicine* 24(3), 122–129. DOI: 10.1053/j.tcam.2009.02.004.

Vail, D.M., Thamm, D. and Liptak, J. (2019) *Withrow and MacEwen's Small Animal Clinical Oncology*. Elsevier, Philadelphia, Pennsylvania.

Vétizou, M., Pitt, J.M., Daillère, R., Lepage, P., Waldschmitt, N. *et al.* (2015) Anticancer immunotherapy by CTLA-4 blockade relies on the gut microbiota. *Science* 350(6264), 1079–1084. DOI: 10.1126/science.aad1329.

Viaud, S., Saccheri, F., Mignot, G., Yamazaki, T., Daillère, R. *et al.* (2013) The intestinal microbiota modulates the anticancer immune effects of cyclophosphamide. *Science* 342(6161), 971–976. DOI: 10.1126/science.1240537.

Vidal, L., Ben Dor, I., Paul, M., Eliakim-Raz, N., Pokroy, E, *et al.* (2013) Oral versus intravenous antibiotic treatment for febrile neutropenia in cancer patients. *Cochrane Database of Systematic Reviews* 2013(10), CD003992. DOI: 10.1002/14651858.CD003992.pub3.

Walther, B., Tedin, K. and Lübke-Becker, A. (2017) Multidrug-resistant opportunistic pathogens challenging veterinary infection control. *Veterinary Microbiology* 200, 71–78. DOI: 10.1016/j.vetmic.2016.05.017.

Weese, J.S., Blondeau, J., Boothe, D., Guardabassi, L.G., Gumley, N, *et al.* (2019) International Society for Companion Animal Infectious Diseases (ISCAID) guidelines for the diagnosis and management of bacterial urinary tract infections in dogs and cats. *Veterinary Journal* 247, 8–25. DOI: 10.1016/j.tvjl.2019.02.008.

Weycker, D., Barron, R., Kartashov, A., Legg, J. and Lyman, G.H. (2014) Incidence, treatment, and consequences of chemotherapy-induced febrile neutropenia in the inpatient and outpatient settings. *Journal of Oncology Pharmacy Practice* 20(3), 190–198. DOI: 10.1177/1078155213492450.

Wiebe, V. and Hamilton, P. (2002) Fluoroquinolone-induced retinal degeneration in cats. *Journal of the American Veterinary Medical Association* 221(11), 1568–1571. DOI: 10.2460/javma.2002.221.1568.

Xu, S., Höglund, M., Håkansson, L. and Venge, P. (2000) Granulocyte colony-stimulating factor (G-CSF) induces the production of cytokines *in vivo. British Journal of Haematology* 108(4), 848–853. DOI: 10.1046/j.1365-2141.2000.01943.x.

Yamamoto, A., Fujino, M., Tsuchiya, T. and Iwata, A. (2011) Recombinant canine granulocyte colony-stimulating factor accelerates recovery from cyclophosphamide-induced neutropenia in dogs. *Veterinary Immunology and Immunopathology* 142(3–4), 271–275. DOI: 10.1016/j.vetimm.2011.05.021.

Zur, G., Gurevich, B. and Elad, D. (2016) Prior antimicrobial use as a risk factor for resistance in selected *Staphylococcus pseudintermedius* isolates from the skin and ears of dogs. *Veterinary Dermatology* 27(6), 468–e125. DOI: 10.1111/vde.12382.

Jocelyn Bisson

16 Antibiotic Mechanism of Action and Resistance

THAWANRUT KIATYINGANGSULEE[1], SHABBIR SIMJEE[2]*, RUNGTIP CHUANCHUEN[3], FAYE SWINBOURNE[4] AND FERGUS ALLERTON[5]

[1]National Institute of Animal Health, Lat Yao, Chatuchak, Bangkok, Thailand; [2]Elanco Animal Health, Bartley Wood Business Park, Hook, UK; [3]Research Unit in Microbial Food Safety and Antimicrobial Resistance, Faculty of Veterinary Science, Chulalongkorn University, Pathum Wan, Bangkok, Thailand; [4]Lumbry Park Veterinary Specialists, Alton, UK; [5]Willows Veterinary Centre & Referral Service, Shirley, Solihull, UK

16.1 Introduction

An understanding of the mechanism of action of antibiotics can help guide optimal selection. A wide array of more than 20 different classes of antimicrobial is available, and the preferred agent must be chosen based on an anticipation of efficacy against the expected microorganisms at the target site. Clinicians should consider the properties of an antibiotic in terms of its spectrum of activity (often linked to the underlying mechanism of action), the ability to penetrate the site of infection (e.g. traverse the blood–brain or blood–prostate barrier), the pharmacokinetic/pharmacodynamic (PK/PD) characteristics (as these will impact dosing decisions) and the potential adverse effect profile, as well as, importantly, their priority-level classification from an antimicrobial resistance (AMR) perspective. This latter consideration is designated by international bodies such as the World Health Organization (WHO) and European Medicines Agency (EMA), and can help practitioners recognize the classes of antibiotics that should be reserved for specific use in human patients.

Given the increasing threat posed to human and animal health by AMR, it is also valuable to understand the machinations of bacterial resistance. This biological arms race can be observed before our very eyes in work performed at the Kishony Laboratory, at Harvard Medical School (Baym *et al.*, 2016). Interested readers are referred to https://hms. harvard.edu/news/bugs-screen (accessed 31 October 2022) for more information. Practitioners can make more informed antibiotic selections if they have an indication of how antibiotic efficacy may be impaired via intrinsic or acquired defences mounted by bacteria. This chapter will describe some of the mechanisms of antibiotic resistance found in bacteria.

16.2 Mechanism of Action

In general, antibiotics have one of four mechanisms of action reflecting their target site (Fig. 16.1 and Table 16.1):

1. They target the structural protective barriers of bacteria (e.g. inhibition of cell-wall synthesis or disruption of the cell membrane).
2. They inhibit protein synthesis.
3. They target bacterial nucleic acids (e.g. inhibition of DNA or RNA synthesis, or DNA degradation).
4. They inhibit biochemical pathways.

Antibiotic dosing regimens are designed to ensure sufficient drug exposure during treatment to effectively eliminate target bacteria. The application of PK/PD principles utilizes an understanding of the distribution and action of a specific antibiotic agent against a given pathogen. These data will allow sophisticated dosing schedules to be designed

---

*Corresponding author: SHABBIR.SIMJEE@elancoah.com

© CAB International 2023. *Infection Control in Small Animal Clinical Practice* (eds F. Allerton and K.L. Bowlt Blacklock)
DOI: 10.1079/9781789244977.0016

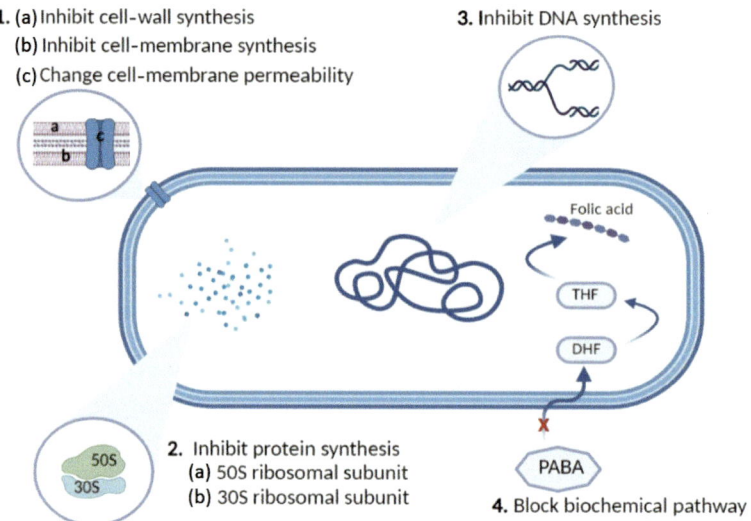

1. (a) Inhibit cell-wall synthesis
   (b) Inhibit cell-membrane synthesis
   (c) Change cell-membrane permeability

3. Inhibit DNA synthesis

Folic acid

THF

DHF

PABA

2. Inhibit protein synthesis
   (a) 50S ribosomal subunit
   (b) 30S ribosomal subunit

4. Block biochemical pathway

Fig. 16.1. Summary of the principle mechanisms of action of antibiotics. DHF, dihydrofolate; PABA, p-aminobenzoic acid; THF, tetrahydrofolate (modified from (Kapoor *et al.*, 2017).

Table 16.1. Summary of different mechanisms of action according to the class of antibiotic.

Mechanism of action	Antibiotics
Antibiotics targeting structural protective barriers	
Antibiotics that target cell-wall synthesis	β-Lactams (penicillin, cephalosporins, carbapenems), glycopeptides (vancomycin, teicoplanin), phosphonic acid
Antibiotics that target cell-membrane synthesis	Polymyxins, lipopeptides, cyclopeptides
Loss of outer-membrane permeability	Polymyxins
Antibiotics inhibiting protein synthesis	
Inhibition of the 30S ribosomal subunit	Aminoglycosides, tetracycline
Inhibition 50S ribosomal subunit mechanism	Macrolides, chloramphenicol, lincosamides, streptogramins, oxazolidinones
Antibiotics targeting nucleic acids	Fluoroquinolones, metronidazole, rifampicin
Antibiotics inhibiting biochemical pathways	Trimethoprim, sulfonamides

that optimize treatment efficacy while minimizing potential adverse effects of antibiotic use (McKellar *et al.*, 2004; Martinez *et al.*, 2012; Papich, 2014). Values such as the lowest concentration of antibiotic that inhibits the growth of the target bacteria (minimum inhibitory concentration (MIC)), peak plasma concentration of antibiotic (C_{max}) and area under the concentration–time curve (AUC) are used to determine optimal dosing regimens (Fig. 16.2). While PK/PD relationships are specific to both the antibiotic agent and pathogen in question, antibiotics can be broadly classified as time dependent or concentration dependent with defined parameters

used to determine optimal dosing schedules for each (McKellar *et al.*, 2004; Martinez *et al.*, 2012; Papich, 2014).

The efficacy of time-dependent agents, such as the β-lactam antibiotics, can be enhanced by increasing the duration of drug exposure. In PK/PD terms, this is typically evaluated as the time that the drug concentration exceeds the MIC for the target pathogen for a certain percentage of the dosing interval ($T >$ MIC). Exceeding MIC by 1–5 multiples for between 40% and 100% of the dosing interval is considered appropriate to achieve clinical efficacy for the majority of time-dependent agents (Levison and

Thawanrut Kiatyingangsulee *et al.*

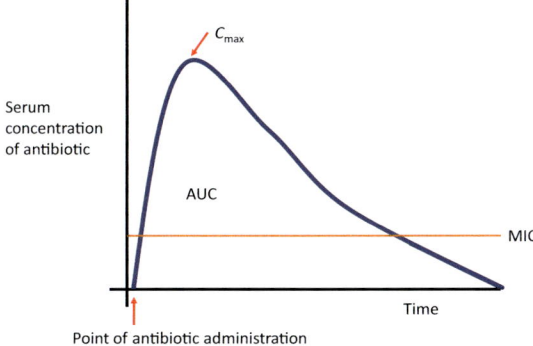

Fig. 16.2. Pharmacokinetic and pharmacodynamic parameters. AUC, area under the curve; C_{max}, peak antibiotic concentration; MIC, Minimum Inhibitory Concentration for a pathogen (modified from (Asín-Prieto *et al.*, 2015).

Levison, 2009). Further increases in the antibiotic concentration above a point of maximal bacterial cell killing action (approximately four times the MIC) has little additional effect, while increasing the dosing frequency can result in improved activity. For concentration-dependent agents, such as the fluoroquinolones, efficacy can be enhanced by increasing the concentration of drug at the target site. Peak plasma concentration to MIC ratio (C_{max}:MIC) or area under the curve to MIC ratio (AUC:MIC) are generally used to determine dosing regimens for concentration-dependent agents, with targets in excess of 100–125 for AUC:MIC and 8–10 for C_{max}:MIC frequently cited to achieve efficacy while minimizing bacterial selection for resistance (McKellar *et al.*, 2004; Papich, 2014).

Suboptimal dosing regimens risk selection for resistant bacterial populations by failing to achieve antibiotic concentrations that are effective against resistant bacteria. Antibiotic concentrations that effectively inhibit susceptible bacteria, but not resistant populations, will serve to amplify the resistant bacterial population (Martinez *et al.*, 2012; Guardabassi *et al.*, 2018). Optimal dosing regimens aim to limit the amount of time that an antibiotic is present at a concentration that will exert this effect, thereby minimizing selection pressure for resistance (Martinez *et al.*, 2012; Guardabassi *et al.*, 2018). The importance of achieving effective drug concentrations for appropriate durations of the dosing interval highlights the need to follow dosing guidelines for a given agent, and to educate owners in terms of compliance with the administration of the correct dose at the correct time. With many current veterinary dosing regimens designed before the application of PK/PD principles, and MIC data not yet available for some clinical isolates, work to revise dosing regimens for veterinary applications is ongoing (Levison and Levison, 2009).

16.2.1 Antibiotics that target the structural protective barriers of bacteria

The bacterial cell wall confers shape and structure to bacteria, protects the microorganism from external threats, including antibiotics, and contains proteins that contribute to the induction of the host immune response. Antibiotics that target the bacterial cell wall include β-lactams, glycopeptides and phosphonic acid (Bush, 2012; Sarkar *et al.*, 2017). Within the β-lactam group, there are several subclasses including narrow- and extended-spectrum penicillins, cephalosporins, monobactams and carbapenems, all of which contain the eponymous central β-lactam ring.

Damage to the integrity of the cell-wall barrier can be achieved via several different pathways.

Antibiotics that target cell-wall synthesis

Peptidoglycan is a vitally important component of the cell wall in most bacteria. Those bacteria that lack a cell wall (e.g. *Mycoplasma* spp.) do not contain peptidoglycan. Crucially, peptidoglycan is not present in eukaryotic cells.

Peptidoglycan consists of alternating residues of β-(1,4)-linked *N*-acetylglucosamine and *N*-acetylmuramic acid (NAM), which form linear glycan or polysaccharide chains. A short peptide chain is attached to each NAM residue and forms cross-links with other peptide chains, creating a three-dimensional mesh-like layer that confers strength and rigidity to the bacterial cell. The cell wall acts to prevent osmotic lysis of the bacterial cell. Cross-linking between the short peptide chains is catalysed by the DD-transpeptidase enzyme. This enzyme, also known as a penicillin-binding protein (PBP), is the target protein of β-lactam antibiotics (see below).

The classification of bacteria as Gram positive or Gram negative reflects differences in the structure of their peptidoglycan cell wall (the greater thickness of the cell wall in Gram-positive bacteria confers different staining properties). The cell membrane of Gram-positive bacteria is surrounded by a tough and rigid cell wall. In contrast, Gram-negative bacteria have a thin cell wall surrounded by a second lipid membrane (the outer membrane). The outer membrane prohibits access of many substances into the bacterium and thus offers extra protection against the effects of antibiotics. The space between the outer membrane and the cell or cytoplasmic membrane is called the periplasmic space.

The synthesis of peptidoglycan can be divided into three stages. The first stage (I) takes place within the cytoplasm and involves the synthesis of peptidoglycan precursors. The precursors must attach to a lipid carrier molecule (bactoprenol) to traverse the cell membrane (stage II), before being incorporated into the existing peptidoglycan matrix (stage III). Each stage of this process can be affected by different antibiotics. Stage I (the cytoplasmic stage) is targeted by antibiotics such as fosfomycin, while stage II (the membrane-associated stage) is affected by antibiotics such as ramoplanin. The last stage (the extracytoplasmic stage) is the target for several antibiotics including β-lactams, glycopeptides and bacitracin (de Kruijff *et al.*, 2008).

Antibiotics can interfere with cell-wall synthesis by several different mechanisms, including:

- inhibition of peptidoglycan synthesis;
- inhibition of the lipid carrier molecule; and
- inhibition of peptidoglycan cross-linkage.

Blumberg and Strominger (1974) first elucidated the mechanism of action of penicillin when they noticed structural similarities between penicillin and part of the peptidoglycan in the bacterial cell wall. β-Lactam antibiotics inhibit the last step of peptidoglycan biosynthesis, which is catalysed by bacterial transpeptidases. By binding to and inhibiting the enzyme that forms the cross-links between the peptide chains, β-lactam antibiotics directly interfere with cell-wall synthesis.

Because of this affinity for penicillin, the bacterial transpeptidases are also known as PBPs. The PBP inhibitory activity of penicillin and other β-lactam antibiotics is derived from their structural, geometric and stereochemical similarity to the enzyme. Importantly, inhibition is irreversible, and the structure of the peptidoglycan molecule is thus permanently compromised. Without an integral cell wall, the bacteria are susceptible to cell lysis and death. β-Lactams are time-dependent antibiotics.

Glycopeptides, such as vancomycin, also target cell-wall synthesis and are used to treat Gram-positive bacterial infections, including methicillin-resistant *Staphylococcus aureus* (MRSA). However, it is important to recognize that this class of antibiotic is not authorized for animal use in many countries and, given its highest priority critically important status, should be reserved for human-only use. Glycopeptides bind strongly and irreversibly to the D-Ala-D-Ala termini of the precursor peptidoglycan subunit at the outer surface of the cytoplasmic membrane, preventing its binding to the transpeptidase and transglycosylase enzymes that are essential for cross-linking (Kapoor *et al.*, 2017).

Antibiotics that target cell-membrane synthesis

The bacterial cell membrane is similar in structure to that of mammalian cells, comprising a phospholipid bilayer containing embedded proteins. However, this structural homogeneity means that the cell membrane is not an ideal target for antibiotics due to the potential toxicity towards the host animal. Antibiotics that target cell-membrane synthesis include polymyxins B and E (colistin). Polymyxins interact with the phospholipids of the cell membrane disrupting its structure. Polymyxin B is most often used for topical treatment in companion animals in the management of ear, eye and skin infections. Colistin is considered a last-resort antibiotic for life-threatening infections, including multidrug-resistant (MDR) bacteria and carbapenem-resistant bacteria (Hansen, 2021), and its use in companion animals is not advised (or even permitted in many countries) from an antibiotic stewardship perspective.

Loss of outer-membrane permeability

Gram-negative selectivity of polymyxins is mediated by the interaction with the outer membrane of Gram-negative bacteria. Polymyxins disrupt the outer membrane, increasing the permeability and leading to an ion imbalance and cell death. However, polymyxins will also permeabilize eukaryotic membranes, leading to swelling and lysis. High levels of renal and neural toxicity have historically limited the use of these medications in people.

16.2.2 Antibiotics that inhibit protein synthesis

Proteins are the building blocks of living cells, and any molecule that affects protein synthesis has the potential to cause cell death. Protein synthesis is completed within the cell by the ribosome, a cellular particle made of RNA and protein. The function of the ribosome is to translate the sequence of messenger RNA (mRNA) into a sequence of amino acids. Ribosomal structure is different between prokaryotes and eukaryotes: the former consists of a 50S and a 30S subunit, while mammalian ribosomes have 60S and 40S subunits. Antibiotics can affect bacterial protein synthesis by acting on the 30S ribosomal subunit and/or the 50S ribosomal subunit (Arenz and Wilson, 2016).

Inhibition of the 30S ribosomal subunit

Two antibiotic classes that affect the 30S ribosomal subunit are the aminoglycosides and tetracyclines.

Aminoglycosides (amikacin, gentamicin, neomycin and streptomycin) inhibit protein synthesis in bacteria by binding irreversibly to the 30S ribosomal subunit. Binding occurs at the aminoacyl site (the A site) of 16S ribosomal RNA within the 30S ribosomal subunit. This causes misreading of the mRNA codons and inhibition of translocation. Aminoglycosides disrupt the elongation of the amino acid chain by promoting failure of translational accuracy (an increased frequency of misreading). They do not interfere with the binding of mRNA to the 30S subunit or the association of the 50S ribosomal subunit. The increased error rate will lead to premature termination of the peptide chain and the incorrect generation of polypeptides that will damage the bacterial cell upon their release. Aminoglycosides also bind to the lipopolysaccharide layer of the cell wall, disrupting its permeability.

One step during the entry of aminoglycosides into the bacterial cell requires oxygen. Consequently, these antibiotics lack activity against anaerobic bacteria. Aminoglycosides are most effective against aerobic Gram-negative bacteria. They have a concentration-dependent killing pattern. Because binding to the 30S ribosomal subunit is irreversible, aminoglycosides also exert a post-antibiotic effect, lasting for multiple hours after the fall in serum concentration. Aminoglycosides have decreased activity at an acid pH, limiting their activity in abscesses.

Tetracyclines (including oxytetracycline, doxycycline and minocycline) inhibit bacterial growth by blocking translation. They bind (reversibly) to the receptor (A) site of the 16S ribosomal RNA portion of the 30S ribosomal subunit and prevent the amino-acyl transfer RNA from binding to the complementary mRNA. Tetracyclines also bind, to some extent, to the 50S ribosomal subunit. They have a broad-spectrum of activity, including efficacy against atypical microorganisms (e.g. *Mycoplasma* spp.).

Inhibition of the 50S ribosomal subunit

Several classes of antibiotic target bacteria at the 50S ribosomal subunit, including the macrolides, lincosamides, chloramphenicol and oxazolidinones.

Macrolides (azithromycin, clarithromycin and erythromycin) inhibit bacterial protein biosynthesis by inhibiting translocation. Translocation is the energy-dependent movement of the ribosome unit along the mRNA by one codon (three bases) and is essential to permit elongation of the protein molecule by adding new amino acids coded by sequential codons. Macrolides bind to the 23S portion of the 50S ribosomal subunit and cause premature dissociation of the transfer RNA. Some macrolides work instead by inhibiting bacterial ribosomal translation. Macrolides are particularly active against Gram-positive cocci.

Chloramphenicol diffuses through the bacterial cell wall and reversibly binds to the 23S portion of the bacterial 50S ribosomal subunit. The binding interferes with peptidyl transferase activity, thereby preventing the transfer of amino acids to the growing peptide chains and blocking peptide bond formation.

Lincosamides (clindamycin and lincomycin) have a similar mechanism of action to macrolides. They bind close to the peptidyl transferase centre on the 23S portion of the 50S subunit of bacterial ribosomes, inhibiting protein synthesis. Lincosamides can be used to treat Gram-positive infections, as well as many anaerobic bacterial infections.

Oxazolidinones and linezolid are novel broad-spectrum antibiotics that bind to the 50S subunit and inhibit protein synthesis. In contrast to the previous antibiotics that interact with the 50S subunit, oxazolidinones and linezolid inhibit both translation and translocation. This class of antibiotic is not authorized for companion animal use.

16.2.3 Antibiotics that affect nucleic acid synthesis

The major classes of antibiotic that interrupt nucleic acid (DNA and RNA) synthesis include the fluoroquinolones, metronidazole and rifampicin (Bhattacharjee, 2016).

Fluoroquinolones (ciprofloxacin, enrofloxacin, marbofloxacin, orbifloxacin and pradofloxacin) act by inhibiting two DNA bacterial type II topoisomerases (DNA gyrase and DNA topoisomerase IV) that are essential for bacterial DNA synthesis. Reversible binding of the antibiotic to the enzyme complexes blocks the resealing of the DNA double-strand break, inhibiting DNA replication. Mammalian cells use topoisomerase II for DNA synthesis, rather than DNA gyrase or topoisomerase IV. Topoisomerase II has a very low affinity for fluoroquinolones, ensuring bacterial specificity while limiting host-cell damage (Hooper, 2001). Fluoroquinolones have a concentration-dependent bacterial killing property and are effective against Gram-negative bacteria (including *Pseudomonas* spp.), as well as having some anti-staphylococcal and anti-streptococcal properties. Four generations of fluoroquinolone have been described (to date) with an increasing spectrum of activity, including superior Gram-positive activity with each subsequent generation, as well as enhanced efficacy against anaerobes and mycobacteria and *Mycoplasma* spp.

Rifampicin (also known as rifampin) inhibits protein synthesis by a very specific inhibition of bacterial DNA-dependent RNA polymerase, thereby blocking the synthesis of mRNA. Rifampicin is not authorized for use in veterinary species but has been proposed as a component of multi-modal therapy for feline tuberculosis (Gunn-Moore *et al.*, 1996).

The mechanism of action of nitroimidazoles (metronidazole) has not yet been fully elucidated. What is known is that metronidazole is able to gain entry to the bacterial cell without the help of any transporting mechanism, entering cells by passive diffusion. Once inside the cell, the metronidazole pro-drug becomes active after being reduced to its nitro group (a free radical entity). Significantly, this reaction occurs only under very low oxygen concentrations – a property that underlies the therapeutic role of metronidazole in managing anaerobic infections.

Various different active intermediates generated by the reduction of metronidazole have been suggested to have toxic activity within bacteria and protozoa. It is likely that multiple different pathways can lead to the generation of these intermediates in microaerophiles and anaerobes. The reduced intermediates of metronidazole bind bacterial DNA, causing damage including strand breaks. This action impairs bacterial nucleic acid synthesis, causing cell death in susceptible organisms.

16.2.4 Antibiotics targeting biochemical pathways

Antibiotics can disrupt cell function by blocking metabolic pathways, impairing the production of metabolites that are essential to the survival of the bacteria. One example of this is the inhibition of folic acid synthesis in bacteria (Fernández-Villa *et al.*, 2019). Mammalian cells obtain sufficient folic acid from dietary ingestion, which explains the selective action of sulfonamides against microorganisms. The folic acid pathway is essential for the synthesis of purines and pyrimidines, and thus DNA.

Trimethoprim is a direct competitor of the enzyme dihydrofolate reductase, thereby blocking the production of tetrahydrofolate from dihydrofolic acid (folic acid). The decreased availability of tetrahydrofolate impairs purine synthesis with knock-on effects on the production of DNA and protein by the bacteria. This antibacterial effect can be optimized by the synergistic use of a sulfonamide with the trimethoprim. Sulfonamides (e.g. sulfamethoxazole or sulfadiazine) directly inhibit the synthesis of folate inside bacteria. Sulfamethoxazole is a structural analogue of *p*-aminobenzoic acid (PABA), the first building block used by bacteria, and thus inhibits the enzyme dihydropteroate synthase. Combination antibiotic therapy involving both a sulfonamide and trimethoprim blocks two steps in the bacterial biosynthesis of essential nucleic acids and proteins, maximizing the lethal potential of these molecules.

16.3 Mechanisms of Resistance

Bacterial AMR can be intrinsic (a naturally occurring phenomenon that pre-dates antibiotic chemotherapy) or acquired (adoption of new resistance pathways that compromise the efficacy of a previously effective antibiotic). Mechanisms that contribute to the intrinsic 'resistome' include structural traits of individual bacteria (e.g. the outer membrane of Gram-negative bacteria blocking entry of the antibiotic into the bacterial cell, or the absence of peptidoglycan in *Mycoplasma* spp.) and the rapid removal of the antibiotic from bacteria via an efflux pump. Intrinsic resistance has been documented in environmental, soil-dwelling bacteria and vastly pre-dates human antibiotic use. The gene encoding resistance to β-lactam, tetracycline and glycopeptide antibiotics was found in metagenome samples of 30,000-year-old permafrost (D'Costa *et al.*, 2011). Knowledge of intrinsic resistance patterns can avoid inherently ineffective antibiotic use (Allerton and Nuttall, 2021). For example, *Bordetella bronchiseptica* shows very low susceptibility to cephalosporins due, at least in part, to an intrinsic reduction in outer-membrane permeability to this antibiotic (Kadlec *et al.*, 2007).

Mechanisms of acquired resistance fall into three main categories (Fig. 16.3 and Table 16.2), and some bacteria may operate more than one protective mechanism simultaneously (Reygaert, 2018):

1. Modifications to the antibiotic itself (chemical alteration or inactivation of the antibiotic).
2. Reduction of intracellular antimicrobial concentrations through the prevention of antibiotic

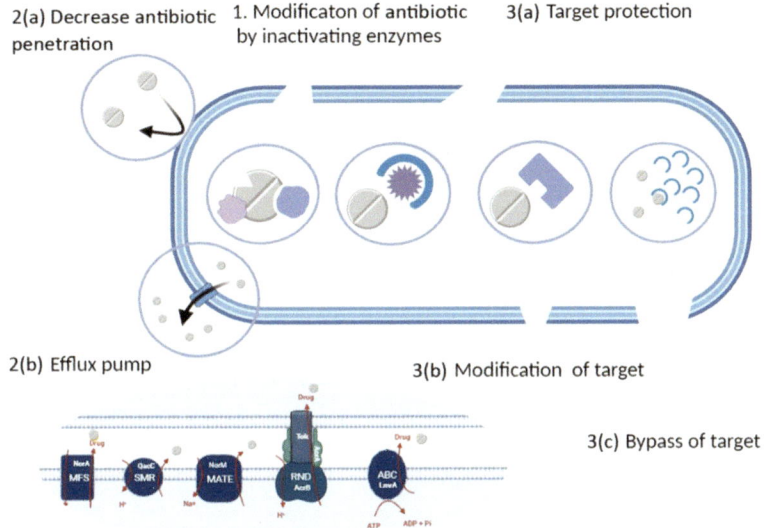

Fig. 16.3. Summary of the mechanisms of antibiotic resistance.

Table 16.2. Summary of different mechanisms of resistance including example antibiotics affected.

Mechanism of resistance	Examples
Modification of the antibiotic molecule	
Alterations of the antibiotic	Aminoglycosides, chloramphenicol, streptogramin, lincosamides
Destruction of the antibiotic	β-Lactams
Decreased antibiotic penetration and efflux	
Decreased permeability	β-Lactams, tetracyclines, some fluoroquinolones
Efflux pumps	Tetracycline, fluoroquinolone
Change in target sites	
Target protection	Tetracyclines, fluoroquinolones, fusidic acid
Modification of the target site	
Mutations of the target site	Fluoroquinolones
Enzymatic alteration of the target site	Macrolides
Complete replacement or bypass of the target site	β-Lactams, sulfonamides-trimethoprim

penetration into and/or increased efflux out of the cell.

3. Modification of the antibiotic target site (e.g. via enzymatic alteration, genetic mutation or pathway bypass).

16.3.1 Modification of the antibiotic

Chemical alteration of the antibiotic

The antibiotics that work by inhibiting bacterial synthesis are the most prone to enzymatic modification that can compromise their efficacy. Modifying enzymes produced by the bacteria are capable of catalysing the acetylation or phosphorylation of aminoglycosides or chloramphenicol and the adenylation of aminoglycosides or lincosamides (Munita and Arias, 2016). The consequent conformational change in the antibiotic structure reduces its ability to bind to its target, imparting decreased activity or complete inactivation of the antibiotic. Aminoglycoside-modifying enzymes modify the hydroxyl or amino groups of the aminoglycoside molecule, causing inactivation. Nearly all types of bacteria could support the genetic machinery required to acquire enzymatic resistance to aminoglycosides. This has led to a wide variety of aminoglycoside-modifying enzymes globally; enzymatic alteration is recognized as the predominant mechanism of aminoglycoside resistance worldwide.

Inactivation of the antibiotic

A little more than 70 years after their first use, β-lactam antibiotics remain the most widely used class of antibiotic across the globe. However, even before their first clinical application in a human patient, β-lactamases had been identified. In fact, there is evidence of their existence in the biological arms race between microorganisms for millions of years (D'Costa *et al.*, 2011). β-Lactamases destroy the amide bond in the β-lactam ring, rendering the β-lactam antibiotic inactive. Multiple (more than 1000) β-lactamases have been described with varying characteristics and spectra of activity dependent on the amino acid configuration around their active site (Paterson and Bonomo, 2005). This region determines the spectrum of β-lactam antibiotics that can be hydrolysed and destroyed by the β-lactamase.

β-Lactamases have been classified into several systems, including the A–D Ambler classification and the 1–4 Bush–Jacoby–Medeiros classification with multiple subgroups. The latter scheme suffers from a complicated nomenclature but is more intuitive from a clinician's perspective because it groups the β-lactamases according to functional similarities (substrate and inhibitor profile). Arguably, the most important and prevalent β-lactamase is TEM-1 because this accounts for over 90% of ampicillin resistance among *Escherichia coli* (Livermore, 1995). TEM-1 was so named because it was first identified from an *E. coli* isolate in a patient from Athens called Temoneira (Datta and Kontomichalou, 1965).

Extended-spectrum β-lactamases (ESBLs) are a subset of the β-lactamases that have the ability to hydrolyse penicillins, third-generation cephalosporins and monobactams, but have little or no activity against carbapenems (Munita and Arias, 2016). Third-generation cephalosporins are classified as 'highest priority critically important antibiotics' because of their critical role in treating life-threatening infections in people. Any and all use of this class of antibiotic in companion animals must be carefully considered because their use could increase the risk of ESBL infections – a phenomenon that has been observed in human hospitals (Pinto Pereira *et al.*, 2004). TEM-1 and TEM-2 are not ESBLs (they are resistant only to penicillins and first- and second-generation cephalosporins). However, their derivatives, including TEM-3 and the majority of other TEM-type β-lactamases, are classified as ESBLs. Most ESBLs (with few exceptions) are susceptible to the effects of β-lactamase inhibitors (e.g. clavulanic acid), which differentiates ESBLs from the AmpC-type β-lactamases that are not inhibited by clavulanic acid.

Group 1 (Ambler Class C) β-lactamases are also known as AmpC enzymes. Group I producer β-lactamases are resistant to β-lactam/β-lactamase inhibitor combinations, penicillins, and first-, second- and third-generation cephalosporins. Enzyme production is induced upon exposure of bacteria to β-lactam antibiotics. Some SHV-type β-lactamases (e.g. SHV-2), some CTX-M enzymes and a few OXA-type β-lactamases (so named because of their oxacillin-hydrolysing abilities) are also ESBLs. Further groups of ESBLs and non-ESBLs have been identified.

16.3.2 Reduction of intracellular antimicrobial concentrations

Prevention of antibiotic penetration into the cell

As discussed above, many antibiotics act on targets located in the cytoplasmic membrane (the inner cell membrane of Gram-negative bacteria) or within the cytoplasm (e.g. the bacterial ribosome). In such cases, membrane permeability is key to efficient antibiotic activity (Ghai and Ghai, 2018). Glycopeptides (e.g. vancomycin) are ineffective against Gram-negative bacteria because of their inability to traverse the outer membrane. To overcome this barrier, hydrophilic antibiotics (β-lactams, tetracyclines and some fluoroquinolones) may enter the bacterial cell via porins (water-filled diffusion channels). There are three mechanisms of porin-mediated antibiotic resistance: (i) alteration of the type of porins expressed; (ii) alteration of the level of porin expression; and (iii) impairment of porin function. Activation of these changes can reduce the membrane permeability, offering low-level bacterial resistance.

Increased antibiotic efflux out of the cell

If an antibiotic molecule can gain access to the interior of the bacterial cell, the bacteria's next defensive option is to rapidly exclude the drug before it can exert its effect. This extrusion process is realized by transport proteins called efflux pumps (Du *et al.*, 2018). Both Gram-positive and Gram-negative bacteria (and eukaryotic organisms) have efflux pumps that may transport just a single substrate or an entire range of structurally dissimilar compounds (including antibiotics of multiple classes) (Webber and Piddock, 2003). By this mechanism, efflux pumps can confer MDR to some bacteria.

Efflux pumps are classified into five major families based on structure, energy source and substrate profile. These are MFS (major facilitator superfamily), SMR (small multidrug resistance), RND (resistance–nodulation–division), ABC (ATP-binding cassette), MATE (multidrug and toxic efflux) and PACE (proteobacterial antimicrobial compound efflux). Importantly, bacteria can express multiple efflux pumps from the same or from different families, conferring a broad spectrum of substrate activity. The intrinsic resistance of *Pseudomonas aeruginosa* to several β-lactams and non-β-lactam antibiotics is consequent to the action of efflux pumps (Li *et al.*, 1994). Acquired resistance can occur following a constitutive increase and permanent upregulation of the expression of efflux pumps. Where bacteria develop increased resistance to multiple antibiotics simultaneously (different from the wild-type bacteria), the mechanism is likely to involve increased antibiotic efflux (Piddock, 2006). Altered efflux can offer fast-acting and effective antibiotic resistance. However, generally this increased resistance (manifested *in vitro* as an increased MIC) is of a considerably lower magnitude than that achieved by the enzymatic inactivation of antibiotics or the alteration of antibiotic target proteins. None the less, induced efflux pumps can increase the MIC above recognized breakpoint concentrations, meaning that the antibiotic is unlikely to be effective. This phenomenon has been described most frequently for fluoroquinolones.

Efflux pumps have at least a contributory role to bacterial resistance against antibiotics, including β-lactams, aminoglycosides, macrolides, fluoroquinolones, chloramphenicol and tetracyclines, but can also transport other substrates including chlorhexidine, other biocides and triclosan. Concerningly, there is a risk that widespread use of such non-antibiotic substrates could impose a selection pressure, favouring the expression of efflux pumps and leading to increased MDR. Furthermore, efflux pumps can also contribute to bacterial pathogenicity by other means. They may also serve to transport proteinaceous toxins and other virulence factors out of the cell, play a role in cell-to-cell communication and contribute to the formation of protective biofilms (Piddock, 2006). The inhibition of efflux pumps represents a promising future therapeutic avenue that could impair this resistance mechanism in some pathogens and increase their antibiotic susceptibility profiles.

16.3.3 Modification of the antibiotic target site

Bacteria can avoid the deleterious effects of antibiotics by interfering with their target site(s). This may be achieved by protecting the target (preventing the antibiotic from reaching its binding site) or by modifying the target site in such a way that it is no longer recognized by the antibiotic (or at least with a much lower affinity). The target binding sites for tetracyclines, fluoroquinolones and fusidic acid can all be blocked by proteins produced by bacteria, thereby compromising their antibiotic effect

(Tomlinson *et al.*, 2016). Target-site protection proteins have been identified in a range of bacterial species, probably reflecting horizontal transfer of the genetic material between bacteria.

Direct modification of the target binding site can reduce antibiotic affinity significantly; this widespread resistance mechanism challenges the efficacy of almost all classes of antibiotic. The target site may be modified by a point mutation of the gene encoding the target site, via enzymatic alteration of the target site, or by replacement or bypass of the target site (Lambert, 2005). As described earlier, antibiotics target specific sites in bacteria, ensuring pathogen specificity and avoiding host toxicity. Alterations to the genetic code for binding sites can lead to an altered configuration and reduced affinity for the antibiotic. Mutational resistance can affect the genes encoding DNA gyrase and topoisomerase IV, leading to fluoroquinolone resistance. Similarly, a point mutation in the gene encoding a bacterial RNA polymerase can distort the rifampin binding pocket, conferring high-level rifampin resistance.

Even if these binding sites have been classically formed (absence of mutation), bacteria can produce enzymes to modify the target site and impair antibiotic binding. Bacteria can produce enzymes capable of catalysing the methylation of the ribosome, leading to macrolide resistance (and cross-resistance to lincosamides given the shared binding site). This enzyme is encoded by the *erm* (erythromycin ribosomal methylation) gene. As the production of unnecessary enzymes would impose a fitness cost to the bacteria, the *erm* gene can be inducible in some pathogens and only activated in the presence of a macrolide (Katz and Ashley, 2005).

Antibiotics are effective when they block essential biochemical processes from occurring in bacteria. This may be achieved by targeting critical steps in these pathways. However, bacteria may evolve new targets that can accomplish the required functionality but that will not bind the antibiotic. By effectively replacing the target site, the bacteria will be resistant to that antibiotic strategy. The classic example of target-site replacement is seen in MRSA (and methicillin-resistant *Staphylococcus pseudintermedius* (MRSP)) due to the acquisition of an alternate PBP (PBP2a). This altered PBP has reduced affinity for β-lactams and a reduced rate of β-lactam-mediated enzyme acylation. PBP2a is encoded by a chromosomal gene (*mecA*) that is often located in a distinct mobile genetic element – the staphylococcal chromosomal cassette (Ubukata *et al.*, 1989). Bacteria that acquire *mecA* will be resistant to all β-lactams (including penicillins and cephalosporins) and carbapenems.

Of significant concern to doctors is the development of vancomycin-resistant enterococci and the potential for serious nosocomial infections. Similar to the β-lactam resistance in MRSA and MRSP, vancomycin resistance in enterococci involves the acquisition of a group of genes (*van* gene clusters). These genes enable the bacteria to produce remodelled peptidoglycan to which vancomycin cannot bind, rendering the antibiotic ineffective.

Finally, bacteria can also look to bypass the metabolic pathway inhibited by an antibiotic by overproducing the antibiotic target. Resistance to folic acid synthesis inhibitors (e.g. trimethoprim-sulfamethoxazole) is achieved by the gross overproduction of key enzymes (dihydropteroic acid synthase and dihydrofolate reductase), overwhelming the antibiotic inhibition and allowing bacterial survival.

16.4 Transfer of Antimicrobial Resistance

A major concern of AMR is its borderless distribution. Resistant mechanisms can rapidly spread from a single location, becoming regional and eventually global as a result of the ability of bacteria to transfer their AMR between different species. The spread of AMR can occur vertically (vertical transmission or vertical gene transfer (VGT)), where resistant bacteria multiply and share their AMR genetic information, including gene mutations, to new generations, or horizontally (horizontal transmission or horizontal gene transfer (HGT)), when resistance genes are transferred from one bacterial species to another.

HGT is considered a major pathway contributing to AMR spread. However, the importance of VGT cannot be underestimated. The different transmission mechanisms could lead to different rates of AMR spread and severity. In fact, the significant involvement of these transmission mechanisms varies with bacterial species and resistant mechanisms. Via VGT, AMR transfer is inherently limited to the same bacterial species. Several classic examples of vertical transmission include the chromosomal mutation in *gyrA* and *parC* genes or quinolone resistance-determining regions in Enterobacteriaceae (Gomez et al., 2017), or the single loci amino acid substitution of Ser83Leu in *gyrA*- and Gly78Cys in *parC*-mediated ciprofloxacin resistance in *Acinetobacter baumannii* (Hamouda and Amyes, 2004).

It is assumed that AMR will gradually spread in bacteria within a certain habitat via vertical transmission. However, AMR can spread much more widely when resistant bacteria themselves are relocated, for example through international travel, import and export of food animals and their products, and via environmental contamination. These factors contribute to the global spread of AMR. In HGT, bacteria can acquire resistance via three different means: (i) the transformation of naked DNA from their environment; (ii) transduction mediated by bacteriophages carrying resistance genes; or (iii) via conjugation from cell-to-cell contact. The latter mechanism plays the most important role in AMR spread and involves the exchange of mobile genetic elements such as plasmids and transposons. HGT can occur both between bacteria of the same species and between different species.

Resistant bacteria can rapidly increase and potentially spread to new environments worldwide. Bacteria can accumulate additional resistance genes from mobile genetic elements. Some plasmids can harbour hundreds of resistance genes. The large plasmid in *Klebsiella pneumoniae* that combines the typical virulence KpVP-1 plasmid with the MDR IncFIIK plasmid harbours many AMR genes such as $bla_{CTX-M-15}$, bla_{TEM}, $aac3'-IIa$, $dfrA1$, $satA2$, bla_{SHV}, $sul1$ and $aadA1$ (Lam et al., 2019). The rapid worldwide spread of highly resistant bacteria across various animal hosts due to HGT has highlighted the need for collaboration via the One Health approach. The *mcr* genes that mediate colistin resistance have been found in various hosts, such as *mcr*-1 in *E. coli* and *K. pneumoniae* isolated from pig (Liu et al., 2016), *mcr*-1 in *E. coli* in humans (Rapoport et al., 2016), *mcr*-1 and *mcr*-2 in *E. coli* and *K. pneumoniae* isolated from wild birds (Ahmed et al., 2019), *mcr*-1 in *E. coli* isolated from chickens (Amin et al., 2020), *mcr*-1 in *Salmonella* spp. isolated from mussels (Lozano-Leon et al., 2019), *mcr*-1 in *E. coli* isolated from vegetables (Manageiro et al., 2020) and *mcr*-1 gene from the metagenome of soil (Anyanwu et al., 2020).

16.5 Conclusions

For millennia, microorganisms have waged war on each other to gain a survival advantage over their competitors. This chapter provides a brief insight into some of the weaponry they use and the counterdefences that have evolved. Veterinarians, like other prescribers, are privileged to be able to wield such tools and utilize them to preserve the health of their patients. By better understanding the mechanisms underpinning the antibiotics we use, and the potential resistance measures in target bacteria, the clinician can ensure that they make their selections wisely and with the optimum chances of success.

References

Ahmed, Z.S., Elshafiee, E.A., Khalefa, H.S., Kadry, M. and Hamza, D.A. (2019) Evidence of colistin resistance genes (mcr-1 and mcr-2) in wild birds and its public health implication in Egypt. *Antimicrobial Resistance & Infection Control* 8(1), 197. DOI: 10.1186/s13756-019-0657-5.

Allerton, F. and Nuttall, T. (2021) Antimicrobial use: importance of bacterial culture and susceptibility testing. *In Practice* 43(9), 500–510. DOI: 10.1002/inpr.139.

Amin, M.B., Sraboni, A.S., Hossain, M.I., Roy, S., Mozmader, T.A.U, et al. (2020) Occurrence and genetic characteristics of mcr-1-positive colistin-resistant *E. coli* from poultry environments in Bangladesh. *Journal of Global Antimicrobial Resistance* 22, 546–552. DOI: 10.1016/j.jgar.2020.03.028.

Anyanwu, M.U., Jaja, I.F. and Nwobi, O.C. (2020) Occurrence and characteristics of mobile colistin resistance (mcr) gene-containing isolates from the environment: a review. *International Journal of Environmental Research and Public Health* 17(3), 1028. DOI: 10.3390/ijerph17031028.

Arenz, S. and Wilson, D.N. (2016) Bacterial protein synthesis as a target for antibiotic inhibition. *Cold Spring Harbor Perspectives in Medicine* 6(9), a025361. DOI: 10.1101/cshperspect.a025361.

Asín-Prieto, E., Rodríguez-Gascón, A. and Isla, A. (2015) Applications of the pharmacokinetic/pharmacodynamic (PK/PD) analysis of antimicrobial agents. *Journal of Infection and Chemotherapy* 21(5), 319–329. DOI: 10.1016/j.jiac.02.001.

Baym, M., Lieberman, T.D., Kelsic, E.D., Chait, R., Gross, R. et al. (2016) Spatiotemporal microbial evolution on antibiotic landscapes. *Science* 353(6304), 1147–1151. DOI: 10.1126/science.aag0822.

Bhattacharjee, M.K. (2016) *Chemistry of Antibiotics and Related Drugs*. Springer, Cham. DOI: 10.1007/978-3-319-40746-3.

Blumberg, P.M. and Strominger, J.L. (1974) Interaction of penicillin with the bacterial cell: penicillin-binding proteins and penicillin-sensitive enzymes. *Bacteriological Reviews* 38(3), 291–335. DOI: 10.1128/br.38.3.291-335.1974.

Bush, K. (2012) Antimicrobial agents targeting bacterial cell walls and cell membranes. *Revue Scientifique et Technique* 31(1), 43–56. DOI: 10.20506/rst.31.1.2096.

Datta, N. and Kontomichalou, P. (1965) Penicillinase synthesis controlled by infectious R factors in *Enterobacteriaceae*. *Nature* 208(5007), 239–241. DOI: 10.1038/208239a0.

D'Costa, V.M., King, C.E., Kalan, L., Morar, M., Sung, W.W.L. *et al*. (2011) Antibiotic resistance is ancient. *Nature* 477(7365), 457–461. DOI: 10.1038/nature10388.

de Kruijff, B., van Dam, V. and Breukink, E. (2008) Lipid II: a central component in bacterial cell wall synthesis and a target for antibiotics. *Prostaglandins, Leukotrienes, and Essential Fatty Acids* 79(3–5), 117–121. DOI: 10.1016/j.plefa.2008.09.020.

Du, D., Wang-Kan, X., Neuberger, A., van Veen, H.W., Pos, K.M *et al*. (2018) Multidrug efflux pumps: structure, function and regulation. *Nature Reviews Microbiology* 16(9), 523–539. DOI: 10.1038/s41579-018-0048-6.

Fernández-Villa, D., Aguilar, M.R. and Rojo, L. (2019) Folic acid antagonists: antimicrobial and immunomodulating mechanisms and applications. *International Journal of Molecular Sciences* 20(20), 4996. DOI: 10.3390/ijms20204996.

Ghai, I. and Ghai, S. (2018) Understanding antibiotic resistance via outer membrane permeability. *Infection and Drug Resistance* 11, 523–530. DOI: 10.2147/IDR.S156995.

Gomez, J.E., Kaufmann-Malaga, B.B., Wivagg, C.N., Kim, P.B., Silvis, M.R. *et al*. (2017) Ribosomal mutations promote the evolution of antibiotic resistance in a multidrug environment. *eLife* 6, e20420. DOI: 10.7554/eLife.20420.

Guardabassi, L., Apley, M., Olsen, J.E., Toutain, P.L. and Weese, S. (2018) Optimization of antimicrobial treatment to minimize resistance selection. *Microbiology Spectrum* 6(3). DOI: 10.1128/microbiolspec.ARBA-0018-2017.

Gunn-Moore, D.A., Jenkins, P.A. and Lucke, V.M. (1996) Feline tuberculosis: a literature review and discussion of 19 cases caused by an unusual mycobacterial variant. *Veterinary Record* 138(3), 53–58. DOI: 10.1136/vr.138.3.53.

Hamouda, A. and Amyes, S.G.B. (2004) Novel gyrA and parC point mutations in two strains of *Acinetobacter baumannii* resistant to ciprofloxacin. *Journal of Antimicrobial Chemotherapy* 54(3), 695–696. DOI: 10.1093/jac/dkh368.

Hansen, G.T. (2021) Continuous evolution: perspective on the epidemiology of carbapenemase resistance among Enterobacterales and other gram-negative bacteria. *Infectious Diseases and Therapy* 10(1), 75–92. DOI: 10.1007/s40121-020-00395-2.

Hooper, D.C. (2001) Mechanisms of action of antimicrobials: focus on fluoroquinolones. *Clinical Infectious Diseases* 32 Suppl 1, S9–S15. DOI: 10.1086/319370.

Kadlec, K., Wiegand, I., Kehrenberg, C. and Schwarz, S. (2007) Studies on the mechanisms of beta-lactam resistance in *Bordetella bronchiseptica*. *Journal of Antimicrobial Chemotherapy* 59(3), 396–402. DOI: 10.1093/jac/dkl515.

Kapoor, G., Saigal, S. and Elongavan, A. (2017) Action and resistance mechanisms of antibiotics: a guide for clinicians. *Journal of Anaesthesiology, Clinical Pharmacology* 33(3), 300–305. DOI: 10.4103/joacp.JOACP_349_15.

Katz, L. and Ashley, G.W. (2005) Translation and protein synthesis: macrolides. *Chemical Reviews* 105(2), 499–528. DOI: 10.1021/cr030107f.

Lambert, P.A. (2005) Bacterial resistance to antibiotics: modified target sites. *Advanced Drug Delivery Reviews* 57(10), 1471–1485. DOI: 10.1016/j.addr.2005.04.003.

Lam, M.M.C., Wyres, K.L., Wick, R.R., Judd, L.M., Fostervold, A., *et al*. (2019) Convergence of virulence and MDR in a single plasmid vector in MDR Klebsiella pneumoniae ST15. *The Journal of Antimicrobial Chemotherapy* 74(5), 1218–1222. DOI: 10.1093/jac/dkz028.

Levison, M.E. and Levison, J.H. (2009) Pharmacokinetics and pharmacodynamics of antibacterial agents. *Infectious Disease Clinics of North America* 23(4), 791–815. DOI: 10.1016/j.idc.2009.06.008.

Liu, Y.-Y., Wang, Y., Walsh, T.R., Yi, L.-X., Zhang, R., *et al*. (2016) Emergence of plasmid-mediated colistin resistance mechanism MCR-1 in animals and human beings in China: a microbiological and molecular biological study. *Lancet Infectious Diseases* 16(2), 161–168. DOI: 10.1016/S1473-3099(15)00424-7.

Livermore, D.M. (1995) beta-Lactamases in laboratory and clinical resistance. *Clinical Microbiology Reviews* 8(4), 557–584. DOI: 10.1128/CMR.8.4.557.

Li, X.Z., Ma, D., Livermore, D.M. and Nikaido, H. (1994) Role of efflux pump(s) in intrinsic resistance of pseudomonas aeruginosa: active efflux as a contributing factor to β-lactam resistance. *Antimicrobial Agents and Chemotherapy* 38, 1742–1752.

Lozano-Leon, A., Garcia-Omil, C., Dalama, J., Rodriguez-Souto, R., Martinez-Urtaza, J, *et al*. (2019) Detection of colistin resistance mcr-1 gene in Salmonella enterica serovar Rissen isolated from mussels, Spain, 2012 to 2016. *Euro Surveillance* 24(16), 1900200. DOI: 10.2807/1560-7917.ES.2019.24.16.1900200.

Manageiro, V., Jones-Dias, D., Ferreira, E. and Caniça, M. (2020) Plasmid-mediated colistin resistance (*mcr-1*) in *Escherichia coli* from non-imported fresh vegetables for human consumption in Portugal. *Microorganisms* 8(3), 429. DOI: 10.3390/microorganisms8030429.

Martinez, M.N., Papich, M.G. and Drusano, G.L. (2012) Dosing regimen matters: the importance of early

Thawanrut Kiatyingangsulee *et al*.

intervention and rapid attainment of the pharmacokinetic/pharmacodynamic target. *Antimicrobial Agents and Chemotherapy* 56(6), 2795–2805. DOI: 10.1128/AAC.05360-11.

McKellar, Q.A., Sanchez Bruni, S.F. and Jones, D.G. (2004) Pharmacokinetic/pharmacodynamic relationships of antimicrobial drugs used in veterinary medicine. *Journal of Veterinary Pharmacology and Therapeutics* 27(6), 503–514. DOI: 10.1111/j.1365-2885.2004.00603.x.

Munita, J.M. and Arias, C.A. (2016) Mechanisms of antibiotic resistance. *Microbiology Spectrum* 4(2). DOI: 10.1128/microbiolspec.VMBF-0016-2015.

Papich, M.G. (2014) Pharmacokinetic-pharmacodynamic (PK-PD) modeling and the rational selection of dosage regimes for the prudent use of antimicrobial drugs. *Veterinary Microbiology* 171(3–4), 480–486. DOI: 10.1016/j.vetmic.2013.12.021.

Paterson, D.L. and Bonomo, R.A. (2005) Extended-spectrum beta-lactamases: a clinical update. *Clinical Microbiology Reviews* 18(4), 657–686. DOI: 10.1128/CMR.18.4.657-686.2005.

Piddock, L.J.V. (2006) Multidrug-resistance efflux pumps - not just for resistance. *Nature Reviews. Microbiology* 4(8), 629–636. DOI: 10.1038/nrmicro1464.

Pinto Pereira, L.M., Phillips, M., Ramlal, H., Teemul, K. and Prabhakar, P. (2004) Third generation cephalosporin use in a tertiary hospital in Port of Spain, Trinidad: need for an antibiotic policy. *BMC Infectious Diseases* 4(1), 59. DOI: 10.1186/1471-2334-4-59.

Rapoport, M., Faccone, D., Pasteran, F., Ceriana, P., Albornoz, E. *et al*. (2016) First description of mcr-1-mediated colistin resistance in human infections caused by *Escherichia coli* in Latin America. *Antimicrobial Agents and Chemotherapy* 60(7), 4412–4413. DOI: 10.1128/AAC.00573-16.

Reygaert, W.C. (2018) An overview of the antimicrobial resistance mechanisms of bacteria. *AIMS Microbiology* 4(3), 482–501. DOI: 10.3934/microbiol.2018.3.482.

Sarkar, P., Yarlagadda, V., Ghosh, C. and Haldar, J. (2017) A review on cell wall synthesis inhibitors with an emphasis on glycopeptide antibiotics. *MedChemComm* 8(3), 516–533. DOI: 10.1039/c6md00585c.

Tomlinson, J.H., Thompson, G.S., Kalverda, A.P., Zhuravleva, A. and O'Neill, A.J. (2016) A target-protection mechanism of antibiotic resistance at atomic resolution: insights into FusB-type fusidic acid resistance. *Scientific Reports* 6, 19524. DOI: 10.1038/srep19524.

Ubukata, K., Nonoguchi, R., Matsuhashi, M. and Konno, M. (1989) Expression and inducibility in *Staphylococcus aureus* of the mecA gene, which encodes a methicillin-resistant *S. aureus*-specific penicillin-binding protein. *Journal of Bacteriology* 171(5), 2882–2885. DOI: 10.1128/jb.171.5.2882-2885.1989.

Webber, M.A. and Piddock, L.J.V. (2003) The importance of efflux pumps in bacterial antibiotic resistance. *Journal of Antimicrobial Chemotherapy* 51(1), 9–11. DOI: 10.1093/jac/dkg050.

17 Responsible Antimicrobial Usage in Small Animal Practice

Martin L. Whitehead*

Chipping Norton Veterinary Hospital, Chipping Norton, Oxon, UK

17.1 Introduction

Antimicrobial resistance (AMR) is widespread worldwide, including in companion animal practice, multidrug-resistant organisms such as methicillin-resistant *Staphylococcus aureus* (MRSA), *Staphylococcus pseudintermedius* (MRSP) and extended-spectrum β-lactamase (ESBL) producing *Enterobacterales*, among others (see Chapter 16, this volume, for more information about resistance mechanisms). MRSA and MRSP may be seen in first-opinion presentations such as otitis, pyoderma, urinary tract infections and wound infections (Perreten *et al.*, 2010; Vincze *et al.*, 2014; Couto *et al.*, 2016; Morris *et al.*, 2017). MRSP is of concern as a nosocomial infection in veterinary practices (Harrison *et al.*, 2014; Perkins *et al.*, 2020; Miranda *et al.*, 2021). MDR Gram-negative bacteria including ESBL-producing organisms may manifest resistance to carbapenems as well as to commonly used β-lactam antibiotics, and also to fluoroquinolones, aminoglycosides, tetracycline and colistin (a polymyxin antibiotic). Gram-negative bacteria are implicated in infections of the urinary tract, skin wounds and abscesses (Rubin and Pitout, 2014; Maeyama *et al.*, 2018; Zogg *et al.*, 2018; Piccolo *et al.*, 2019; Pepin-Puget *et al.*, 2020; Salgado-Caxito *et al.*, 2021; Singleton *et al.*, 2021a). All these and other MDR bacteria are carried by some healthy pets (Miranda *et al.*, 2021).

AMR is a consequence of natural selection among bacteria – bacteria that survive the presence of antibiotics in their environment proliferate at the expense of those that do not. Therefore, some degree of AMR is unavoidable if antimicrobials are used to any extent. AMR reduces the future utility of antimicrobials, and its primary harms are increased mortality and morbidity, and their associated increased costs, in human healthcare. The same harms apply in the veterinary arena. AMR contamination is widespread in the environment, and this further harms public health (Martins and Rabinowitz, 2020; EMA, 2021), as well as having direct ecological effects (Grenni *et al.*, 2018; Kraemer *et al.*, 2019; Serwecińska, 2020; EMA, 2021). Total antimicrobial usage in companion animal practice is small compared with human healthcare or food-animal production and practice (Woolhouse *et al.*, 2015; Boeckel *et al.*, 2017; EMA, 2020a), and by extension, companion animal practice probably contributes far less to the global load of AMR. Nevertheless, it does contribute to that load and, of course, antimicrobial use in companion animals contributes directly to development of AMR in companion animals (Pomba *et al.*, 2016; Schmidt *et al.*, 2018a; Werner *et al.*, 2020; Nielsen *et al.*, 2021). In addition, pets can be reservoirs of MDR bacteria and AMR genes, and pets and their family members can exchange bacteria, including AMR genes and MDR bacteria (Manian, 2003; Johnson *et al.*, 2008; Westgarth *et al.*, 2008; EMA, 2015; Pomba *et al.*, 2016; Zhang *et al.*, 2016; Belas *et al.*, 2020; Toombs-Ruane *et al.*, 2020; Hackmann *et al.*, 2021; Menezes *et al.*, 2022), most vividly demonstrated by pet reptile-associated salmonellosis in humans (Varma *et al.*, 2006; Hoelzer *et al.*, 2011; Murphy and Oshin, 2014; Mughini-Gras *et al.*, 2016; Corrente *et al.*, 2017; Sodagari *et al.*, 2020; Marin *et al.*, 2021).

AMR, and its associated harms, can be minimized by:

- reducing the overall usage of antimicrobials, including by preventing infectious diseases,

*martin@chippingnortonvets.co.uk

by confirming that any disease treated with antimicrobials actually has a bacterial/fungal aetiology, and not using antimicrobials to treat self-limiting diseases;

- using those antimicrobials that have a lower risk of potentiating AMR, e.g. using narrow- rather than broad-spectrum antimicrobials, and avoiding antimicrobials that have a higher chance of prompting *de novo* mutations (e.g. fluoroquinolones and rifampicin);
- reducing, especially, the usage of those antimicrobials regarded as 'highest priority critically important' antimicrobials (HPCIAs) in human medicine (EMA, 2019; WHO, 2019); and
- optimizing usage of those antimicrobials that are used, i.e. minimizing misuse of antimicrobials.

17.2 Responsible Antimicrobial Usage

The term 'responsible' (a.k.a. 'appropriate', 'judicious', 'prudent' or 'rational') antimicrobial usage places emphasis on usage that minimizes the potential for development of AMR. However, responsible usage also includes selecting the correct antimicrobials to cure – and sometimes prevent (e.g. in severely immunocompromised patients, or peri-operatively for certain surgical procedures) – microbial disease while minimizing adverse effects of those drugs. Responsible antimicrobial use not only reduces the development of AMR, thus safeguarding the future effectiveness of antimicrobials, but also reduces the here-and-now morbidity and mortality of antimicrobial therapy, with their associated costs.

The World Health Organization (WHO) defines responsible use of medicines as 'the activities, capabilities and existing resources of health-system stakeholders being aligned to ensure (human) patients receive the right medicines at the right time, use them appropriately, and benefit from them' (WHO, 2012). Rephrased for veterinary practice: 'Responsible use of antimicrobials is the activities, capabilities and resources of a veterinary practice being aligned to ensure patients receive the right antimicrobials at the right time, veterinarians and clients use those antimicrobials appropriately, and the antimicrobials benefit the patients.'

This definition emphasizes not only the key proximate components of responsible usage – the right antimicrobial at the right time, used appropriately and actually benefitting the patient – but also

the many factors affecting the process of bringing about responsible usage, such as how veterinarians make prescribing decisions, and how their own capabilities and their societal, professional and individual practice environments enable or constrain their usage of antimicrobials.

Societal context, the veterinary profession as a whole, and individual practice 'culture' and circumstances, each influence the occurrence of microbial disease and thus the need for antimicrobial use, for example by the quality of animal husbandry and nutrition, the degree of preventative medicine including vaccination, and the rigour of practice hygiene and infection control, respectively. In addition, veterinarians' societal, professional and practice environments each unavoidably affect individual veterinarians' antimicrobial usage. For example, some governments have regulations to restrict the use of specific antimicrobials in companion animals: in the Netherlands, France, Sweden and Germany, fluoroquinolones and third- and fourth-generation cephalosporins should only be used after culture and susceptibility (C&S) testing (Hopman *et al.*, 2019a; Prouillac, 2021; Wierup *et al.*, 2021; Moerer *et al.*, 2022). Government regulation affects which antimicrobials are commonly used in practice by influencing which antimicrobials become authorized for use in certain species and under certain conditions, and different countries' veterinary professional regulatory bodies may or may not hold positions or provide guidance on aspects of antimicrobial usage, while other national veterinary bodies may provide guidance on antimicrobial usage (Allerton *et al.*, 2021), which may be more, or less, effectively propagated to practices. The socio-economic demographic of different practices' client bases may also influence what testing is done to determine whether antimicrobial treatment is actually required and, if so, which antimicrobials are used, and factors within individual practices other than responsible usage – commercial deals with suppliers, profitability, practice 'culture' of usage, time pressure – can influence which antimicrobials are available for use, or which antimicrobials tend to be used for specific conditions.

17.3 Antimicrobial Stewardship

Antimicrobial stewardship is an organizational, systematic approach to promoting and monitoring responsible use of antimicrobials to preserve their future effectiveness (NICE, 2015; Dyar *et al.*, 2017). Stewardship involves raising awareness of AMR, and educating and persuading prescribers of antimicrobials to reduce and improve their prescribing. Stewardship measures can be put in place at any level from government or (inter)national veterinary bodies down to individual practices, and may be very general or focus on highly specific areas of antimicrobial usage.

Broadly, prescribing can be reduced by strategies that limit either supply and/or demand for antimicrobials. In human medicine, national stewardship interventions in various countries have successfully reduced and improved the supply (i.e. prescribing and dispensing, of antimicrobials) by measures such as antibiotic-usage advisory committees or management teams, clinical guidelines and prescribing restrictions (Lim *et al.*, 2020). These measures, by reducing prescription, have reduced consumption of antimicrobials. However, national interventions targeting inappropriate demand for antibiotics, such as educational campaigns targeted at healthcare profesionals and/or the public, have shown inconsistent evidence of effectiveness (Lim *et al.*, 2020).

In human healthcare, specific stewardship interventions in hospitals and primary practices have been shown to reduce and improve antimicrobial usage (Hallsworth *et al.*, 2016; Meeker *et al.*, 2016; Schuts *et al.*, 2016; Baur *et al.*, 2017; Davey *et al.*, 2017; McNulty *et al.*, 2018), although suboptimal prescribing persisted. As a rule of thumb, interventions that make good usage easier and/or poor usage harder in practice – that (in behavioural economics parlance) increase the 'friction' of poor usage – tend to be more effective than efforts to educate and persuade (Schuts *et al.*, 2016; Crayton *et al.*, 2020; Lim *et al.*, 2020).

In the veterinary sphere, the food-producing animal sector has had the most attention, as it uses the greatest amount of antimicrobials, and contributes most to AMR development, and the associated public health risks (Woolhouse *et al.*, 2015; Boeckel *et al.*, 2017; EMA, 2020a). Some governments have regulations to limit antimicrobial use in food-producing animals (Mevius and Heederik, 2014; More, 2020; European Parliament, 2022), and in the UK, the threat of government intervention (O'Neill, 2016) led to voluntary measures by the agricultural sector that substantially reduced usage in food-producing animals (RUMA, 2021; VMD, 2022).

Specific interventions in farm-animal practice have shown that overall antimicrobial use (Rojo-Gimeno *et al.*, 2016; Collineau *et al.*, 2017; Postma *et al.*, 2017; Schmenger *et al.*, 2020) or the use of HPCIAs (Turner *et al.*, 2018; Hubbuch *et al.*, 2021) can be greatly decreased with no apparent detriment to animal welfare or production, although again some suboptimal prescribing persisted.

Veterinary bodies in various countries have produced guidelines for antimicrobial usage in small animal practice (reviewed for the European Union (EU) by Allerton *et al.*, 2021). Only a few attempts have been made to assess whether such guidelines or other interventions improve antimicrobial use in companion animals (Weese, 2006; Ekiri *et al.*, 2019; Moerer *et al.*, 2022; Taylor *et al.*, 2022). Simply introducing greater traceability of prescriptions was associated with reduced use of some HPCIAs (Chirollo *et al.*, 2021). There is evidence that the Danish national guidelines have contributed to improved antimicrobial usage (Jessen *et al.*, 2017). Specific educational and advisory stewardship interventions targeted at companion animal practices have been associated with improved antimicrobial usage (Sarrazin *et al.*, 2017; Hopman *et al.*, 2019a; Hubbuch *et al.*, 2020; Lehner *et al.*, 2020; Singleton *et al.*, 2021b; Hardefeldt *et al.*, 2022; Walker *et al.*, 2022), although much suboptimal prescribing continued, and some interventions, unexpectedly, appeared to be associated with worsening of some specific aspects of antimicrobial usage (Sarrazin *et al.*, 2017; Walker *et al.*, 2022).

17.4 Antimicrobial Usage in Small Animal Practice

Antimicrobial usage in companion animal practice is not well quantified. Some countries (e.g. EMA, 2020a) record annual tonnage total veterinary sales of antimicrobial classes, and in some countries, sales for companion animals are – imperfectly – separated out from sales for equids and farm livestock (VMD, 2020). However, total sales are not identical to actual usage, and these figures include only antimicrobial products authorized for animals, excluding products authorized for humans.

Nevertheless, it is clear that antimicrobial usage deviating from recommended responsible usage is common in companion animal practice, with overuse of antimicrobials in general, overuse of HPCIAs in particular, and misuse of antimicrobials all common in the UK (Mateus *et al.*, 2011, 2014; Radford *et al.*, 2011; Hughes *et al.*, 2012; Summers *et al.*, 2014; Buckland *et al.*, 2016; Burke *et al.*, 2017; Singleton *et al.*, 2017, 2019a, 2021b; Walker *et al.*, 2022), other Western countries (Weese, 2006; Escher *et al.*, 2011; Shea *et al.*, 2011; Wayne *et al.*, 2011; Kvaale *et al.*, 2012; Murphy *et al.*, 2012; Pleydell *et al.*, 2012; de Briyne *et al.*, 2013; Jacob *et al.*, 2015; Banfield Pet Hospital, 2017; Barbarossa *et al.*, 2017; Barzelai and Whittem, 2017; Hardefeldt *et al.*, 2017b; Jessen *et al.*, 2017; Sarrazin *et al.*, 2017; Gómez-Poveda and Moreno, 2018; Sørensen *et al.*, 2018; Van Cleven *et al.*, 2018; Ekakoro and Okafor, 2019; Hopman *et al.*, 2019a, b, c; Norris *et al.*, 2019; Schmitt *et al.*, 2019; Hardefeldt *et al.*, 2020; Hur *et al.*, 2020; Joosten *et al.*, 2020; Lutz *et al.*, 2020; Robbins *et al.*, 2020; Scarborough *et al.*, 2020; Valiakos *et al.*, 2020; Goggs *et al.*, 2021; Schnepf *et al.*, 2021; Hur *et al.*, 2022; Taylor *et al.*, 2022) and other countries (Tanaka *et al.*, 2017; Galarce *et al.*, 2021; Gómez-Beltrán *et al.*, 2021; Makita *et al.*, 2021).

In the UK, EU, USA, Australia and Japan, there is a preponderance of use of penicillins and other β-lactam antibiotics in both cats and dogs, with amoxicillin-clavulanate the most commonly prescribed antibiotic (Odensvik *et al.*, 2001; Watson and Maddison, 2001; Rantala *et al.*, 2004; Hölsö *et al.*, 2005; Weese, 2006; Regula *et al.*, 2009; Thomson *et al.*, 2009; Escher *et al.*, 2011; Mateus *et al.*, 2011; Radford *et al.*, 2011; Wayne *et al.*, 2011; Baker *et al.*, 2012; Hughes *et al.*, 2012; Kvaale *et al.*, 2012; Murphy *et al.*, 2012; Pleydell *et al.*, 2012; Mateus *et al.*, 2014; Summers *et al.*, 2014; Buckland *et al.*, 2016; Fowler *et al.*, 2016; Banfield Pet Hospital, 2017; Barbarossa *et al.*, 2017; Hardefeldt *et al.*, 2017b; Sarrazin *et al.*, 2017; Singleton *et al.*, 2017; Tanaka *et al.*, 2017; Gómez-Poveda and Moreno, 2018; Ekakoro and Okafor, 2019; Hopman *et al.*, 2019a, b; Norris *et al.*, 2019; EMA, 2020a; Hur *et al.*, 2020; Joosten *et al.*, 2020; Lutz *et al.*, 2020; Mendez and Moreno, 2020; Robbins *et al.*, 2020; VMD, 2020, VMD, 2022; Attauabi *et al.*, 2021; Chirollo *et al.*, 2021; Galarce *et al.*, 2021; Goggs *et al.*, 2021; Makita *et al.*, 2021; Prouillac, 2021; Schnepf *et al.*, 2021; Urban *et al.*, 2021; Moerer *et al.*, 2022; Walker *et al.*, 2022). The fact that amoxicillin-clavulanate, a broad-spectrum antibiotic, is in many countries the most prescribed antibiotic indicates widespread suboptimal usage of antimicrobials, because narrow-spectrum antimicrobials should be utilized where possible.

Widespread high usage of potentiated β-lactams as first-line treatments risks selection and spread of MDR – including ESBL-producing – bacteria (Grønvold *et al.*, 2010; Schmidt *et al.*, 2018a; Werner *et al.*, 2020).

In addition to these very high rates of usage of critically important antimicrobials, HPCIAs are also commonly prescribed in many countries, particularly fluoroquinolones and third-generation cephalosporins (Heuer *et al.*, 2005; Escher *et al.*, 2011; Mateus *et al.*, 2011; Radford *et al.*, 2011; Baker *et al.*, 2012; Hughes *et al.*, 2012; Kvaale *et al.*, 2012; Murphy *et al.*, 2012; Pleydell *et al.*, 2012; de Briyne *et al.*, 2013; Buckland *et al.*, 2016; Fowler *et al.*, 2016; Banfield Pet Hospital, 2017; Barbarossa *et al.*, 2017; Burke *et al.*, 2017; Chipangura *et al.*, 2017; Sarrazin *et al.*, 2017; Singleton *et al.*, 2017; Gómez-Poveda and Moreno, 2018; Hardefeldt *et al.*, 2018; Van Cleven *et al.*, 2018; Ekakoro and Okafor, 2019; Hopman *et al.*, 2019a, c; Stallwood *et al.*, 2019; EMA, 2020a; Hardefeldt *et al.*, 2020; Joosten *et al.*, 2020; Lutz *et al.*, 2020; Robbins *et al.*, 2020; Singleton *et al.*, 2020b; Valiakos *et al.*, 2020; Chirollo *et al.*, 2021; Galarce *et al.*, 2021; Goggs *et al.*, 2021; Gómez-Beltrán *et al.*, 2021; Schnepf *et al.*, 2021; Weese *et al.*, 2021; RUMA, 2022; Walker *et al.*, 2022), despite their importance in human medicine. HPCIA usage is proportionally higher in cats than in dogs, largely because of the use of cefovecin, a third-generation cephalosporin marketed as a very convenient long-acting preparation (Mateus *et al.*, 2011; Buckland *et al.*, 2016; Burke *et al.*, 2017; Singleton *et al.*, 2017; Hardefeldt *et al.*, 2018, 2020, Stallwood *et al.*, 2019; Hur *et al.*, 2020; Goggs *et al.*, 2021; Schnepf *et al.*, 2021; Hur *et al.*, 2022; Walker *et al.*, 2022).

Because C&S testing is generally relatively little used prior to antibiotic prescribing, even prior to prescribing HPCIAs (Thomson *et al.*, 2009; Escher *et al.*, 2011; Wayne *et al.*, 2011; Hughes *et al.*, 2012; de Briyne *et al.*, 2013; Mateus *et al.*, 2014; Fowler *et al.*, 2016; Barbarossa *et al.*, 2017; Burke *et al.*, 2017; Chipangura *et al.*, 2017; Gómez-Poveda and Moreno, 2018; Van Cleven *et al.*, 2018; Stallwood *et al.*, 2019; Hardefeldt *et al.*, 2020; Robbins *et al.*, 2020; Valiakos *et al.*, 2020; Chirollo *et al.*, 2021; Galarce *et al.*, 2021; Prouillac, 2021), amoxicillin-clavulanate, other broad-spectrum antimicrobials and HPCIAs must be routinely prescribed empirically. Indeed, it is likely that veterinarians prescribe these antimicrobials empirically precisely because their broad spectrum of action provides them with a sense of security in their prescribing. Some EU countries have introduced regulations to minimize use of HPCIAs in companion animals without appropriate C&S results (Hopman *et al.*, 2019a; Wierup *et al.*, 2021; Moerer *et al.*, 2022). Such regulation may reduce use of HPCIAs but further increase the use of other broad-spectrum antimicrobials that do not require prior C&S testing (Moerer *et al.*, 2022; Walker *et al.*, 2022).

Surveys of small animal veterinarians and studies in which data have been extracted from practice management systems have shown marked variation in the number of antimicrobial prescriptions among practices (Regula *et al.*, 2009; Radford *et al.*, 2011; Singleton *et al.*, 2017; Hopman *et al.*, 2019a), a correlation between the numbers of prescriptions for dogs and cats across practices (Radford *et al.*, 2011; Singleton *et al.*, 2017) and marked variation in the proportion of antimicrobials prescribed that are HPCIAs (Tompson *et al.*, 2020), suggesting that some of the variation is due to practice/practitioner factors rather than animal and disease factors. Preliminary data also show marked variation in the numbers of antibiotic prescriptions among individual practitioners seeing similar caseloads within a single practice, and correlation across practitioners between the amounts used in dogs and cats, again suggesting that some of the variation may be due to practitioner factors rather than animal and disease factors (Tompson *et al.*, 2020; Whitehead, 2020). These findings suggest that some practices and some veterinarians may be prescribing less responsibly than others, as is the case for primary-care practices and physicians in human healthcare (Pinder *et al.*, 2015; Schmidt *et al.*, 2018b; Borek *et al.*, 2022; Van Staa *et al.*, 2022).

Antimicrobial usage appears to be particularly poor for pets other than dogs and cats. In the UK, by far the most commonly used antibiotic in pet rabbits is enrofloxacin (Radford *et al.*, 2011), in contrast to dogs and cats. Enrofloxacin also appears disproportionately heavily used for backyard poultry (Singleton *et al.*, 2020a), and – along with other HPCIAs – in other exotic pets (Hedley *et al.*, 2021). Enrofloxacin, despite being an HPCIA, may be used so heavily in these species in the UK because enrofloxacin products are specifically authorized for 'exotic animals (small mammals, reptiles and avian species)' in general, whereas only one other antibiotic product has an authorized indication in any exotic species, and that with very specific

indications in only three species (Hedley *et al.*, 2021; NOAH, 2021). This is an example of regulation directly negatively (with regard to responsible usage) impacting antimicrobial-prescribing decisions in practice. The UK veterinary medicines regulator (the Veterinary Medicines Directorate) explicitly allows veterinarians to prescribe off-license in the interests of reducing AMR. However, there is still a strong tendency among many UK veterinarians to use a product authorized for a particular species and indication, even though other products with less risk of AMR development may be suitable.

Box 17.1 lists examples of actual or potential concerns about antimicrobial usage in UK small animal practice that may be encouraging the development of AMR, most of which will also apply to other countries. This suboptimal usage includes: 'defensive prescribing', including the use of antimicrobials for conditions for which they are not indicated, such as most cases of feline lower urinary tract diseases, subclinical bacteriuria (Weese *et al.*, 2019), uncomplicated acute diarrhoea (Marks *et al.*, 2011; Werner *et al.*, 2020) or vomiting, kennel cough (Lappin *et al.*, 2017), sneezing, most burst cat-bite abscesses, and prophylactic use around most routine clean surgeries (Vasseur *et al.*, 1985; Brown *et al.*, 1997; Eugster *et al.*, 2004; Knights *et al.*, 2012; Currie *et al.*, 2018; Williams, 2018) and uncomplicated dental work, including most extractions (Bellows *et al.*, 2019); use of HPCIAs or other broad-spectrum and HPCIAs when they are not indicated; frequent prescribing of HPCIAs and other broad-spectrum antimicrobials without C&S testing (see above); and, when HPCIAs are used, failure to record the justification for doing so in patients' clinical records (Shea *et al.*, 2011; Burke *et al.*, 2017; Hardefeldt *et al.*, 2020; Hur *et al.*, 2022).

17.4.1 Changes in antimicrobial usage over the last decade

Companion animal antimicrobial overall usage, and HPCIA usage, has reduced over the last decade in the UK (Singleton *et al.*, 2017, 2019b; VMD, 2019, VMD, 2020, VMD, 2022; RUMA, 2022; Walker *et al.*, 2022), Denmark (Jessen *et al.*, 2017; Attauabi *et al.*, 2021), the Netherlands (Hopman *et al.*, 2019b) and Australia (Hardefeldt *et al.*, 2018). From 2014 to 2018, total antibiotic sales for UK companion animals declined by about

Martin L. Whitehead

Antimicrobials are commonly misused and overused in veterinary practice, driving selection of resistant infections (see references in text):

- Prescribing behaviour often does not match available prescribing guidelines, e.g. the PROTECT ME poster in the UK (BSAVA/SAMSoc, 2018).
- Gram-negative infections are often unnecessarily treated with antibiotics, particularly gastrointestinal, urinary tract and respiratory tract infections.
- Other common infections overtreated with antibiotics include canine infectious tracheobronchitis (usually viral) and feline abscesses.
- Other common overuses of antimicrobials include feline lower urinary tract disease (often sterile), acute vomiting or diarrhoea, and surgical prophylaxis.
- Antimicrobials of a higher tier than necessary are often used, including highest priority critically important antimicrobials (HPCIAs) – especially cefovecin in cats, and enrofloxacin in pet rabbits, small mammals, birds and reptiles.
- Higher-tier antimicrobials are often used empirically, rather than on the basis of culture and susceptibility (C&S) results.
- Veterinarians often fail to record any justification for the use of higher-tier antimicrobials on patient records.
- Prescribing behaviour varies significantly among individual veterinary practices and among individual veterinarians within practices.
- C&S testing is underutilized, and can improve responsible usage of antimicrobials.

Broad-spectrum antimicrobials and HPCIAs are often prescribed without support from C&S testing.

- Cytology alongside culture is underutilized in veterinary practice and can improve responsible usage of antimicrobials.
- Some veterinarians' interpretation of some types of cytology may be poor, which can lead to incorrect antimicrobial prescribing.
- When antibiotics have been prescribed empirically while awaiting C&S test results, veterinarians often fail to stop the antibiotic course, or to de-escalate (i.e. change to a lower tier) the antibiotic, when this is indicated by the C&S results.
- Audit and surveillance of veterinary multidrug resistance is minimal (in veterinary practices and diagnostic laboratories) and needs to be improved.
- There is a lack of studies designed to inform the duration of treatment of many infections with antimicrobials. Many courses of antimicrobial treatment are longer than necessary, increasing the risk of antimicrobial resistance development.
- There is a lack of studies designed to provide evidence in support of not treating many infections with antimicrobials.

[a]Most of these concerns were raised during a meeting of practising veterinarians and veterinary laboratory staff to discuss ways to reduced antimicrobial resistance, held at Willows Referrals, Solihull, UK, November 2019.

16%, and of the HPCIAs, fluoroquinolone use declined by 35%, but third- and fourth-generation cephalosporin use showed no clear trend (VMD, 2019). These declines are associated with increased awareness and concern around AMR in the profession, increased emphasis on this topic in veterinary school teaching and continuing professional education, prescribing guidance by national veterinary bodies and other efforts to reduce usage, although the relative contributions of various factors to the reduced usage are unquantified.

These substantial and ongoing declines in antimicrobial usage constitute further evidence for how widespread suboptimal antimicrobial prescribing has been. Clearly, much companion animal antimicrobial usage has not been 'responsible' and, despite ongoing improvement, this remains the case.

17.5 Factors that Influence Antimicrobial Prescribing

As noted above, antimicrobial usage is influenced by numerous societal, regulatory and professional factors external to individual practices, over most of which individual practices or veterinarians have little or no influence. Those factors will not be discussed further, and the focus of the rest of this chapter is on factors operating at the level of individual practices and veterinarians to influence antimicrobial prescribing, and the extent to which this prescribing matches responsible antimicrobial usage. Individual practices or veterinarians have the potential to improve many of these factors. These factors can be divided into 'clinical and patient' factors, and 'non-clinical, higher-level' factors (Mateus *et al.*, 2014; Pinder *et al.*, 2015; Currie *et al.*, 2018; Hopman *et al.*, 2018; King *et al.*, 2018; Monnier *et al.*, 2018; Smith *et al.*, 2018; Singleton *et al.*, 2020b; Tompson *et al.*, 2020; Charani *et al.*, 2021), as listed in Table 17.1. Individual veterinarians and practices can consider these elements when planning how to reduce and improve their antimicrobial usage. Many of these elements are self-explanatory. The remainder of this article provides discussion around how to improve some of these elements in practice.

17.5.1 Clinical and patient-level elements

The clinical and patient-level elements involved in responsible antimicrobial prescribing are outlined in Table 17.1A–D. Veterinarians in general are very aware of these direct, proximate factors influencing their prescribing – these issues are taught at veterinary school, in clinical continuing professional development, and are covered in standard clinical texts and journal review articles. Nevertheless, with regard to AMR, veterinarians often prescribe antimicrobials in ways contrary to those indicated by the available scientific knowledge and clinical considerations, i.e. they often do not follow recommendations and guidelines for responsible prescribing. Why not?

17.5.2 Non-clinical, higher-level elements

Suboptimal prescribing occurs for many reasons, and studies in which companion animal veterinarians have been surveyed or interviewed have assessed 'barriers' to responsible antimicrobial prescribing (de Briyne *et al.*, 2013; Mateus *et al.*, 2014; Hardefeldt *et al.*, 2017a; Currie *et al.*, 2018; Hopman *et al.*, 2018; King *et al.*, 2018; Smith *et al.*, 2018; Norris *et al.*, 2019; Tompson *et al.*, 2020, 2021; Alcantara *et al.*, 2021; Servia-Dopazo *et al.*, 2021), many of which are listed in Box 17.2.

As is clear from Table 17.1 and Box 17.2, numerous non-clinical factors influence prescribing decisions in general (Hajjaj *et al.*, 2010), including in relation to antimicrobials, in both human and veterinary medicine (Brookes-Howell *et al.*, 2012; Mateus *et al.*, 2014; Pinder *et al.*, 2015; Horwood

et al., 2016; Hardefeldt *et al.*, 2017a; Currie *et al.*, 2018; King *et al.*, 2018; Lum *et al.*, 2018; Smith *et al.*, 2018; Krockow *et al.*, 2019; Borek *et al.*, 2020; Tompson *et al.*, 2020; Servia-Dopazo *et al.*, 2021; Tompson *et al.*, 2021). They include practice-level factors, such as the (un)availability (Mateus *et al.*, 2014; Jessen *et al.*, 2017) and ease of accessibility or ease of use of the various antimicrobial products within a practice (Mateus *et al.*, 2011), business factors including time constraints, and – importantly – practice 'culture' and psychosocial factors, including social norms around antibiotic usage in a practice and 'prescribing etiquette' (Hulscher *et al.*, 2010; Charani *et al.*, 2011, 2013). If a veterinarian's colleagues use antimicrobials in a certain way, that veterinarian may feel – consciously or unconsciously – pressure (which may not be deliberate or explicit on the part of the veterinarian's colleagues) to prescribe in a similar way, especially if their colleague(s) is/are more senior (Mateus *et al.*, 2014), as has been demonstrated in human healthcare (Charani *et al.*, 2011, 2013, 2021; Mattick *et al.*, 2014; Papoutsi *et al.*, 2017; Tompson *et al.*, 2020). This can be a problem if more senior veterinarians have less responsible prescribing behaviour on average, which may be the case (Hopman *et al.*, 2018; King *et al.*, 2018), and as has been reported for doctors in human primary care (Schmidt *et al.*, 2018b; Fernandez-Lazaro *et al.*, 2019).

Non-clinical factors also include individual-veterinarian factors, such as preferences and attitudes, e.g. veterinarians vary in their degree of knowledge and/or concern about AMR, in their 'uncertainty avoidance' (their anxiety about 'missing something'), in their need to 'do something' rather than adopt a wait-and-see approach, in the degree to which they practice 'defensive medicine' and in their inclination to meet clients' requests for antimicrobials (Cheng and Worth, 2015). Antimicrobial usage may vary with years since gradation (Hopman *et al.*, 2018). These and other individual-veterinarian factors may lead to substantial between-veterinarian differences in overall prescribing, even for veterinarians seeing similar caseloads in the same practice (Fig. 17.1).

Clients are a further source of non-clinical factors influencing veterinarians' prescribing behaviour. Practices' client bases vary in sociodemographic factors, which can influence expectations of veterinary care. Practices serving lower socioeconomic status clients may be more restricted in the diagnostic tests they can carry out and the

Martin L. Whitehead

Table 17.1. Elements of responsible antimicrobial use in practice to optimize patient outcome by treating or preventing microbial infections, while limiting development of AMR so as to conserve future efficacy of antimicrobials. Modified from Table 2 of Monnier *et al.* (2018), adapted for veterinary practice.

CLINICAL and PATIENT-LEVEL ELEMENTS

A. Avoid unnecessary usage

1. *Correct diagnosis*: Including use of microbiology diagnostic tools, particularly cytology and C&S, to confirm the diagnosis. Is the disease bacterial?

2. *Indication*: Use antimicrobials only to prevent or cure infections for which antimicrobial treatment provides a proven benefit. Not all bacterial diseases require antimicrobial treatment, e.g. many cases of diarrhoea.

3. *Alternative treatments*: Consider if alternative, non-antimicrobial treatments may be effective, e.g. antiseptics rather than antimicrobials for some topical infections, diet change or glucocorticoids rather than antibiotics for some chronic enteropathies.

B. The right antimicrobial at the correct dose for the shortest duration

4. *Antibacterial activity*: Select antimicrobials based on their antimicrobial activity.

5. *Antimicrobial spectrum*: Select antimicrobials with the narrowest possible antimicrobial spectrum.

6. *Dosing, PK/PD and interval*: Dose and dosing frequency of antimicrobial treatment to be based on available knowledge of PK/PD to ensure sufficient free concentration(s) of antimicrobial at the site(s) of infection.

7. *Duration*: Use the shortest possible evidence-based duration of the antimicrobial treatment.

8. *Route*: Select the optimal route (e.g. parenteral, oral, topical) based on antibiotic, location, severity or type of infection, and patient characteristics.

9. Timing: Start treatment in a timely manner.

10. *Compliance*: Maximize client and patient compliance.

11. *De-escalation*: If culture results after starting empirical treatment suggest an antimicrobial is not needed, stop treatment, or if they suggest a narrower-spectrum antimicrobial is sufficient, change the treatment.

C. Minimize patient harm resulting from usage of the antimicrobial

12. *Interactions*: Select antimicrobials to minimize potentially harmful interactions with other medications.

13. *Toxicity*: Select antimicrobials with the least toxicity profile for the species.

14. *Other unintended consequences*: Select antimicrobials with the lowest risk of secondary infections.

D. Documentation

15. *Documentation*: Fully document the antibiotic regimen, including the indication, in the clinical record. In particular, if an HPCIA has been used, the justification for its use should be recorded.

16. *Document any antimicrobial lack of efficacy in the clinical record*.

NON-CLINICAL, HIGHER-LEVEL ELEMENTS

E. Access and Availability

17. *Access and availability*: Ensure access to and routine availability of quality antimicrobials, including lower-tier antimicrobials without a veterinary licence if useful for minimizing risk of AMR. Also, prevent usage, or put barriers to easy usage, of those antimicrobial products that might encourage development of AMR. Both facilitating and restricting availability of antimicrobials can be achieved at societal or individual practice level (see Box 17.5).

F. Clinical governance

18. *Oversight*: One or more members of the practice team should be recognized as responsible for overseeing practice antimicrobial usage.

19. *Educate healthcare professionals*: Ensure your and your colleagues' knowledge of antimicrobial usage is up to date.

20. *Treatment guidelines*: Follow national or international treatment guidelines – ideally evidence-based, but if not, 'theoretically' based or based on expert consensus.

21. *Expertise and resources*: Use available infectious disease expertise and resources, including that at veterinary commercial laboratories.

Continued

Table 17.1. Continued

22. *AMR surveillance*: If available, use local or regional antibiotic resistance surveillance data to guide empirical antimicrobial prescribing (Scarborough *et al.*, 2020; Klinker *et al.*, 2021).

23. *Audit*: Quality improvement.

24. *Report suspected lack of efficacy to the regulatory authorities.*

G. Clients and the public

25. *Educate your clients and the public* about AMR.

26. *Educate your clients and the public* about reducing disease risk by good husbandry, nutrition and preventative medicine, including vaccination.

H. Waste disposal

27. *Waste disposal*: Safely dispose of unused antimicrobials and waste products containing antimicrobials to prevent selection of AMR in the environment.

I. Prevent unnecessary disease and thus antimicrobial use

28. *By preventative medicine*, including husbandry advice and vaccination.

29. *By strict infection control in the practice.*

AMR, antimicrobial resistance; C&S, culture and susceptibility; HPCIA, highest priority critically important' antimicrobial; PK/PD, pharmacokinetic/pharmacodynamics.

---

antimicrobial products or other medications they can use. Individual clients vary in expectations and attitudes, which can influence veterinarians' prescribing, an example being an expectation of antimicrobial treatment for some diseases (Currie *et al.*, 2018; Hopman *et al.*, 2018; King *et al.*, 2018; Tompson *et al.*, 2020), although sometimes that client 'expectation' may itself be a mistaken perception by the veterinarian (King *et al.*, 2018; Smith *et al.*, 2018), as is sometimes also the case for doctors (Boiko *et al.*, 2020).

Some recognized barriers to responsible prescribing are largely outside the abilities of practising veterinarians to overcome. For instance, the shorter the duration of antimicrobial courses, the less the potential for AMR development (Llewelyn *et al.*, 2017), but the shortest clinically effective duration of antimicrobial treatment of many veterinary diseases is unknown to veterinary science (Weese *et al.*, 2015, Weese *et al.*, 2021; Allerton *et al.*, 2022). The 'data-sheet' dosages of most antimicrobials have been developed with the aim of determining clinical efficacy, largely without consideration of AMR (Courvalin, 2008; Weese *et al.*, 2015; Lloyd and Page, 2018). In human medicine, many recent studies of various diseases have shown shorter durations of antimicrobial treatment to be clinically non-inferior to previously used longer durations of the same antimicrobial (e.g. Crotty *et al.*, 2015; Hanretty and Gallagher, 2018; Spellberg and Rice, 2019; Wilson *et al.*, 2019; Smith *et al.*, 2020; Palin *et al.*, 2021), and recommended durations of

treatment for many diseases in humans are shorter than those for similar diseases in veterinary species (e.g. Weese *et al.*, 2015; Lee *et al.*, 2021). It is often unclear why recommended treatment durations are longer for veterinary patients than humans, and it is likely that many veterinary treatment-course durations could be shortened without impairing efficacy (Weese *et al.*, 2015). No studies have yet directly compared shorter versus longer course durations of the same antimicrobial in companion animals, although Westropp *et al.* (2012) and Clare *et al.* (2014) demonstrated that short courses of one antibiotic were clinically non-inferior to longer courses of another for canine urinary tract infections. Shortening course durations reduces the overall exposure of commensal bacteria to the antimicrobials, thereby reducing risk of AMR developing. However, determining the shortest efficacious course durations for antimicrobials for veterinary diseases will require much research.

In many cases presented to veterinarians, it is not clear whether the illness has a bacterial, viral or non-infectious cause, and – as in human medicine – antimicrobials are often used to treat diseases that have no bacterial involvement, with much 'defensive' or 'just-in-case' prescribing (Currie *et al.*, 2018; Smith *et al.*, 2018). If there were more in-house, rapid, inexpensive diagnostic tests that could reliably confirm or rule out bacterial involvement in such cases, unnecessary antimicrobial treatment of animals without bacterial illness could be greatly reduced. Similarly, reliable point-of-care microbial

Box 17.2. Some in-practice barriers to responsible antimicrobial prescribing.

EXAMPLES OF BARRIERS NOT AMENABLE TO BEING OVERCOME FROM WITHIN A PRACTICE

- Lack of rapid 'patient-side' diagnostic tests to confirm bacterial involvement.
    - Such tests are starting to appear for, e.g. urinary tract infections, but their reliability is not yet clear.
- Lack of specific knowledge in veterinary science regarding optimal treatment to reduce antimicrobial resistance (AMR), e.g. the optimal duration of treatment of many diseases by specific antimicrobials is unknown. Antimicrobial-prescribing guidelines themselves are not perfect due to the lack of such evidence.
- Socio-economic status of the practice's client base.

BARRIERS AMENABLE TO CHANGE WITHIN PRACTICES

Lack of confirmation of diagnoses and of clinical need for antimicrobials

- Use available diagnostic tests more frequently, in particular cytology and culture and susceptibility (C&S).

Antimicrobial product factors

- Marketing authorizations encouraging irresponsible prescribing, e.g. HPCIA products that are highly convenient to use.
    - Increase the 'friction' of using these products within the practice (see Box 17.5).
- No veterinary-authorized products containing antimicrobials useful with respect to minimizing AMR for the relevant species/indication.
    - In the UK, veterinarians can prescribe off license in the interest of minimizing AMR.

Incorrect dose of chosen antimicrobials

- Avoid under- or overdosing, e.g. by weighing patients and ensuring suitable scales in all consult rooms (Walker et al., 2022).

Individual (implicit) veterinarian factors

- Lack of up-to-date knowledge/training regarding AMR.
- Previous experiences with antimicrobials, preferences for antimicrobial use ('habit').
- Attitude to AMR (complacency in antimicrobial usage).
- Attitude to 'risk' when prescribing ('fear'/'self-confidence') – 'defensive prescribing'.
    - Identify suboptimal usage by audit and provide feedback and/or training.

Business factors

- Accessibility/availability of different antimicrobials in the practice
    - Ensure lower-tier/narrow-spectrum antimicrobials are available to use.
    - Increase the 'friction' of using highest priority critically important antimicrobials (see Table 17.5).
- Time pressure: shorter consults discourage use of diagnostics, and discussion of AMR with clients.
    - Can consult durations be increased, or gaps provided in consult schedules to allow more diagnostics to be done?
- Availability of diagnostic tests in the practice, including cytology and C&S.
- Commercial imperative – veterinarian concern that clients might go to another practice if antibiotics are not prescribed.

Practice culture, interaction with colleagues, psychosocial factors

- Management/senior vets' attitude towards AMR.
- Practice's 'social norms' of prescribing.
- Direct peer pressure (good or bad) from colleagues, particularly from senior or older colleagues.
- Observed prescribing behaviour (good or bad) of colleagues.
- Lack of antimicrobial stewardship governance structures and resources.
    - Are professional antimicrobial-prescribing guidelines available in the practice?
    - Does the practice have an antimicrobial-prescribing policy (based on guidelines)?
    - Can suboptimal prescribing be demonstrated by audit?

Client factors/interaction with clients

- Real or perceived-by-veterinarians (Smith et al., 2018; Stallwood et al., 2019) pressure from clients for antibiotics.
- Clients unable or unwilling to pay for diagnostics.
- Vets' perception that some clients are not able or willing to pay for diagnostics (Stallwood et al., 2019).
    - Effective communication with and education of clients about antimicrobial usage and AMR.

Poor infection control in veterinary practices

- Improve infection control (see other chapters in this book).

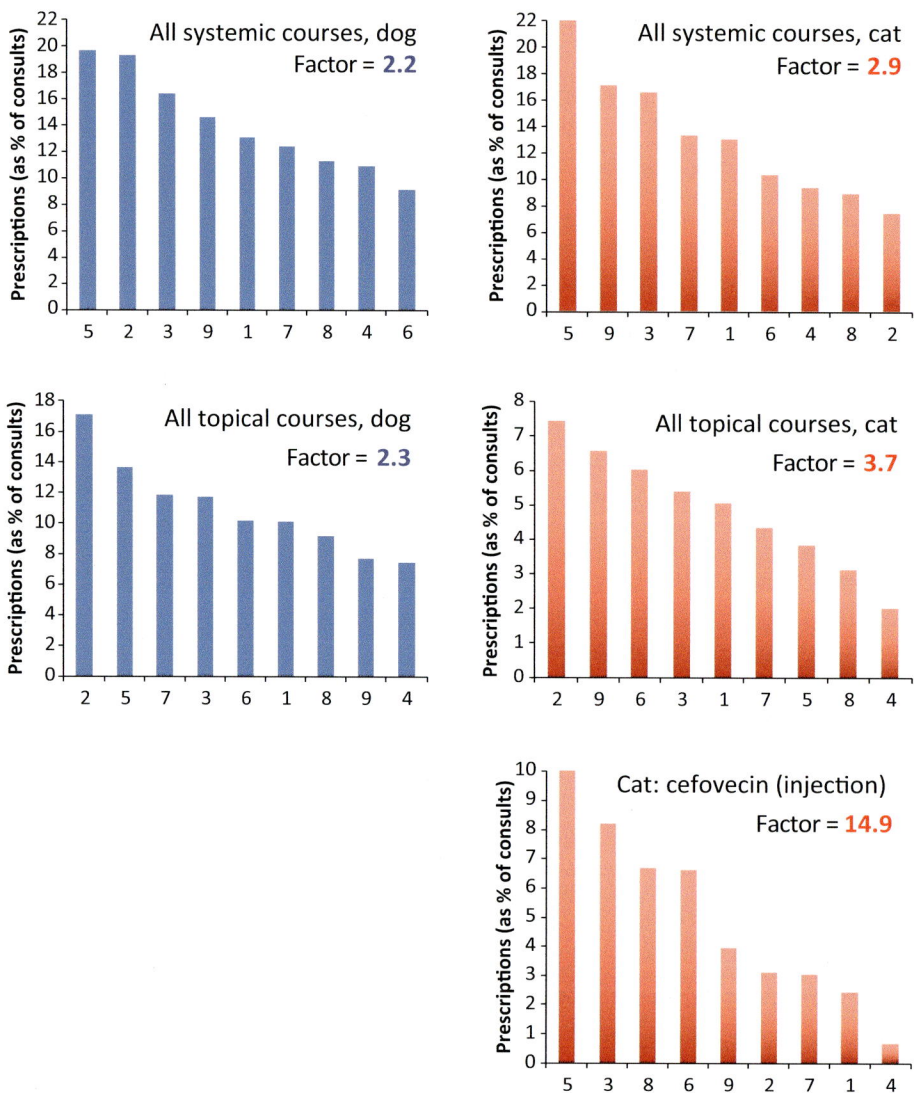

Fig. 17.1. Bar charts showing the number of antibiotic courses prescribed for dogs (blue, left) and cats (red, right) by each of nine veterinarians (1–9) in the author's veterinary hospital, over the 18-month period starting 1 January 2018. Veterinarians are anonymized (*x*-axes), and these data are shown with their permission. Numbers of prescriptions are expressed as % of consults done by each veterinarian, excluding vaccination consults, for dogs and cats, respectively. Data are provided for systemic courses (top), topical courses (i.e. skin, ear and eye antibiotic preparations) (middle) and long-acting cefovecin injections (bottom right). The factor given in each chart is the difference between the lowest- and highest-prescribing veterinarian. Veterinarian 4 was a new graduate.

identification and susceptibility tests could greatly improve responsible prescribing, by allowing more targeted antimicrobial selection. Some such tests are becoming available (e.g. for urine testing), although it is not clear that they are yet reliable enough to guide treatment on their own, in part due to lack of standardization. Samples testing positive, and strains testing resistant, by such tests should therefore be sent to accredited laboratories for validation.

Martin L. Whitehead

Box 17.3. Suggested measures to improve antimicrobial prescribing in veterinary practices: general.

- Use antibiotic-prescribing guidelines such as the UK's small animal PROTECT ME poster (BSAVA/SAMSoc, 2018). This is especially important for use of highest priority critically important antimicrobials (HPCIAs).
- Create a practice protocol for prescribing antimicrobials, particularly for common conditions and for use of HPCIAs. Have an easy-to-access summary of this protocol available in the consulting rooms and preparation room.
- Display a poster in each consulting room, ward and preparation room listing the antibiotics in the different tiers and highlighting HPCIAs.
- Instead of organizing the practice dispensary in alphabetic order only, separate by antimicrobial tier (e.g. first-line, second-line, 'reserve') and organize in alphabetical order within each tier.
- Create a practice summary of antimicrobial resistance patterns for the most commonly cultured organisms in the practice.

- Animals should be weighed when prescribing to avoid underdosing. Ensure that suitable weighing scales are available.
- Use non-prescription forms for clients, explaining that their animals' condition will not benefit from antimicrobial therapy.
- Provide 'delayed prescriptions', as used by National Health Service General Practitioner practices; rather than start the antimicrobials immediately, the client can have them within a few days if the animal is not better, without being seen again.
- Have a practice WhatsApp or e-mail group to allow discussion of antibiotic choice for individual cases, around the time of prescribing.
- Appoint an 'antibiotic guardian', similar to the 'infection-control champion' already in some practices.
- Encourage vets to attend continuing professional development on antimicrobial resistance and antimicrobial stewardship.

17.6 In-Practice Measures to Reduce and Improve Antimicrobial Usage

Many in-practice barriers to responsible prescribing (Box 17.2) are at least potentially amenable to being reduced or overcome by individual veterinarians or practices, and Table 17.1 and Box 17.2 indicate that there are many ways in which antimicrobial prescribing could potentially be improved in practice. Others (Guardabassi and Prescott, 2015; Lloyd and Page, 2018) have described the sorts of measures that would be required for implementation in veterinary practices of antimicrobial stewardship programmes akin to those used in human hospitals in many countries. Full implementation of such programmes would be impractical for economic and time reasons in all but the largest veterinary practices, but introducing selected measures in individual practices should lead to substantial improvements in responsible antimicrobial usage. Boxes 17.3–17.6 suggest measures that could be considered, some of which are discussed below. Some of these measures are easy to implement, others more difficult or time consuming – and this will vary across companion animal practices. A key determinant to success of implementation will be the attitude of management and/or senior veterinarians towards AMR. Many practices have already implemented some of these measures, but there is little evidence to show how effective the various suggested measures might be at reducing antimicrobial usage in veterinary practice. This final section of the chapter suggests five examples of, arguably, 'low-hanging fruit' in terms of in-practice actions to improve antimicrobial prescribing.

17.6.1 More accurate diagnosis: greater use of easily available diagnostic tests

Antimicrobials should be used to treat or prevent only microbial diseases, and presumptive and incorrect diagnoses are perhaps the major driver of antimicrobial overuse in humans and animals (O'Neill, 2015). Incorrect diagnosis can occur because of lack of knowledge, because diagnostic tests were not undertaken or diagnostic test results were inaccurate (Sørensen et al., 2018), or because of poor or irrational clinical decision making despite all relevant information and test results being to hand (Canfield et al., 2016; Sørensen et al., 2018). Although new diagnostic tests would

Box 17.4. Suggested measures to improve antimicrobial prescribing in veterinary practices: culture and susceptibility (C&S) testing and cytology.

- Increase use of C&S testing.
- Ensure sampling technique and sample handling are optimal.
- Increase use of cytology alongside C&S testing to assist determination of whether isolated organisms actually require antimicrobial treatment.
- For in-house cytology, ensure veterinarians or nurses are appropriately trained in interpretation of the samples.
- Ensure veterinarians are providing the information on C&S submission forms that diagnostic laboratories require to provide the best advice in their C&S reports.
- De-escalate antimicrobial therapy whenever indicated. For cases treated empirically while awaiting C&S, if the C&S results indicate that antimicrobial therapy was unnecessary, stop the therapy; if the C&S results indicate that a lower-tier antimicrobial than the one empirically selected would be appropriate, change to the lower-tier antimicrobial.

Box 17.5. Suggested measures to improve antimicrobial prescribing in veterinary practices: reducing use of HPCIAs.

- Ensure suitable lower-tier antimicrobials are available to use in the practice.
- Where there are no veterinary-licensed formulations of lower-tier antimicrobials such as trimethoprim-sulfonamide, oxytetracycline or amoxicillin, then have unlicensed products available to use, where appropriate.
- Keep HPCIAs such as fluoroquinolones and third- and fourth-generation cephalosporins in a marked cupboard, separate from other antibiotics. Perhaps keep that cupboard locked, as for controlled drugs.
- Require a vet prescribing HPCIAs to record the prescription in a logbook, with a signature.
- Require veterinarians prescribing HPCIAs to record on the animal's clinical notes the justification for doing so, rather than using a lower-tier antimicrobial.
- Require the antibiotic guardian, clinical director or another vet to approve prescriptions of HPCIAs, if that usage does not match the practice's antimicrobial-usage policy or does not have supporting C&S results.
- If C&S results indicate that an infection being treated with an HPCIA is sensitive to a lower-tier antimicrobial, de-escalate the treatment (i.e. change to the lower-tier antimicrobial).
- Where appropriate, use lower-tier antimicrobials rather than licensed enrofloxacin or other HPCIA products for 'exotic' pets (Hedley et al., 2021).

---

improve diagnosis, and thus antimicrobial prescribing, diagnostic tests that are already readily available – in particular, cytology and C&S – are underused. If these tests were used more frequently to confirm bacterial involvement in disease causation and to identify the bacteria involved and their antimicrobial susceptibility, then prescribing could greatly improve, in terms of both reduced unnecessary usage, and more accurate targeting of the antimicrobials to reduce usage of HPCIAs and broad-spectrum antimicrobials where lower-tier and narrow-spectrum antimicrobials would be effective (Allerton and Nuttall, 2021). Box 17.4

suggests measures around C&S testing and cytology that may improve antimicrobial prescribing.

It is not always possible or practical to obtain appropriate samples, but where such samples can be obtained, cytology helps determine whether microbes are involved in the disease process at all (e.g. are microbes present, and if so are they just incidental contaminants or colonizers?). This information can provide some indication of which antimicrobials may be most appropriate (e.g. differentiating bacteria from yeasts in otitis externa, or Gram staining of bacteria). The usefulness of cytology will depend on the veterinarians' competence

Martin L. Whitehead

> **Box 17.6.** Suggested measures to improve antimicrobial prescribing in veterinary practices: audit & adapt.
>
> - Audit and benchmark individual veterinarians' antibiotic usage, e.g. by counting the number of antibiotic prescriptions and/or the number of HPCIA prescriptions every few months, as is done in many UK National Health Service general practices (https://openprescribing.net/; accessed 31 October 2022).
> - Periodically review a subset of each veterinarian's recent antimicrobial prescriptions, particularly of HPCIAs, to assess whether they are using antimicrobials responsibly, according to guidelines.
> - Annually count and record the practice's total purchases, or prescriptions, of certain antimicrobials for companion animals, e.g. those most commonly used, and HPCIAs, to monitor long-term usage trends.
> - In the UK, use mySAVSNet AMR (www.liverpool.ac.uk/savsnet/my-savsnet-amr/; accessed 31 October 2022) to compare the practice's antimicrobial prescribing with other companion animal practices.
> - Audit other aspects of prescribing practice relevant to antimicrobial usage, e.g. how often the prescribed dose was correct according to the data sheet for the animal's body weight, if weight was recorded; whether antimicrobial course durations for the same antimicrobial and condition vary over time or across veterinarians; how often veterinarians performed cytology prior to prescription of antimicrobials for skin lesions or otitis externa; how often veterinarians carried out C&S testing prior to prescribing HPCIAs; or how often the justification for prescription of HPCIAs was recorded on the patient's clinical record.
> - Monitor practice AMR patterns, as seen in C&S results, over time for commonly cultured conditions.
> - Discuss audit and benchmarking with the 'antibiotic guardian' equivalent at your local human primary-care practice.

at interpretation of cytology, and there is evidence that some veterinarians may lack some of these requisite skills (Sørensen *et al.*, 2018). Using cytology more, and improving competence at cytology, may optimize antimicrobial usage.

C&S can further improve antimicrobial usage. Culture aids determination of whether pathogenic organisms are contributing to the disease process, and susceptibility testing aids selection of the most appropriate antimicrobial(s) to treat that organism in that patient. The reliability of the results is dependent on the quality of sample collection, particularly the use of aseptic technique, where possible submitting the actual specimens (e.g. fluid or biopsy) for culture rather than swabs, and on rapid submission. Cytology aids interpretation of the clinical significance of the bacteria cultured. Telling the laboratory (on the submission form) the clinical signs and the site sampled can aid laboratory staff in giving better advice regarding treatment.

In some cases, obtaining suitable samples for C&S and/or cytology may be expensive, difficult or impossible. Some samples do not require routine C&S testing – for faeces and anal gland samples, culture is rarely indicated. For infections to be treated topically, such as many otitis externa or superficial pyoderma cases, culture for pathogen identification may be helpful, but antimicrobial susceptibility testing provides information regarding systemic concentrations of antibiotics only. Clinical breakpoints do not exist for antimicrobials used topically, for which *in vivo* concentrations are typically far higher, so results of *in vitro* tests assessing much lower systemic concentrations can be meaningless for infections treated topically, and may not predict clinical response.

Nevertheless, for many conditions in which suitable samples for cytology and/or C&S can be obtained, more frequent use of these tests to confirm bacterial involvement and guide antimicrobial choice could greatly improve antimicrobial usage. However, barriers exist that reduce usage of these tests (Box 17.2), including factors implicit to individual veterinarians, such as their knowledge and attitude regarding AMR and their previous experience of antimicrobial usage, and factors implicit to the practice the veterinarian works in, such as time pressure (longer consults would allow more time for investigations and to explain the benefit of those investigations to the clients), the availability of the tests in-practice, the cost of the tests, the socio-economic status of the clients (will they pay for the tests?), and the delay between sampling and C&S results.

Some of these barriers are amenable, at least potentially, to modification by individual veterinarians and practices. Can some consults be made longer? Could there be a break in consults to allow some diagnostic tests to be done? How easily available are the tests in the practice: For example, how easily accessible is the microscope, are the appropriate stains available, and can the practice's veterinary nurses stain the slides? Would training in cytology be helpful? Could a lower mark-up be put on C&S tests, perhaps allowing more tests to be done? Could the commercial laboratory provide a courier to get C&S samples there sooner?

17.6.2 Use professional guidelines and create a practice prescribing policy

Much information is available to guide responsible antimicrobial prescribing in veterinary practice. Much of this guidance is general, for instance the European Medicines Agency scheme, which categorizes antibiotics for use in animals by their potential for contribution to development of problematic AMR (categories A: avoid usage, B: restrict usage, C: use with caution, D: use with prudence) (EMA, 2020b), the British Veterinary Association's seven-point plan for the use of antimicrobials in veterinary practice that lays out general principles of responsible antimicrobial usage (BVA, 2019), and the Federation of European Companion Animal Veterinary Associations *Advice on the Responsible Use of Antimicrobials* (FECAVA, 2018). Articles discussing the principles of antimicrobial stewardship programmes in practice are available (Guardabassi and Prescott, 2015; Lloyd and Page, 2018). Very specific information regarding antimicrobial usage in certain conditions is available in expert reviews, such as the International Society for Companion Animal Infectious Disease expert reviews for superficial bacterial folliculitis (Hillier *et al.*, 2014), respiratory disease (Lappin *et al.*, 2017) and urinary tract infections (Weese *et al.*, 2019) (all available at https://iscaid.org/; accessed 31 October 2022), the American College of Veterinary Internal Medicine consensus statements on enteropathogenic diarrhoea (Marks *et al.*, 2011) and Lyme borreliosis

(Littman *et al.*, 2018) in dogs and cats, and other expert reviews (e.g. Morris *et al.*, 2017; Cerquetella *et al.*, 2020).

Some veterinary organizations have created easy-to-follow, practical guidelines for use in everyday companion animal practice that have effectively done most of the literature review and thinking required for practising veterinarians to determine – given the current state of knowledge – which bacteria or potentially bacterial common conditions do not require antimicrobial treatment, and which antimicrobials would constitute responsible usage for the treatment of those common conditions that do require antimicrobial treatment. Following such guidelines allows veterinarians to address most of the elements of Table 17.1A and B. An example is the British Small Animal Veterinary Association/ Small Animal Medicine Society PROTECT ME scheme (BSAVA/SAMSoc, 2018), the core of which is a poster that can be hung on a wall in a practice, indicating which antimicrobials could be used for a variety of common conditions, and allowing practices to easily create their own antimicrobial 'prescribing policy' for these conditions.

Allerton *et al.* (2021) provided an overview of EU antimicrobial-usage guidelines for companion animals (including PROTECT ME). Box 17.7, modified from Allerton *et al.* (2021), lists key recommendations common across many of those guidelines. Practice prescribing policies incorporating such recommendations have the potential to greatly improve the profession's antimicrobial prescribing.

17.6.3 Access and availability of antimicrobial products in practice, and measures to reduce usage of HPCIAs

A fundamental component of antimicrobial-prescribing guidelines is that some antimicrobials, particularly narrow-spectrum antimicrobials, should be used more commonly whereas broader-spectrum, and particularly HPCIAs including fluoroquinolones and third- and fourth-generation cephalosporins, should be used less commonly.

Some older, lower-tier antibiotics that are useful in companion animal medicine appear to be relatively little used in most EU countries (EMA, 2020a), such as oxytetracycline and trimethoprim-sulfonamide. In some countries, this low usage is associated with a lack of veterinary products of that antibiotic class authorized for the relevant species and indications

(Odensvik *et al.*, 2001). In contrast, as noted above, the third-generation cephalosporin cefovecin is overused in cats, reflecting the convenience of the 14-day depot injection. Similarly, enrofloxacin is overused in rabbits (Radford *et al.*, 2011), 'small furries', birds (Singleton *et al.*, 2020a) and reptiles (Hedley *et al.*, 2021), probably because enrofloxacin products are authorized for general usage in those species (Hedley *et al.*, 2021; NOAH, 2021). These are examples of factors outside of practice that powerfully influence antimicrobial usage by veterinarians, to the detriment of responsible usage.

To some extent, these factors can be overcome by using unauthorized products. In the UK, the veterinary medicines regulator (the Veterinary Medicines Directorate) has clarified that veterinarians can use the Prescribing Cascade to deviate from the use of authorized antimicrobial products for reasons of reducing development of AMR, although the extent to which companion animal veterinarians do so is unknown.

More generally, some practices may stock certain antimicrobials and not others, thereby limiting the choices made by their veterinarians (Mateus *et al.*, 2014). It is important to ensure that suitable lower-tier antimicrobials are available in practice.

As noted above, some EU countries have regulated to reduce veterinary use of HPCIAs, requiring use of fluoroquinolones and third- and fourth-generation cephalosporins to be supported by prior

C&S results. Other measures to reduce inappropriate use of HPCIAs are listed in Box 17.5. Some of these are based on increasing the 'friction' involved in prescribing them, making them more difficult or time consuming to use than other antimicrobials. For example, requiring them to be 'signed out', or requiring senior (or multi) vet approval for their use.

In future, it is to be hoped that practice management software will automatically display a warning message whenever an HPCIA is prescribed and require the veterinarian to state on the notes why the HPCIA is being prescribed instead of a lower-tier antimicrobial.

17.6.4 Not using antimicrobials when they are not required

As in human medicine (Hecker *et al.*, 2003; Llor and Bjerrum, 2014; Davey *et al.*, 2017; Chua *et al.*, 2019; Ray *et al.*, 2019), some companion animal veterinarians commonly use antimicrobials when they are not necessary. Examples include the following:

- Prophylaxis for routine soft-tissue surgical procedures (Knights *et al.*, 2012; Currie *et al.*, 2018; Williams, 2018) and uncomplicated dental work, including most extractions (Bellows *et al.*, 2019).

- Treating conditions for which antimicrobials are not indicated, including most cases of uncomplicated diarrhoea (including uncomplicated haemorrhagic diarrhoea), vomiting, feline lower urinary tract disease, subclinical bacteriuria, kennel cough, nasal discharge and sneezing. Not providing antimicrobials can be aided by providing clients with a 'no-antibiotic prescription' form, such as that available from the British Small Animal Veterinary Association (BSAVA) (Fig. 17.2), similar to those used by UK National Health Service (NHS) primary-care practices for a variety of common infectious conditions.
- Treating self-limiting diseases in patients that are not very ill. Many cases of infectious diseases, bacterial or otherwise, are self-limiting, and often a wait-and-see approach is appropriate if this will not compromise the patient's welfare. This can be aided by providing a 'no antibiotic prescription required' form, or a delayed ('backup') prescription allowing the owner to collect antimicrobials without needing the animal to be seen again if it has not improved after a few days (NICE, 2016). Delayed prescriptions have been shown to reduce antimicrobial use in human respiratory infections (Spurling et al., 2017).
- Treating identified bacteria that are commensals or contaminants, and are not actually contributing to the disease.
- Too long a duration of antimicrobial treatment. As noted above, in human medicine, recommended antibiotic treatment durations have been decreasing over the last couple of decades and are generally shorter than recommended antimicrobial courses in veterinary medicine. There is evidence that course durations have also been declining in veterinary medicine, at least for some conditions (e.g. Weese et al., 2021). However, in veterinary medicine, there is little evidence for any antimicrobial or bacterial disease to indicate how short courses should be to provide clinical efficacy while minimizing risk of AMR, and data-sheet recommendations are based on considerations of efficacy rather than minimizing AMR, which are not necessarily the same. It is important that veterinarians avoid too short a duration of treatment to clear the infection. In general, antimicrobials should not be continued past clinical and microbiological cure.
- Continuing antimicrobial treatment after C&S or other results obtained after treatment has commenced have indicated that the disease is not bacterial. In such cases, antimicrobials should be stopped immediately – not doing so exposes commensal bacteria to the antimicrobials for longer than necessary, encouraging the development of AMR. Some patients undoubtedly require early, and thus empirical, antimicrobial treatment, but sometimes that treatment turns out to be unnecessary. In human medicine, a UK Public Health England initiative is 'Start smart then focus', meaning give early effective antibiotics and then 'review and revise' 24–72 h later on the basis of test results (PHE, 2015). However, despite studies indicating that 20–30% of prescriptions could have been stopped at review, in 2017 less than 10% were stopped. An initiative to address this deficit in human hospitals is the Antibiotic Review Kit for Hospitals (Walker et al., 2019).

17.6.5 Clinical governance: oversight, audit, benchmarking and prescription review with feedback to veterinarians

Oversight

One of the most important factors allowing improvement of prescribing behaviour, as is the case for other aspects of practice, is clinical governance. Governance requires oversight – someone responsible for that aspect of practice. One or more members of the practice clinical team should be recognized as responsible for overseeing practice antimicrobial usage and for improving that usage – an 'antimicrobial guardian' – in the same way that many practices have an 'infection-control champion'. Importantly, those persons should be a member of, or have the clear-and-visible support of, senior staff or management. If senior staff or management do not support efforts to improve – in antimicrobial prescribing as well as other aspects of practice – such efforts may have little effect.

Audit and benchmarking

Improving performance is often easier if current performance is quantified. At its simplest level, audit is measuring current behaviour and comparing it against a standard. A simple audit may be to count the average number of antimicrobial prescriptions per consult over a period of time, perhaps splitting the count by antimicrobial class and specifically counting HPCIA prescriptions, and comparing

Martin L. Whitehead

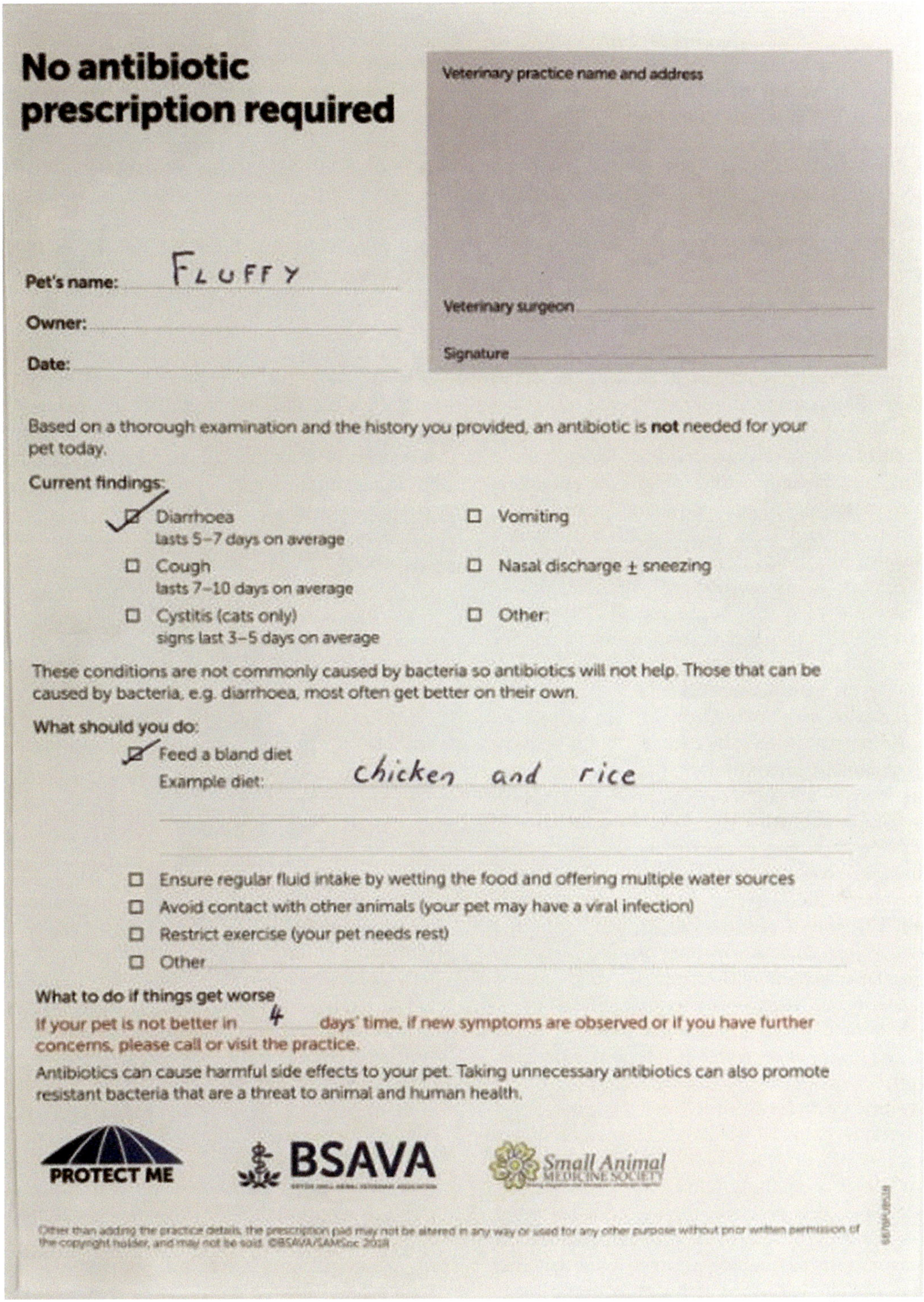

No antibiotic prescription required

Veterinary practice name and address

Veterinary surgeon

Signature

Pet's name: FLUFFY

Owner:

Date:

Based on a thorough examination and the history you provided, an antibiotic is **not** needed for your pet today.

Current findings:

- ☑ Diarrhoea
  lasts 5–7 days on average
- ☐ Cough
  lasts 7–10 days on average
- ☐ Cystitis (cats only)
  signs last 3–5 days on average
- ☐ Vomiting
- ☐ Nasal discharge ± sneezing
- ☐ Other:

These conditions are not commonly caused by bacteria so antibiotics will not help. Those that can be caused by bacteria, e.g. diarrhoea, most often get better on their own.

What should you do:

- ☑ Feed a bland diet
  Example diet: chicken and rice
- ☐ Ensure regular fluid intake by wetting the food and offering multiple water sources
- ☐ Avoid contact with other animals (your pet may have a viral infection)
- ☐ Restrict exercise (your pet needs rest)
- ☐ Other

What to do if things get worse

If your pet is not better in 4 days' time, if new symptoms are observed or if you have further concerns, please call or visit the practice.

Antibiotics can cause harmful side effects to your pet. Taking unnecessary antibiotics can also promote resistant bacteria that are a threat to animal and human health.

PROTECT ME BSAVA Small Animal Medicine Society

Other than adding the practice details, the prescription pad may not be altered in any way or used for any other purpose without prior written permission of the copyright holder, and may not be sold. ©BSAVA/SAMSoc 2018

Fig. 17.2. The British Small Animal Veterinary Association's 'No antibiotic prescription required' form.

the results with those of other, anonymized practices (i.e. benchmarking). This is done in human healthcare for hospitals (Fitzpatrick and Edwards, 2008; Ibrahim and Polk, 2014) and primary-care practices, for example by the UK's NHS (Wang *et al.*, 2009; Ahluwalia *et al.*, 2018; Devine *et al.*, 2022; see https://openprescribing.net/, accessed 31 October 2022). For companion animal veterinarians in the UK, this can be done using the mySAVS-Net AMR website (www.liverpool.ac.uk/savsnet/my-savsnet-amr/; accessed 31 October 2022), the results of which have shown large variation among practices in the numbers of prescriptions (Singleton *et al.*, 2017), suggesting that, notwithstanding some variation in practice circumstances, some practices have substantial scope to improve their prescribing behaviour.

A similar process can be carried out for individual veterinarians seeing broadly similar case portfolios within a practice – again, as done in primary-care practices in the UK's NHS. Figure 17.1 shows the results for the nine permanent veterinarians (anonymized) in the author's hospital, separately for dogs and cats, for the 18 months starting 1 January 2018. In each antimicrobial category (systemic, or topical for skin, ears or eyes), some vets prescribed antibiotics far more than others, and especially in the case of the HPCIA cefovecin. The case portfolios seen by each vet will not have been absolutely identical but, nevertheless, these results indicate substantial scope to reduce antibiotic usage by adjusting the prescribing behaviour of higher-prescribing veterinarians to match that of lower-prescribing veterinarians (Whitehead, 2020). Interestingly, by far the 'lowest' prescriber of HPCIAs was a recent graduate (and not the author!). One benefit of this process was the increased engagement of the hospital's veterinarians with responsible usage once they saw the results.

Such simple prescription counts can be very useful, especially if repeated at intervals – perhaps annually – to assess any changes in prescribing behaviour (including after any 'interventions' aimed at improving prescribing). They can indicate where the practice's or individual veterinarians' antimicrobial-prescribing behaviour is, or is not, approaching best-practice usage, and to what extent. However, they provide little information on the reasons why antimicrobial prescribing deviated from recommended usage, if it did so – and some such deviations can be justified by reasons other than considerations of AMR (e.g. was a long-acting,

higher-tier preparation given when a lower-tier antimicrobial would have been suitable from the efficacy and AMR perspectives, because the cat could not be tableted at home?). To assess such factors requires prescription review. For example, assess the last 10 or 20 prescriptions of HPCIAs within the practice, or the last 10 antimicrobial prescriptions by each veterinarian in the practice, and discuss among the veterinarians how appropriate that prescribing has been, and whether it matched prescribing guidelines, such as PROTECT ME or the practice's prescribing policy. If audit demonstrates that veterinarians are consistently prescribing in ways inconsistent with guidelines, feedback can be given and the reasons investigated, and education or training provided if necessary. Such prescribing review with feedback to the prescriber has improved antimicrobial prescribing in human medicine (Hallsworth *et al.*, 2016; Meeker *et al.*, 2016; Davey *et al.*, 2017).

Prescription review is aided if the justification for every use of antibiotic, especially HPCIAs, is recorded on the patients' clinical notes. Unfortunately, this is frequently not the case (Shea *et al.*, 2011; Burke *et al.*, 2017; Hardefeldt *et al.*, 2020; Hur *et al.*, 2020), as in human medicine (Saini *et al.*, 2022).

Suggested measures to improve prescribing with benchmarking and audit are summarized in Box 17.6.

17.7 Conclusion

Veterinarians often do not prescribe antimicrobials responsibly, as a result of many factors that influence antimicrobial-prescribing decisions by individual veterinarians. Although some, such as societal, regulatory and professional factors, are beyond the control of individual veterinary practices or individual veterinarians, other factors – both clinical and non-clinical – are within the control of practices or individual veterinarians to a greater or lesser extent. The more practices and veterinarians that address some of these factors, the more antimicrobial-prescribing behaviour within the companion animal profession will improve. Veterinarians should not let 'perfect be the enemy of the good', and adopting just some measures, such as increasing use of C&S testing and cytology to improve the diagnoses of microbial diseases, following recommended prescribing guidelines via a practice prescribing policy, ensuring access to lower-tier antimicrobials and increasing the friction of use of HPCIAs, de-escalating antimicrobial treatment when indicated and carrying out basic audit of antimicrobial prescribing, including benchmarking and prescription review with feedback to the veterinarians, should go a long way towards improving responsible antimicrobial usage.

References

Ahluwalia, S., Sadak, M. and Ashworth, M. (2018) Antimicrobial prescribing in post-graduate training practices: a cross-sectional study of prescribing data in general practices in England. *Education for Primary Care* 29(3), 139–143. DOI: 10.1080/14739879.2018.1430515.

Alcantara, G.L.C., Pinello, K.C., Severo, M. and Niza-Ribeiro, J. (2021) Antimicrobial resistance in companion animals - Veterinarians' attitudes and prescription drivers in Portugal. *Comparative Immunology, Microbiology and Infectious Diseases* 76, 101640. DOI: 10.1016/j.cimid.2021.101640.

Allerton, F. and Nuttall, T. (2021) Antimicrobial use: importance of bacterial culture and susceptibility testing. *In Practice* 43(9), 500–510. DOI: 10.1002/inpr.139.

Allerton, F., Prior, C., Bagcigil, A.F., Broens, E. and Callens, B. (2021) Overview and evaluation of existing guidelines for rational antimicrobial use in small-animal veterinary practice in Europe. *Antibiotics* 10(4), 409. DOI: 10.3390/antibiotics10040409.

Allerton, F., Pouwels, K.B., Bazelle, J., Caddy, S., Cauvin, A. *et al.* (2022) Prospective trial of different antimicrobial treatment durations for presumptive canine urinary tract infections. *BMC Veterinary Research* 17(1), 229. DOI: 10.1186/s12917-021-02974-y.

Attauabi, M., BorckHøg, B. and Müller-Pebody, B. (eds) (2021) *DANMAP 2020. Use of Antimicrobial Agents and Occurrence of Antimicrobial Resistance in Bacteria from Food Animals, Food and Humans in Denmark*. National Food Institute/Statens Serum Institut, Denmark. Available at: www.ssi.dk/-/media/arkiv/subsites/antibiotikaresistens/danmap_2020_07102021_version-2_low.pdf?la=da (accessed 28 October 2022).

Baker, S.A., Van-Balen, J., Lu, B., Hillier, A. and Hoet, A.E. (2012) Antimicrobial drug use in dogs prior to admission to a veterinary teaching hospital. *Journal of the American Veterinary Medical Association* 241(2), 210–217. DOI: 10.2460/javma.241.2.210.

Banfield Pet Hospital (2017) Veterinary emerging topics report: are we doing our part to prevent superbugs? Antimicrobial usage patterns among companion animal veterinarians. Available at: www.banfieldexchange.com/VET-Report (accessed October 2022).

Barbarossa, A., Rambaldi, J., Miraglia, V., Giunti, M., Diegoli, G *et al.* (2017) Survey on antimicrobial prescribing patterns in small animal veterinary practice in Emilia Romagna, Italy. *Veterinary Record* 181(3), 69. DOI: 10.1136/vr.104128.

Barzelai, I.D. and Whittem, T. (2017) Survey of systemic antimicrobial prescribing for dogs by Victorian veterinarians. *Australian Veterinary Journal* 95(10), 375–385. DOI: 10.1111/avj.12637.

Baur, D., Gladstone, B.P., Burkert, F., Carrara, E., Foschi, F *et al.* (2017) Effect of antibiotic stewardship on the incidence of infection and colonisation with antibiotic-resistant bacteria and *Clostridium difficile* infection: a systematic review and meta-analysis. *Lancet Infectious Diseases* 17(9), 990–1001. DOI: 10.1016/S1473-3099(17)30325-0.

Belas, A., Menezes, J., Gama, L.T. and Pomba, C. (2020) Sharing of clinically important antimicrobial resistance genes by companion animals and their human household members. *Microbial Drug Resistance* 26(10), 1174–1185. DOI: 10.1089/mdr.2019.0380.

Bellows, J., Berg, M.L., Dennis, S., Harvey, R., Lobprise, H.B. *et al.* (2019) 2019 AAHA dental care guidelines for dogs and cats. *Journal of the American Animal Hospital Association* 55(2), 49–69. DOI: 10.5326/JAAHA-MS-6933.

Boeckel, T.P.V., Glennon, E.E., Chen, D., Gilbert, M., Robinson, T.P., *et al.* (2017) Reducing antimicrobial use in food animals. *Science* 357(6358), 1350–1352. DOI: 10.1126/science.aao1495.

Boiko, O., Gulliford, M.C. and Burgess, C. (2020) Revisiting patient expectations and experiences of antibiotics in an era of antimicrobial resistance: qualitative study. *Health Expectations* 23(5), 1250–1258. DOI: 10.1111/hex.13102.

Borek, A.J., Anthierens, S., Allison, R., Mcnulty, C.A.M. and Anyanwu, P.E. (2020) Social and contextual influences on antibiotic prescribing and antimicrobial stewardship: a qualitative study with clinical commissioning group and general practice professionals. *Antibiotics* 9(12), 859. DOI: 10.3390/antibiotics9120859.

Borek, A.J., Pouwels, K.B., van Hecke, O., Robotham, J.V., Butler, C.C. *et al.* (2022) Role of locum GPs in antibiotic prescribing and stewardship: a mixed-methods study. *British Journal of General Practice* 72(715), e118–e127. DOI: 10.3399/BJGP.2021.0354.

Brookes-Howell, L., Hood, K., Cooper, L., Little, P., Verheij, T. *et al.* (2012) Understanding variation in primary medical care: a nine-country qualitative study of clinicians' accounts of the non-clinical factors that shape antibiotic prescribing decisions for lower respiratory tract infection. *BMJ Open* 2(4), e000796. DOI: 10.1136/bmjopen-2011-000796.

Brown, D.C., Conzemius, M.G., Shofer, F. and Swann, H. (1997) Epidemiologic evaluation of postoperative wound infections in dogs and cats. *Journal* of the *American Veterinary Medical Association* 210, 1302–1306.

BSAVA/SAMSoc (2018) *PROTECT ME. British Small Animal Veterinary Association/Small Animal Medicine Society*. Quedgeley, UK. Available at: www.bsava.co m/Resources/Veterinary-resources/PROTECT-ME/ (accessed 28 October 2022).

Buckland, E.L., O'Neill, D., Summers, J., Mateus, A., Church, D *et al.* (2016) Characterisation of antimicrobial usage in cats and dogs attending UK primary care companion animal veterinary practices. *Veterinary Record* 179(19), 489. DOI: 10.1136/vr.103830.

Burke, S., Black, V., Sánchez-Vizcaíno, F., Radford, A., Hibbert, A. *et al.* (2017) Use of cefovecin in a UK population of cats attending first-opinion practices as recorded in electronic health records. *Journal of Feline Medicine and Surgery* 19(6), 687–692. DOI: 10.1177/1098612X16656706.

BVA (2019) *Responsible Use of Antimicrobials in Veterinary Practice 7-Point Plan*. British Veterinary Association, London. Available at: www.bva.co.uk/re sources-support/medicines/responsible-use-of-antim icrobials-in-veterinary-practice-poster/ (accessed 10 May 2022).

Canfield, P.J., Whitehead, M.L., Johnson, R., O'Brien, C.R. and Malik, R. (2016) Case-based clinical reasoning in feline medicine: 2: managing cognitive error. *Journal of Feline Medicine and Surgery* 18(3), 240–247. DOI: 10.1177/1098612X16631233.

Cerquetella, M., Rossi, G., Suchodolski, J.S., Schmitz, S.S., Allenspach, K *et al.* (2020) Proposal for rational antibacterial use in the diagnosis and treatment of dogs with chronic diarrhoea. *Journal of Small Animal Practice* 61(4), 211–215. DOI: 10.1111/jsap.13122.

Charani, E., Edwards, R., Sevdalis, N., Alexandrou, B., Sibley, E. *et al.* (2011) Behavior change strategies to influence antimicrobial prescribing in acute care: a systematic review. *Clinical Infectious Diseases* 53(7), 651–662. DOI: 10.1093/cid/cir445.

Charani, E., Castro-Sanchez, E., Sevdalis, N., Kyratsis, Y., Drumright, L. *et al.* (2013) Understanding the determinants of antimicrobial prescribing within hospitals: the role of "prescribing etiquette." *Clinical Infectious Diseases* 57(2), 188–196. DOI: 10.1093/cid/cit212.

Charani, E., McKee, M., Ahmad, R., Balasegaram, M., Bonaconsa, C *et al.* (2021) Optimising antimicrobial use in humans - review of current evidence and an interdisciplinary consensus on key priorities for research. *Lancet Regional Health. Europe* 7, 100161. DOI: 10.1016/j.lanepe.2021.100161.

Cheng, A.C. and Worth, L.J. (2015) Cultural dimensions relevant to antimicrobial stewardship: the contribution of individualism and power distance to perioperative prescribing practices in European hospitals. *Healthcare Infection* 20(3–4), 124–127. DOI: 10.1071/HI15010.

Chipangura, J.K., Eagar, H., Kgoete, M., Abernethy, D. and Naidoo, V. (2017) An investigation of antimicrobial usage patterns by small animal veterinarians in South Africa. *Preventive Veterinary Medicine* 136, 29–38. DOI: 10.1016/j.prevetmed.2016.11.017.

Chirollo, C., Nocera, F.P., Piantedosi, D., Fatone, G., Della Valle, G. *et al.* (2021) Data on before and after the traceability system of veterinary antimicrobial prescriptions in small animals at the university veterinary teaching hospital of Naples. *Animals* 11(3), 913. DOI: 10.3390/ani11030913.

Chua, K.P., Fischer, M.A. and Linder, J.A. (2019) Appropriateness of outpatient antibiotic prescribing among privately insured US patients: ICD-10-CM based cross sectional study. *British Medical Journal* 364, k5092. DOI: 10.1136/bmj.k5092.

Clare, S., Hartmann, F.A., Jooss, M., Bachar, E., Wong, Y.Y. *et al.* (2014) Short- and long-term cure rates of short-duration trimethoprim-sulfamethoxazole treatment in female dogs with uncomplicated bacterial cystitis. *Journal of Veterinary Internal Medicine* 28(3), 818–826. DOI: 10.1111/jvim.12324.

Collineau, L., Rojo-Gimeno, C., Léger, A., Backhans, A., Loesken, S. *et al.* (2017) Herd-specific interventions to reduce antimicrobial usage in pig production without jeopardising technical and economic performance. *Preventive Veterinary Medicine* 144, 167–178. DOI: 10.1016/j.prevetmed.2017.05.023.

Corrente, M., Sangiorgio, G., Grandolfo, E., Bodnar, L., Catella, C. *et al.* (2017) Risk for zoonotic Salmonella transmission from pet reptiles: a survey on knowledge, attitudes and practices of reptile-owners related to reptile husbandry. *Preventive Veterinary Medicine* 146, 73–78. DOI: 10.1016/j.prevetmed.2017.07.014.

Courvalin, P. (2008) Can pharmacokinetic-pharmacodynamic parameters provide dosing regimens that are less vulnerable to resistance? *Clinical Microbiology and Infection* 14(11), 989–994. DOI: 10.1111/j.1469-0691.2008.02081.x.

Couto, N., Monchique, C., Belas, A., Marques, C., Gama, L.T *et al.* (2016) Trends and molecular mechanisms of antimicrobial resistance in clinical staphylococci isolated from companion animals over a 16 year period. *Journal of Antimicrobial Chemotherapy* 71(6), 1479–1487. DOI: 10.1093/jac/dkw029.

Crayton, E., Richardson, M., Fuller, C., Smith, C., Liu, S. *et al.* (2020) Interventions to improve appropriate antibiotic prescribing in long-term care facilities: a systematic review. *BMC Geriatrics* 20(1), 237. DOI: 10.1186/s12877-020-01564-1.

Crotty, M.P., Meyers, S., Hampton, N., Bledsoe, S., Ritchie, D.J *et al.* (2015) Impact of antibacterials on subsequent resistance and clinical outcomes in adult patients with viral pneumonia: an opportunity for stewardship. *Critical Care* 19, 404. DOI: 10.1186/s13054-015-1120-5.

Martin L. Whitehead

Currie, K., King, C., Nuttall, T., Smith, M. and Flowers, P. (2018) Expert consensus regarding drivers of antimicrobial stewardship in companion animal veterinary practice: a Delphi study. *Veterinary Record* 182(24), 691. DOI: 10.1136/vr.104639.

Davey, P., Marwick, C.A., Scott, C.L., Charani, E., McNeil, K. *et al.* (2017) Interventions to improve antibiotic prescribing practices for hospital inpatients. *Cochrane Database of Systematic Reviews* 2(2), CD003543. DOI: 10.1002/14651858.CD003543.pub4.

de Briyne, N., Atkinson, J., Pokludová, L., Borriello, S.P. and Price, S. (2013) Factors influencing antibiotic prescribing habits and use of sensitivity testing amongst veterinarians in Europe. *Veterinary Record* 173, 475. DOI: 10.1136/vr.101454.

Devine, P., O'Kane, M. and Bucholc, M. (2022) Trends, variation, and factors influencing antibiotic prescribing: a longitudinal study in primary care using a multilevel modelling approach. *Antibiotics* 11, 17. DOI: 10.3390/antibiotics11010017.

Dyar, O.J., Huttner, B., Schouten, J. and Pulcini, C. (2017) What is antimicrobial stewardship? *Clinical Microbiology and Infection* 23(11), 793–798. DOI: 10.1016/j.cmi.2017.08.026.

Ekakoro, J.E. and Okafor, C.C. (2019) Antimicrobial use practices of veterinary clinicians at a veterinary teaching hospital in the United States. *Veterinary and Animal Science* 7, 100038. DOI: 10.1016/j.vas.2018.09.002.

Ekiri, A., Haesler, B., Mays, N., Staerk, K. and Mateus, A. (2019) *Impact of Guidelines and Recommendations on The Level and Patterns of Antimicrobial Use in Livestock and Companion Animals*. Policy Innovation Research Unit Publication 2019-25-A8. Available at: https://piru.ac.uk/assets/files/App%208%20Impact%20of%20guidelines%20on%20patterns%20of%20AMU%20in%20livestock%20and%20companion%20animals%20(Ekiri%20et%20al)%20December%2019.pdf (accessed 28 October 2022).

EMA (2015) *Risk of Antimicrobial Resistance Transfer From Companion Animals*. European Medicines Agency, Amsterdam, Netherlands. Available at: www.ema.europa.eu/en/risk-antimicrobial-resistance-transfer-companion-animals (accessed 28 October 2022).

EMA (2019) *Categorisation of Antibiotics in the European*. European Medicines Agency, Amsterdam, Netherlands. Available at: www.ema.europa.eu/en/documents/report/categorisation-antibiotics-european-union-answer-request-european-commission-updating-scientific_en.pdf (accessed 28 October 2022).

EMA (2020a) *Sales of Veterinary Antimicrobial Agents in 31 Countries in 2018: Tenth ESVAC Report*. European Medicines Agency, Amsterdam, Netherlands. Available at: www.ema.europa.eu/en/news/10th-esvac-report-shows-continued-decrease-sales-veterinary-antibiotics (accessed 28 October 2022).

EMA (2020b) *Categorisation of Antibiotics Used in Animals Responsible Use to Protect Public and Animal Health*. European Medicines Agency, Amsterdam, Netherlands. Available at: www.ema.europa.eu/en/news/categorisation-antibiotics-used-animals-promotes-responsible-use-protect-public-animal-health (accessed 28 October 2022).

EMA (2021) *Antimicrobial Resistance in the Environment: Considerations for Current and Future Risk Assessment of Veterinary Medicinal*. European Medicines Agency, Amsterdam, Netherlands. Available at: www.ema.europa.eu/en/antimicrobial-resistance-environment-considerations-current-future-risk-assessment-veterinary (accessed 28 October 2022).

Escher, M., Vanni, M., Intorre, L., Caprioli, A., Tognetti, R *et al.* (2011) Use of antimicrobials in companion animal practice: a retrospective study in a veterinary teaching hospital in Italy. *Journal of Antimicrobial Chemotherapy* 66(4), 920–927. DOI: 10.1093/jac/dkq543.

Eugster, S., Schawalder, P., Gaschen, F. and Boerlin, P. (2004) A prospective study of postoperative surgical site infections in dogs and cats. *Veterinary Surgery* 33(5), 542–550. DOI: 10.1111/j.1532-950X.2004.04076.x.

European Parliament (2022) Council of the European Union, Regulation (EU) 2019/6 of the European parliament and of the council of 11 december 2018 on veterinary medicinal products and repealing directive 2001/82/EC. Available at: https://eur-lex.europa.eu/legal-content/EN/TXT/?uri=CELEX%3A02019R0006-20220128 (accessed 28 October 2022).

FECAVA (2018) *Advice on the Responsible Use of Antimicrobials*. Federation of European Companion Animal Veterinary Associations, Brussels. Available at: www.fecava.org/policies-actions/guidelines/ (accessed 10 May 2022).

Fernandez-Lazaro, C.I., Brown, K.A., Langford, B.J., Daneman, N., Garber, G. *et al.* (2019) Late-career physicians prescribe longer courses of antibiotics. *Clinical Infectious Diseases* 69(9), 1467–1475. DOI: 10.1093/cid/ciy1130.

Fitzpatrick, R.W. and Edwards, C.M.C. (2008) Evaluation of a tool to benchmark hospital antibiotic prescribing in the United Kingdom. *Pharmacy World & Science* 30(1), 73–78. DOI: 10.1007/s11096-007-9147-6.

Fowler, H., Davis, M.A., Perkins, A., Trufan, S., Joy, C. *et al.* (2016) A survey of veterinary antimicrobial prescribing practices, Washington State 2015. *The Veterinary Record* 179(25), 651. DOI: 10.1136/vr.103916.

Galarce, N., Arriagada, G., Sánchez, F., Venegas, V., Cornejo, J. *et al.* (2021) Antimicrobial use in companion animals: assessing veterinarians' prescription patterns through the first national survey in Chile. *Animals* 11(2), 348. DOI: 10.3390/ani11020348.

Goggs, R., Menard, J.M., Altier, C., Cummings, K.J., Jacob, M.E. *et al.* (2021) Patterns of antimicrobial drug use in veterinary primary care and specialty practice: a 6-year multi-institution study. *Journal of Veterinary Internal Medicine* 35(3), 1496–1508. DOI: 10.1111/jvim.16136.

Gómez-Beltrán, D.A., Schaeffer, D.J., Ferguson, D.C., Monsalve, L.K. and Villar, D. (2021) Antimicrobial prescribing practices in dogs and cats by colombian veterinarians in the City of Medellin. *Veterinary Sciences* 8(5), 73. DOI: 10.3390/vetsci8050073.

Gómez-Poveda, B. and Moreno, M.A. (2018) Antimicrobial prescriptions for dogs in the capital of Spain. *Frontiers in Veterinary Science* 5, 309. DOI: 10.3389/fvets.2018.00309.

Grenni, P., Ancona, V. and Barra Caracciolo, A. (2018) Ecological effects of antibiotics on natural ecosystems: a review. *Microchemical Journal* 136, 25–39. DOI: 10.1016/j.microc.2017.02.006.

Grønvold, A.-M.R., L'abée-Lund, T.M., Sørum, H., Skancke, E., Yannarell, A.C. *et al.* (2010) Changes in fecal microbiota of healthy dogs administered amoxicillin. *FEMS Microbiology Ecology* 71(2), 313–326. DOI: 10.1111/j.1574-6941.2009.00808.x.

Guardabassi, L. and Prescott, J.F. (2015) Antimicrobial stewardship in small animal veterinary practice: from theory to practice. *Veterinary Clinics of North America. Small Animal Practice* 45(2), 361–376. DOI: 10.1016/j.cvsm.2014.11.005.

Hackmann, C., Gastmeier, P., Schwarz, S., Lübke-Becker, A., Bischoff, P. *et al.* (2021) Pet husbandry as a risk factor for colonization or infection with MDR organisms: a systematic meta-analysis. *Journal of Antimicrobial Chemotherapy* 76(6), 1392–1405. DOI: 10.1093/jac/dkab058.

Hajjaj, F.M., Salek, M.S., Basra, M.K.A. and Finlay, A.Y. (2010) Non-clinical influences on clinical decision-making: a major challenge to evidence-based practice. *Journal of the Royal Society of Medicine* 103(5), 178–187. DOI: 10.1258/jrsm.2010.100104.

Hallsworth, M., Chadborn, T., Sallis, A., Sanders, M., Berry, D. *et al.* (2016) Provision of social norm feedback to high prescribers of antibiotics in general practice: a pragmatic national randomised controlled trial. *Lancet* 387(10029), 1743–1752. DOI: 10.1016/S0140-6736(16)00215-4.

Hanretty, A.M. and Gallagher, J.C. (2018) Shortened courses of antibiotics for bacterial infections: a systematic review of randomized controlled trials. *Pharmacotherapy* 38(6), 674–687. DOI: 10.1002/phar.2118.

Hardefeldt, L.Y., Gilkerson, J.R., Billman-Jacobe, H., Stevenson, M.A., Thursky, K. *et al.* (2017a) Barriers to and enablers of implementing antimicrobial stewardship programs in veterinary practices. *Journal of Veterinary Internal Medicine* 32(3), 1092–1099. DOI: 10.1111/jvim.15083.

Hardefeldt, L.Y., Holloway, S., Trott, D.J., Shipstone, M., Barrs, V.R. *et al.* (2017b) Antimicrobial prescribing in dogs and cats in Australia: results of the Australasian infectious disease advisory panel survey. *Journal of Veterinary Internal Medicine* 31(4), 1100–1107. DOI: 10.1111/jvim.14733.

Hardefeldt, L.Y., Selinger, J., Stevenson, M.A., Gilkerson, J.R., Crabb, H. *et al.* (2018) Population wide assessment of antimicrobial use in dogs and cats using a novel data source - a cohort study using pet insurance data. *Veterinary Microbiology* 225, 34–39. DOI: 10.1016/j.vetmic.2018.09.010.

Hardefeldt, L., Hur, B., Verspoor, K., Baldwin, T., Bailey, K.E. *et al.* (2020) Use of cefovecin in dogs and cats attending first-opinion veterinary practices in Australia. *Veterinary Record* 187(11), e95. DOI: 10.1136/vr.105997.

Hardefeldt, L.Y., Hur, B., Richards, S., Scarborough, R., Browning, G.F. *et al.* (2022) Antimicrobial stewardship in companion animal practice: an implementation trial in 135 general practice veterinary clinics. *JAC-Antimicrobial Resistance* 4(1), dlac015. DOI: 10.1093/jacamr/dlac015.

Harrison, E.M., Weinert, L.A., Holden, M.T.G., Welch, J.J., Wilson, K. *et al.* (2014) A shared population of epidemic methicillin-resistant *Staphylococcus aureus* 15 circulates in humans and companion animals. *MBio* 5(3), e00985–13. DOI: 10.1128/mBio.00985-13.

Hecker, M.T., Aron, D.C., Patel, N.P., Lehmann, M.K. and Donskey, C.J. (2003) Unnecessary use of antimicrobials in hospitalized patients: current patterns of misuse with an emphasis on the antianaerobic spectrum of activity. *Archives of Internal Medicine* 163(8), 972–978. DOI: 10.1001/archinte.163.8.972.

Hedley, J., Whitehead, M.L., Munns, C., Pellett, S., Abou-Zahr, T *et al.* (2021) Antibiotic stewardship for reptiles. *Journal of Small Animal Practice* 62(10), 829–839. DOI: 10.1111/jsap.13402.

Heuer, O.E., Jensen, V.F. and Hammerum, A.M. (2005) Antimicrobial drug consumption in companion animals. *Emerging Infectious Diseases* 11(2), 344–345. DOI: 10.3201/eid1102.040827.

Hillier, A., Lloyd, D.H., Weese, J.S., Blondeau, J.M., Boothe, D. *et al.* (2014) Guidelines for the diagnosis and antimicrobial therapy of canine superficial bacterial folliculitis (Antimicrobial Guidelines Working Group of the International Society for Companion Animal Infectious Diseases). *Veterinary Dermatology* 25(3), 163–e43. DOI: 10.1111/vde.12118.

Hoelzer, K., Moreno Switt, A.I. and Wiedmann, M. (2011) Animal contact as a source of human non-typhoidal salmonellosis. *Veterinary Research* 42(1), 34. DOI: 10.1186/1297-9716-42-34.

Hölsö, K., Rantala, M., Lillas, A., Eerikäinen, S., Huovinen, P. *et al.* (2005) Prescribing antimicrobial agents for dogs and cats via university pharmacies in Finland--patterns and quality of information. *Acta Veterinaria Scandinavica* 46(1–2), 87–93. DOI: 10.1186/1751-0147-46-87.

Hopman, N.E.M., Hulscher, M.E.J.L., Graveland, H., Speksnijder, D.C., Wagenaar, J.A. *et al.* (2018) Factors influencing antimicrobial prescribing by Dutch companion animal veterinarians: a qualitative study. *Preventive Veterinary Medicine* 158, 106–113. DOI: 10.1016/j.prevetmed.2018.07.013.

Hopman, N.E.M., van Dijk, M.A.M., Broens, E.M., Wagenaar, J.A., Heederik, D.J.J. *et al.* (2019a) Quantifying antimicrobial use in dutch companion animals. *Frontiers in Veterinary Science* 6, 158. DOI: 10.3389/fvets.2019.00158.

Hopman, N.E.M., Portengen, L., Heederik, D.J.J., Wagenaar, J.A., Van Geijlswijk, I.M. *et al.* (2019b) Time trends, seasonal differences and determinants of systemic antimicrobial use in companion animal clinics (2012–2015). *Veterinary Microbiology* 235, 289–294. DOI: 10.1016/j.vetmic.2019.07.016.

Hopman, N.E.M., Portengen, L., Hulscher, M.E.J.L., Heederik, D.J.J., Verheij, T.J.M. *et al.* (2019c) Implementation and evaluation of an antimicrobial stewardship programme in companion animal clinics: a stepped-wedge design intervention study. *PloS One* 14(11), e0225124. DOI: 10.1371/journal.pone.0225124.

Horwood, J., Cabral, C., Hay, A.D. and Ingram, J. (2016) Primary care clinician antibiotic prescribing decisions in consultations for children with RTIs: a qualitative interview study. *British Journal of General Practice* 66(644), e207–13. DOI: 10.3399/bjgp16X683821.

Hubbuch, A., Schmitt, K., Lehner, C., Hartnack, S., Schuller, S. *et al.* (2020) Antimicrobial prescriptions in cats in Switzerland before and after the introduction of an online antimicrobial stewardship tool. *BMC Veterinary Research* 16(1), 229. DOI: 10.1186/s12917-020-02447-8.

Hubbuch, A., Peter, R., Willi, B., Hartnack, S., Müntener, C. *et al.* (2021) Comparison of antimicrobial prescription patterns in calves in Switzerland before and after the launch of online guidelines for prudent antimicrobial use. *BMC Veterinary Research* 17(1), 2. DOI: 10.1186/s12917-020-02704-w.

Hughes, L.A., Williams, N., Clegg, P., Callaby, R., Nuttall, T. *et al.* (2012) Cross-sectional survey of antimicrobial prescribing patterns in UK small animal veterinary practice. *Preventive Veterinary Medicine* 104(3–4), 309–316. DOI: 10.1016/j.prevetmed.2011.12.003.

Hulscher, M.E.J.L., van der Meer, J.W.M. and Grol, R.P.T.M. (2010) Antibiotic use: how to improve it? *International Journal of Medical Microbiology* 300(6), 351–356. DOI: 10.1016/j.ijmm.2010.04.003.

Hur, B.A., Hardefeldt, L.Y., Verspoor, K.M., Baldwin, T. and Gilkerson, J.R. (2020) Describing the antimicrobial usage patterns of companion animal veterinary practices; free text analysis of more than 4.4 million consultation records. *PloS One* 15(3), e0230049. DOI: 10.1371/journal.pone.0230049.

Hur, B., Hardefeldt, L.Y., Verspoor, K.M., Baldwin, T. and Gilkerson, J.R. (2022) Evaluating the dose, indication and agreement with guidelines of antimicrobial use in companion animal practice with natural language processing. *JAC-Antimicrobial Resistance* 4(1), dlab194. DOI: 10.1093/jacamr/dlab194.

Ibrahim, O.M. and Polk, R.E. (2014) Antimicrobial use metrics and benchmarking to improve stewardship outcomes: methodology, opportunities, and challenges. *Infectious Disease Clinics of North America* 28(2), 195–214. DOI: 10.1016/j.idc.2014.01.006.

Jacob, M.E., Hoppin, J.A., Steers, N., Davis, J.L., Davidson, G. *et al.* (2015) Opinions of clinical veterinarians at a US veterinary teaching hospital regarding antimicrobial use and antimicrobial-resistant infections. *Journal of the American Veterinary Medical Association* 247(8), 938–944. DOI: 10.2460/javma.247.8.938.

Jessen, L.R., Sørensen, T.M., Lilja, Z.L., Kristensen, M., Hald, T. *et al.* (2017) Cross-sectional survey on the use and impact of the Danish national antibiotic use guidelines for companion animal practice. *Acta Veterinaria Scandinavica* 59(1), 81. DOI: 10.1186/s13028-017-0350-8.

Johnson, J.R., Owens, K., Gajewski, A. and Clabots, C. (2008) *Escherichia coli* colonization patterns among human household members and pets, with attention to acute urinary tract infection. *Journal of Infectious Diseases* 197(2), 218–224. DOI: 10.1086/524844.

Joosten, P., Ceccarelli, D., Odent, E., Sarrazin, S. and Graveland, H. (2020) Antimicrobial usage and resistance in companion animals: a cross-sectional study in three European Countries. *Antibiotics* 9(2), 87. DOI: 10.3390/antibiotics9020087.

King, C., Smith, M., Currie, K., Dickson, A., Smith, F. *et al.* (2018) Exploring the behavioural drivers of veterinary surgeon antibiotic prescribing: a qualitative study of companion animal veterinary surgeons in the UK. *BMC Veterinary Research* 14(1), 332. DOI: 10.1186/s12917-018-1646-2.

Klinker, K.P., Hidayat, L.K., DeRyke, C.A., DePestel, D.D., Motyl, M. *et al.* (2021) Antimicrobial stewardship and antibiograms: importance of moving beyond traditional antibiograms. *Therapeutic Advances in Infectious Disease* 8, 20499361211011372. DOI: 10.1177/20499361211011373.

Knights, C.B., Mateus, A. and Baines, S.J. (2012) Current British veterinary attitudes to the use of perioperative antimicrobials in small animal surgery. *Veterinary Record* 170(25), 646. DOI: 10.1136/vr.100292.

Kraemer, S.A., Ramachandran, A. and Perron, G.G. (2019) Antibiotic pollution in the environment: from microbial ecology to public policy. *Microorganisms* 7(6), 180. DOI: 10.3390/microorganisms7060180.

Krockow, E.M., Colman, A.M., Chattoe-Brown, E., Jenkins, D.R., Perera, N *et al.* (2019) Balancing the risks to individual and society: a systematic review and synthesis of qualitative research on antibiotic prescribing behaviour in hospitals. *Journal of Hospital Infection* 101(4), 428–439. DOI: 10.1016/j.jhin.2018.08.007.

Kvaale, M.K., Grave, K., Kristoffersen, A.B. and Norström, M. (2012) The prescription rate of antibacterial agents in dogs in Norway - geographical patterns and trends during the period 2004–2008. *Journal of Veterinary Pharmacology and Therapeutics* 36(3), 285–291. DOI: 10.1111/j.1365-2885.2012.01425.x.

Lappin, M.R., Blondeau, J., Boothe, D., Breitschwerdt, E.B., Guardabassi, L. *et al.* (2017) Antimicrobial use guidelines for treatment of respiratory tract disease in dogs and cats: Antimicrobial Guidelines Working Group of the International Society for Companion Animal Infectious Diseases. *Journal of Veterinary Internal Medicine* 31(2), 279–294. DOI: 10.1111/jvim.14627.

Lee, R.A., Centor, R.M., Humphrey, L.L., Jokela, J.A., Andrews, R. *et al.* (2021) Appropriate use of short-course antibiotics in common infections: best practice advice from the American College of Physicians. *Annals of Internal Medicine* 174(6), 822–827. DOI: 10.7326/M20-7355.

Lehner, C., Hubbuch, A., Schmitt, K., Schuepbach-Regula, G., Willi, B. *et al.* (2020) Effect of antimicrobial stewardship on antimicrobial prescriptions for selected diseases of dogs in Switzerland. *Journal of Veterinary Internal Medicine* 34(6), 2418–2431. DOI: 10.1111/jvim.15906.

Lim, J.M., Singh, S.R., Duong, M.C., Legido-Quigley, H., Hsu, L.Y. *et al.* (2020) Impact of national interventions to promote responsible antibiotic use: a systematic review. *Journal of Antimicrobial Chemotherapy* 75(1), 14–29. DOI: 10.1093/jac/dkz348.

Littman, M.P., Gerber, B., Goldstein, R.E., Labato, M.A., Lappin, M.R. *et al.* (2018) ACVIM consensus update on Lyme borreliosis in dogs and cats. *Journal of Veterinary Internal Medicine* 32, 887–903. DOI: 10.1111/jvim.15085.

Llewelyn, M.J., Fitzpatrick, J.M., Darwin, E.D., Tonkin-Crine, S. and Gorton, C. (eds) (2017) The antibiotic course has had its day. *British Medical Journal* 358, j3418. DOI: 10.1136/bmj.j3418.

Llor, C. and Bjerrum, L. (2014) Antimicrobial resistance: risk associated with antimicrobial overuse and initiatives to reduce the problem. *Therapeutic Advances in Drug Safety* 5, 229–241. DOI: 10.1177/2042098614554919.

Lloyd, D.H. and Page, S.W. (2018) Antimicrobial stewardship in veterinary medicine. In: Schwarz, S., Cavaco, L.M. and Shen, J. (eds) *Antimicrobial Resistance in Bacteria from Livestock and Companion Animals*. American Society for Microbiology, Washington, DC, pp. 675–698. DOI: 10.1128/microbiolspec. ARBA-0023-2017.

Lum, E.P.M., Page, K., Whitty, J.A., Doust, J. and Graves, N. (2018) Antibiotic prescribing in primary healthcare: Dominant factors and trade-offs in decision-making. *Infection, Disease & Health* 23(2), 74–86. DOI: 10.1016/j.idh.2017.12.002.

Lutz, B., Lehner, C., Schmitt, K., Willi, B., Schüpbach, G. *et al.* (2020) Antimicrobial prescriptions and adherence to prudent use guidelines for selected canine diseases in Switzerland in 2016. *Veterinary Record Open* 7(1), e000370. DOI: 10.1136/vetreco-2019-000370.

Maeyama, Y., Taniguchi, Y., Hayashi, W., Ohsaki, Y., Osaka, S. *et al.* (2018) Prevalence of ESBL/AmpC genes and specific clones among the third-generation cephalosporin-resistant Enterobacteriaceae from canine and feline clinical specimens in Japan. *Veterinary Microbiology* 216, 183–189. DOI: 10.1016/j.vetmic.2018.02.020.

Makita, K., Sugahara, N., Nakamura, K., Matsuoka, T., Sakai, M. *et al.* (2021) Current status of antimicrobial drug use in Japanese companion animal clinics and the factors associated with their use. *Frontiers in Veterinary Science* 8, 705648. DOI: 10.3389/fvets.2021.705648.

Manian, F.A. (2003) Asymptomatic nasal carriage of mupirocin-resistant, methicillin-resistant *Staphylococcus aureus* (MRSA) in a pet dog associated with MRSA infection in household contacts . *Clinical Infectious Diseases* 36(2), e26–e28. DOI: 10.1086/344772.

Marin, C., Lorenzo-Rebenaque, L., Laso, O., Villora-Gonzalez, J. and Vega, S. (2021) Pet reptiles: a potential source of transmission of multidrug-resistant salmonella. *Frontiers in Veterinary Science* 7, 613718. DOI: 10.3389/fvets.2020.613718.

Marks, S.L., Rankin, S.C., Byrne, B.A. and Weese, J.S. (2011) Enteropathogenic bacteria in dogs and cats: diagnosis, epidemiology, treatment, and control. *Journal of Veterinary Internal Medicine* 25(6), 1195–1208. DOI: 10.1111/j.1939-1676.2011.00821.x.

Martins, A.F. and Rabinowitz, P. (2020) The impact of antimicrobial resistance in the environment on public health. *Future Microbiology* 15(9), 699–702. DOI: 10.2217/fmb-2019-0331.

Mateus, A., Brodbelt, D.C., Barber, N. and Stärk, K.D.C. (2011) Antimicrobial usage in dogs and cats in first opinion veterinary practices in the UK. *Journal of Small Animal Practice* 52, 515–521. DOI: 10.1111/j.1748-5827.2011.01098.x.

Mateus, A.L.P., Brodbelt, D.C., Barber, N. and Stärk, K.D.C. (2014) Qualitative study of factors associated with antimicrobial usage in seven small animal veterinary practices in the UK. *Preventive Veterinary Medicine* 117(1), 68–78. DOI: 10.1016/j. prevetmed.2014.05.007.

Mattick, K., Kelly, N. and Rees, C. (2014) A window into the lives of junior doctors: narrative interviews exploring antimicrobial prescribing experiences. *Journal of Antimicrobial Chemotherapy* 69, 2274–2283. DOI: 10.1093/jac/dku093.

McNulty, C., Hawking, M., Lecky, D., Jones, L., Owens, R. *et al*. (2018) Effects of primary care antimicrobial stewardship outreach on antibiotic use by general practice staff: pragmatic randomized controlled trial of the TARGET antibiotics workshop. *Journal of Antimicrobial Chemotherapy* 73, 1423–1432. DOI: 10.1093/jac/dky004.

Meeker, D., Linder, J.A., Fox, C.R., Friedberg, M.W., Persell, S.D. *et al*. (2016) Effect of behavioral interventions on inappropriate antibiotic prescribing among primary care practices. *JAMA* 315(6), 562. DOI: 10.1001/jama.2016.0275.

Mendez, M. and Moreno, M.A. (2020) Quantifying antimicrobial exposures in dogs from a longitudinal study. *Frontiers in Veterinary Science* 7, 545. DOI: 10.3389/fvets.2020.00545.

Menezes, J., Frosini, S.M., Moreira da Silva, J., Amaral, A., Loeffler, A. *et al*. (2022) Characterisation of ESBL/pAMPc-producing *Escherichia coli* isolated from healthy companion animals and humans in Portugal and the United Kingdom 2018–2020: a shared dynamic. In: *European Congress of Clinical Microbiology and Infectious Diseases, 23–26 April 2022, Lisbon, Portugal*. Abstract P0936.

Mevius, D. and Heederik, D. (2014) Reduction of antibiotic use in animals "let's go Dutch." *Journal Für Verbraucherschutz Und Lebensmittelsicherheit* 9(2), 177–181. DOI: 10.1007/s00003-014-0874-z.

Miranda, C., Silva, V., Igrejas, G. and Poeta, P. (2021) Impact of European pet antibiotic use on enterococci and staphylococci antimicrobial resistance and human health. *Future Microbiology* 16(3), 185–201. DOI: 10.2217/fmb-2020-0119.

Moerer, M., Merle, R. and Bäumer, W. (2022) A cross-sectional study of veterinarians in Germany on the impact of the TÄHAV amendment 2018 on antimicrobial use and development of antimicrobial resistance in dogs and cats. *Antibiotics* 11(4), 484. DOI: 10.3390/antibiotics11040484.

Monnier, A.A., Eisenstein, B.I., Hulscher, M.E., Gyssens, I.C and DRIVE-AB WP1 group (2018) Towards a global definition of responsible antibiotic use: results of an international multidisciplinary consensus procedure. *Journal of Antimicrobial Chemotherapy* 73(suppl_6), vi3–vi16. DOI: 10.1093/jac/dky114.

More, S.J. (2020) European perspectives on efforts to reduce antimicrobial usage in food animal production. *Irish Veterinary Journal* 73, 2. DOI: 10.1186/s13620-019-0154-4.

Morris, D.O., Loeffler, A., Davis, M.F., Guardabassi, L. and Weese, J.S. (2017) Recommendations for approaches to meticillin-resistant staphylococcal infections of small animals: diagnosis, therapeutic considerations and preventative measures. *Veterinary Dermatology* 28(3), 304–e69. DOI: 10.1111/vde.12444.

Mughini-Gras, L., Heck, M. and van Pelt, W. (2016) Increase reptile-associated human salmonellosis and shift toward adulthood in the age groups at risk, the Netherlands, 1985 to 2014. *Eurosurveillance* 21, 30324. DOI: 10.2807/1560-7917.ES.2016.21.34.30324.

Murphy, C.P., Reid-Smith, R.J., Boerlin, P., Weese, J.S., Prescott, J.F. *et al*. (2012) Out-patient antimicrobial drug use in dogs and cats for new disease events from community companion animal practices in Ontario. *Canadian Veterinary Journal* 53, 291–298.

Murphy, D. and Oshin, F. (2014) Reptile-associated salmonellosis in children aged under 5 years in South West England. *Archives of Diseases in Childhood* 100, 364–365. DOI: 10.1136/archdischild-2014-306134.

NICE (2015) *Antimicrobial Stewardship; Systems and Processes for Effective Antimicrobial Medicine Use*. NICE guideline NG15. National Institute for Clinical Excellence, London. Available at: www.nice.org.uk/guidance/ng15 (accessed 29 October 2022).

NICE (2016) *Antimicrobial Stewardship. Back-up (Delayed) Prescribing*. QualityStandard QS121. National Institute for Clinical Excellence, London. Available at: www.nice.org.uk/guidance/qs121/chapter/quality-statement-2-back-up-delayed-prescribing (accessed 29 October 2022).

Nielsen, S.S., Bicout, D.J., Calistri, P., Canali, E., Drewe, J.A *et al*. (2021) Assessment of animal diseases caused by bacteria resistant to antimicrobials: dogs and cats. *EFSA Journal* 19(6), e06680. DOI: 10.2903/j.efsa.2021.6680.

NOAH (2021) Compendium of data sheets for animal medicines 2021. National Office of Animal Health, Enfield, UK. Available at: www.noahcompendium.co.uk/ (accessed 29 October 2022).

Norris, J.M., Zhuo, A., Govendir, M., Rowbotham, S.J., Labbate, M. *et al*. (2019) Factors influencing the behaviour and perceptions of Australian veterinarians towards antibiotic use and antimicrobial resistance. *PLoS One* 14(10), e0224844. DOI: 10.1371/journal.pone.0224844.

Odensvik, K., Grave, K. and Greko, C. (2001) Antibacterial drugs prescribed for dogs and cats in Sweden and Norway 1990–1998. *Acta Veterinaria Scandinavica* 42, 189–198. DOI: 10.1186/1751-0147-42-189.

O'Neill, J. (2015) *Rapid Diagnostics: Stopping Unnecessary Use of Antibiotics*. Review on Antimicrobial Resistance, HM Government, UK. Available at: https://amr-review.org/sites/default/files/

Paper-Rapid-Diagnostics-Stopping-Unnecessary-Prescription-Low-Res.pdf (accessed 29 October 2022).

O'Neill, J. (2016) *Tackling Drug-Resistant Infections Globally: Final Report and Recommendations*. Review on Antimicrobial Resistance, HM Government, UK. Available at: https://amr-review.org (accessed 29 October 2022).

Palin, V., Welfare, W., Ashcroft, D.M. and van Staa, T.P. (2021) Shorter and longer courses of antibiotics for common infections and the association with reductions of infection-related complications including hospital admissions. *Clinical Infectious Diseases* 73, 1805–1812. DOI: 10.1093/cid/ciab159.

Papoutsi, C., Mattick, K., Pearson, M., Brennan, M., Briscoe, S. *et al.* (2017) Social and professional influences on antimicrobial prescribing for doctors-in-training: a realist review. *Journal of Antimicrobial Chemotherapy* 72, 2418–2430. DOI: 10.1093/jac/dkx194.

Pepin-Puget, L., Garch, F.E., Bertrand, X., Valot, B. and Hocquet, D. (2020) Genome analysis of *Enterobacteriaceae* with non-wild type susceptibility to third-generation cephalosporins recovered from diseased dogs and cats in Europe. *Veterinary Microbiology* 242, 108601. DOI: 10.1016/j.vetmic.2020.108601.

Perkins, A.V., Sellon, D.C., Gay, J.M., Lofgren, E.T., Moore, D.A., Jones, L.P. and Davis, M.A. (2020) Prevalence of methicillin-resistant *Staphylococcus pseudintermedius* on hand-contact and animal-contact surfaces in companion animal community hospitals. *Canadian Veterinary Journal* 61, 613–620.

Perreten, V., Kadlec, K., Schwarz, S., Andersson, U.G., Finn, M. *et al.* (2010) Clonal spread of methicillin-resistant *Staphylococcus pseudintermedius* in Europe and North America: an international multicentre study. *Journal of Antimicrobial Chemotherapy* 65, 1145–1154. DOI: 10.1093/jac/dkq078.

PHE (2015) *Antimicrobial Stewardship: Start Smart – Then Focus*. Public Health England, London. Available at: www.gov.uk/government/publications/antimicrobial-stewardship-start-smart-then-focus (accessed 29 October 2022).

Piccolo, F.L., Belas, A., Foti, M., Fisichella, V., Catia, M. *et al.* (2019) Detection of multidrug resistance and extended-spectrum/plasmid-mediated AmpC β-lactamase genes in *Enterobacteriaceae* isolates from diseased cats in Italy. *Journal of Feline Medicine and Surgery* 22, 613–622. DOI: 10.1177/1098612X19868029.

Pinder, R., Sallis, A., Berry, D. and Chadborn, T. (2015) *Behaviour Change and Antibiotic Prescribing In Healthcare Settings: Literature Review and Behavioural Analysis*. Public Health England and Department of Health Report No. 2014719. Available at: www.gov.uk/government/publications/antibiotic-prescribing-and-behaviour-change-in-healthcare-settings (accessed 29 October 2022).

Pleydell, E.J., Souphavanh, K., Hill, K.E., French, N.P. and Prattley, D.J. (2012) Descriptive epidemiological study of the use of antimicrobial drugs by companion animal veterinarians in New Zealand. *New Zealand Veterinary Journal* 60, 115–122. DOI: 10.1080/00480169.2011.643733.

Pomba, C., Rantala, M., Greko, C., Baptiste, K.E., Catry, B. *et al.* (2016) Public health risk of antimicrobial resistance transfer from companion animals. *Journal of Antimicrobial Chemotherapy* 72, dkw481. DOI: 10.1093/jac/dkw481.

Postma, M., Vanderhaeghen, W., Sarrazin, S., Maes, D. and Dewulf, J. (2017) Reducing antimicrobial usage in pig production without jeopardizing production parameters. *Zoonoses and Public Health* 64(1), 63–74. DOI: 10.1111/zph.12283.

Prouillac, C. (2021) Use of antimicrobials in a French veterinary teaching hospital: a retrospective study. *Antibiotics* 10(11), 1369. DOI: 10.3390/antibiotics10111369.

Radford, A.D., Noble, P.J., Coyne, K.P., Gaskell, R.M., Jones, P.H *et al.* (2011) Antibacterial prescribing patterns in small animal veterinary practice identified via SAVSNET: the small animal veterinary surveillance network. *Veterinary Record* 169(12), 310. DOI: 10.1136/vr.d5062.

Rantala, M., Hölsö, K., Lillas, A., Huovinen, P. and Kaartinen, L. (2004) Survey of condition-based prescribing of antimicrobial drugs for dogs at a veterinary teaching hospital. *Veterinary Record* 155(9), 259–262. DOI: 10.1136/vr.155.9.259.

Ray, M.J., Tallman, G.B., Bearden, D.T., Elman, M.R. and McGregor, J.C. (2019) Antibiotic prescribing without documented indication in ambulatory care clinics: national cross sectional study. *British Medical Journal* 367, l6461. DOI: 10.1136/bmj.l6461.

Regula, G., Torriani, K., Gassner, B., Stucki, F. and Müntener, C.R. (2009) Prescription patterns of antimicrobials in veterinary practices in Switzerland. *Journal of Antimicrobial Chemotherapy* 63(4), 805–811. DOI: 10.1093/jac/dkp009.

Robbins, S.N., Goggs, R., Lhermie, G., Lalonde-Paul, D.F. and Menard, J. (2020) Antimicrobial prescribing practices in small animal emergency and critical care. *Frontiers in Veterinary Science* 7, 110. DOI: 10.3389/fvets.2020.00110.

Rojo-Gimeno, C., Postma, M., Dewulf, J., Hogeveen, H., Lauwers, L. *et al.* (2016) Farm-economic analysis of reducing antimicrobial use whilst adopting improved management strategies on farrow-to-finish pig farms. *Preventive Veterinary Medicine* 129, 74–87. DOI: 10.1016/j.prevetmed.2016.05.001.

Rubin, J.E. and Pitout, J.D.D. (2014) Extended-spectrum β-lactamase, carbapenemase and AmpC producing *Enterobacteriaceae* in companion animals. *Veterinary Microbiology* 170(1–2), 10–18. DOI: 10.1016/j.vetmic.2014.01.017.

Martin L. Whitehead

RUMA (2021) Targets task force report 2020. Responsible Use of Medicines in Agriculture Alliance. Leominster, UK. Available at: www.ruma.org.uk/reports/ (accessed 15 November 2022).

RUMA (2022) Annual Progress Report 2022. Responsible use of Medicines Alliance - Companion Animal & Equine. Leominster, UK. Available at: https://rumacae.org.uk/reports/ (accessed 29 March 2023).

Saini, S., Leung, V., Si, E., Ho, C., Cheung, A. *et al.* (2022) Documenting the indication for antimicrobial prescribing: a scoping review. *BMJ Quality & Safety* bmjqs-2021-014582. DOI: 10.1136/bmjqs-2021-014582.

Salgado-Caxito, M., Benavides, J.A., Adell, A.D., Paes, A.C. and Moreno-Switt, A.I. (2021) Global prevalence and molecular characterization of extended-spectrum β-lactamase-producing *Escherichia coli* in dogs and cats - A scoping review and meta-analysis. *One Health* 12, 100236. DOI: 10.1016/j.onehlt.2021.100236.

Sarrazin, S., Vandael, F., Van Cleven, A., De Graef, E., De Rooster, H. *et al.* (2017) The impact of antimicrobial use guidelines on prescription habits in fourteen Flemish small animal practices. *Vlaams Diergeneeskundig Tijdschrift* 86(3), 173–182. DOI: 10.21825/vdt.v86i3.16287.

Scarborough, R., Bailey, K., Galgut, B., Williamson, A. and Hardefeldt, L. (2020) Use of local antibiogram data and antimicrobial importance ratings to select optimal empirical therapies for urinary tract infections in dogs and cats. *Antibiotics* 9(12), 924. DOI: 10.3390/antibiotics9120924.

Schmenger, A., Leimbach, S., Wente, N., Zhang, Y., Biggs, A.M. *et al.* (2020) Implementation of a targeted mastitis therapy concept using an on-farm rapid test: antimicrobial consumption, cure rates and compliance. *Veterinary Record* 187(10), 401. DOI: 10.1136/vr.105674.

Schmidt, V.M., Pinchbeck, G., McIntyre, M., Nuttall, T., McEwan, N. *et al.* (2018a) Routine antibiotic therapy in dogs increases the detection of antimicrobial-resistant faecal *Escherichia coli*. *Journal of Antimicrobial Chemotherapy* 73, 3305–3316. DOI: 10.1093/jac/dky352.

Schmidt, M.L., Spencer, M.D. and Davidson, L.E. (2018b) Patient, provider, and practice characteristics associated with inappropriate antimicrobial prescribing in ambulatory practices. *Infection Control and Hospital Epidemiology* 39(3), 307–315. DOI: 10.1017/ice.2017.263.

Schmitt, K., Lehner, C., Schuller, S., Schüpbach-Regula, G., Mevissen, M. *et al.* (2019) Antimicrobial use for selected diseases in cats in Switzerland. *BMC Veterinary Research* 15(1), 94. DOI: 10.1186/s12917-019-1821-0.

Schnepf, A., Kramer, S., Wagels, R., Volk, H.A. and Kreienbrock, L. (2021) Evaluation of antimicrobial usage in dogs and cats at a veterinary teaching hospital in Germany in 2017 and 2018. *Frontiers in Veterinary Science* 8, 689018. DOI: 10.3389/fvets.2021.689018.

Schuts, E.C., Hulscher, M.E.J.L., Mouton, J.W., Verduin, C.M., Stuart, J.W.T.C. *et al.* (2016) Current evidence on hospital antimicrobial stewardship objectives: a systematic review and meta-analysis. *Lancet Infectious Diseases* 16(7), 847–856. DOI: 10.1016/S1473-3099(16)00065-7.

Servia-Dopazo, M., Taracido-Trunk, M. and Figueiras, A. (2021) Non-clinical factors determining the prescription of antibiotics by veterinarians: a systematic review. *Antibiotics* 10(2), 133. DOI: 10.3390/antibiotics10020133.

Serwecińska, L. (2020) Antimicrobials and antibiotic-resistant bacteria: a risk to the environment and to public Health. *Water* 12(12), 3313. DOI: 10.3390/w12123313.

Shea, A., McCarthy, R. and Lindenmayer, J. (2011) Therapeutic antibiotic use patterns in dogs: observations from a veterinary teaching hospital. *Journal of Small Animal Practice* 52, 310–318. DOI: 10.1111/j.1748-5827.2011.01072.x.

Singleton, D.A., Sánchez-Vizcaíno, F., Dawson, S., Jones, P.H., Noble, P.J.M. *et al.* (2017) Patterns of antimicrobial agent prescription in a sentinel population of canine and feline veterinary practices in the United Kingdom. *Veterinary Journal* 224, 18–24. DOI: 10.1016/j.tvjl.2017.03.010.

Singleton, D.A., Noble, P.J.M., Sánchez-Vizcaíno, F., Dawson, S., Pinchbeck, G.L. *et al.* (2019a) Pharmaceutical prescription in canine acute diarrhoea: a longitudinal electronic health record analysis of first opinion veterinary practices. *Frontiers in Veterinary Science* 6, 218. DOI: 10.3389/fvets.2019.00218.

Singleton, D.A., Stavisky, J., Jewell, C., Smyth, S., Brant, B. *et al.* (2019b) Small animal disease surveillance 2019: respiratory disease, antibiotic prescription and canine infectious respiratory disease complex. *Veterinary Record* 184(21), 640–645. DOI: 10.1136/vr.l3128.

Singleton, D.A., Ball, C., Rennie, C., Coxon, C., Ganapathy, K. *et al.* (2020a) Backyard poultry cases in UK small animal practices: Demographics, health conditions and pharmaceutical prescriptions. *Veterinary Record* 188, e71. DOI: 10.1002/vetr.71.

Singleton, D.A., Pinchbeck, G.L., Radford, A.D., Arsevska, E., Dawson, S. *et al.* (2020b) Factors associated with prescription of antimicrobial drugs for dogs and cats, United Kingdom, 2014–2016. *Emerging Infectious Diseases* 26(8), 1778–1791. DOI: 10.3201/eid2608.191786.

Singleton, D.A., Pongchaikul, P., Smith, S., Bengtsson, R.J., Baker, K. *et al.* (2021a) Temporal, spatial, and genomic analyses of *Enterobacteriaceae* clinical antimicrobial resistance in companion animals reveals phenotypes and genotypes of one health concern. *Frontiers in Microbiology* 12, 700698. DOI: 10.3389/fmicb.2021.700698.

Singleton, D.A., Rayner, A., Brant, B., Smyth, S., Noble, P.-J.M. *et al.* (2021b) A randomised controlled trial to reduce highest priority critically important antimicrobial prescription in companion animals. *Nature Communications* 12, 1593. DOI: 10.1038/s41467-021-21864-3.

Smith, B.J., Heriot, G. and Buising, K. (2020) Antibiotic treatment of common infections: more evidence to support shorter durations. *Current Opinion in Infectious Diseases* 33(6), 433–440. DOI: 10.1097/QCO.0000000000000680.

Smith, M., King, C., Davis, M., Dickson, A., Park, J. *et al.* (2018) Pet owner and vet interactions: exploring the drivers of AMR. *Antimicrobial Resistance and Infection Control* 7, 46. DOI: 10.1186/s13756-018-0341-1.

Sodagari, H.R., Habib, I., Shahabi, M.P., Dybing, N.A., Wang, P. *et al.* (2020) A review of the public health challenges of *Salmonella* and turtles. *Veterinary Sciences* 7(2), 56. DOI: 10.3390/vetsci7020056.

Sørensen, T.M., Bjørnvad, C.R., Cordoba, G., Damborg, P., Guardabassi, L. *et al.* (2018) Effects of diagnostic work-up on medical decision-making for canine urinary tract infection: an observational study in danish small animal practices. *Journal of Veterinary Internal Medicine* 32(2), 743–751. DOI: 10.1111/jvim.15048.

Spellberg, B. and Rice, L.B. (2019) Duration of antibiotic therapy: shorter is better. *Annals of Internal Medicine* 171(3), 210–211. DOI: 10.7326/M19-1509.

Spurling, G.K.P., Del Mar, C.B., Dooley, L., Clark, J. and Askew, D.A. (2017) Delayed antibiotic prescriptions for respiratory infections. *Cochrane Database of Systematic Reviews* 9, CD004417. DOI: 10.1002/14651858.CD004417.pub5.

Stallwood, J., Shirlow, A. and Hibbert, A. (2019) A UK-based survey of cat owners' perceptions and experiences of antibiotic usage. *Journal of Feline Medicine and Surgery* 22, 69–76. DOI: 10.1177/1098612X19826353.

Summers, J.F., Hendricks, A. and Brodbelt, D.C. (2014) Prescribing practices of primary-care veterinary practitioners in dogs diagnosed with bacterial pyoderma. *BMC Veterinary Research* 10(1), 240. DOI: 10.1186/s12917-014-0240-5.

Tanaka, N., Takizawa, T., Miyamoto, N., Funayama, S., Tanaka, R. *et al.* (2017) Real world data of a veterinary teaching hospital in Japan: a pilot survey of prescribed medicines. *Veterinary Record Open* 4, e000218. DOI: 10.1136/vetreco-2016-000218.

Taylor, D.D., Martin, J.N. and Scallan Walter, E.J. (2022) Survey of companion animal veterinarians' antimicrobial drug prescription practices and awareness of antimicrobial drug use guidelines in the United States. *Zoonoses and Public Health* 69, 277–285. DOI: 10.1111/zph.12915.

Thomson, K., Rantala, M.H.J., Viita-Aho, T.K., Vainio, O.M. and Kaartinen, L.A. (2009) Condition-based use of antimicrobials in cats in Finland: results from two surveys. *Journal of Feline Medicine and Surgery* 11, 462–466. DOI: 10.1016/j.jfms.2008.10.005.

Tompson, A.C., Chandler, C.I.R., Mateus, A.L.P., O'Neill, D.G., Chang, Y.-M. *et al.* (2020) What drives antimicrobial prescribing for companion animals? A mixed-methods study of UK veterinary clinics. *Preventive Veterinary Medicine* 183, 105117. DOI: 10.1016/j.prevetmed.2020.105117.

Tompson, A.C., Mateus, A.L.P., Brodbelt, D.C. and Chandler, C.I.R. (2021) Understanding antibiotic use in companion animals: a literature review identifying avenues for further efforts. *Frontiers in Veterinary Science* 8: 719547.

Toombs-Ruane, L.J., Benschop, J., French, N.P., Biggs, P.J., Midwinter, A.C. *et al.* (2020) Carriage of extended-spectrum-β-lactamase- and AmpC β-lactamase-producing *Escherichia coli* strains from humans and pets in the same households. *Applied and Environtal Microbiolology* 86, e01613–20. DOI: 10.1128/AEM.01613-20.

Turner, A., Tisdall, D., Barrett, D.C., Wood, S., Dowsey, A. *et al.* (2018) Ceasing the use of the highest priority critically important antimicrobials does not adversely affect production, health or welfare parameters in dairy cows. *Veterinary Record* 183, 67.

Urban, D., Chevance, A. and Moulin, G. (2021) *Sales Survey of Veterinary Medicinal Products Containing Antimicrobials in France in 2020. Annual Report.* French Agency for Food, Environmental and Occupational Health & Safety, French Agency for Veterinary Medicinal Products, Javené, France. Available at: www.anses.fr/en/system/files/ANMV-Ra-Antibiotiques2020EN.pdf

Valiakos, G., Pavlidou, E., Zafeiridis, C., Tsokana, C.N. and Del Rio Vilas, V.J. (2020) Antimicrobial practices among small animal veterinarians in Greece: a survey. *One Health Outlook* 2, 7. DOI: 10.1186/s42522-020-00013-8.

Van Cleven, A., Sarrazin, S., de Rooster, H., Paepe, D., Van der Meeren, S. *et al.* (2018) Antimicrobial prescribing behaviour in dogs and cats by Belgian veterinarians. *Veterinary Record* 182(11), 324. DOI: 10.1136/vr.104316.

Van Staa, T., Li, Y., Gold, N., Chadborn, T., Welfare, W. *et al.* (2022) Comparing antibiotic prescribing between clinicians in UK primary care: an analysis in a cohort study of eight different measures of antibiotic prescribing. *BMJ Quality & Safety* 31(11), 831–838. DOI: 10.1136/bmjqs-2020-012108.

Varma, J.K., Marcus, R., Stenzel, S.A., Hanna, S.S., Gettner, S. *et al.* (2006) Highly resistant *Salmonella* Newport-MDRAmpC transmitted through the domestic US food supply: a FoodNet case-control study of sporadic *Salmonella* Newport infections, 2002-2003.

Martin L. Whitehead

Journal of Infectious Diseases 194(2), 222–230. DOI: 10.1086/505084.

Vasseur, P.B., Paul, H.A., Enos, L.R. and Hirsh, D.C. (1985) Infection rates in clean surgical procedures: a comparison of ampicillin prophylaxis vs a placebo. *Journal of the American Veterinary Medical Association* 187(8), 825–827.

Vincze, S., Stamm, I., Kopp, P.A., Hermes, J., Adlhoch, C. *et al.* (2014) Alarming proportions of methicillin-resistant *Staphylococcus aureus* (MRSA) in wound samples from companion animals, Germany 2010-2012. *PloS One* 9(1), e85656. DOI: 10.1371/journal.pone.0085656.

VMD (2019) UK veterinary antibiotic resistance and sales surveillance report 2018. Veterinary Medicines Directorate, Addlestone, UK. Available at: www.gov.uk/government/publications/veterinary-antimicrobial-resistance-and-sales-surveillance-2018 (accessed 29 October 2022).

VMD (2020) UK veterinary antibiotic resistance and sales surveillance report 2019. Veterinary Medicines Directorate, Addlestone, UK. Available at: www.gov.uk/government/publications/veterinary-antimicrobial-resistance-and-sales-surveillance-2019 (accessed 29 October 2022).

VMD (2022) UK Veterinary Antibiotic Resistance and Sales Surveillance Report 2021. Veterinary Medicines Directorate, Addlestone, UK. Available at: www.gov.uk/government/publications/veterinary-antimicrobial-resistance-and-sales-surveillance-2021 (accessed 15 November 2022).

Walker, A.S., Budgell, E., Laskawiec-Szkonter, M., Sivyer, K., Wordsworth, S. *et al.* (2019) Antibiotic Review Kit for Hospitals (ARK-Hospital): study protocol for a stepped-wedge cluster-randomised controlled trial. *Trials* 20, 421. DOI: 10.1186/s13063-019-3497-y.

Walker, B., Sánchez-Vizcaíno, F. and Barker, E. (2022) Effect of an antimicrobial stewardship intervention on the prescribing behaviours of companion animal veterinarians: a pre-post study. *Veterinary Record* 190, e1485. DOI: 10.1002/vetr.1485.

Wang, K.Y., Seed, P., Schofield, P., Ibrahim, S. and Ashworth, M. (2009) Which practices are high antibiotic prescribers? A cross-sectional analysis. *British Journal of General Practice* 59, e315–e320. DOI: 10.3399/bjgp09X472593.

Watson, A.D.J. and Maddison, J.E. (2001) Systemic drug use in dogs in Australia. *Australian Veterinary Journal* 79, 740–746. DOI: 10.1111/j.1751-0813.2001.tb10888.x.

Wayne, A., McCarthy, R. and Lindenmayer, J. (2011) Therapeutic antibiotic use patterns in dogs: observations from a veterinary teaching hospital. *Journal of Small Animal Practice* 52(6), 310–318. DOI: 10.1111/j.1748-5827.2011.01072.x.

Weese, J.S. (2006) Investigation of antimicrobial use and the impact of antimicrobial use guidelines in a small animal veterinary teaching hospital: 1995–2004. *Journal of the American Veterinary Medical Association* 228, 553–558. DOI: 10.2460/javma.228.4.553.

Weese, J.S., Giguère, S., Guardabassi, L., Morley, P.S., Papich, M. *et al.* (2015) ACVIM consensus statement on therapeutic antimicrobial use in animals and antimicrobial resistance. *Journal of Veterinary Internal Medicine* 29, 487–498. DOI: 10.1111/jvim.12562.

Weese, J.S., Blondeau, J.M., Boothe, D., Guardabassi, L., Gumley, N. *et al.* (2019) International Society for Companion Animal Infectious Diseases (ISCAID) guidelines for the diagnosis and management of bacterial urinary tract infections in dogs and cats. *Veterinary Journal* 247, 8–25. DOI: 10.1016/j.tvjl.2019.02.008.

Weese, J.S., Webb, J., Balance, D., McKee, T., Stull, J.W. *et al.* (2021) Evaluation of antimicrobial prescriptions in dogs with suspected bacterial urinary tract disease. *Journal of Veterinary Internal Medicine* 35, 2277–2286. DOI: 10.1111/jvim.16246.

Werner, M., Suchodolski, J.S., Straubinger, R.K., Wolf, G. and Steiner, J.M. (2020) Effect of amoxicillin-clavulanic acid on clinical scores, intestinal microbiome, and amoxicillin-resistant *Escherichia coli* in dogs with uncomplicated acute diarrhoea. *Journal of Veterinary Internal Medicine* 34, 1166–1176. DOI: 10.1111/jvim.15775.

Westgarth, C., Pinchbeck, G.L., Bradshaw, J.W.S., Dawson, S., Gaskell, R.M. *et al.* (2008) Dog–human and dog–dog interactions of 260 dog-owning households in a community in Cheshire. *Veterinary Record* 162, 436–442. DOI: 10.1136/vr.162.14.436.

Westropp, J.L., Sykes, J.E., Irom, S., Daniels, J.B., Smith, A. *et al.* (2012) Evaluation of the efficacy and safety of high dose short duration enrofloxacin treatment regimen for uncomplicated urinary tract infections in dogs. *Journal of Veterinary Internal Medicine* 26, 506–512. DOI: 10.1111/j.1939-1676.2012.00914.x.

Whitehead, M.L. (2020) Benchmarking antibiotic prescribing by individual veterinary surgeons within a practice. In: *BSAVA Congress Proceedings 2020*, BSAVA, Birmingham, UK, p. 433.

WHO (2012) *The Pursuit of Responsible Use of Medicines: Sharing and Learning from Country Experiences*. World Health Organization, Geneva, Switzerland. Available at: https://apps.who.int/iris/handle/10665/75828

WHO (2019) *Critically Important Antimicrobials for Human Medicine: 6th Revision*. World Health Organization, Geneva, Switzerland. Available at: www.who.int/publications/i/item/9789241515528

Wierup, M., Wahlström, H. and Bengtsson, B. (2021) Successful prevention of antimicrobial resistance in animals – a retrospective country case study of Sweden. *Antibiotics* 10, 129. DOI: 10.3390/antibiotics10020129.

Williams, J. (2018) The why and how of antimicrobial prophylaxis. *BSAVA Companion* 11, 4–7. DOI: 10.22233/20412495.1118.4.

Wilson, H.L., Daveson, K. and Del Mar, C.B. (2019) Optimal antimicrobial duration for common bacterial infections. *Australian Prescriber* 42, 5–9. DOI: 10.18773/%20austprescr.2019.001.

Woolhouse, M., Ward, M., van Bunnik, B. and Farrar, J. (2015) Antimicrobial resistance in humans, livestock and the wider environment. *Philosophical Transactions of the Royal Society B Biological Sciences* 370, 20140083. DOI: 10.1098/rstb.2014.0083.

Zhang, X.-F., Doi, Y., Huang, X., Li, H.-Y., Zhong, L.-L. *et al.* (2016) Possible transmission of mcr-1-harboring *Escherichia coli* between companion animals and human. *Emerging Infectious Diseases* 22, 1679–1681. DOI: 10.3201/eid2209.160464.

Zogg, A.L., Simmen, S., Zurfluh, K., Stephan, R., Schmitt, S.N. *et al.* (2018) High prevalence of extended-spectrum β-lactamase producing Enterobacteriaceae among clinical isolates from cats and dogs admitted to a veterinary hospital in Switzerland. *Frontiers in Veterinary Science* 5, 62. DOI: 10.3389/fvets.2018.00062.

Martin L. Whitehead

18 Antimicrobial Use and Resistance Surveillance in Companion Animals

DAVID A. SINGLETON*, NICOLA J. WILLIAMS AND ALAN D. RADFORD

University of Liverpool, Liverpool, L69 3BX, UK

18.1 Introduction

Antimicrobial resistance (AMR) is a multifactorial issue, demanding a multi-pronged and interdisciplinary approach across animal, human and environmental health if we are to limit its impact. A 2016 global review on AMR provided a series of wide-ranging recommendations for tackling this global health threat, encompassing improved diagnostic capabilities, surveillance, wider implementation and development of vaccines, and enhanced educational efforts, among others (O'Neill, 2016). However, given the key role antimicrobial use plays in the development and dissemination of AMR (Trott *et al.*, 2004; Magalhães *et al.*, 2010; Cantón and Bryan, 2012; Cuny *et al.*, 2015; Lei *et al.*, 2017), this report also recommended greater efforts at surveying and understanding the use of antimicrobials in people and animals, which may contribute to effective antimicrobial stewardship (O'Neill, 2016). These aims are now being acted upon, at both national and international levels (VMD, 2015), particularly in the medical (PHE, 2021) and agricultural (VMD, 2021) sectors.

While in the veterinary sector efforts to survey antimicrobial use and resistance have hitherto largely concentrated on livestock, there have been an increasing number of attempts to survey antimicrobial prescription (Buckland *et al.*, 2016; Singleton *et al.*, 2017; Bollig *et al.*, 2022) and resistance trends (Marques *et al.*, 2016) in companion animals. However, these have been relatively sporadic and generally restricted to academic publications. There remains a need to establish technology-driven methodologies capable of providing consistent, ongoing surveillance that is easily accessible to practising veterinary surgeons. Similarly, although efforts at encouraging stewardship, such as the PROTECT ME antimicrobial-prescribing guidance (BSAVA/SAMSoc, 2018), have provided a valuable resource for practitioners, there is a paucity of evidence underpinning such guidance. This chapter will discuss methods and efforts for surveying antimicrobial use and resistance surveillance in veterinary species. Although some examples will be based on agricultural species, the chapter will primarily focus on companion animals. Some examples of how such surveillance may be used to enact antimicrobial stewardship will also be given.

18.2 Antimicrobial Prescription

Although the term 'antimicrobial' can be used to describe a number of pharmaceutical agents capable of killing or inhibiting the growth of a range of microbial pathogens, here we use the term to refer to pharmaceutical agents that possess specific action against bacterial cells (Pankey and Sabath, 2004), targeting essential components of bacterial cell metabolism (Coates *et al.*, 2002). Antimicrobials could be considered the single most important pharmaceutical family prescribed to both humans and animals, and their discovery has been credited with revolutionizing both medical and veterinary health (O'Neill, 2016). However, due to the global emergence of AMR, and the subsequent reduction of treatment options available, significant attention has been drawn to the manner in which we are currently prescribing these important agents (O'Neill, 2016). Antimicrobial use has been recognized as

*Corresponding author: D.A.Singleton@liverpool.ac.uk

© CAB International 2023. *Infection Control in Small Animal Clinical Practice* (eds F. Allerton and K.L. Bowlt Blacklock)
DOI: 10.1079/9781789244977.0018

the key driver of AMR (Cantón and Bryan, 2012); hence, gaining further understanding on how they are used, and examining ways in which such use can be optimized to reduce AMR development and transmission risk, remains a critical aim of global AMR surveillance (O'Neill, 2016). Antimicrobials are commonly prescribed in first-opinion and referral companion animal practice (Rantala *et al.*, 2004a; Buckland *et al.*, 2016; Singleton *et al.*, 2017; van Cleven *et al.*, 2018; Bollig *et al.*, 2022), and thus it is important that companion animals are included in global, shared and One Health-focused efforts to ensure prescribing actions are undertaken responsibly.

18.3 Antimicrobial Use and Prescription Surveillance

The decision to prescribe an antimicrobial is understood to be complex, extending beyond the probability of a patient suffering from a bacterial infection alone (Mateus *et al.*, 2014). Hence, the approaches employed to effectively survey antimicrobial prescription and use are correspondingly diverse, including both quantitative (Mateus *et al.*, 2011; Radford *et al.*, 2011; Hughes *et al.*, 2012; Hawker *et al.*, 2014; Buckland *et al.*, 2016; Singleton *et al.*, 2017; Gómez-Poveda and Moreno, 2018; Hardefeldt *et al.*, 2018; van Cleven *et al.*, 2018; Hopman *et al.*, 2019c; Schmitt *et al.*, 2019; Hur *et al.*, 2020; Joosten *et al.*, 2020; Lutz *et al.*, 2020; Galarce *et al.*, 2021; Goggs *et al.*, 2021; Bollig *et al.*, 2022; Taylor *et al.*, 2022) and qualitative (de Briyne *et al.*, 2013; Teixeira Rodrigues *et al.*, 2013; Mateus *et al.*, 2014; Currie *et al.*, 2018; King *et al.*, 2018; Smith *et al.*, 2018; Dickson *et al.*, 2019; Tompson *et al.*, 2020) research methodologies. Although such attempts have previously largely been driven by academic institutions, as the global importance of AMR is being further realized, surveillance is increasingly being coordinated by national governmental or inter-governmental groups, such as the European Surveillance of Veterinary Antimicrobial Consumption (ESVAC) group of the European Medicines Agency (EMA) (ESVAC, 2021). Such groups have placed increasing emphasis on standardizing surveillance across species and countries to provide the best, unbiased measure of the impact that antimicrobial prescription is having on AMR development and spread.

Before proceeding further, it should be noted that, within the context of pharmaceutical agent surveillance, the terms 'prescription' and 'use' are not necessarily synonymous. The term 'use' is utilized when there is reasonable confidence that the patient(s) in question actually took the pharmaceutical agent, i.e. the prescriber administered the agent themselves or observed it being administered. While all 'used' pharmaceutical agents are initially prescribed in the UK, some formulations such as oral tablets frequently have some level of uncertainty as to whether the entire course (or indeed any of the course) was actually taken by the patient, especially when surveying at scale. As a result, for ease of understanding, we will henceforth use the term 'prescription' to cover either of these eventualities.

18.3.1 Quantifying antimicrobial prescription

A number of methodologies have been utilized to quantify antimicrobial prescription in companion animals, ranging from overall weight of antimicrobial sold (VMD, 2021) to survey-based approaches (Hughes *et al.*, 2012; de Briyne *et al.*, 2014; Gómez-Poveda and Moreno, 2018; Joosten *et al.*, 2020; Lutz *et al.*, 2020; Odoi *et al.*, 2021; Bollig *et al.*, 2022; Taylor *et al.*, 2022), in-person interviews (Mateus *et al.*, 2014; Hopman *et al.*, 2018; Dickson *et al.*, 2019), direct observation of consultations (Robinson *et al.*, 2015), ethnography (Tompson *et al.*, 2020), use of prescription journals (Murphy *et al.*, 2012), use of pet insurance data (Hardefeldt *et al.*, 2018) and use of electronic health records (EHRs), both in first-opinion practice (Mateus *et al.*, 2011; Radford *et al.*, 2011; Buckland *et al.*, 2016; Hopman *et al.*, 2019a, c; Schmitt *et al.*, 2019; Singleton *et al.*, 2019a, c, d; Bollig *et al.*, 2022) and referral practice (German *et al.*, 2010; Wayne *et al.*, 2011; Goggs *et al.*, 2021).

Antimicrobial sales by weight

Provision of a measure of the overall weight of antimicrobial sold by pharmaceutical manufacturers to veterinary prescribers, available via the UK Veterinary Medicine Directorate's Veterinary Antimicrobial Resistance and Sales Surveillance (VARSS) report (VMD, 2021), represents the widest-scale, regular survey of antimicrobial sales in the UK. At the time of writing, the latest VARSS report described data collected in 2020, noting a

David A. Singleton *et al.*

49% total reduction in the quantity of antimicrobial agent sold for animal species since 2014. In food-producing species, sales of highest priority critically important antimicrobials (HPCIAs) (WHO, 2019) have also decreased by some 79% since 2014, although in both cases it should be noted that decreases were most pronounced between 2014 and 2017, with a more static picture being apparent since then. For dogs and cats, a 23% reduction in total antimicrobial sales was also observed between 2014 and 2020, with HPCIA sales decreasing by 34% over the same time period (VMD, 2021). In contrast to food-producing species, observed decreases appeared to be most pronounced in companion animals between 2017 and 2020.

More widely, across 31 European countries submitting data on antimicrobial sales by weight, large variations in sales by weight of antimicrobial sold per population correction unit (PCU) can be observed across all veterinary species, with countries ranging between 2.3 mg PCU^{-1} (Norway) and 393.9 mg PCU^{-1} (Cyprus) in 2020. Nevertheless, for 25 countries submitting data between 2011 and 2020, an aggregated reduction of 43% in total antimicrobial sales was observed, with Antimicrobial Advice Ad Hoc Expert Group (AMEG) Category B antimicrobials (broadly comparative to HPCIAs) also showing pronounced decreases over this time period (ESVAC, 2021). In the USA, reductions in total 'medically important' antimicrobial sales have also been observed (23% between 2011 and 2020), although in this case, reports were unfortunately restricted to food-producing species alone (FDA, 2021). However, at a global scale, antimicrobial sales for food-producing animals are predicted to increase by some 11% between 2019 and 2030, suggesting a need for wider action on reducing antimicrobial sales worldwide (Tiseo et al., 2020).

While these insights are of some use to gauge the national and international picture on companion animal antimicrobial sales, there are a number of limitations. First, species authorization is used to attribute the relative share of sales to individual or groups of species (i.e. all oral tablet sales are attributed to companion animals). It is unknown which species these antimicrobials are actually prescribed to 'off licence' under the veterinary cascade system (VMD, 2013), and indeed, of those authorized for dog and cat use only, how much of the total volume can be attributed to each individual species. Additionally, the VMD and other organizations utilize a range of benchmarking measures, such as defined daily dose (DDD) and defined course dose (DCD), which remain inaccessible to companion animal surveillance. These measures are used to directly compare different species, taking into account dosage variation between species and substances (EMA, 2015, 2016). However, they depend on knowledge of the population structure of the species being surveyed, including demographics and average animal weight. Although methods to estimate the pet populations are in development (Murray et al., 2015; Aegerter et al., 2017), securing a definitive value is rare, limiting the potential of such measures to be used at national or international scales. Similarly, unlike other animal species, weight variability among dog breeds is large (Rimbault et al., 2013), limiting our current ability to extrapolate overall volume of companion animal-only authorized antimicrobials to a measure of DDD or DCD. It should be noted, however, that in the UK, the VMD has recently attempted to summarize antimicrobial sales by weight in dogs and cats, using an annual pet population survey and weight data from animals attending first-opinion clinics. Interestingly, this did corroborate the broader decreasing trends discussed earlier (VMD, 2020). As such, although such attempts remain heavily caveated, with improved pet population size and demographic data, such approaches may gain enhanced utility in the future.

In addition to the limitations noted above, it should also be noted that sales surveillance currently generally focuses on antimicrobials intended for systemic (oral, injectable, intramammary and intrauterine) administration alone (VMD, 2015). Topical antimicrobial therapies are commonly prescribed to companion animals (Holso et al., 2005; Mateus et al., 2011; Summers et al., 2014; Singleton et al., 2017, 2019b, 2020b), and have been shown to achieve much higher local concentrations than are possible with systemic antimicrobials alone. As such, topical antimicrobials might present an important alternative or adjunct to systemic antibiosis (Lazar et al., 2014), although topical use has also been associated with selection for resistance (Fintelmann et al., 2011; Scott et al., 2019). Finally, it should be noted that efforts at surveillance by these methods are typically led by government agencies. Due to a need for relatively tightly regulated antimicrobial procurement and monitoring requirements to produce meaningful, regular outputs at this scale, such surveillance is typically restricted to high-income countries (Tiseo et al., 2020). Given that the impact of AMR is predicted to fall most heavily on low- and middle-income countries (LMICs) (Barzelai and Whittem, 2017), more equitable approaches for surveying antimicrobial use are likely to be needed for all species.

Survey-based approaches

While measurement of antimicrobial sales to prescribers does hold value, there is significant interest in how such products are actually being prescribed to individual animals under care. Hence, surveys targeting practising veterinary surgeons have been deployed at both national (Hughes et al., 2012; Pleydell et al., 2012; Barzelai and Whittem, 2017; Gómez-Poveda and Moreno, 2018; van Cleven et al., 2018; Joosten et al., 2020; Galarce et al., 2021; Odoi et al., 2021; Bollig et al., 2022; Taylor et al., 2022) and European (de Briyne et al., 2014) levels. In these surveys, veterinary surgeons reported that certain clinical conditions, such as skin disease, respiratory disease and urinary tract infections, are common indications for antibiosis in both dogs and cats (de Briyne et al., 2014; Barzelai and Whittem, 2017; van Cleven et al., 2018), with such decisions also frequently being empirical in nature (Hardefeldt et al., 2017). HPCIA use has been reported as being more frequent in cats compared with dogs, specifically use of third-generation cephalosporins (de Briyne et al., 2014; Hardefeldt et al., 2017). Compared against the relevant products' summary of product characteristics (SPC), inappropriate dosage was also reported as being relatively frequent (Hughes et al., 2012), as was variability among prescribers over treatment-course length, with both of these findings being risk factors for resistance development (Barzelai and Whittem, 2017).

The use of surveys has offered the opportunity to summarize the opinions of large populations of veterinary surgeons in a systematic manner, providing high-quality and consistent data for analyses. Such surveys have provided crucial insights into, for example, knowledge and attitudes surrounding bacterial diagnostic tests (de Briyne et al., 2013), and utilization of antimicrobial-prescribing guidance (Hughes et al., 2012). However, as the surveys generally ask veterinary surgeons to describe what they would do when faced with hypothetical scenarios, when it comes to quantifying antimicrobial prescription, reporting bias is of some concern.

Indeed, a recent practitioner study deployed a survey prior to summarizing actual antimicrobial-prescribing practices in the same study population, revealing that these practitioners tended to actually prescribe differently compared with their self-described prescribing habits as recorded within the survey (Bollig et al., 2022). While this does provide a fascinating insight into practitioner behaviour, it does suggest that surveys may better be utilized in summarizing practitioners' opinions on AMR, and to build consensus on antimicrobial steward-ship approaches most likely to result in an impact on AMR (Currie et al., 2018). It also suggests a need to report on prescribing decisions as they are being made, rather than in concept or in simulated scenarios.

EHRs

HEALTH INFORMATICS IN COMPANION ANIMALS. An EHR can be defined as a secure digital longitudinal repository of patient data provided in a standardized format, with the purpose of expanding accessibility to include a wide range of authorized users, thus improving care efficiency (Hayrinen et al., 2008). The precise content of the EHR can vary, and might include information pertaining to the direct clinical history of the patient or, often separately, diagnostic test results held by a diagnostic laboratory (Raman et al., 2018). EHR data can range from structured data, for example signalment information (age, sex) or fixed-answer questionnaire responses (Sánchez-Vizcaíno et al., 2015), to semi-structured data, for instance animal breed or prescribed medications (Anholt et al., 2014a; Buckland et al., 2016; Singleton et al., 2017; Hur et al., 2019, 2020) and largely unstructured data, such as clinical free text (Anholt et al., 2014b). EHRs are now widely used in veterinary and medical practice (Robinson and Hooker, 2006), and the advent of such technologies has the potential to revolutionize the manner by which epidemiologists and health informaticians approach health surveillance, in both humans (Raman et al., 2018) and animals (O'Neill et al., 2014a; Sánchez-Vizcaíno et al., 2015).

However, while such approaches have started to provide outputs of real impact to human and animal health (O'Neill et al., 2014a), there are a number of data integrity, epidemiological and ethical challenges that need resolving, both in general and particularly in the companion animal sector. The increase in popularity of EHRs has given rise to

David A. Singleton et al.

a large number of companies providing practice management system (PMS) software to veterinary practices, and veterinary diagnostic laboratories developing their own bespoke laboratory information management systems (LIMS) (O'Neill *et al.*, 2014a). Practically, this limits the ability of EHR data collection projects to rapidly assimilate large numbers of practices and diagnostic laboratories into any health surveillance scheme, and also raises questions regarding data equivalence between PMSs when repurposing such data for surveillance. To attempt to mitigate such issues, the use of 'extensible mark-up language' (XML) schema as a means to define a standardized structure and content of an EHR regardless of PMS within the veterinary sector has been proposed by the Veterinary XML (VetXML) Consortium. This schema has been integrated into some LIMS, and has also been successfully trialled on veterinary practice EHR data (Jones-Diette *et al.*, 2016), although it is currently unclear whether such schemas will be adopted at scales great enough for population-level companion animal health surveillance.

A further important consideration is that of patient – or in the veterinary sector, client – consent and privacy (Birnbaum *et al.*, 2018; Raman *et al.*, 2018). Particularly due to the application of the General Data Protection Regulations (GDPR) across the European Union (EU), there is heightened concern that current consent procedures, in particular opt-out consent, might not fully comply with current legislation. Hence, if such regulations are firmly applied, they might hinder the potential of EHR data collection projects to provide insights of real epidemiological value (Rumbold and Pierscionek, 2017). These regulations have also further highlighted the importance of ensuring EHR anonymity. It has been found that simply deleting the name and address is not sufficient to ensure de-identification in the majority of cases (Rumbold and Pierscionek, 2017); this is particularly true for the clinical free-text component of EHRs, which frequently contain personal identifiers such as phone numbers. Although use of clinical free text offers perhaps the greatest detail relating to a clinical case, concerns have also been raised regarding the variable quality of information provided within such fields (Raman *et al.*, 2018). While this variability has been observed in companion animal EHRs, it has not prevented clinical free text from being able to provide valuable insights for routine surveillance (Anholt *et al.*, 2014b), responses to specific disease

outbreaks (Radford *et al.*, 2021) and clinical governance (Burke *et al.*, 2017; Hardefeldt *et al.*, 2020). The continued development of text-mining technologies also offers an exciting opportunity to efficiently apply such free-text-based health surveillance at scale in medical and veterinary health surveillance (Duz *et al.*, 2017; Hur *et al.*, 2019; Noble *et al.*, 2021).

In addition to free-text analyses, there have been other attempts within companion animal health surveillance to further augment the EHR, most notably in the UK with the use of compulsory questionnaires by the Small Animal Veterinary Surveillance Network (SAVSNET) (Sánchez-Vizcaíno *et al.*, 2015; Singleton *et al.*, 2019c), and the use of voluntary veterinary nomenclature (VeNom) coding by the Veterinary Companion Animal Surveillance System (VetCompass) (O'Neill *et al.*, 2014a). Both of these complementary projects collect first-opinion EHR practice data from a range of voluntarily contributing veterinary practices; SAVSNET also collects EHR veterinary diagnostic laboratory data from multiple laboratories (Sánchez-Vizcaíno *et al.*, 2017).

SAVSNET augments every practice-provided EHR through the use of an embedded inline frame (iframe), an HTML element that allows an external webpage to be embedded into an HTML document within compliant PMSs (Fig. 18.1); this webpage is used to ask the consulting veterinary professional to record the main reason why the animal has presented for consultation from a short pre-selected list encompassing preventative healthcare reasons (e.g. vaccination), investigation of disease (e.g. respiratory, gastrointestinal), and post-operative check consultations. Further to this, in randomly selected consultations, the consulting veterinary professional can be asked to complete a further questionnaire to provide additional details pertaining to the investigation and management of the case in question. Opt-out client consent is employed, with client information posters being displayed prominently in the waiting rooms of participating veterinary practices (Sánchez-Vizcaíno *et al.*, 2017). Regarding EHR data supplied by veterinary diagnostic laboratories, a different approach is employed. Specific consent is sought from each laboratory, with no standardized data formats being required prior to participation. For both aims, veterinary practices and diagnostic laboratories are recruited by convenience. This approach has been demonstrated most frequently through SAVSNET's

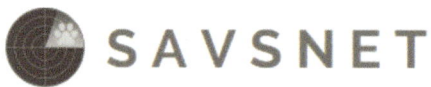

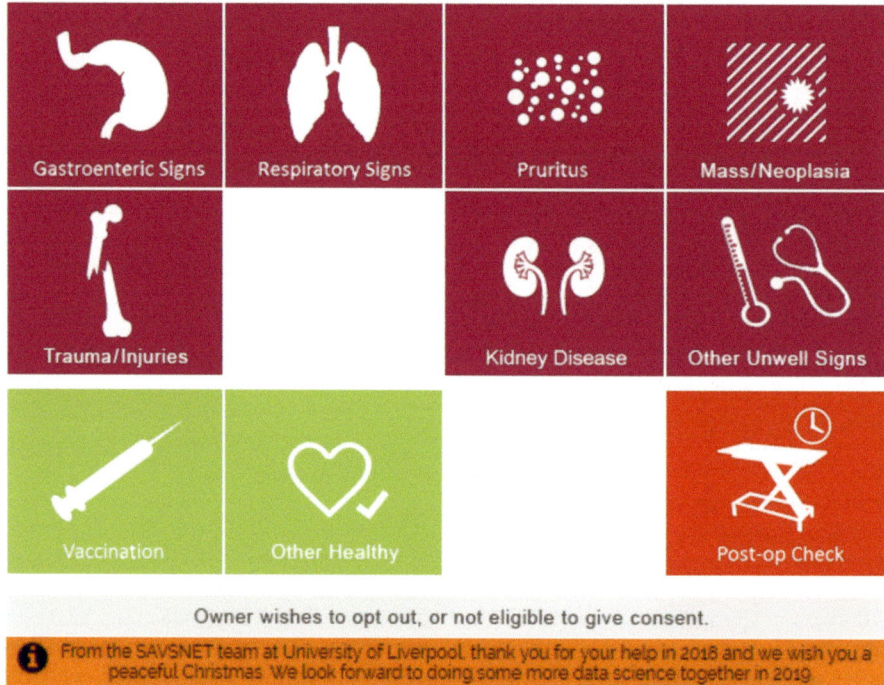

Fig. 18.1. The SAVSNET window, an inline frame (iframe) embedded into each compliant PMS, which appears at the conclusion of every consultation. The iframe contains a range of options that mandatorily require the consulting veterinary professional to provide a main reason the animal presented for examination, or an option to opt out of data collection. In a randomized subset of consultations, some syndromes may contain a further short questionnaire pertaining to the selected complaint. Reproduced with permission from the University of Liverpool, Liverpool, UK.

quarterly health surveillance reports published in *The Veterinary Record* (Sánchez-Vizcaíno *et al.*, 2015, 2016; Arsevska *et al.*, 2017, 2018a; Singleton *et al.*, 2019a, b, d; Collins *et al.*, 2021).

In contrast, VeNom coding enables consultations to be placed within a hierarchical ontology summarizing the presentation, any diagnoses made and any treatments provided within the relevant consultation, enabling surveillance from syndromic classification to diagnosis-level precision (O'Neill *et al.*, 2014a, b, O'Neill *et al.*, 2014c). As with SAVSNET, VetCompass also recruits veterinary practices by convenience. Each of these approaches has distinct advantages and disadvantages. For instance, while

SAVSNET enables broad classification of every recorded consultation, to gain further granularity researchers would rely on clinical free-text mining for most cases, the quality of which can be variable (Burke *et al.*, 2017). Similarly, although VeNom coding might provide greater granularity, the voluntary nature of data collection has resulted in limited uptake of the coding scheme (Jones-Diette *et al.*, 2016). Furthermore, although estimates have been attempted (Aegerter *et al.*, 2017), the lack of definitive pet population demographic data in the UK currently limits the ability of both projects to draw firm conclusions on the representativeness of their findings.

David A. Singleton *et al.*

Asides from these two UK projects, there are a growing number of active companion animal health surveillance projects throughout the world, notably in Australia (McGreevy *et al.*, 2017), Canada (Anholt *et al.*, 2014b), the Netherlands (Hopman *et al.*, 2019c), New Zealand (Muellner *et al.*, 2016), Spain (Gómez-Poveda and Moreno, 2018), Switzerland (Schmitt *et al.*, 2019) and the USA (Raghavan *et al.*, 2007; CAVSNET, 2022), among others. It is likely that important global health issues such as AMR will prompt further international interest in companion animal health surveillance, in terms of both antimicrobial prescription (O'Neill, 2016) and resistance (Marques *et al.*, 2016), paving the way for truly international companion animal health surveillance.

Using EHRs to quantify antimicrobial prescription.

EHRs have been increasingly utilized in first-opinion (Mateus *et al.*, 2011; Radford *et al.*, 2011; Jones *et al.*, 2014; Summers *et al.*, 2014; Buckland *et al.*, 2016; Burke *et al.*, 2017; Hopman *et al.*, 2019a, c; Schmitt *et al.*, 2019; Singleton *et al.*, 2019a, c; Hardefeldt *et al.*, 2020; Bollig *et al.*, 2022) and referral/university-based (Prescott *et al.*, 2002; Holso *et al.*, 2005; German *et al.*, 2010; Wayne *et al.*, 2011; Goggs *et al.*, 2021) veterinary practices to quantify antimicrobial prescription in companion animals. These studies focused initially on referral/university-based animal populations, although it was recognized that these cases might not be representative of the wider veterinary-visiting population and not representative of the majority of antimicrobials prescribed on a national level (German *et al.*, 2010). Hence, attention has moved towards utilizing EHRs contributed by first-opinion practices, although this has brought some unique challenges, such as PMS compatibility and EHR data quality variation, as noted earlier. While such challenges have so far limited EHR-based antimicrobial prescription studies to subnational scales, a growing number of countries (Buckland *et al.*, 2016; Singleton *et al.*, 2017; Gómez-Poveda and Moreno, 2018; van Cleven *et al.*, 2018; Hopman *et al.*, 2019a, c; Hur *et al.*, 2020; Hardefeldt *et al.*, 2020; Bollig *et al.*, 2022) are managing to utilize increasing volumes of EHR data to describe companion animal antimicrobial prescription across a range of conditions (Summers *et al.*, 2014; Singleton *et al.*, 2019a, b, c, d; Bollig *et al.*, 2022), administration routes (Buckland *et al.*, 2016; Hur *et al.*, 2020; Bollig *et al.*, 2022) and authorization categories (Bollig *et al.*, 2022).

So far, EHR studies have corroborated several findings suggested by survey-based studies and antimicrobial sales reports, and have also produced novel findings of relevance to AMR. EHRs collected from multiple first-opinion practices were first used to characterize antimicrobial prescription in 2011. Radford *et al.* (2011) utilized data collected over 3 months in 2010 from 16 veterinary practices in the UK, and found antimicrobial prescription to be common, with systemic antimicrobial prescription occurring in 35% of dog, 49% of cat and 37% of rabbit consultations, where the animal presented for investigation and/or treatment of ill health. The β-lactam class was found to be the most commonly prescribed class to dogs and cats, and fluoroquinolones the most commonly prescribed to rabbits, although considerable variation among contributing veterinary practices was observed (Radford *et al.*, 2011). Mateus *et al.* (2011) also found, utilizing 2007 data from 11 veterinary practices, that β-lactams were the most popular class in dogs and cats. This study also reported antimicrobial prescription to have occurred in 45% of dogs and 33% of cats over a 1-year period, the majority of which were systemic antimicrobials (77% of canine and 89% of feline prescriptions).

More recently, Buckland *et al.* (2016) published a study of significantly increased scope, utilizing data supplied by some 374 veterinary practices in the UK, using data collected between 2012 and 2014. This revealed that systemic antimicrobials were prescribed to 25% of dogs and 21% of cats throughout the study period, with β-lactams remaining the most commonly prescribed antimicrobial class. However, while potentiated penicillins remained the most commonly prescribed β-lactam subclass between 2011 and 2014 for dogs, for cats, third-generation cephalosporins became the most commonly prescribed β-lactam subclass (Buckland *et al.*, 2016), extended-spectrum penicillins having been the most common previously (Mateus *et al.*, 2011; Radford *et al.*, 2011). As third-generation cephalosporins are classed as HPCIAs (WHO, 2019), this finding has significant relevance for antimicrobial stewardship. This latter finding was corroborated by Singleton *et al.* (2017) utilizing data from 216 UK veterinary practices. Similar trends have also been observed outside the UK. For example, in Australia in a study utilizing data from 137 veterinary practices, third-generation cephalosporins were also the most common β-lactam subclass prescribed to cats (Hur *et al.*, 2020).

Further studies have also sought to quantify antimicrobial prescription in the context of specific clinical conditions, such as canine acute diarrhoea (Singleton *et al.*, 2019c) and canine pyoderma (Summers *et al.*, 2014), or by specific antimicrobial agent, for example feline cefovecin prescription (Burke *et al.*, 2017; Hardefeldt *et al.*, 2020). These studies have begun to compare prescribing decisions against existing clinical evidence, the SPC and/or prescribing guidance, and by doing so have been able to comment on the appropriateness of identified prescription trends. For example, Burke *et al.* (2017) was able to conclude that of 1148 consultations in which cefovecin was prescribed, prescription complied with authorized indications for use (as described within the SPC) in 70% of cases (Burke *et al.*, 2017). Although such studies are of clear importance in the context of antimicrobial stewardship, it is unknown whether EHR-based studies could contribute more directly to clinical evidence. For example, while small-scale, referral population-based interventional studies have questioned the necessity of antibiosis for acute canine diarrhoea (Mortier *et al.*, 2015), there is uncertainty over whether such findings would necessarily translate to the wider, largely first-opinion, canine community. Large-scale observational trials utilizing EHRs have been extensively utilized to define the population benefit or absence of a range of pharmaceutical therapies in the medical field (Benchimol *et al.*, 2015; Page *et al.*, 2017). However, to date, this important developing area remains largely unexplored in veterinary medicine.

These studies have also begun to explore temporal variation in antimicrobial-prescribing habits. For example, a recent UK study utilizing EHR data collected by SAVSNET found that overall antimicrobial prescription frequency decreased by around 33% between 2014 and 2020, and HPCIA prescriptions decreased by 54% in dogs and 43% in cats over the same time period (VMD, 2021). This validates findings suggested by antimicrobial wholesale data (VMD, 2020, 2021), lending further evidence to suggest, in the assumed absence of large-scale changes in the demographics of the UK pet population, that companion animal-treating veterinary surgeons are changing their approach to, and frequency of, antimicrobial prescription. Although antimicrobial-prescribing guidance is available (BSAVA/SAMSoc, 2018), such changes

in the UK are in the absence of any statutory legislation restricting antimicrobial access to companion animals, potentially demonstrating the power of voluntary social change in enhancing antimicrobial stewardship efforts (Singleton *et al.*, 2021b). Interestingly, decreases in antimicrobial prescription frequency have also been noted across different broad clinical presentations, for example, gastroenteric (Singleton *et al.*, 2019a) and respiratory disease (Singleton *et al.*, 2019d). Although the questionnaire-based approach to ascertaining broad clinical presentation in these examples did not allow precise determination of clinical conditions, these findings are in line with emerging clinical evidence questioning, for instance, the value of using antimicrobials to manage gastroenteric conditions (Mortier *et al.*, 2015).

Although so far we have discussed relatively large-scale attempts at surveying antimicrobial prescription as part of wider EHR surveillance efforts, it should be noted that, as discussed earlier, establishing routine, long-term, wide-scale surveillance does come with significant challenges and expense. As such, there is an increasing number of more pragmatic attempts that have sought to focus on the issue of antimicrobial prescription alone that have encouraged veterinary practices to engage with prescription surveillance over short periods of time – even as short as a single day per year (Radford *et al.*, 2017; Bollig *et al.*, 2022). Although these approaches do carry limitations – for example, questions over how representative the chosen day(s) might be of normal prescribing practices within the particular veterinary practice – these efforts do provide a more readily accessible gateway for antimicrobial prescription surveillance. This might encourage practitioners to take a 'first step' towards reflective practice, stewardship intervention and involvement with longer-term surveillance projects, ensuring more equitable involvement in attempts to mitigate the impact of AMR.

Other surveillance methods

Other techniques to quantify antimicrobial prescription include the use of specific auditing tools, such as a prescription journal (Murphy *et al.*, 2012) and direct observation of consultations (Robinson *et al.*, 2017). In 2012, Murphy *et al.* (2012) distributed prescription journals, in paper or electronic format, to 82 veterinary surgeons practising in Ontario, Canada, who were required to complete the journal for a subset of cases over the course of a year. This study reported similar prescription trends to those reported in EHR- and survey-based studies, including common prescription of β-lactams, and frequent prescription for respiratory conditions and urinary tract infections. Regarding direct observation, Robinson *et al.* (2017) directly observed 1720 consultations conducted by 62 veterinary surgeons. It was found that antimicrobials were the most common prescription, comprising 30% of total prescription events.

While both approaches could be regarded as relatively labour intensive on the part of the veterinary surgeon and/or researcher, it has been shown that EHRs often only record a portion of total discussions and actions taken during a companion animal consultation. Although pharmaceutical prescriptions do tend to be recorded relatively more accurately (Jones-Diette *et al.*, 2017), these methodologies can provide high-quality evidence on relatively small subsets of the prescribing population, and could form useful and complementary adjuncts to wider-scale surveys. Indeed, a recent study utilized both EHRs and in-person ethnographic study within veterinary practices belonging to large practice groups (Tompson *et al.*, 2020). While in this case the study was focused on characterizing rather than quantifying antimicrobial prescription, this conjoined approach may well have laid the groundwork for future mixed-approach quantitative studies. Future methodological developments may also seek to combine various strategies, such as using technology-based approaches to deploy surveys in a more targeted way at the point of prescription to maximize surveillance efficiency. Such adaptations might minimize reporting bias while providing structured data, reducing the challenge of analysing results.

18.3.2 Characterizing antimicrobial prescription

Although quantifying antimicrobial prescription is clearly of importance, further understanding of the complexities of prescription decision making remains a key goal of AMR surveillance and research, particularly with regard to the development of effective antimicrobial stewardship strategies.

Considering this, survey-based (Hughes *et al.*, 2012; de Briyne *et al.*, 2013, 2014; Barzelai and Whittem, 2017; Gómez-Poveda and Moreno, 2018; van Cleven *et al.*, 2018; Joosten *et al.*, 2020; Galarce *et al.*, 2021; Odoi *et al.*, 2021; Bollig *et al.*, 2022; Taylor *et al.*, 2022) and EHR-focused (Prescott *et al.*, 2002; Rantala *et al.*, 2004a; Holso *et al.*, 2005; Mateus *et al.*, 2011; Radford *et al.*, 2011; Summers *et al.*, 2014; Buckland *et al.*, 2016; Hopman *et al.*, 2019a, c; Schmitt *et al.*, 2019; Singleton *et al.*, 2019c, 2020a; Bollig *et al.*, 2022) studies have revealed clinical conditions more likely to result in antimicrobial prescription (Rantala *et al.*, 2004a; Holso *et al.*, 2005; Radford *et al.*, 2011; Hughes *et al.*, 2012; Murphy *et al.*, 2012; de Briyne *et al.*, 2014; Jones *et al.*, 2014; Summers *et al.*, 2014; Burke *et al.*, 2017; Barzelai and Whittem, 2017; Singleton *et al.*, 2017; van Cleven *et al.*, 2018; Hardefeldt *et al.*, 2020; Singleton *et al.*, 2020b), associations between client or animal demographics and antimicrobial prescription likelihood (Radford *et al.*, 2011; Hughes *et al.*, 2012; Murphy *et al.*, 2012; Jones *et al.*, 2014; Buckland *et al.*, 2016; Singleton *et al.*, 2019c, 2020b; Tompson *et al.*, 2020), and more general attitudes towards antimicrobial prescription and AMR (Hughes *et al.*, 2012; de Briyne *et al.*, 2013; van Cleven *et al.*, 2018). However, so far, perhaps most progress has been made through more qualitative approaches, using in-person interview methods (Mateus *et al.*, 2014; Currie *et al.*, 2018; Hopman *et al.*, 2018; King *et al.*, 2018; Smith *et al.*, 2018; Dickson *et al.*, 2019) and ethnography (Tompson *et al.*, 2020).

Qualitative approaches

In-person interviews have been used extensively in human medicine to explore factors potentially influencing antimicrobial prescription decision making (Teixeira Rodrigues *et al.*, 2013); such studies focusing on companion animal prescribing, however, are relatively scarce (Mateus *et al.*, 2014; Hopman *et al.*, 2018; King *et al.*, 2018; Smith *et al.*, 2018; Dickson *et al.*, 2019). A 2014 study conducted face-to-face interviews, utilizing a semi-structured questionnaire and four hypothetical clinical scenarios, with 21 veterinary surgeons practising in the UK (Mateus *et al.*, 2014). This study identified several themes guiding the prescription decision-making process, broadly grouped into 'intrinsic' and 'extrinsic' factors. Of intrinsic factors, the veterinary surgeon's knowledge of infectious diseases was identified as being of particular importance, as was a personal preference for particular antimicrobials, based largely on previous experience.

Regarding identified 'extrinsic factors', veterinary surgeons reported choosing antimicrobials based on perceived efficacy, spectrum of activity (generally preferring broad-spectrum antimicrobials), ease of administration, duration of therapy and drug availability in their workplace. Some veterinary surgeons practising in low and mixed socio-economic status areas also reported cost as influencing choices, although most veterinary surgeons also stated that they offered the same therapeutic options to all owners regardless of the owner's perceived socio-economic status. Veterinary surgeons also reported being influenced by their colleagues, although older participants suggested their antimicrobial prescription to be more frequent compared with their younger colleagues. Difficulties surrounding justifying the necessity and cost of diagnostic testing appeared to be an important factor in prescribing, as was lack of time for a more thorough case work-up. Most veterinary surgeons were given clinical freedom to decide on prescriptions themselves, with limited awareness of, or actual presence of, internal practice prescribing protocols or external prescribing guidance such as PROTECT ME (BSAVA/SAMSoc, 2018).

Considering other extrinsic factors, where veterinary surgeons perceived potential compliance difficulties, they were more likely to prescribe long-acting injectable agents. Similarly, if the owner expressed unwillingness to pay for therapy, veterinary surgeons would frequently change to a cheaper alternative. Meeting client expectations was identified as an important factor, although participants disagreed over the level of impact it had on guiding prescription choices. However, if owners had a negative experience with a specific antimicrobial (whether their pet or themselves), participants would often alter their choice. Finally, regarding the animal itself, previous clinical history was of importance, as was species, weight, age and presenting clinical signs (Mateus et al., 2014).

A more recent study of 18 Dutch veterinary surgeons in 2015, again via semi-structured face-to-face interviews, corroborated many of these findings (Hopman et al., 2018). However, an interesting divergence of opinion was noted regarding the role companion animal antimicrobial prescribing might play in the context of AMR. Some recognized their personal duty to prescribe responsibly, whereas others suggested that the contribution to AMR from the companion animal sector was so small as to render stewardship largely unnecessary. Dutch law places heavier restrictions on veterinary antimicrobial prescribing; for instance, third- or fourth-generation cephalosporins can only be prescribed if an antimicrobial susceptibility test (AST) indicates resistance to all other antimicrobials. As such, participants indicated the influence of legal restrictions to have significant impact on their decision making. Participants also reported a public health responsibility; for instance, the presence of children in the animal's home might prompt prescription for fear of zoonotic transmission. Regarding the clinical condition itself, participants reported an increased likelihood of prescription in animals displaying more severe clinical signs, especially pyrexia; the presence of comorbidities might also increase antimicrobial prescription likelihood (Hopman et al., 2018).

A further UK study that interviewed 16 companion animal-treating veterinary surgeons identified five key components of antimicrobial-prescribing behaviour: (i) confirming clinical need for antimicrobials; (ii) responding to clients; (iii) confirming diagnosis; (iv) dose, duration and type of antimicrobial; and (v) preventing infection around surgical interventions (King et al., 2018). Interestingly, this study placed stronger emphasis on client influence than Mateus et al. (2014), where interviewees were initially found to be split in their opinions over whether clients played any meaningful role in antimicrobial prescription decision making. King et al. (2018) suggested that, although it was not common for clients to expressly request antimicrobials, it was the perception of the interviewed veterinary surgeons that providing an antimicrobial prescription would be more likely to ensure client satisfaction, and therefore retain business, than if they did not provide a prescription (King et al., 2018). Perceived patient pressure has also been linked to increased likelihood of an antimicrobial prescription in the medical sector (McKay et al., 2016). However, when patients presenting to primary-care practices with an acute cough were actually asked about their expectations and hopes for an antimicrobial prescription following a consultation, only modest levels of agreement were revealed between patient expectation and actual receipt of an antimicrobial prescription (Coenen et al., 2013). This suggests that clinicians are not particularly good at identifying client expectations or hopes for an antimicrobial prescription, indicating a need for improved communication between clinicians and their patients/clients (Smith *et al.*, 2018).

Other interview-based studies have also assessed AMR knowledge and harnessed related opinions of pet owners (Smith *et al.*, 2018; Dickson *et al.*, 2019). These studies revealed poor understanding of AMR, although participants did show awareness of problematic antimicrobial use. Unfortunately, while this awareness sometimes related to AMR risk, it more commonly referred to direct health risks to those receiving antimicrobial therapy (i.e. adverse events), or that the recipients themselves could develop resistance to an antimicrobial. While this would suggest a need for improved client education, Dickson *et al.* (2019) also revealed that the close relationship enjoyed between pets and their owners frequently translated to a perception of 'guardianship' when it came to seeking veterinary care and/or antimicrobial therapy for their pets. In other words, owners felt a personal responsibility for ensuring the welfare of their pets, such that a wait-and-see approach was often felt to be 'too risky' for their animal. This was true even when the wider risks of AMR were considered, which was felt to be a rather remote issue in comparison to the immediacy of their pet's ill health (Smith *et al.*, 2018).

As with survey-based approaches, interview-based approaches can also be associated with enhanced risk of reporting bias compared with observation of actual prescribing practices. Whereas use of EHRs does largely mitigate this issue, they do not contain a complete description of all interactions held within a veterinary appointment (Robinson *et al.*, 2015; Jones-Diette *et al.*, 2017). Tompson *et al.* (2020) utilized an ethnographic approach to examine interactions between owners and veterinary surgeons in relation to antimicrobial prescription decision making. This study further corroborated findings from other studies, indicating a tension where prescribers (and to a lesser extent, owners) are trying to balance the immediate welfare needs of the animal under their care against the somewhat more remote and less tangible issue of AMR. In such situations, a decision that might appear to contravene responsible use guidance may actually 'make sense' in the particular situation once the veterinary surgeon has also assessed the owner's frailty, mobility or financial hardship; it is likely that none of these complexities would be consistently recorded in an EHR, for instance (Tompson *et al.*, 2020). It should be noted that,

although this study did also utilize EHR data, due to anonymization requirements the EHR analysis was not able to be directly linked to the ethnographic analysis (Tompson *et al.*, 2020). With appropriate ethical and consent controls in place, future studies may wish to more closely link such research techniques to associate actual prescribing practices more directly with the expressed attitudes of study participants.

Survey-based approaches

Researchers have also utilized surveys to characterize companion animal antimicrobial prescription. An interesting approach was recently explored by Currie *et al.* (2018), who sought to gain an 'expert consensus' on companion animal antimicrobial prescription, specifically seeking to identify the most important prescribing behaviours that need to change to achieve effective stewardship, and the key barriers preventing such change from occurring. A two-stage online Delphi survey was deployed, a technique recognized as effective for gaining expert consensus (Hasson *et al.*, 2000), which was completed by 16 participants. Findings indicated that experts agreed that antimicrobial prescription in companion animals had an important impact on AMR. They further agreed that poor antimicrobial choice was the most important AMR contributory factor, whether that included unnecessary prescriptions, over-reliance on broad-spectrum antimicrobials or HPCIAs being used as first-line therapies (Currie *et al.*, 2018). Although the results of Mateus *et al.* (2014) showed mixed opinions, experts considered client expectation of an antimicrobial prescription to have an important influence on prescription decision making and hence resistance (Mateus *et al.*, 2014; Currie *et al.*, 2018).

Considering other survey-based studies, as discussed earlier, clinical condition has a significant impact on antimicrobial prescription likelihood, as evidenced by both surveys and EHR-based studies (Rantala *et al.*, 2004b; Radford *et al.*, 2011; Hughes *et al.*, 2012; Murphy *et al.*, 2012; de Briyne *et al.*, 2013, 2014; Summers *et al.*, 2014; Barzelai and Whittem, 2017; Burke *et al.*, 2017; van Cleven *et al.*, 2018; Singleton *et al.*, 2017, 2019c, 2020b; Hardefeldt *et al.*, 2020; Bollig *et al.*, 2022). Similarly, Hughes *et al.* (2012) found that surveyed veterinary surgeons considered clinical signs to be the most important factor when deciding to prescribe an antimicrobial, followed by bacterial culture, ease of administration, financial constraints, cytology and, lastly, client expectations. Despite patient pressure being a recognized issue in human medicine (Lewis and Tully, 2011) that sometimes results in unnecessary prescriptions (Little *et al.*, 2004), it would appear, as also revealed via qualitative study, that opinion remains split as to the influence of client expectations on prescribing in companion animal practice.

On an international scale, a European-wide survey of veterinary surgeons belonging to all sectors also reported veterinary surgeons to consider 'owner demand' to be of relatively low importance. In this survey, AST results were ranked as the most important guiding factor for antimicrobial choice among companion animal-treating veterinary surgeons, followed by perceived AMR risk, administration ease, the SPC and legal restrictions (de Briyne *et al.*, 2013). Finally, a 2018 survey of veterinary surgeons practising in Belgium reported the three most important influencing factors in decision making to be clinical presentation, owner compliance and ease of administration. This study also reported owner expectations to be one of the least important factors, along with financial restrictions (van Cleven *et al.*, 2018). To summarize, while surveys appear to corroborate some factors revealed during qualitative study, generally agreeing on the most important factors that influence antimicrobial prescription, there appears to be some disagreement over factors considered by some to be of lesser importance or, perhaps, more controversial.

EHRs

Although relatively limited, several factors thought to be related to antimicrobial prescription decision making have been explored through use of actual prescribing data, focusing largely on animal intrinsic factors. For instance, Radford *et al.* (2011) revealed decreasing odds of a dog or cats being prescribed an antimicrobial (on a per-consultation basis) as they increased in age. Of perhaps some relevance here, this study also revealed considerable prescription frequency variation among practices contributing data (Radford *et al.*, 2011), something later confirmed by larger studies (Buckland *et al.*, 2016; Singleton *et al.*, 2017).

More recently, Singleton *et al.* (2020b) utilized data from 178 veterinary practices to examine animal factors, owner factors and veterinary practice factors in relation to antimicrobial prescription likelihood. This study confirmed a complex interplay of all three major factors suggested by an earlier qualitative study (Mateus *et al.*, 2014), with animals who had previous evidence of preventative medicine interaction (i.e. vaccination, neutering) or who were insured being associated with a lower likelihood of antimicrobial prescription. Although some of these factors could be linked with biologically plausible reasons to explain such variant prescription risk, it is perhaps more probable that previous engagement with preventative healthcare services might select for clients more likely to promptly seek veterinary attention earlier or to pursue diagnostic options rather than empirical antimicrobial prescription (Singleton *et al.*, 2020b). Although a comparatively minor factor, this study also associated veterinary practice membership of a clinical standards scheme with less frequent antimicrobial prescription, potentially highlighting the important role that both owner and veterinary practitioner education may play in ensuring effective antimicrobial stewardship (Singleton *et al.*, 2020b).

Considering animal intrinsic factors further, considerable breed variation in antimicrobial prescription risk was observed in this and a more recent study (Tompson *et al.*, 2020). Interestingly, while increased age has been associated with decreased odds of antimicrobial prescription (Radford *et al.*, 2011; Singleton *et al.*, 2020b), a converse increased odds of HPCIA prescription with increased age has also been seen (Singleton *et al.*, 2020b; Tompson *et al.*, 2020). Such age-based variability has also been linked with sex, with, for example, younger male cats being more commonly associated with antimicrobial prescription (Singleton *et al.*, 2020b). Such variations may suggest that specific behaviours or morphologies associated with particular age or sex characteristics could alter the risk of bacterial infection between and within species (Huerta *et al.*, 2011), but also potentially changing relationships with veterinary care. For instance, increased odds of HPCIA prescription with age might be associated with increasingly fractious responses to veterinary intervention increasing the likelihood of an easy-to-administer, long-acting, injectable HPCIA being given in older animals (Burke *et al.*, 2017). However, currently many of these findings remain associations alone, with their actual causative impact yet to be assessed.

Finally, regarding EHR-based studies exploring specific clinical conditions, Jones *et al.* (2014)

reported antimicrobial prescription to be more likely in haemorrhagic diarrhoea cases, indicating that case severity might have an influence on prescription likelihood (Jones *et al.*, 2014). This finding was reinforced in a later study, which associated those cases identified by the veterinary practitioner as being of increased severity, as well as those cases with increased body temperature and haemorrhagic diarrhoea, with increased likelihood of an antimicrobial prescription being made (Singleton *et al.*, 2019c). This had been identified previously in an interview-based study (Hopman *et al.*, 2018), although an earlier study found no association between reported respiratory disease severity and antimicrobial prescription likelihood in dogs and cats (Murphy *et al.*, 2012). In summary, as with qualitative- and survey-based approaches, while a multitude of potentially contributory factors have been identified, there have so far been comparatively limited attempts to seek to prioritize which factors are of greatest importance for antimicrobial stewardship (Currie *et al.*, 2018), and, crucially, to act on those recommendations.

18.4 Approaches to Antimicrobial Resistance Diagnosis

To consider approaches to AMR surveillance, we must first consider approaches to laboratory-based resistance diagnosis. The two most widely used methods by which bacterial isolates are phenotypically assessed for resistance are agar disc diffusion and calculation of minimum inhibitory concentration via broth or agar dilution (Biemer, 1973). Both of these methods are widely utilized in veterinary diagnostic laboratories (Marques *et al.*, 2016; Singleton *et al.*, 2021a), and while broad equivalence between both methods has been demonstrated (Andrews, 2001), it should be borne in mind that this equivalence is not consistent for all bacterial species and antimicrobials (Gaudreau and Gilbert, 1997; Nicodemo *et al.*, 2004).

Variation between veterinary diagnostic laboratories also exists with regard to AST interpretation (Marques *et al.*, 2016; Singleton *et al.*, 2021a). Following both methods, isolates are classified as sensitive, intermediate or resistant to the antimicrobial in question through use of numerical 'breakpoints', the intention of this being to provide a prediction of how effective the antimicrobial might be at treating the bacterial infection *in vivo* (Roca *et al.*, 2015). Devising appropriate breakpoints is a multifactorial process taking into account an array of considerations such as recently identified resistance trends and mechanisms, the animal species for which treatment is intended, the pharmacodynamics and pharmacokinetics of the tested antimicrobial, and the bacterial species being tested, among others (Kahlmeter *et al.*, 2003). Breakpoints were initially devised at a national level for medical use, for example through the British Society of Antimicrobial Chemotherapy (BSAC) (Andrews, 2001); however, considering the complexities involved in determining such values, sometimes considerable variation among countries was observed, resulting in calls for greater international breakpoint harmonization (Kahlmeter *et al.*, 2003). Currently, two such more international guidelines are commonly used: the European Committee on Antimicrobial Susceptibility Testing (EUCAST) guidance (Leclercq *et al.*, 2013), and the US-led Clinical and Laboratory Standards Institute (CLSI) guidance (Roca *et al.*, 2015). Unfortunately, discrepancies still remain between these two schemes, meaning that there is still some way to go before truly international unified AMR surveillance can be achieved (Roca *et al.*, 2015).

Considering breakpoints devised for veterinary species specifically, the Veterinary Committee on Antimicrobial Susceptibility Testing (VetCAST), a subcommittee of EUCAST (Toutain *et al.*, 2017), and CLSI (CLSI, 2008) have begun to provide some guidance. However, due to a relative paucity of veterinary data necessary to determine breakpoints, such summaries are incomplete, frequently relying on human breakpoints or species-independent epidemiological cut-off values (Toutain *et al.*, 2017). In practical terms, this dearth of evidence and variation in approach to diagnosing AMR has resulted in veterinary diagnostic laboratories utilizing a variety of techniques and interpretations, including their own in-house interpretations in some cases (Marques *et al.*, 2016). While such issues do pose a challenge to effective companion animal AMR surveillance, extensive efforts are currently under way to improve harmonization between veterinary diagnostic laboratories, hopefully enhancing AMR surveillance capacity in the future (ENOVAT, 2022).

A key barrier to the application of ASTs in clinical practice is the time it takes for a result to be made available to the clinician, which can be in excess of 1 week (de Briyne *et al.*, 2013). As a result, recent research has focused on developing new methods to characterize resistant isolates more rapidly within a clinically relevant time frame. So far, mass spectrometry (e.g. matrix-assisted laser desorption/ionization time-of-flight mass spectrometry (MALDI-TOF MS); Burckhardt and Zimmermann, 2018; Idelevich et al., 2018) and molecular techniques (Roca et al., 2015) have generated particular interest, both for direct clinical application and for surveillance. While the significant potential of molecular techniques, particularly whole-genome sequencing, for AMR surveillance (Koser et al., 2014), outbreak investigation (McGann et al., 2016) and routine diagnostic microbiology (Rossen et al., 2018) is widely recognized, such approaches have only comparatively recently begun to be utilized regularly in companion animal health, being largely restricted to academic publications (Radford et al., 2021; Singleton et al., 2021a).

18.4.1 AMR surveillance

AMR surveillance can be classified into two branches: (i) surveillance of resistance carriage; and (ii) surveillance of resistance in clinically affected animals or humans. Both branches have been explored in veterinary species, with some studies considering phenotypic resistance (Trott et al., 2004; Leite-Martins et al., 2014; Marques et al., 2016; Arsevska et al., 2018b; Conner et al., 2018; Singleton et al., 2021a) and others utilizing genotypic methods, including single-gene (Loeffler et al., 2011; Wedley et al., 2011; Damborg et al., 2015; Schmidt et al., 2015, 2018a, 2018b; Ventrella et al., 2017), multiple-gene (Damborg et al., 2011; Pires Dos Santos et al., 2016; Zhang et al., 2016; Ventrella et al., 2017; Wedley et al., 2017; Zogg et al., 2018), or whole-genome (Harrison et al., 2014; McCarthy et al., 2015; Zhang et al., 2018; Scott et al., 2019; Singleton et al., 2021a) identification methodologies. Besides prevalence of resistance, studies have also sought to identify risk factors associated with resistance, such as antimicrobial therapy, via retrospective observational studies (Loeffler et al., 2011; Leite-Martins et al., 2014; Schmidt et al., 2015; Wedley et al., 2017; Singleton et al., 2021a) and prospective experimental trials (Trott et al., 2004; Damborg et al., 2011; Schmidt et al., 2018a, b). Studies have also demonstrated probable interspecies resistance transfer (Guardabassi et al., 2004; Loeffler and Lloyd, 2010; Harrison et al., 2014; Zhang et al., 2016), with these findings having clear implications for antimicrobial stewardship.

As with antimicrobials, bacterial species have also been classified by the World Health Organization (WHO) into AMR priority groups (critical, high and medium), with the aim of focusing global surveillance and research initiatives. The critically important bacteria are all Gram negative and include carbapenem-resistant *Acinetobacter baumannii*, carbapenem-resistant *Pseudomonas aeruginosa*, and carbapenem- or third-generation cephalosporin-resistant *Enterobacterales*. Of Gram-positive bacteria, the highest-ranking species include vancomycin-resistant *Enterococcus faecium* and methicillin-resistant *Staphylococcus aureus* or vancomycin-resistant *Staphylococcus aureus*, both being considered high priority (Tacconelli et al., 2018). Although this prioritization exercise is focused on human health, there are several bacterial species (arguably, especially the *Enterobacterales*) of direct relevance to veterinary health.

AMR surveillance has also been used to make predictions about what the future might hold for resistant infections. For example, Van Boeckel et al. (2019) utilized point prevalence surveys to extrapolate findings for farmed animals across LMICs. They revealed a steady increase in resistance over the past 20 years, with particular hotspots of resistance being identified in Asia, which is home to over half of the world's population of pigs and chickens. Interestingly, comparatively few AMR hotspots were identified in Africa, a region of the world already shown to possess the greatest burden of deaths from resistant infections in people (Murray et al., 2022).

In many ways, this apparent contradiction serves to demonstrate the complexities of understanding and tackling AMR. In this case, many African countries have only limited access to antimicrobials for human use (MacPherson et al., 2021), meaning that when faced with a bacterial infection resistant to widely available 'first-line' antimicrobials, prescribers may well not have access to 'second-line' antimicrobials, which may otherwise be more readily accessible in higher-income countries. In this case, one could argue that *any* resistant infection presents a risk for mortality in many LMICs, rather than just the multidrug-resistant infections that are of particular concern to clinicians in higher-income countries. Interestingly, Van Boeckel et al. (2019) suggested that a more permissive attitude should be taken towards regulating the use of antimicrobials in Africa, as a heavy-handed approach may unfairly hamper such countries' farming and economic development (Van Boeckel *et al.*, 2019). It is for this reason that the global action plan on AMR recommended that individual countries should develop their own plans, as it was recognized that tackling AMR should be viewed in conjunction with the particular situation of each country (WHO, 2015).

18.5 Antimicrobial Stewardship

Antimicrobial stewardship can be defined as any effort to optimize use of antimicrobials, with the primary aim of decreasing selection pressure for AMR but also of reducing adverse events resulting from antimicrobial use and delivering cost-effective therapy (Morris *et al.*, 2012). It is clear that for a prescriber to achieve these aims, they must possess extensive general and local knowledge concerning aetiology, antimicrobial consumption and resistance trends, and treatment efficacy (Fishman, 2006). Thus, while the responsibility for antimicrobial stewardship rests most firmly with the prescriber, it is clear that a truly multi-disciplinary approach that also includes educators, academics, diagnostic services, policy makers and pharmaceutical companies is necessary to ensure that the prescriber can make truly informed and responsible prescription choices. In medicine, antimicrobial stewardship has already been widely incorporated into the daily routine of clinicians, in some cases also demonstrating a reduction in AMR or antimicrobial prescription-related infections (e.g. *Clostridioides difficile*) at a local level (Thursky *et al.*, 2006; Talpaert *et al.*, 2011; Gerber *et al.*, 2013; Martinez-Gonzalez *et al.*, 2017).

In veterinary species, stewardship is less well developed. Currie *et al.* (2018) conducted an expert consensus-building study seeking to identify barriers and opportunities for enacting antimicrobial stewardship in companion animals. This study identified a range of aspects that could contribute to stewardship, including optimizing dosage and reducing reliance on broad-spectrum antimicrobials, improved veterinarian–client communication, improved access to AMR educational material and improved infection-control processes, among others. They also suggested that development of both local and national mechanisms by which antimicrobial prescription audits, with feedback to clinicians, can be achieved would represent a key goal of antimicrobial stewardship efforts (Currie *et al.*, 2018).

This study demonstrates once more that there are no single 'best' approaches to tackling AMR, and accordingly, in veterinary species, there are a growing number of efforts utilizing a range of different tactics, including legislated (Dutil *et al.*, 2010; Hesp *et al.*, 2019; Chirollo *et al.*, 2021; Moerer *et al.*, 2022), prescribing guidance-focused (Jessen *et al.*, 2017; Hopman *et al.*, 2019b; Hubbuch *et al.*, 2020; Hardefeldt *et al.*, 2022; Hur *et al.*, 2022), education-centred (Hardefeldt *et al.*, 2022; Hopman *et al.*, 2021) and audit/benchmarking-based (Hopman *et al.*, 2019b; Hardefeldt *et al.*, 2020; Singleton *et al.*, 2021b; Walker *et al.*, 2022) approaches to help ensure that antimicrobials are being used more responsibly. While many of these utilize 'before and after' style assessment methods, there are also some instances where randomized controlled trials have been implemented (Hopman *et al.*, 2019b; Hardefeldt *et al.*, 2022; Singleton *et al.*, 2021b), suggesting that veterinary attempts to devise and assess stewardship interventions are becoming increasingly sophisticated and robust.

Considering legislated approaches, perhaps the most effective – but also the bluntest – stewardship tool is to ban the use of particular antimicrobials, either in whole species or for particular purposes (i.e. prophylactic or in-feed use). In 2016, following the identification in commercially farmed pigs from China of *mcr-1*, a plasmid-mediated gene conferring colistin resistance (Liu *et al.*, 2016), some countries implemented a complete ban on the use of colistin as feed additives in animals (Olaitan *et al.*, 2021), whereas others implemented a voluntary withdrawal of colistin from the veterinary market (Ribeiro *et al.*, 2021). These actions have, for example, led to a 70% reduction in the use of colistin in Europe (ESVAC, 2021), with one study demonstrating a sharp reduction in *mcr* gene identification in chicken meat approximately 8 months after voluntary colistin withdrawal in Portugal (Ribeiro *et al.*, 2021). While most likely effective at reducing resistance carriage, care does have to be taken in how such sharp tools are implemented, particularly with regard to economic development, farming sustainability and, above all, animal welfare. A recent controversy erupted across the EU when a motion was put forward suggesting that a wide range of antimicrobials should be effectively banned for use in animals, including some that are commonly used (European Parliament, 2021). In this case, even strong proponents of responsible antimicrobial use raised concerns regarding the potentially damaging effect such a ban might have on animal welfare (StopAMR, 2021). In this case, the motion was voted down (FACE, 2021), with a revised proposition banning a more limited range of antimicrobials (e.g. vancomycin) recently put to public consultation (European Commission, 2022).

Beyond outright bans, legislation has also been used to implement antimicrobial use/sales reduction targets (Hesp et al., 2019), improved traceability and monitoring of antimicrobial use/prescription (Chirollo et al., 2021) and stricter requirements (e.g. an AST supporting antimicrobial choice) for prescription of HPCIAs (Moerer et al., 2022). Such approaches have resulted in rapid initial reductions in both antimicrobial use and resistance carriage (Hesp et al., 2019). However, whereas such approaches do seem able to produce rapid changes, there is some evidence to suggest that, for antimicrobial use, rates of initial success are hard to maintain (Hesp et al., 2019), potentially suggesting that legislated approaches may not be the most effective means for engaging practitioners in stewardship efforts. It could also reflect the fact that there may be a natural lower 'limit' to the frequency with which antimicrobials can be prescribed to animals, reflective of actual underlying bacterial infection trends. In such cases, improved biosecurity and other adjunctive methods may actually be more effective than a continued focus on antimicrobial use reduction alone (O'Neill, 2016). It should also be remembered that reduced antimicrobial use is not de facto evidence for increased responsible use, nor is it a guarantee of reduced AMR prevalence. As such, it could be argued that legislated antimicrobial use reduction targets are too blunt for sustainable improvements in the longer term.

Interestingly, however, legislated direction to increase the use of ASTs prior to prescribing HPCIAs in companion animals has been associated with an increase in the number of veterinary surgeons reporting that they had changed their AST and antimicrobial prescription habits (Moerer et al., 2022). It is well known that any antimicrobial prescription decision should be based on knowledge of the bacterial species causing infection and its associated susceptibility profile (i.e. via bacterial culture and ASTs). However, in practice, antimicrobial prescription is frequently empirical (de Briyne et al., 2013; Burke et al., 2017), with frequent prescription of broad-spectrum antimicrobials (Buckland et al., 2016; Singleton et al., 2017); this would seem to be clearly at odds with the aims of antimicrobial stewardship. As such, while promoting the use of bacterial diagnostic testing has been noted as a key aim of antimicrobial stewardship (Currie et al., 2018), it has not been clear for some time how this might be achieved practically.

As discussed earlier, there are universal issues regarding the often-considerable time taken for an AST to be completed. This presents difficulties when justifying this course of action to clients; in veterinary medicine, this difficulty is likely to be compounded by the need to also justify the cost of diagnostic tests to the client (de Briyne et al., 2013; Bourély et al., 2018). While developing rapid diagnostic methods remains an active research area (Rossen et al., 2018), there is work to be done to encourage practitioners to engage with existing bacterial diagnostics more frequently. It is possible that introducing legal requirements for the use of ASTs could provide a justification for the use of ASTs that a client cannot object to. However, it should also be noted in the aforementioned study that, even though 63% of veterinarians reported using ASTs more frequently, 17% reported that they did not, in spite of legislation (Moerer et al., 2022). As such, even when one arguably uses the 'strongest tool' to direct practitioners towards more responsible use, achieving 100% compliance is likely to be some way off. Hence, beyond legislated approaches, others have investigated the impact that voluntary interventions might have on encouraging improved antimicrobial stewardship.

Chief among voluntary approaches is the development and implementation of antimicrobial prescription guidance, including devising practice-level antimicrobial use policies. A range of organizations have developed such advice for companion animal prescribers (FECAVA, 2013; Jessen et al., 2017; BSAVA/SAMSoc, 2018; Hur et al., 2019; Hubbuch et al., 2020; Hardefeldt et al., 2022), with evidence to suggest that prescribing guidance is becoming increasingly widely used in practice (Jessen et al., 2017). The fact that prescribing guidance is frequently recommended as part of multifaceted stewardship intervention packages (Hopman et al., 2019b; Hardefeldt et al., 2022; Singleton et al., 2021b) has meant that assessing the precise impact of prescribing guidance alone is often difficult. However, one guidance-alone observational study did present a mixed picture of reduced antimicrobial prescription post-intervention but no clear increased compliance with the guidance itself (Hubbuch et al., 2020). Large-scale observational approaches utilizing EHRs for assessing the impact of prescribing guidance can be difficult due to the complexities of language contained with free-text clinical notes; however, Hur et al. (2019) developed a sophisticated tool to enable such an approach to take place. The authors were able to use this tool to demonstrate that compliance with dosage recommendations on prescribing guidance were followed in the majority of cases where complete information was available; however, only 40% of cases had such complete information available (Hur et al., 2019). Nevertheless, it is hoped that studies such as this may prompt improvements in clinical record quality, enabling novel approaches such as this to take on greater clinical significance. It should also be noted that a generalized lack of veterinary clinical evidence means that prescribing guidance is often based on relatively poor evidence and/or expert opinion or consensus. Luckily, there are wide-scale efforts currently in development that seek to address these limitations (ENOVAT, 2022), and we would invite the reader to 'watch this space'.

Considering education-based approaches, although as with prescribing guidance this is frequently incorporated within multifaceted interventions, Hopman et al. (2021) used education as a primary intervention (although information on prescribing guidance, for example, was still a part of the education package delivered). Course participants reported heightened awareness of AMR, and also reported that they used antimicrobials more responsibly as a result of attendance (Hopman et al., 2021). This study was a pilot, with wider implementation and systematic evaluation planned.

Finally, with increasingly widespread use and analysis of EHRs, audit and benchmarking-focused stewardship interventions are becoming more widely implemented. These range from small-scale, accessible approaches whereby practitioners are encouraged to (manually, if necessary) submit achievable volumes of data for benchmarking (Radford et al., 2017; Bollig et al., 2022) to wide-scale studies involving tens or hundreds of veterinary practices (Hopman et al., 2019b; Singleton et al., 2021b; Hardefeldt et al., 2022; Walker et al., 2022). These interventions are generally rooted in behaviour change theory – specifically, the idea that establishing departure from a 'social norm' (in this case, higher prescribing rates compared with their peers) may provide a motivator to reflect on, and change, approaches to antimicrobial prescription (Hallsworth et al., 2016).

So far, these approaches have shown some promise, although as stated above, discerning the precise impact of audit and benchmarking alone in a multifactorial intervention study remains challenging. For example, Hopman et al. (2019b) found a 15% decrease in total antimicrobial usage in 44 Dutch companion animal veterinary practices in response to an intervention including audit and case reflection. Similarly, Hardefeldt et al. (2022), implementing an education-only arm as a control group against two varying intensity intervention groups found reductions of 36% across all practices during the intervention period, with the low- and high-intervention groups being associated with reductions of 4% and 6% compared with the control education-only group. This latter study found relatively greater reductions among practices that were more frequent antimicrobial prescribers compared with others included in the trial, suggesting that practitioners may respond to being identified as outside the 'social norm' of antimicrobial prescribing. However, as enhanced reductions were also seen in the control education-only group who did not receive any auditing or benchmarking intervention, it is also possible that the room for improvement was simply greater in such practices.

This considered, a recent trial by the authors that targeted above-average HPCIA prescribing practices within a large UK practice group, and utilized a 'true' control group where no intervention was delivered against two varying intensity intervention groups, found that cats in the heavy intervention group were associated with a 40% decrease in HPCIA prescription frequency post-intervention (Singleton et al., 2021b). This finding suggests that efficient stewardship might best be achieved by using benchmarking as part of not only the intervention itself but also when selecting practices for intervention. However, whereas HPCIA prescription frequency decreased markedly post-intervention, overall antimicrobial prescription decreases were less marked and were accompanied by a notable (although not significant) increase in the prescription of clavulanic acid-potentiated amoxicillin. Interestingly, another UK study uncovered similar results, although in this case the increase in clavulanic acid-potentiated amoxicillin prescription was significant (Walker et al., 2022). Like the HPCIAs, use of clavulanic acid-potentiated amoxicillin has been associated with resistance development (Schmidt et al., 2018a) and is only infrequently prescribed to humans (PHE, 2021), although it is commonly prescribed to dogs and cats (Singleton *et al.*, 2017). As such, it would appear that care needs to be taken when seeking to establish targeted interventions, as in these cases focusing on HPCIAs could well have reduced resistance development risk on the one hand only to enhance or at least sustain broader β-lactam resistance risk on the other (Singleton *et al.*, 2021b).

18.6 Conclusion

While the importance of antimicrobial prescription and resistance surveillance in veterinary species has been recognized previously, technological and practical limitations have in the past limited both of them to small groups of veterinary practices, farms or singular veterinary diagnostic laboratories. However, recent advances have enabled increasingly sophisticated surveillance tools (particularly EHRs) to be utilized at scale, enabling innovative stewardship interventions to be developed, trialled, evaluated and implemented in veterinary practice. Although several challenges remain before such developments could be considered 'mature' or 'routine', at least in high-income countries, the road to effective, widespread antimicrobial prescription and resistance surveillance conjoined with stewardship intervention appears increasingly clear. There now remains one major challenge ahead – implementing similar schemes in LMICs, where the burden of resistant infections is predicted to fall most heavily.

References

Aegerter, J., Fouracre, D. and Smith, G.C. (2017) A first estimate of the structure and density of the populations of pet cats and dogs across Great Britain. *PloS One* 12(4), e0174709. DOI: 10.1371/journal.pone.0174709.

Andrews, J.M. (2001) The development of the BSAC standardized method of disc diffusion testing. *Journal of Antimicrobial Chemotherapy* 48(Suppl. 1), 29–42. DOI: 10.1093/jac/48.suppl_1.29.

Anholt, R.M., Berezowski, J., Ribble, C.S., Russell, M.L. and Stephen, C. (2014a) Using informatics and the electronic medical record to describe antimicrobial use in the clinical management of diarrhea cases at 12 companion animal practices. *PloS One* 9(7), e103190. DOI: 10.1371/journal.pone.0103190.

Anholt, R.M., Berezowski, J., Jamal, I., Ribble, C. and Stephen, C. (2014b) Mining free-text medical records for companion animal enteric syndrome surveillance.

Preventive Veterinary Medicine 113(4), 417–422. DOI: 10.1016/j.prevetmed.2014.01.017.

Arsevska, E., Singleton, D., Sánchez-Vizcaíno, F., Williams, N., Jones, P.H. *et al.* (2017) Small animal disease surveillance: GI disease and salmonellosis. *Veterinary Record* 181(9), 228–232. DOI: 10.1136/vr.j3642.

Arsevska, E., Priestnall, S.L., Singleton, D.A., Jones, P.H., Smyth, S *et al.* (2018a) Small animal disease surveillance: respiratory disease 2017. *Veterinary Record* 182(13), 369–373. DOI: 10.1136/vr.k1426.

Arsevska, E., Singleton, D.A., Jewell, C., Paterson, S., Jones, P.H *et al.* (2018b) Small animal disease surveillance: pruritus and Pseudomonas skin infections. *Veterinary Record* 183(6), 182–187. DOI: 10.1136/vr.k3462.

Barzelai, I.D. and Whittem, T. (2017) Survey of systemic antimicrobial prescribing for dogs by Victorian veterinarians. *Australian Veterinary Journal* 95(10), 375–385. DOI: 10.1111/avj.12637.

Benchimol, E.I., Smeeth, L., Guttmann, A., Harron, K., Moher, D. *et al.* (2015) The reporting of studies conducted using observational routinely-collected health data (RECORD) statement. *PLoS Medicine* 12(10), e1001885. DOI: 10.1371/journal.pmed.1001885.

Biemer, J.J. (1973) Antimicrobial susceptibility testing by the Kirby-Bauer disc diffusion method. *Annals of Clinical Laboratory Science* 3(2), 135–140.

Birnbaum, D., Gretsinger, K., Antonio, M.G., Loewen, E. and Lacroix, P. (2018) Revisiting public health informatics: patient privacy concerns. *International Journal of Health Governance* 23, 149–159.

Bollig, E.R., Granick, J.L., Webb, T.L., Ward, C. and Beaudoin, A.L. (2022) A quarterly survey of antibiotic prescribing in small animal and equine practices – Minnesota and North Dakota, 2020. *Zoonoses Public Health* 69, 864–874.

Bourély, C., Fortané, N., Calavas, D., Leblond, A. and Gay, E. (2018) Why do veterinarians ask for antimicrobial susceptibility testing? A qualitative study exploring determinants and evaluating the impact of antibiotic reduction policy. *Preventive Veterinary Medicine* 159, 123–134.

BSAVA/SAMSoc (2018) *BSAVA/SAMSoc Guide to Responsible Use of Antibacterials: PROTECT ME.* British Small Animal Veterinary Association/Small Animal Medicine Society, Quedgeley, UK. Available at: www.bsavalibrary.com/content/book/10.22233/9781910443644 (accessed 30 October 2022).

Buckland, E.L., O'Neill, D., Summers, J., Mateus, A., Church, D. *et al.* (2016) Characterisation of antimicrobial usage in cats and dogs attending UK primary care companion animal veterinary practices. *Veterinary Record* 179, 489. DOI: 10.1136/vr.103830.

Burckhardt, I. and Zimmermann, S. (2018) Susceptibility testing of bacteria using Maldi-Tof mass spectrometry.

David A. Singleton *et al.*

Frontiers in Microbiology 9, 1744. DOI: 10.3389/fmicb.2018.01744.

Burke, S., Black, V., Sánchez-Vizcaíno, F., Radford, A., Hibbert, A. *et al.* (2017) Use of cefovecin in a UK population of cats attending first-opinion practices as recorded in electronic health records. *Journal of Feline Medicine and Surgery* 19(6), 687–692. DOI: 10.1177/1098612X16656706.

Cantón, R. and Bryan, J. (2012) Global antimicrobial resistance: from surveillance to stewardship. Part 1: surveillance and risk factors for resistance. *Expert Review of Anti-Infective Therapy* 10(11), 1269–1271. DOI: 10.1586/eri.12.120.

CAVSNET (2022) Companion Animal Veterinary Surveillance Network (CAVSNET). Available at: https://cavsnet.umn.edu/about-cavsnet (accessed 30 October 2022).

Chirollo, C., Nocera, F.P., Piantedosi, D., Fatone, G., Della Valle, G. *et al.* (2021) Data on before and after the traceability system of veterinary antimicrobial prescriptions in small animals at the University Veterinary Teaching Hospital of Naples. *Animals* 11(3), 913. DOI: 10.3390/ani11030913.

CLSI (2008) *Performance Standards for Antimicrobial Disk and Dilution Susceptibility Tests for Bacteria Isolated from Animals: Approved Standard*, 3rd edn. Clinical and Laboratory Standards Institute, Malvern, Pennsylvania.

Coates, A., Hu, Y., Bax, R. and Page, C. (2002) The future challenges facing the development of new antimicrobial drugs. *Nature Reviews Drug Discovery* 1, 895–910. DOI: 10.1038/nrd940.

Coenen, S., Francis, N., Kelly, M., Hood, K., Nuttall, J *et al.* (2013) Are patient views about antibiotics related to clinician perceptions, management and outcome? A multi-country study in outpatients with acute cough. *PloS One* 8(10), e76691. DOI: 10.1371/journal.pone.0076691.

Collins, M., Singleton, D.A., Noble, P.J.M., Pinchbeck, G.L., Smith, S *et al.* (2021) Small animal disease surveillance 2020/21: SARS-cov-2, syndromic surveillance and an outbreak of acute vomiting in UK dogs. *Veterinary Record* 188(8), 304. DOI: 10.1002/vetr.427.

Conner, J.G., Smith, J., Erol, E., Locke, S., Phillips, E. *et al.* (2018) Temporal trends and predictors of antimicrobial resistance among *staphylococcus* spp. isolated from canine specimens submitted to a diagnostic laboratory. *PLoS One* 13, e0200719.

Cuny, C., Wieler, L.H. and Witte, W. (2015) Livestock-associated MRSA: the impact on humans. *Antibiotics* 4, 521–543. DOI: 10.3390/antibiotics4040521.

Currie, K., King, C., Nuttall, T., Smith, M. and Flowers, P. (2018) Expert consensus regarding drivers of antimicrobial stewardship in companion animal veterinary practice: a Delphi study. *Veterinary Record* 182, 691. DOI: 10.1136/vr.104639.

Damborg, P., Gaustad, I.B., Olsen, J.E. and Guardabassi, L. (2011) Selection of CMY-2 producing *escherichia coli* in the faecal flora of dogs treated with cephalexin. *Veterinary Microbiology* 151, 404–408.

Damborg, P., Morsing, M.K., Petersen, T., Bortolaia, V. and Guardabassi, L. (2015) CTX-M-1 and CTX-M-15-producing *Escherichia coli* in dog faeces from public gardens. *Acta Veterinaria Scandinavica* 57, 83. DOI: 10.1186/s13028-015-0174-3.

de Briyne, N., Atkinson, J., Pokludova, L., Borriello, S.P. and Price, S. (2013) Factors influencing antibiotic prescribing habits and use of sensitivity testing amongst veterinarians in Europe. *Veterinary Record* 173, 475. DOI: 10.1136/vr.101454.

de Briyne, N., Atkinson, J., Pokludova, L. and Borriello, S.P. (2014) Antibiotics used most commonly to treat animals in Europe. *Veterinary Record* 175, 325. DOI: 10.1136/vr.102462.

Dickson, A., Smith, M., Smith, F., Park, J., King, C *et al.* (2019) Understanding the relationship between pet owners and their companion animals as a key context for antimicrobial resistance-related behaviours: an interpretative phenomenological analysis. *Health Psychology and Behavioral Medicine* 7(1), 45–61. DOI: 10.1080/21642850.2019.1577738.

Dutil, L., Irwin, R., Finley, R., Ng, L.K., Avery, B *et al.* (2010) Ceftiofur resistance in Salmonella enterica serovar Heidelberg from chicken meat and humans, Canada. *Emerging Infectious Diseases* 16(1), 48–54. DOI: 10.3201/eid1601.090729.

Duz, M., Marshall, J.F. and Parkin, T. (2017) Validation of an improved computer-assisted technique for mining free-text electronic medical records. *JMIR Medical Informatics* 5, e17.

EMA (2015) *Principles on Assignment of Defined Daily Dose for Animals (DDDvet) and Defined Course Dose for Animals (DCDvet)*. European Medicines Agency, Amsterdam, Netherlands. Available at: www.ema.europa.eu/docs/en_GB/document_library/Scientific_guideline/2015/06/WC500188890.pdf (accessed 30 October 2022).

EMA (2016) *Defined Daily Doses for Animals (DDDvet) and Defined Course Doses for Animals (DCDvet)*. European Medicines Agency, Amsterdam, Netherlands. Available at: www.ema.europa.eu/docs/en_GB/document_library/Other/2016/04/WC500205410.pdf (accessed 30 October 2022).

ENOVAT (2022) European Network for the Optimisation of Veterinary Antimicrobial Therapy (ENOVAT). Available at: https://enovat.eu/ (accessed 30 October 2022).

ESVAC (2021) *Sales of Veterinary Antimicrobial Agents in 31 European Countries in 2019 and 2020*. European Surveillance of Veterinary Antimicrobial Consumption, European Medicines Agency, Amsterdam, Netherland. Available at: www.ema.europa.eu/en/documents/report/

sales-veterinary-antimicrobial-agents-31-european-countries-2019-2020-trends-2010-2020-eleventh_en. pdf (accessed 30 October 2022).

European Commission (2022) *Commission Implementing Regulation (EU)*. European Commission, Brussels. Available at: https://members.wto.org/crnattachments/2022/SPS/EEC/22_2956_00_e.pdf (accessed 30 October 2022).

European Parliament (2021) *Motion for a Resolution*. European Parliament, Strasbourg, France. Available at: www.europarl.europa.eu/doceo/document/B-9-2021-0424_EN.pdf (accessed 30 October 2022).

FACE (2021) European Parliament rejects problematic motion on antimicrobials. European Federation for Hunting and Conservation (FACE), Brussels, Belgium. Available at: www.face.eu/2021/09/european-parliament-rejects-problematic-motion-on-antimicrobials/ (accessed 30 October 2022).

FDA (2021) *Summary Report On Antimicrobials Sold or Distributed for Use in Food-Producing Animals*. US Food and Drug Administration, Silver Spring, Maryland. Available at: www.fda.gov/media/154820/download (accessed 30 October 2022).

FECAVA (2013) *FECAVA Recommendations for Appropriate Antimicrobial Therapy*. Federation of European Companion Animal Veterinary Associations, Paris. Available at: www.fecava.org/wp-content/uploads/2020/01/FECAVA-Recommendations-for-Appropriate-Antimicrobial-ENGLISH-1.pdf (accessed 30 October 2022).

Fintelmann, R.E., Hoskins, E.N., Lietman, T.M., Keenan, J.D., Gaynor, B.D *et al*. (2011) Topical fluoroquinolone use as a risk factor for *in vitro* fluoroquinolone resistance in ocular cultures. *Archives of Ophthalmology* 129, 399–402.

Fishman, N. (2006) Antimicrobial stewardship. *American Journal of Infection Control* 34, S55–S63. DOI: 10.1016/j.ajic.2006.05.237.

Galarce, N., Arriagada, G., Sánchez, F., Venegas, V., Cornejo, J. *et al*. (2021) Antimicrobial use in companion animals: assessing veterinarians' prescription patterns through the first National Survey in Chile. *Animals* 11, 348.

Gaudreau, C. and Gilbert, H. (1997) Comparison of disc diffusion and agar dilution methods for antibiotic susceptibility testing of *Campylobacter jejuni* subsp. *jejuni* and *Campylobacter coli*. *Journal of Antimicrobial Chemotherapy* 39, 707–712.

Gerber, J.S., Prasad, P.A., Fiks, A.G., Localio, A.R., Grundmeier, R.W *et al*. (2013) Effect of an outpatient antimicrobial stewardship intervention on broad-spectrum antibiotic prescribing by primary care pediatricians: a randomized trial. *Journal of the American Medical Association* 309(22), 2345–2352. DOI: 10.1001/jama.2013.6287.

German, A.J., Halladay, L.J. and Noble, P.J. (2010) First-choice therapy for dogs presenting with diarrhoea in clinical practice. *Veterinary Record* 167, 810–814. DOI: 10.1136/vr.c4090.

Goggs, R., Menard, J.M., Altier, C., Cummings, K.J., Jacob, M.E *et al*. (2021) Patterns of antimicrobial drug use in veterinary primary care and specialty practice: a 6-year multi-institution study. *Journal of Veterinary Internal Medicine* 35(3), 1496–1508. DOI: 10.1111/jvim.16136.

Gómez-Poveda, B. and Moreno, M.A. (2018) Antimicrobial prescriptions for dogs in the capital of spain. *Frontiers in Veterinary Science* 5, 309. DOI: 10.3389/fvets.2018.00309.

Guardabassi, L., Loeber, M.E. and Jacobson, A. (2004) Transmission of multiple antimicrobial-resistant *staphylococcus intermedius* between dogs affected by deep pyoderma and their owners. *Veterinary Microbiology* 98, 23–27.

Hallsworth, M., Chadborn, T., Sallis, A., Sanders, M., Berry, D. *et al*. (2016) Provision of social norm feedback to high prescribers of antibiotics in general practice: a pragmatic national randomised controlled trial. *Lancet* 387, 1743–1752. DOI: 10.1016/S0140-6736(16)00215-4.

Hardefeldt, L., Hur, B., Verspoor, K., Baldwin, T., Bailey, K.E, *et al*. (2020) Use of cefovecin in dogs and cats attending first-opinion veterinary practices in Australia. *Veterinary Record* 187, e95–e95. DOI: 10.1136/vr.105997.

Hardefeldt, L.Y., Holloway, S., Trott, D.J., Shipstone, M., Barrs, V.R, *et al*. (2017) Antimicrobial prescribing in dogs and cats in Australia: results of the Australasian infectious disease advisory panel survey. *Journal of Veterinary Internal Medicine* 31, 1100–1107. DOI: 10.1111/jvim.14733.

Hardefeldt, L.Y., Selinger, J., Stevenson, M.A., Gilkerson, J.R., Crabb, H. *et al*. (2018) Population wide assessment of antimicrobial use in dogs and cats using a novel data source–a cohort study using pet insurance data. *Veterinary Microbiology* 225, 34–39.

Hardefeldt, L.Y., Hur, B., Richards, S., Scarborough, R., Browning, G.F. *et al*. (2022) Antimicrobial stewardship in companion animal practice: an implementation trial in 135 general practice veterinary clinics. *JAC Antimicrobial Resistance* 4, dlac015. DOI: 10.1093/jacamr/dlac015.

Harrison, E.M., Weinert, L.A., Holden, M.T., Welch, J.J., Wilson, K. *et al*. (2014) A shared population of epidemic methicillin-resistant *Staphylococcus aureus* 15 circulates in humans and companion animals. *MBio* 5, e00985–13. DOI: 10.1128/mBio.00985-13.

Hasson, F., Keeney, S. and McKenna, H. (2000) Research guidelines for the Delphi survey technique. *Journal of Advanced Nursing* 32, 1008–1015.

Hawker, J.I., Smith, S., Smith, G.E., Morbey, R., Johnson, A.P. *et al*. (2014) Trends in antibiotic prescribing in primary care for clinical syndromes subject to national recommendations to reduce antibiotic resistance,

UK 1995–2011: analysis of a large database of primary care consultations. *Journal of Antimicrobial Chemotherapy* 69, 3423–3430.

Hayrinen, K., Saranto, K. and Nykanen, P. (2008) Definition, structure, content, use and impacts of electronic health records: a review of the research literature. *International Journal of Medical Informatics* 77, 291–304. DOI: 10.1016/j.ijmedinf.2007.09.001.

Hesp, A., Veldman, K., van der Goot, J., Mevius, D. and van Schaik, G. (2019) Monitoring antimicrobial resistance trends in commensal *escherichia coli* from livestock, The Netherlands, 1998 to 2016. *Eurosurveillance* 24, 1800438.

Holso, K., Rantala, M., Lillas, A., Eerikäinen, S., Huovinen, P. *et al.* (2005) Prescribing antimicrobial agents for dogs and cats via university pharmacies in Finland – patterns and quality of information. *Acta Veterinaria Scandinavica* 46, 87–93.

Hopman, N.E.M., Hulscher, M.E.J.L., Graveland, H., Speksnijder, D.C., Wagenaar, J.A *et al.* (2018) Factors influencing antimicrobial prescribing by Dutch companion animal veterinarians: a qualitative study. *Preventive Veterinary Medicine* 158, 106–113.

Hopman, N.E.M., Wagenaar, J.A., van Geijlswijk, I.M. and Broens, E.M. (2021) Development and pilot of an interactive online course on antimicrobial stewardship in companion animals. *Antibiotics* 10, 610.

Hopman, N.E.M., Portengen, L., Heederik, D.J.J., Wagenaar, J.A., van Geijlswijk, I.M. *et al.* (2019a) Time trends, seasonal differences and determinants of systemic antimicrobial use in companion animal clinics (2012–2015). *Veterinary Microbiology* 235, 289–294.

Hopman, N.E.M., Portengen, L., Hulscher, M.E.J.L., Heederik, D.J.J., Verheij, T.J.M. *et al.* (2019b) Implementation and evaluation of an antimicrobial stewardship programme in companion animal clinics: a stepped-wedge design intervention study. *PLoS One* 14, e0225124.

Hopman, N.E.M., van Dijk, M.A.M., Broens, E.M., Wagenaar, J.A., Heederik, D.J.J. *et al.* (2019c) Quantifying antimicrobial use in Dutch companion animals. *Frontiers in Veterinary Science* 6, 158.

Hubbuch, A., Schmitt, K., Lehner, C., Hartnack, S., Schuller, S. *et al.* (2020) Antimicrobial prescriptions in cats in Switzerland before and after the introduction of an online antimicrobial stewardship tool. *BMC Veterinary Research* 16, 229. DOI: 10.1186/s12917-020-02447-8.

Huerta, B., Maldonado, A., Ginel, P.J., Tarradas, C., Gómez-Gascón, L. *et al.* (2011) Risk factors associated with the antimicrobial resistance of staphylococci in canine pyoderma. *Veterinary Microbiology* 150, 302–308. DOI: 10.1016/j.vetmic.2011.02.002.

Hughes, L.A., Williams, N., Clegg, P., Callaby, R., Nuttall, T. *et al.* (2012) Cross-sectional survey of antimicrobial prescribing patterns in UK small animal veterinary practice. *Preventive Veterinary Medicine* 104, 309–316. DOI: 10.1016/j.prevetmed.2011.12.003.

Hur, B., Hardefeldt, L.Y., Verspoor, K., Baldwin, T. and Gilkerson, J.R. (2019) Using natural language processing and VetCompass to understand antimicrobial usage patterns in Australia. *Australian Veterinary Journal* 97, 298–300.

Hur, B., Hardefeldt, L.Y., Verspoor, K.M., Baldwin, T. and Gilkerson, J.R. (2022) Evaluating the dose, indication and agreement with guidelines of antimicrobial use in companion animal practice with natural language processing. *JAC Antimicrobial Resistance* 4, dlab194.

Hur, B.A., Hardefeldt, L.Y., Verspoor, K.M., Baldwin, T. and Gilkerson, J.R. (2020) Describing the antimicrobial usage patterns of companion animal veterinary practices; free text analysis of more than 4.4 million consultation records. *PLoS One* 15(3), e0230049. DOI: 10.1371/journal.pone.0230049.

Idelevich, E.A., Sparbier, K., Kostrzewa, M. and Becker, K. (2018) Rapid detection of antibiotic resistance by MALDI-TOF mass spectrometry using a novel direct-on-target microdroplet growth assay. *Clinical Microbiology and Infection* 24, 738–743. DOI: 10.1016/j.cmi.2017.10.016.

Jessen, L.R., Sorensen, T.M., Lilja, Z.L., Kristensen, M., Hald, T. *et al.* (2017) Cross-sectional survey on the use and impact of the Danish national antibiotic use guidelines for companion animal practice. *Acta Veterinaria Scandinavica* 59, 81. DOI: 10.1186/s13028-017-0350-8.

Jones-Diette, J.S., Brennan, M.L., Cobb, M., Doit, H. and Dean, R.S. (2016) A method for extracting electronic patient record data from practice management software systems used in veterinary practice. *BMC Veterinary Research* 12, 239.

Jones-Diette, J., Robinson, N.J., Cobb, M., Brennan, M.L. and Dean, R.S. (2017) Accuracy of the electronic patient record in a first opinion veterinary practice. *Preventive Veterinary Medicine* 148, 121–126. DOI: 10.1016/j.prevetmed.2016.11.014.

Jones, P.H., Dawson, S., Gaskell, R.M., Coyne, K.P., Tierney, A. *et al.* (2014) Surveillance of diarrhoea in small animal practice through the Small Animal Veterinary Surveillance Network (SAVSNET). *Veterinary Journal* 201, 412–418. DOI: 10.1016/j.tvjl.2014.05.044.

Joosten, P., Ceccarelli, D., Odent, E., Sarrazin, S., Graveland, H. *et al.* (2020) Antimicrobial usage and resistance in companion animals: a cross-sectional study in three European Countries. *Antibiotics* 9, 87. DOI: 10.3390/antibiotics9020087.

Kahlmeter, G., Brown, D.F., Goldstein, F.W., MacGowan, A.P., Mouton, J.W. *et al.* (2003) European harmonization of MIC breakpoints for antimicrobial susceptibility testing of bacteria. *Journal of Antimicrobial Chemotherapy* 52, 145–148.

King, C., Smith, M., Currie, K., Dickson, A., Smith, F. *et al.* (2018) Exploring the behavioural drivers of veterinary surgeon antibiotic prescribing: a qualitative study of companion animal veterinary surgeons in the UK. *BMC Veterinary Research* 14, 332.

Koser, C.U., Ellington, M.J. and Peacock, S.J. (2014) Whole-genome sequencing to control antimicrobial resistance. *Trends in Genetics* 30, 401–407. DOI: 10.1016/j.tig.2014.07.003.

Lazar, H.L., Ketchedjian, A., Haime, M., Karlson, K. and Cabral, H. (2014) Topical vancomycin in combination with perioperative antibiotics and tight glycemic control helps to eliminate sternal wound infections. *Journal of Thoracic and Cardiovascular Surgery* 148, 1035–1040.

Leclercq, R., Canton, R., Brown, D.F., Giske, C.G., Heisig, P. *et al.* (2013) EUCAST expert rules in antimicrobial susceptibility testing. *Clinical Microbiology and Infection* 19, 141–160. DOI: 10.1111/j.1469-0691.2011.03703.x.

Lei, L., Wang, Y., Schwarz, S., Walsh, T.R., Ou, Y. *et al.* (2017) *mcr-1* in *Enterobacteriaceae*from *Companion Animals*, Beijing,China, 2012–2016. *Emerging Infectious Diseases* 23, 710–711.

Leite-Martins, L.R., Mahu, M.I., Costa, A.L., Mendes, A., Lopes, E. *et al.* (2014) Prevalence of antimicrobial resistance in enteric *Escherichia coli* from domestic pets and assessment of associated risk markers using a generalized linear mixed model. *Preventive Veterinary Medicine* 117, 28–39.

Lewis, P.J. and Tully, M.P. (2011) The discomfort caused by patient pressure on the prescribing decisions of hospital prescribers. *Research in Social and Administrative Pharmacy* 7, 4–15. DOI: 10.1016/j.sapharm.2010.02.002.

Little, P., Dorward, M., Warner, G., Stephens, K., Senior, J *et al.* (2004) Importance of patient pressure and perceived pressure and perceived medical need for investigations, referral, and prescribing in primary care: nested observational study. *British Medical Journal* 328, 444.

Liu, Y.Y., Wang, Y., Walsh, T.R., Yi, L.-X., Zhang, R. *et al.* (2016) Emergence of plasmid-mediated colistin resistance mechanism MCR-1 in animals and human beings in China: a microbiological and molecular biological study. *Lancet Infectious Diseases* 16, 161–168.

Loeffler, A. and Lloyd, D.H. (2010) Companion animals: a reservoir for methicillin-resistant *Staphylococcus aureus* in the community? *Epidemiology and Infection* 138, 595–605.

Loeffler, A., Pfeiffer, D.U., Lindsay, J.A., Magalhães, R.J.S. and Lloyd, D.H. (2011) Prevalence of and risk factors for MRSA carriage in companion animals: a survey of dogs, cats and horses. *Epidemiology and Infection* 139, 1019–1028. DOI: 10.1017/S095026881000227X.

Lutz, B., Lehner, C., Schmitt, K., Willi, B., Schüpbach, G. *et al.* (2020) Antimicrobial prescriptions and adherence to prudent use guidelines for selected canine diseases in Switzerland in 2016. *Veterinary Record Open* 7, e000370. DOI: 10.1136/vetreco-2019-000370.

MacPherson, E.E., Reynolds, J., Sanudi, E., Nkaombe, A., Phiri, C. *et al.* (2021) Understanding antimicrobial resistance through the lens of antibiotic vulnerabilities in primary health care in rural Malawi. *Global Public Health*. Available at: https://doi.org/10.1080/17441692.2021.2015615

Magalhães, R.J.S., Loeffler, A., Lindsay, J., Rich, M., Roberts, L, *et al.* (2010) Risk factors for methicillin-resistant *Staphylococcus aureus* (MRSA) infection in dogs and cats: a case–control study. *Veterinary Research* 41, 55.

Marques, C., Gama, L.T., Belas, A., Bergström, K., Beurlet, S. *et al.* (2016) European multicenter study on antimicrobial resistance in bacteria isolated from companion animal urinary tract infections. *BMC Veterinary Research* 12, 213. DOI: 10.1186/s12917-016-0840-3.

Martinez-Gonzalez, N.A., Coenen, S., Plate, A., Colliers, A., Rosemann, T *et al.* (2017) The impact of interventions to improve the quality of prescribing and use of antibiotics in primary care patients with respiratory tract infections: a systematic review protocol. *BMJ Open* 7, e016253. DOI: 10.1136/bmjopen-2017-016253.

Mateus, A., Brodbelt, D.C., Barber, N. and Stärk, K.D.C. (2011) Antimicrobial usage in dogs and cats in first opinion veterinary practices in the UK. *Journal of Small Animal Practice* 52, 515–521. DOI: 10.1111/j.1748-5827.2011.01098.x.

Mateus, A.L., Brodbelt, D.C., Barber, N. and Stärk, K.D.C. (2014) Qualitative study of factors associated with antimicrobial usage in seven small animal veterinary practices in the UK. *Preventive Veterinary Medicine* 117, 68–78. DOI: 10.1016/j.prevetmed.2014.05.007.

McCarthy, A.J., Harrison, E.M., Stanczak-Mrozek, K., Leggett, B., Waller, A, *et al.* (2015) Genomic insights into the rapid emergence and evolution of MDR in *Staphylococcus pseudintermedius*. *Journal of Antimicrobial Chemotherapy* 70, 997–1007. DOI: 10.1093/jac/dku496.

McGann, P., Bunin, J.L., Snesrud, E., Singh, S., Maybank, R. *et al.* (2016) Real time application of whole genome sequencing for outbreak investigation – what is an achievable turnaround time? *Diagnostic Microbiology and Infectious Disease* 85, 277–282. DOI: 10.1016/j.diagmicrobio.2016.04.020.

McGreevy, P., Thomson, P., Dhand, N.K., Raubenheimer, D., Masters, S. *et al.* (2017) VetCompass Australia: a national big data collection system for veterinary science. *Animals* 7, 74.

McKay, R., Mah, A., Law, M.R., McGrail, K. and Patrick, D.M. (2016) Systematic review of factors associated with antibiotic prescribing for respiratory tract infections. *Antimicrobial Agents and Chemotherapy* 60, 4106–4118. DOI: 10.1128/AAC.00209-16.

Moerer, M., Merle, R. and Bäumer, W. (2022) A cross-sectional study of veterinarians in Germany on the impact of the ÄHAV amendment 2018 on antimicrobial use and development of antimicrobial resistance in dogs and cats. *Antibiotics* 11, 484.

Morris, A.M., Brener, S., Dresser, L., Daneman, N., Dellit, T.H. *et al.* (2012) Use of a structured panel process to define quality metrics for antimicrobial stewardship programs. *Infection Control & Hospital Epidemiology* 33, 500–506.

Mortier, F., Strohmeyer, K., Hartmann, K. and Unterer, S. (2015) Acute haemorrhagic diarrhoea syndrome in dogs: 108 cases. *Veterinary Record* 176, 627. DOI: 10.1136/vr.103090.

Muellner, P., Muellner, U., Gates, M.C., Pearce, T., Ahlstrom, C. *et al.* (2016) Evidence in practice – a pilot study leveraging companion animal and equine health data from primary care veterinary clinics in New Zealand. *Frontiers in Veterinary Science* 3, 116. DOI: 10.3389/fvets.2016.00116.

Murphy, C.P., Reid-Smith, R.J., Boerlin, P., Weese, J.S., Prescott, J.F. *et al.* (2012) Out-patient antimicrobial drug use in dogs and cats for new disease events from community companion animal practices in Ontario. *Canadian Veterinary Journal* 53, 291–298.

Murray, C.J.L., Ikuta, K.S., Sharara, F., Swetschinski, L., Aguilar, G.R. *et al.* (2022) Global burden of bacterial antimicrobial resistance in 2019: a systematic analysis. *Lancet* 399, 629–655.

Murray, J.K., Gruffydd-Jones, T.J., Roberts, M.A. and Browne, W.J. (2015) Assessing changes in the UK pet cat and dog populations: numbers and household ownership. *Veterinary Record* 177, 259. DOI: 10.1136/vr.103223.

Nicodemo, A.C., Araujo, M.R., Ruiz, A.S. and Gales, A.C. (2004) *In vitro* susceptibility of *Stenotrophomonas maltophilia* isolates: comparison of disc diffusion, Etest and agar dilution methods. *Journal of Antimicrobial Chemotherapy* 53, 604–608.

Noble, P.J.M., Appleton, C., Radford, A.D. and Nenadic, G. (2021) Using topic modelling for unsupervised annotation of electronic health records to identify an outbreak of disease in UK dogs. *PLoS One* 16, e0260402.

Odoi, A., Samuels, R., Carter, C.N. and Smith, J. (2021) Antibiotic prescription practices and opinions regarding antimicrobial resistance among veterinarians in Kentucky, USA. *PLoS One* 16, e0249653. DOI: 10.1371/journal.pone.0249653.

Olaitan, A.O., Dandachi, I., Baron, S.A., Daoud, Z., Morand, S. *et al.* (2021) Banning colistin in feed additives: a small step in the right direction. *Lancet Infectious Diseases* 21, 29–30. DOI: 10.1016/S1473-3099(20)30915-4.

O'Neill, D.G., Church, D.B., McGreevy, P.D., Thomson, P.C. and Brodbelt, D.C. (2014c) Prevalence of disorders recorded in cats attending primary-care veterinary practices in england. *Veterinary Journal* 202, 286–291.

O'Neill, J. (2016) *Tackling Drug-Resistant Infections Globally: Final Report and Recommendations*. Review on Antimicrobial Resistance. Available at: http://amr-review.org/ (accessed 30 October 2022).

O'Neill, D.G., Church, D.B., McGreevy, P.D., Thomson, P.C. and Brodbelt, D.C. (2014a) Approaches to canine health surveillance. *Canine Genetics and Epidemiology* 1, 2. DOI: 10.1186/2052-6687-1-2.

O'Neill, D., Church, D.B., McGreevy, P.D., Thomson, P.C. and Brodbelt, D.C. (2014b) Prevalence of disorders recorded in dogs attending primary-care veterinary practices in England. *PLoS One* 9, e90501.

Page, N., Baysari, M.T. and Westbrook, J.I. (2017) A systematic review of the effectiveness of interruptive medication prescribing alerts in hospital CPOE systems to change prescriber behavior and improve patient safety. *International Journal of Medical Informatics* 105, 22–30. DOI: 10.1016/j.ijmedinf.2017.05.011.

Pankey, G.A. and Sabath, L.D. (2004) Clinical relevance of bacteriostatic versus bactericidal mechanisms of action in the treatment of Gram-positive bacterial infections. *Clinical Infectious Diseases* 38, 864–870.

PHE (2021) *English Surveillance Programme for Antimicrobial Utilisation and Resistance (ESPAUR)*. Public Health England, London. Available at: https://assets.publishing.service.gov.uk/government/uploads/system/uploads/attachment_data/file/1069632/espaur-report-2020-to-2021-16-Nov-FINAL-v2.pdf (accessed 30 October 2022).

Pires Dos Santos, T., Damborg, P., Moodley, A. and Guardabassi, L. (2016) Systematic review on global epidemiology of methicillin-resistant *Staphylococcus pseudintermedius*: inference of population structure from multilocus sequence typing data. *Frontiers in Microbiology* 7, 1599.

Pleydell, E.J., Souphavanh, K., Hill, K.E., French, N.P. and Prattley, D.J. (2012) Descriptive epidemiological study of the use of antimicrobial drugs by companion animal veterinarians in New Zealand. *New Zealand Veterinary Journal* 60, 115–122. DOI: 10.1080/00480169.2011.643733.

Prescott, J.F., Hanna, W.J., Reid-Smith, R. and Drost, K. (2002) Antimicrobial drug use and resistance in dogs. *Canadian Veterinary Journal* 43, 107–116.

Radford, A., Singleton, D., Jones, P, *et al.* (2017) Prescribing antibiotics in small animals practices. *Veterinary Record* 181, 71.

Radford, A.D., Noble, P.J., Coyne, K.P., Gaskell, R.M., Jones, P.H. *et al.* (2011) Antibacterial prescribing patterns in small animal veterinary practice identified via SAVSNET: the small animal veterinary surveillance network. *Veterinary Record* 169, 310.

Radford, A.D., Singleton, D.A., Jewell, C., Appleton, C., Rowlingson, B. *et al*. (2021) Outbreak of severe vomiting in dogs associated with a canine enteric coronavirus, United Kingdom. *Emerging Infectious Diseases* 27, 517–528. DOI: 10.3201/eid2702.202452.

Raghavan, M., Glickman, N., Moore, G., Caldanaro, R., Lewis, H. *et al*. (2007) Prevalence of and risk factors for canine tick infestation in the United States, 2002–2004. *Vector-Borne and Zoonotic Diseases* 7, 65–75. DOI: 10.1089/vbz.2006.0570.

Raman, S.R., Curtis, L.H., Temple, R., Andersson, T., Ezekowitz, J. *et al*. (2018) Leveraging electronic health records for clinical research. *American Heart Journal* 202, 13–19. DOI: 10.1016/j.ahj.2018.04.015.

Rantala, M., Hölsö, K., Lillas, A., Huovinen, P. and Kaartinen, L. (2004a) Survey of condition-based prescribing of antimicrobial drugs for dogs at a veterinary teaching hospital. *Veterinary Record* 155, 259–262. DOI: 10.1136/vr.155.9.259.

Rantala, M., Lahti, E., Kuhalampil, J., Pesonen, S., Järvinen, A.K. *et al*. (2004b) Antimicrobial resistance in *Staphylococcus* spp., *Escherichia coli* and *Enterococcus* spp. in dogs given antibiotics for chronic dermatological disorders, compared with nontreated control dogs. *Acta Veterinaria Scandinavica* 45, 37–45.

Ribeiro, S., Mourão, J., Novais, A., Campos, J., Peixe, L. *et al*. (2021) From farm to fork: colistin voluntary withdrawal in Portuguese farms reflected in decreasing occurrence of *mcr-1*-carrying *Enterobacteriaceae* from chicken meat. *Environmental Microbiology* 23, 7563–7577.

Rimbault, M., Beale, H.C., Schoenebeck, J.J., Hoopes, B.C., Allen, J.J. *et al*. (2013) Derived variants at six genes explain nearly half of size reduction in dog breeds. *Genome Research* 23, 1985–1995. DOI: 10.1101/gr.157339.113.

Robinson, D. and Hooker, H. (2006) The UK veterinary profession in 2006: the findings of a survey of the profession conducted by the Royal College of Veterinary Surgeons. Royal College of Veterinary Surgeons, London. Available at: www.rcvs.org.uk/news-and-views/publications/rcvs-survey-of-the-professions-2006/ (accessed 30 October 2022).

Robinson, N.J., Brennan, M.L., Cobb, M. and Dean, R.S. (2015) Capturing the complexity of first opinion small animal consultations using direct observation. *Veterinary Record* 176, 48.

Robinson, N.J., Brennan, M.L., Cobb, M. and Dean, R.S. (2017) Common decisions made and actions taken during small-animal consultations at eight first-opinion practices in the United Kingdom. *Preventive Veterinary Medicine* 139, 1–9. DOI: 10.1016/j.prevetmed.2016.12.002.

Roca, I., Akova, M., Baquero, F., Carlet, J., Cavaleri, M. *et al*. (2015) The global threat of antimicrobial resistance: science for intervention. *New Microbes and New Infections* 6, 22–29. DOI: 10.1016/j.nmni.2015.02.007.

Rossen, J.W.A., Friedrich, A.W., Moran-Gilad, J. and ESCMID Study Group for Genomic and Molecular Diagnostics (ESCMID) (2018) Practical issues in implementing whole-genome-sequencing in routine diagnostic microbiology. *Clinical Microbiology and Infection* 24, 355–360.

Rumbold, J.M. and Pierscionek, B. (2017) The effect of the general data protection regulation on medical research. *Journal of Medical Internet Research* 19, e47. DOI: 10.2196/jmir.7108.

Sánchez-Vizcaíno, F., Jones, P.H., Menacere, T., Heayns, B., Wardeh, M. *et al*. (2015) Small animal disease surveillance. *Veterinary Record* 177, 591–594. DOI: 10.1136/vr.h6174.

Sánchez-Vizcaíno, F., Singleton, D., Jones, P.H.H., Heayns, B., Wardeh, M. *et al*. (2016) Small animal disease surveillance: pruritus, and coagulase-positive staphylococci. *Veterinary Record* 179, 352–355.

Sánchez-Vizcaíno, F., Noble, P.M., Jones, P.H., Menacere, T., Buchan, I. *et al*. (2017) Demographics of dogs, cats, and rabbits attending veterinary practices in great britain as recorded in their electronic health records. *BMC Veterinary Research* 13, 218. DOI: 10.1186/s12917-017-1138-9.

Schmidt, V.M., Pinchbeck, G.L., Nuttall, T., McEwan, N., Dawson, S. *et al*. (2015) Antimicrobial resistance risk factors and characterisation of faecal *E. coli* isolated from healthy Labrador retrievers in the United Kingdom. *Preventive Veterinary Medicine* 119, 31–40.

Schmidt, V.M., Pinchbeck, G., McIntyre, K.M., Nuttall, T., McEwan, N *et al*. (2018a) Routine antibiotic therapy in dogs increases the detection of antimicrobial-resistant faecal *Escherichia coli*. *Journal of Antimicrobial Chemotherapy* 73, 3305–3316.

Schmidt, V.M., Pinchbeck, G., Nuttall, T., Shaw, S., McIntyre, K.M. *et al*. (2018b) Impact of systemic antimicrobial therapy on mucosal staphylococci in a population of dogs in Northwest England. *Veterinary Dermatology* 29, 192–e70. DOI: 10.1111/vde.12538.

Schmitt, K., Lehner, C., Schuller, S., Schüpbach-Regula, G., Mevissen, M. *et al*. (2019) Antimicrobial use for selected diseases in cats in Switzerland. *BMC Veterinary Research* 15, 94. DOI: 10.1186/s12917-019-1821-0.

Scott, A., Pottenger, S., Timofte, D., Moore, M., Wright, L. *et al*. (2019) Reservoirs of resistance: polymyxin resistance in veterinary-associated companion animal isolates of *Pseudomonas aeruginosa*. *Veterinary Record* 185, 206. DOI: 10.1136/vr.105075.

Singleton, D.A., Noble, P.J., Radford, A.D., Brant, B., Pinchbeck, G.L. *et al*. (2020a) Prolific vomiting in dogs. *Veterinary Record* 186, 191.

Singleton, D.A., Pinchbeck, G.L., Radford, A.D., Arsevska, E., Dawson, S. *et al*. (2020b) Factors associated with prescription of antimicrobial drugs for dogs and cats, United Kingdom, 2014–2016. *Emerging Infectious Diseases* 26(8), 1778–1791. DOI: 10.3201/eid2608.191786.

Singleton, D.A., Arsevska, E., Smyth, S., Barker, E.N., Jewell, C. *et al.* (2019a) Small animal disease surveillance: gastrointestinal disease, antibacterial prescription and *Tritrichomonas* foetus. *Veterinary Record* 184, 211–216.

Singleton, D.A., McGarry, J., Torres, J.R., Killick, D., Jewell, C. *et al.* (2019b) Small animal disease surveillance 2019: pruritus, pharmacosurveillance, skin tumours and flea infestations. *Veterinary Record* 185, 470–475. DOI: 10.1136/vr.l6074.

Singleton, D.A., Noble, P.J.M., Sánchez-Vizcaíno, F., Dawson, S., Pinchbeck, G.L. *et al.* (2019c) Pharmaceutical prescription in canine acute diarrhoea: a longitudinal electronic health record analysis of first opinion veterinary practices. *Frontiers in Veterinary Science* 6, 218. DOI: 10.3389/fvets.2019.00218.

Singleton, D.A., Stavisky, J., Jewell, C., Smyth, S., Brant, B. *et al.* (2019d) Small animal disease surveillance 2019: respiratory disease, antibiotic prescription and canine infectious respiratory disease complex. *Veterinary Record* 184, 640–645.

Singleton, D.A., Sánchez-Vizcaíno, F., Dawson, S., Jones, P.H., Noble, P.J.M. *et al.* (2017) Patterns of antimicrobial agent prescription in a sentinel population of canine and feline veterinary practices in the United Kingdom. *Veterinary Journal* 224, 18–24. DOI: 10.1016/j.tvjl.2017.03.010.

Singleton, D.A., Pongchaikul, P., Smith, S., Bengtsson, R.J., Baker, K. *et al.* (2021a) Temporal, spatial, and genomic analyses of *Enterobacteriaceae* clinical antimicrobial resistance in companion animals reveals phenotypes and genotypes of one health concern. *Frontiers in Microbiology* 12, 2160. DOI: 10.3389/fmicb.2021.700698.

Singleton, D.A., Rayner, A., Brant, B., Smyth, S., Noble, P.M. *et al.* (2021b) A randomised controlled trial to reduce highest priority critically important antimicrobial prescription in companion animals. *Nature Communications* 12, 1593.

Smith, M., King, C., Davis, M., Dickson, A., Park, J. *et al.* (2018) Pet owner and vet interactions: exploring the drivers of AMR. *Antimicrobial Resistance & Infection Control* 7, 46.

StopAMR (2021) Do veterinarians lobby against restrictions on use of critically important antibiotics for human use only? stopAMR blog, 9 September. Available at: www.stopamr.eu/blog/policy/do-veterinarians-lobby-against-restrictions-on-use-of-critically-important-antibiotics-for-human-use-only (accessed 30 October 2022).

Summers, J.F., Hendricks, A. and Brodbelt, D.C. (2014) Prescribing practices of primary-care veterinary practitioners in dogs diagnosed with bacterial pyoderma.
BMC Veterinary Research 10, 240. DOI: 10.1186/s12917-014-0240-5.

Tacconelli, E., Carrara, E., Savoldi, A., Harbarth, S., Mendelson, M. *et al.* (2018) Discovery, research, and development of new antibiotics: the WHO priority list of antibiotic-resistant bacteria and tuberculosis. *Lancet Infectious Diseases* 18, 318–327. DOI: 10.1016/S1473-3099(17)30753-3.

Talpaert, M.J., Gopal Rao, G., Cooper, B.S. and Wade, P. (2011) Impact of guidelines and enhanced antibiotic stewardship on reducing broad-spectrum antibiotic usage and its effect on incidence of *clostridium difficile* infection. *Journal of Antimicrobial Chemotherapy* 66, 2168–2174. DOI: 10.1093/jac/dkr253.

Taylor, D.D., Martin, J.N. and Scallan Walter, E.J. (2022) Survey of companion animal veterinarians antimicrobial drug prescription practices and awareness of antimicrobial drug use guidelines in the United States. *Zoonoses Public Health* 69, 277–285.

Teixeira Rodrigues, A., Roque, F., Falcão, A., Figueiras, A. and Herdeiro, M.T. (2013) Understanding physician antibiotic prescribing behaviour: a systematic review of qualitative studies. *International Journal of Antimicrobial Agents* 41, 203–212. DOI: 10.1016/j.ijantimicag.2012.09.003.

Thursky, K.A., Buising, K.L., Bak, N., Macgregor, L., Street, A.C. *et al.* (2006) Reduction of broad-spectrum antibiotic use with computerized decision support in an intensive care unit. *International Journal for Quality in Health Care* 18(3), 224–231. DOI: 10.1093/intqhc/mzi095.

Tiseo, K., Huber, L., Gilbert, M., Robinson, T.P. and van Boeckel, T.P. (2020) Global trends in antimicrobial use in food animals from 2017 to 2030. *Antibiotics* 9, 918. DOI: 10.3390/antibiotics9120918.

Tompson, A.C., Chandler, C.I.R., Mateus, A.L.P., O'Neill, D.G., Chang, Y.M. *et al.* (2020) What drives antimicrobial prescribing for companion animals? A mixed-methods study of UK veterinary clinics. *Preventive Veterinary Medicine* 183, 105117. DOI: 10.1016/j.prevetmed.2020.105117.

Toutain, P.-L., Bousquet-Mélou, A., Damborg, P., Ferran, A.A., Mevius, D. *et al.* (2017) En route towards European clinical breakpoints for veterinary antimicrobial susceptibility testing: a position paper explaining the VetCAST approach. *Frontiers in Microbiology* 8, 2344. DOI: 10.3389/fmicb.2017.02344.

Trott, D.J., Filippich, L.J., Bensink, J.C., Downs, M.T., McKenzie, S.E. *et al.* (2004) Canine model for investigating the impact of oral enrofloxacin on commensal coliforms and colonization with multidrug-resistant *Escherichia coli*. *Journal of Medical Microbiology* 53(Pt 5), 439–443. DOI: 10.1099/jmm.0.05473-0.

Van Boeckel, T.P., Pires, J., Silvester, R., Zhao, C., Song, J. *et al.* (2019) Global trends in antimicrobial resistance in animals in low- and middle-income countries.

Science 365(6459), eaaw1944. DOI: 10.1126/science.aaw1944.

van Cleven, A., Sarrazin, S., de Rooster, H., Paepe, D., van der Meeren, S. *et al.* (2018) Antimicrobial prescribing behaviour in dogs and cats by Belgian veterinarians. *Veterinary Record* 182, 324. DOI: 10.1136/vr.104316.

Ventrella, G., Moodley, A., Grandolfo, E., Parisi, A., Corrente, M, *et al.* (2017) Frequency, antimicrobial susceptibility and clonal distribution of methicillin-resistant staphylococcus pseudintermedius in canine clinical samples submitted to a veterinary diagnostic laboratory in italy: a 3-year retrospective investigation. *Veterinary Microbiology* 211, 103–106. DOI: 10.1016/j.vetmic.2017.09.015.

VMD (2013) *Availability of Animal Medicines*. Veterinary Medicines Directorate, London. Available at: www.gov.uk/government/publications/availability-of-animal-medicines (accessed 30 October 2022).

VMD (2015) Combined report on antimicrobial resistance in people and animals. *Veterinary Record* 177, 111–112.

VMD (2020) *UK Veterinary Antibiotic Resistance and Sales Surveillance Report*. Veterinary Medicines Directorate, London. Available at: https://assets.publishing.service.gov.uk/government/uploads/system/uploads/attachment_data/file/950126/UK-VARSS_2019_Report__2020-TPaccessible.pdf (accessed 30 October 2022).

VMD (2021) *UK Veterinary Antibiotic Resistance and Sales Surveillance Report*. Veterinary Medicines Directorate, London. Available at: https://assets.publishing.service.gov.uk/government/uploads/system/uploads/attachment_data/file/1072796/03.05.22_VARSS_Main_Report__Final_Accessible_version__3_.pdf (accessed 30 October 2022).

Walker, B., Sánchez-Vizcaíno, F. and Barker, E.N. (2022) Effect of an antimicrobial stewardship intervention on the prescribing behaviours of companion animal veterinarians: a pre-post study. *Veterinary Record* 190, e1485.

Wayne, A., McCarthy, R. and Lindenmayer, J. (2011) Therapeutic antibiotic use patterns in dogs: observations from a veterinary teaching hospital. *Journal of Small Animal Practice* 52, 310–318. DOI: 10.1111/j.1748-5827.2011.01072.x.

Wedley, A.L., Maddox, T.W., Westgarth, C., Coyne, K.P., Pinchbeck, G.L. *et al.* (2011) Prevalence of antimicrobial-resistant *Escherichia coli* in dogs in a cross-sectional, community-based study. *Veterinary Record* 168, 354. DOI: 10.1136/vr.d1540.

Wedley, A.L., Dawson, S., Maddox, T.W., Coyne, K.P., Pinchbeck, G.L. *et al.* (2017) Carriage of antimicrobial resistant *Escherichia coli* in dogs: Prevalence, associated risk factors and molecular characteristics. *Veterinary Microbiology* 199, 23–30. DOI: 10.1016/j.vetmic.2016.11.017.

WHO (2015) *Global Action Plan on Antimicrobial Resistance*. World Health Organization, Geneva, Switzerland. Available at: http://apps.who.int/iris/bitstream/handle/10665/193736/9789241509763_eng.pdf?sequence=1 (accessed 30 October 2022).

WHO (2019) *Critically Important Antimicrobials for Human Medicine*. 6th revision. World Health Organization, Geneva, Switzerland. Available at: www.who.int/publications/i/item/9789241515528 (accessed 30 October 2022).

Zhang, P.L.C., Shen, X., Chalmers, G., Reid-Smith, R.J., Slavic, D. *et al.* (2018) Prevalence and mechanisms of extended-spectrum cephalosporin resistance in clinical and fecal *Enterobacteriaceae* isolates from dogs in Ontario, Canada. *Veterinary Microbiology* 213, 82–88.

Zhang, X.-F., Doi, Y., Huang, X., Li, H.-Y., Zhong, L.-L, *et al.* (2016) Possible transmission of mcr-1-harboring *Escherichia coli* between companion animals and humans. *Emerging Infectious Diseases* 22(9), 1679–1681. DOI: 10.3201/eid2209.160464.

Zogg, A.L., Zurfluh, K., Schmitt, S., Nüesch-Inderbinen, M. and Stephan, R. (2018) Antimicrobial resistance, multilocus sequence types and virulence profiles of ESBL producing and non-ESBL producing uropathogenic *Escherichia coli* isolated from cats and dogs in Switzerland. *Veterinary Microbiology* 216, 79–84.

19 Antibiotic Use in Surgical Patients

FAYE SWINBOURNE*

Lumbry Park Veterinary Specialists, Selborne Road, Alton, Hampshire, UK

19.1 Introduction

Antibiotics may be used in the surgical patient with either prophylactic or therapeutic intent. Prophylactic use of an antibiotic refers to its administration in the absence of infection with the aim of reducing the risk of subsequent infection. In surgical patients, this typically relates to the use of antibiotics before the start of surgery to reduce the bacterial burden at the surgical site and consequently decrease the risk of infection developing in the post-operative period. Therapeutic antibiotic use refers to the treatment of an established bacterial infection. Understanding whether antibiotic use in an individual is under the guise of prevention or treatment of infection is essential because this will influence decision making in relation to key components of the antibiotic regimen. While the use of antibiotic agents in surgical patients can reduce post-operative infection risk and improve treatment outcomes for individuals undergoing surgery, there are potential adverse effects of antibiotic use that can have implications for the individual patient and wider population. Consequently, the judicious use of antibiotics in surgical patients is key to balancing effective treatment with good antimicrobial stewardship.

This chapter will review the prophylactic and therapeutic use of antibiotics in surgical patients, including indications for use, appropriate agent selection and considerations for the dosing regimen. There will be an emphasis on the overall goals of maximizing the efficacy of antibiotic use, reducing unnecessary antibiotic use and minimizing the potential for adverse effects, with development of bacterial resistance a key concern. The potential consequences of inappropriate antibiotic use and suggestions to optimize stewardship in surgical patients are included. Infection prevention and control of the surgical patient is multi-faceted, and readers are directed to specific chapters in Sections 2 and 3 of this volume for further information relating to the concepts discussed in this chapter.

19.2 Prophylactic Antibiotic Use in Surgical Patients

19.2.1 Bacterial contamination of the surgical site and infection risk

All surgical patients will be exposed to bacterial contamination of the surgical site. The magnitude of bacterial contamination and nature of the contaminants will depend on numerous factors, including the location and type of surgical procedure, measures taken during preparation of the patient to reduce the bacterial burden of the skin microbiome, intraoperative steps to minimize contamination and host factors such as the systemic health of the patient. Potential sources of bacterial contamination of a surgical site can be broadly categorized as those originating from the patient's own resident microbial flora (endogenous) and those present in the external environment (exogenous). Native microbial populations residing on the patient's skin and mucous membranes, and those within internal body systems such as the gastrointestinal, urogenital and respiratory tracts, have the potential to contaminate otherwise sterile, unpopulated locations within the body when the integrity of these structures is breached by a surgical incision. While endogenous bacteria do not cause disease at their native site in healthy individuals, they are considered opportunistic pathogens, having the potential to exert a pathogenic effect and cause infection either when introduced to a non-native site, if the normal resident microbial equilibrium is disrupted, or if host defences are impaired. Environmental

*faye.swinbourne@cvsvets.com

contaminants may originate from the hospital environment (including contact with contaminated equipment or hospital personnel) or they may colonize the patient prior to admission (having been acquired from the patient's home environment or the wider community). Currently, the most prevalent pathogen associated with the development of infection following surgical intervention in dogs and cats is *Staphylococcus pseudintermedius* (Vasseur *et al.*, 1988; Weese *et al.*, 2012; Nazarali *et al.*, 2014; Turk *et al.*, 2015; Windahl *et al.*, 2015). Opportunistic staphylococci such as *S. pseudintermedius* originate from the patient's skin microbiome. When a surgical procedure involves entry into a body cavity that houses a commensal population, other pathogens are likely to be implicated in the development of infection post-operatively. For example, Gram-negative bacilli such as *Escherichia coli* are most commonly isolated from infections of the surgical site following gastrointestinal procedures in dogs and cats (Williams *et al.*, 2020).

Once a critical level of contamination of the surgical site occurs, there is the potential for infection to result, and the threshold for this in an individual patient or surgical site will be dependent on several factors. To an extent, the innate host defences will serve to address bacterial contamination, but this relies on an immunocompetent host and may be influenced by local tissue health at the surgical site as well as bacterial load and virulence. When the host defences are overwhelmed, multiplication of bacterial contaminants can proceed unchecked, providing an opportunity for infection to become established. Development of a post-operative surgical-site infection (SSI) can have significant implications for the patient in terms of associated morbidity and a need for ongoing treatment. Management of SSIs also carries a financial burden for the client, which can vastly exceed that of the primary surgical intervention in some instances (Nicoll *et al.*, 2014; Espinel-Rupérez *et al.*, 2019).

It is logical that the degree of bacterial contamination at a surgical site correlates positively with the risk of infection development; however, a linear association cannot be assumed, because specific patient, procedure and environmental factors can influence contamination and subsequent progression to infection (Vasseur *et al.*, 1988). Occurrence of SSIs in dogs and cats undergoing surgery varies widely: reported SSI rates range from 2% to 5% for clean procedures and up to 20% for dirty procedures (Vasseur *et al.*, 1988; Brown *et al.*, 1997;

Nicholson *et al.*, 2002; Eugster *et al.*, 2004; Turk *et al.*, 2015; Garcia Stickney and Thieman Mankin, 2018). It is common for the veterinary literature to report varied rates of SSIs for a given procedure (see Chapter 10, this volume, for more details), and this is the result of differing peri-operative protocols, patient factors and SSI detection methods among studies, with prospective studies employing active surveillance measures more likely to detect SSIs (Turk *et al.*, 2015; Garcia Stickney and Thieman Mankin, 2018). Numerous proposed risk factors for SSIs are reported in the literature, and studies reporting significant factors in dogs and cats are often conflicting. Duration of surgery has consistently been recognized as a risk factor for SSIs in dogs and cats, with infection risk doubling for procedures taking 90 minutes to complete rather than 60 minutes, or with every 70 minutes of surgical time (Brown *et al.*, 1997; Eugster *et al.*, 2004). Other reported risk factors for SSIs include duration of anaesthesia independent of surgery time, clipping of hair before induction of anaesthesia, wound classification, surgeon experience, use of a surgical implant, intraoperative hypotension and patient factors including age, sex, American Society of Anaesthesiologists (ASA) score and concurrent endocrinopathy (Vasseur *et al.*, 1988; Brown *et al.*, 1997; Beal *et al.*, 2000; Nicholson *et al.*, 2002; Eugster *et al.*, 2004; Turk *et al.*, 2015; Thieman Mankin and Cohen, 2020). Additional factors that are believed to negatively impact host immune function and contribute to SSI risk in human surgical patients, such as peri-operative hypothermia and hyperglycaemia, have also been investigated in veterinary patients, but clear associations are yet to be determined (Beal *et al.*, 2000; Espinel-Rupérez *et al.*, 2019).

Pre-operative preparation of the patient including skin antisepsis to reduce the bacterial burden of the cutaneous microbiome, intraoperative techniques to minimize contamination of the surgical site and adherence to a strict aseptic technique are principal strategies for reduction of SSIs. Even with a robust approach to these infection control measures, it is unrealistic to attempt to eliminate all bacterial contaminants from a surgical site and the aim should be to significantly reduce bacterial numbers rather than to create a sterile environment. The prophylactic use of antibiotics in surgical patients is an additional measure that can be implemented to reduce bacterial contamination of the surgical site and consequently infection risk. Antibiotic use for

Box 19.1. Principles of surgical antimicrobial prophylaxis.

- Avoid the use of antibiotics for clean surgical procedures unless there is a specific indication (e.g. procedure lasts more than 90 minutes, use of an implant, patient comorbidities).
- Considerations for antibiotic agent selection should include:
  - activity against the bacterial species most likely to contaminate the surgical site;
  - minimal activity against non-target bacterial species to limit impact on selection pressure for emergence of antimicrobial resistance; and
  - low risk of adverse reaction or toxicity to the patient.

- Administer the first dose of antibiotic within 60 minutes before the first incision in order to achieve effective concentrations of antibiotic at the surgical site before bacterial contamination occurs.
- Redosing of antibiotics should be performed if the duration of the procedure extends beyond two half-lives of the agent administered to ensure effective concentrations of antibiotic at the surgical site for the duration of the procedure.
- Do not administer antibiotics beyond closure of the surgical incision unless there is a specific indication to do so (e.g. a major break in aseptic technique intraoperatively).

---

this indication should be viewed as an adjunct to the principal strategies of infection control and never as a substitute for meticulous preparation of the patient or adherence to a strict aseptic technique.

19.2.2 Principles of surgical antimicrobial prophylaxis

The use of prophylactic antibiotics in designated surgical patients is practised in both human and veterinary medicine with the aim of reducing the bacterial burden at the surgical site and consequently the risk of SSIs (Bratzler *et al.*, 2013; BSAVA/SAMSoc, 2018). The principles of surgical antimicrobial prophylaxis are summarized in Box 19.1.

Experimental studies in the late 1950s and early 1960s demonstrated that systemic antibiotic administration suppressed the development of infection in dermal lesions inoculated with staphylococci, with maximal suppression of infection noted when antibiotic was given before the bacteria were introduced (Miles, 1956; Miles *et al.*, 1957; Burke, 1961). The same studies showed that systemic antibiotic administration had no effect on the suppression of infection when inoculated bacteria had been present in the tissue for over 3 hours before the antibiotic was first administered. These findings support the use of antibiotic prophylaxis to reduce the development of infection and highlight the importance of effective antibiotic tissue concentrations before contamination occurs. Such principles form the basis of surgical antimicrobial prophylaxis

and are supported in the clinical setting: large, prospective trials in human surgical patients confirm that antibiotic administration pre-operatively is optimal in reducing the incidence of wound infection and delaying the administration of antibiotic until the post-operative period has minimal to no effect on infection prevention (Stone *et al.*, 1976; Classen *et al.*, 1992). Comparable veterinary studies investigating the timing of prophylactic antibiotic administration on SSI rates in dogs and cats are lacking; however, it is reasonable to assume that the importance of timely initiation of antibiotics in relation to the start of surgery is transferable.

While it is widely accepted that surgical antimicrobial prophylaxis reduces infection risk and that antibiotic initiation must be commenced before the start of the surgical procedure, the indications for prophylaxis in each patient undergoing a specific surgical procedure are less clear. There is a need to balance the interests of the individual patient against the potential adverse effects of antibiotic use for the individual and the wider population. Any form of antibiotic use can contribute to selection for resistant bacteria. The overall goal should be to optimize the peri-operative management of surgical patients while avoiding unnecessary antibiotic use. This approach will preserve the efficacy of available antibiotic agents and minimize the development of resistance. The prophylactic use of antibiotics in surgical patients is valid when there is either an elevated risk of infection or when the consequences of infection could be severe for the patient (Bratzler *et al.*, 2013). An example of the latter is

Table 19.1. Wound classification system (adapted from National Research Council, 1964), anticipated level of bacterial contamination and intent of antibiotic use for each classification.

Wound classification	Level of bacterial contamination anticipated at surgical site	Examples of surgical procedures	Intent of antibiotic use
Clean	Minimal; generally considered to be adequately controlled by a combination of appropriate patient preparation, aseptic technique and innate host defence mechanisms	Castration, simple skin mass excision, splenectomy, elective orthopaedic procedure	Not indicated (unless predefined factors present, e.g. procedure >90 minutes, use of a surgical implant, infection would have catastrophic consequences for the patient)
Clean-contaminated	Minimal–moderate; the result of controlled entry into a hollow viscus or a minor break in aseptic technique	Gastrotomy, enterotomy, enterectomy (without gross spillage of luminal content)	Prophylactic (no indication for continued antimicrobial prophylaxis administration post-operatively)
Contaminated	Moderate–marked; the result of significant contamination from spillage of the content of a hollow viscus or a major break in aseptic technique. Also acute, traumatic wounds with non-purulent inflammation present	Gross spillage of intestinal content at enterotomy, infected urine at cystotomy	Prophylactic (antimicrobial prophylaxis administration may be continued for 24–48 hours post-operatively depending on the magnitude and nature of the contamination)
Dirty	Marked; the result of the presence of a perforated hollow viscus pre-operatively, abscessation with necrotic tissue and/or pus or faecal contamination. Also traumatic wounds with purulent inflammation present	Septic peritonitis, pyothorax	Therapeutic (antibiotic is administered peri-operatively and continued post-operatively to treat established infection)

joint prosthesis, where an SSI is likely to result in significant clinical implications, the requirement for a protracted antibiotic course(s) and substantial patient morbidity. The use of a wound classification system to categorize surgical wounds in terms of anticipated degree of bacterial contamination, and therefore infection risk, can serve as a guide to determine whether antimicrobial prophylaxis may be indicated in a given patient.

19.2.3 Wound classification to guide antibiotic use in surgical patients

The premise that the degree of bacterial contamination at a surgical site is likely to correlate with infection risk can be used to subjectively quantify the likelihood of infection for a given surgical procedure. This concept forms the basis of wound classification, a system adapted from human medicine and employed to predict infection risk and consequently the appropriateness of antimicrobial prophylaxis (National Research Council, 1964). There are four

broad categories of wound classification; clean, clean-contaminated, contaminated and dirty. Table 19.1 provides an overview of the wound classification categories, the level of bacterial contamination anticipated for each category and the intent of antibiotic use.

Clean surgical procedures

A clean surgical procedure is considered as elective, without entry into the gastrointestinal, urogenital or respiratory tracts, and with no inflammation or break in aseptic technique. Prophylactic antibiotic use is *not indicated* for clean surgical procedures. Appropriate preparation of the patient and attention to strict asepsis throughout should minimize bacterial contamination of the surgical site to such an extent that the host defences are able to address the minimal bacterial burden that results. In dogs and cats, there are occasional exceptions to the recommendation that prophylaxis should be withheld for clean surgical procedures, although they are principally extrapolated from human guidelines due to the paucity of evidence supporting specific antibiotic recommendations in veterinary medicine. Use of a surgical implant and the potential for infection to have catastrophic consequences for the patient are accepted as reasonable justifications for prophylactic antibiotic use in clean procedures (Bratzler *et al.*, 2013). For example, the placement of a joint prosthesis would fulfil both criteria. The presence of a surgical implant provides a surface for bacterial adhesion and biofilm formation, which facilitates bacteria to evade host immune defences and antimicrobial actions, increasing infection risk (Costerton *et al.*, 1995; Clutterbuck *et al.*, 2007). Lengthy surgical procedures are also generally considered grounds for antimicrobial prophylaxis due to increased exposure and the potential for contamination of the surgical site, although it is unclear at what point a procedure is deemed to be of sufficient duration to warrant prophylaxis.

In a study investigating surgical wound infection rates in over 2000 surgical procedures in dogs and cats, Vasseur *et al.* (1988) concluded that the administration of antibiotic prophylactically significantly reduced the frequency of infection in clean surgical procedures, but this effect was not observed in surgical procedures lasting less than 90 minutes or those that were performed by experienced surgeons. This led to the recommendation that antibiotics should be administered prophylactically in dogs and cats undergoing clean surgical procedures expected to last more than 90 minutes. In addition to recommendations relating to the surgical procedure, any patient with a perceived risk factor for an SSI undergoing a clean surgical procedure warrants consideration for the use of prophylaxis, particularly when factors exist that may negatively impact their immune status (e.g. concurrent endocrinopathy or use of immunosuppressive therapy). When determining whether prophylactic antibiotics are required for each patient, the risk of infection and potential consequences of infection should be weighed against the negative effects of indiscriminate antibiotic use, for both the individual and the wider population. It is worth highlighting that all routine neutering procedures are classified as clean surgical procedures. While the reproductive tract is transected during ovariectomy and ovariohysterectomy, contamination of the surgical site from microbial flora of the healthy reproductive tract is expected to be negligible, and consequently antimicrobial prophylaxis is not indicated for these procedures.

Support for withholding antimicrobial prophylaxis in veterinary patients undergoing clean surgical procedures comes from studies that favourably compare administration of a placebo with the use of prophylaxis, or that report low rates of SSIs without the administration of antibiotic. Vasseur *et al.* (1985) prospectively compared the infection rates in dogs and cats undergoing clean surgical procedures following random assignment to an ampicillin prophylaxis group or a placebo (saline administration) group. No difference in infection rate was detected between the two groups; however, no animals in the placebo group developed infection, and there is the potential that relatively low case numbers resulted in an underpowered study that failed to detect a potential difference between the groups. Other prospective, randomized trials comparing antimicrobial prophylaxis with a placebo in dogs and cats undergoing predominantly clean surgical procedures did not identify a benefit of prophylaxis in reducing infection rates (Holmberg, 1985; Daude-Lagravei *et al.*, 2001).

A recent prospective study assessing risk factors for SSIs associated with clean surgical procedures included 1550 dogs undergoing a variety of soft-tissue, orthopaedic and neurological procedures, 36% of which received antimicrobial prophylaxis (Stetter *et al.*, 2021). No association between the use of prophylaxis and SSI development was detected, with acceptable levels of overall SSIs reported, providing further support for avoiding prophylaxis in patients undergoing clean surgical procedures. However, recommendations regarding antimicrobial prophylaxis could not be made in relation to specific procedures due to limited numbers in the subgroups. A separate study incorporating active surveillance measures (follow-up patient examination and owner interview) to detect SSIs in dogs after hemilaminectomy or laminectomy without the administration of prophylactic antibiotics reported an extremely low SSI rate of 0.6% (Dyall and Schmökel, 2018). It should be noted that a large proportion of the patients included in both of these studies underwent procedures without placement of a surgical implant and with relatively short surgical durations. Currently, use of a surgical implant is widely considered to be grounds for the administration of prophylaxis due to the challenges of treating an SSI in the presence of implanted foreign material (Bratzler *et al.*, 2013; BSAVA/SAMSoc,

2018). Further research is needed to clarify the indications for prophylaxis in the presence of a surgical implant for given procedures. Studies have reported SSI rates following clean surgeries involving placement of orthopaedic implants in dogs and cats without the use of antimicrobial prophylaxis, and results are promising. Stabilization of simple, closed radial and ulnar fractures in small-breed dogs and cats with a titanium locking plate system was associated with a 3% SSI rate (Schmökel et al., 2021). Use of titanium implants for tibial tuberosity advancement in small-breed dogs resulted in SSIs in 2% of dogs (Dyall and Schmökel, 2017). The significance of the use of titanium implants and the patient demographic is unknown, and findings may not be transferable to other implant materials and patient populations.

In contrast to literature that refutes the benefit of antimicrobial prophylaxis to reduce infection rates for clean surgical procedures, there are veterinary studies that support the use of prophylaxis. A prospective, randomized controlled trial investigating the effect of antimicrobial prophylaxis versus a saline placebo in dogs undergoing elective orthopaedic surgery reported a significantly higher infection rate in dogs receiving the placebo, and the study was terminated once this effect was identified (Whittem et al., 1999).

A potential explanation for discrepancies in findings between study conclusions relating to antimicrobial prophylaxis is likely to be due to interstudy variability in terms of case inclusion, peri-operative protocols and criteria for SSI detection. While guidelines relating to surgical antimicrobial prophylaxis serve as a useful framework to aid decision making, the presence of confounding factors (patient, surgeon or procedure derived) have the potential to impact infection risk and may alter the justification for prophylactic antibiotic use on a case-by-case basis.

Clean-contaminated surgical procedures

A clean-contaminated surgical procedure is one that involves entry into the gastrointestinal, urogenital or respiratory tract under controlled conditions without major contamination from excessive spillage of luminal contents. Oropharyngeal procedures are also considered clean-contaminated. A minor break in aseptic technique, for example surgical glove perforation, in an otherwise clean surgical procedure would result in the procedure being reclassified as clean-contaminated. Prophylactic antibiotic use is generally indicated for clean-contaminated procedures with the aim of reducing the degree of bacterial contamination that is anticipated given the nature of the surgery. Effective antibiotic concentrations should be present within the tissues for the duration of the surgical procedure while there is the potential for contamination of the surgical site. Generally, there is no indication for antibiotic administration to be continued once the surgical incision has been closed.

The inclusion of a wide variety of surgical procedures under the category clean-contaminated creates significant challenges in terms of providing blanket recommendations for prophylactic antibiotic use, and is a probable explanation for the varying evidence to support prophylaxis for this category of surgery (Brown et al., 1997; Daude-Lagravei et al., 2001; Nicholson et al., 2002). As an example, uncomplicated cystotomy carries minimal risk of contamination of the surgical site, and as such, antimicrobial prophylaxis is arguably not necessary. However, a colorectal procedure, also classed as clean-contaminated, carries the risk of significant contamination from the heavy Gram-negative bacilli and anaerobic commensal populations of the large intestine, and consequently prophylaxis is clearly appropriate. Despite the presence of significant oral commensal populations, antimicrobial prophylaxis is not generally indicated for routine dental scaling unless the patient has a concurrent disease meaning that transient bacteraemia associated with the dental procedure poses a systemic threat (Greene and Marks, 2012; Bellows et al., 2019).

Placement of a surgical drain has been proposed as a possible risk factor for post-operative infection in dogs and cats, with the presence of foreign material serving to facilitate bacterial colonization (Eugster et al., 2004). It has been suggested by some that clean procedures be reclassified as clean-contaminated if a surgical drain is used; however, guidelines from the Centers for Disease Control and Prevention (CDC) and National Institute for Health and Care Excellence (NICE) do not consider the use of drains when classifying surgical wounds (see Chapter 10, this volume). The risk period for bacterial colonization of the drain is predominantly post-operative, and efforts are better directed towards minimizing colonization rather than the implementation of antimicrobial prophylaxis. Measures to minimize drain colonization include use of a closed, active suction drain rather than an open, passive (e.g. Penrose) drain, exiting the drain distant to the surgical incision, covering the drain exit site post-operatively, using personal protective equipment when handling the drain and removing the drain as soon as is clinically appropriate. The prolonged retention of a surgical wound drain post-operatively has been associated with SSI development in humans, and bacterial colonization of a drain increases substantially with drain indwelling time (Felippe *et al.*, 2007; Pennington *et al.*, 2019). These findings can likely be extrapolated to veterinary patients and it is prudent to remove surgical drains once no longer functional or required.

The considerable variation within and overlap between wound classification categories is an inherent limitation of the system and highlights its use as a guide for determining indications for antimicrobial prophylaxis, with an additional requirement for consideration of factors that may impact infection risk in an individual patient (Vasseur *et al.*, 1988; Brown *et al.*, 1997). There is a need for further veterinary studies to help to define the specific requirements for antimicrobial prophylaxis in the broad category of clean-contaminated surgical wounds. An inability to definitively determine the risk of intraoperative contamination pre-operatively and the relatively common scenario of operating in the absence of laboratory results (e.g. cystotomy prior to receiving a urine culture result) may limit the true instances when antibiotic use can be withheld with confidence for clean-contaminated procedures.

Contaminated surgical procedures

A contaminated surgical procedure may be the result of gross spillage of luminal contents from a hollow viscera, a major break in aseptic technique or operating in the presence of non-purulent inflammation (which may be encountered with an acute, traumatic wound). Antibiotics are used with prophylactic intent for contaminated procedures with the aim of limiting progression of contamination to established infection. Effective antibiotic concentrations should be present at least until the end of surgery with consideration for the extension of prophylaxis post-operatively, depending on the magnitude and nature of the inoculum given the source of contamination. Decision making relating to the duration of prophylaxis administration is discussed further in later sections of this chapter.

Dirty surgical procedures

A dirty surgical procedure is defined as surgery in the presence of established infection and may include pre-existing viscus perforation, abscessation, faecal contamination or a traumatic wound with purulent inflammation. Antibiotics are administered with therapeutic intent to treat the infection. Therapy is likely to consist of initiation of antibiotic administration at the time the infection is diagnosed and extension into the post-operative period, with the duration of treatment dictated by the underlying disease process and clinical response to treatment. The administration of antibiotic with therapeutic intent is discussed in more detail later in section 19.3.

19.2.4 Antibiotic regimens for prophylactic purposes

The basis for most guidelines relating to surgical antimicrobial prophylaxis balances efficacy of the antibiotic regime to minimize infection risk with potential negative effects of antibiotic use for this purpose (Bratzler *et al.*, 2013; Berríos-Torres *et al.*, 2017). Guidelines for the use of antimicrobial prophylaxis in dogs and cats undergoing surgery are mostly derived from recommendations for human surgical patients, where there is limited robust evidence for many of the widely accepted practices relating to prophylaxis (Berríos-Torres *et al.*, 2017; BSAVA/SAMSoc, 2018). There is a clear need for further, high-quality research in both the veterinary and human field to: (i) better define optimal prophylaxis regimes, including agent selection, intraoperative redosing regimes and the necessary duration of therapy; and (ii) identify strategies that will preserve antimicrobial efficacy while minimizing adverse effects.

Agent selection

An antibiotic agent administered for the purpose of antimicrobial prophylaxis should be effective against the bacterial species most likely to contaminate the surgical site for the given procedure. In dogs and cats, the target bacterial species are typically the microbial flora of the skin, principally *Staphylococcus* spp. Surgery that involves entry into the gastrointestinal tract risks contamination from diverse, intralumial commensal populations, with Gram-negative bacilli such as *E. coli* and anaerobes

Table 19.2. Likely bacteria encountered by anatomic location of surgical intervention in dogs and cats and suggested antimicrobial prophylaxis.

Anatomic location of surgical intervention	Bacteria most commonly encountered	Suggested antibiotic agent for surgical antimicrobial prophylaxis
Skin (to include skin reconstruction and elective orthopaedic/neurological surgery with implant placement)	*Staphylococcus* spp.	First-generation cephalosporin
Oropharynx	Gram-positive cocci, e.g. *Staphylococcus* and *Streptococcus* spp. Anaerobes Gram-negative organisms, e.g. *Pasteurella* spp.	First-generation cephalosporin *or* clindamycin *or* ampicillin
Upper gastrointestinal (gastroduodenal)	Gram-positive cocci Enteric Gram-negative bacilli, e.g. *Escherichia coli*	First-generation cephalosporin
Lower gastrointestinal	Enteric Gram-negative bacilli, e.g. *E. coli* Anaerobes Gram-positive cocci, e.g. *Enterococcus* spp.	Second-generation cephalosporin
Hepatobiliary	Enteric Gram-negative bacilli, e.g. *E. coli* Anaerobes, e.g. *Clostridium* spp., *Streptococcus* spp.	Second-generation cephalosporin
Urogenital	Gram-negative organisms e.g. *E. coli*, *Proteus* spp. Gram-positive cocci, e.g. *Staphylococcus*, *Streptococcus* and *Enterococcus* spp. Anaerobes	First-generation cephalosporin *or* ampicillin

predominating in the distal small intestine and colon (Greene and Marks, 2012). Bacterial counts within the colon far exceed those of the stomach and proximal small intestine, and consequently surgical procedures involving large intestinal entry are considered higher risk for contamination than those involving more proximal sites. Potential contaminants from entry into the lower urinary tract include *E. coli* and *Enterococcus* spp., and these isolates may be present even in the absence of lower urinary tract signs (Garcia *et al.*, 2020). Table 19.2 provides a summary of the likely bacteria encountered by anatomic location of surgical intervention in dogs and cats and suggested agents for antimicrobial prophylaxis.

Use of a single, bactericidal antibiotic agent is usually sufficient for the purpose of prophylaxis unless there is a clear indication to use a combination of agents. β-Lactam antibiotics (including penicillins and cephalosporins) are common choices for prophylaxis because they have good efficacy against the common contaminants encountered during surgery in dogs and cats, and are associated with a low risk of patient toxicity. A first-generation cephalosporin (e.g. cefazolin) is a suitable choice for a surgical procedure that does not involve entry into a hollow viscus because potential contaminants are likely to be Gram-positive cocci originating from the microbial flora of the skin.

Use of a second-generation cephalosporin is appropriate for procedures that involve entry into the lower gastrointestinal tract because additional coverage against Gram-negative bacilli is required. For situations where effective anaerobic cover is likely to be required (e.g. oropharyngeal procedures, colorectal procedures), the use of amoxicillin-clavulanate may be preferable. Alternatively, metronidazole can be used in combination with a

Faye Swinbourne

first-generation cephalosporin to increase anaerobic cover. Where a first-generation cephalosporin is not readily available, it is acceptable to substitute a second-generation cephalosporin. This practice should be avoided when a first-generation agent is available due to the increased potential for effects on non-target bacterial species associated with the use of a second-generation cephalosporin and implications for the development of bacterial resistance. Antibiotic agents that are considered to have a particularly broad spectrum of activity, are deemed critically important for human health or have rapidly developing resistance profiles are not appropriate for prophylactic use. Third- and fourth-generation cephalosporins and fluoroquinolones are examples of such agents, and their use for prophylactic purposes should be avoided.

An antibiotic agent suitable for surgical antimicrobial prophylaxis, with availability as an intravenous (IV) preparation and with a veterinary product authorization does not currently exist. Therefore, preparations with a human licence tend to be used in dogs and cats under the Veterinary Medicine Regulations Cascade (VMD, 2013). Consideration for potential adverse effects on the patient when using any medication is important. Adverse reactions to antibiotic agents commonly used for surgical prophylaxis in dogs and cats in the UK have been reported in anaesthetised patients (Norgate and Bruniges, 2016; Gosling and Martínez-Taboada, 2018; Leigh et al., 2019). Amoxicillin-clavulanate agents have been implicated more commonly than second-generation cephalosporins, with one study reporting adverse events in 36% and 2% of surgical patients receiving these agents, respectively (Gosling and Martínez-Taboada, 2018). Such reactions are suspected to be anaphylactic in origin and typically manifest as urticarial reactions involving the lips, face and periocular regions, often with concurrent hypotension. Resolution of these signs can be expected in most patients following discontinuation of antibiotic administration and with provision of an antihistamine agent, IV fluids and medical management of the hypotension where indicated. While an uneventful recovery is generally expected when patients suffering adverse reactions receive appropriate symptomatic treatment, infrequent fatal outcomes have been described anecdotally, and an awareness of the potential for adverse reactions, including how to recognize and manage them promptly, is important when using such agents.

Route of antibiotic administration

IV administration of antibiotics is preferred for prophylaxis because this route is likely to provide the most rapid and predictable peak serum and tissue antibiotic concentrations (Boothe and Boothe, 2015). Oral administration of antibiotics for the purpose of prophylaxis is not recommended, as peak concentrations may be lower and tissue distribution less predictable. Concurrent intramuscular or subcutaneous administration may play a role in extending the duration of action of an IV-administered agent, potentially reducing the need or frequency for redosing intraoperatively; however, clear guidelines for optimal administration regimes have not yet been established for commonly used agents in dogs and cats (Albarellos et al., 2016; Gonzalez et al., 2017).

The local application of antibiotics directly to a surgical site with the aim of reducing SSI risk has been described for a variety of surgical procedures in humans, with some studies demonstrating a significant reduction in SSI incidence and others reporting no benefit or an increase in the development of infection (McHugh et al., 2011; Bratzler et al., 2013). Current guidelines in human medicine state that the prophylactic use of topical antibiotics cannot be recommended at this time because the safety and efficacy of this route of delivery has not been clearly established (Bratzler et al., 2013). An exception is the use of antibiotic-loaded bone cement for the prevention of an SSI following total joint replacement in people, which is approved for routine use in primary joint arthroplasty in some countries but reserved for high-risk patients or for revision arthroplasty in others (Leta et al., 2021). The sequelae of prosthetic joint infection, including a potential requirement for prosthesis removal/replacement and prolonged antibiotic administration, drive the desire to minimize prosthesis-related infection. However, the efficacy of antibiotic-loaded bone cement in reducing prosthetic joint infection is debated, with concerns raised regarding the potential for toxicity and selection for bacterial resistance (Sebastian et al., 2020). These reservations are applicable to veterinary patients, and the prophylactic application of local antibiotics should be viewed with caution until our understanding of the efficacy of this practice and the potential for adverse effects are better defined in all species.

Timing of antibiotic administration

The initiation of antibiotic administration for the purpose of prophylaxis should aim to achieve effective plasma and tissue concentrations of antibiotic before the start of surgery because the potential for bacterial contamination of the surgical site starts when the first incision is made. Both experimental and clinical studies have consistently demonstrated the importance of this concept, with a decline in the beneficial effect of antibiotic administration demonstrated when antibiotics are administered after contamination of the tissue has already occurred (Burke, 1961; Stone et al., 1976; Shapiro and Sacks, 1982; van Kasteren et al., 2007). The optimal timing of antibiotic administration pre-operatively has not been clearly defined in veterinary or human patients. A systematic review and meta-analysis assessing the effect of timing of antibiotic initiation in over 54,000 human surgical patients concluded that there was no significant difference in SSI rates when antibiotic was administered 0–60 or 60–120 minutes prior to the first incision (de Jonge et al., 2017). In the same study, the risk of an SSI almost doubled when antibiotics were administered after the first incision and was five times higher when administered more than 120 minutes prior to the first incision. The optimal timing of antibiotic administration is likely to be dependent on factors such as the dose administered and tissue distribution, and may differ among individuals. Administration within 60 minutes before the first incision is the broadly accepted recommendation for the initiation of surgical antimicrobial prophylaxis (Bratzler et al., 2013; BSAVA/SAMSoc, 2018). This time point may coincide with the induction of anaesthesia in veterinary patients, which can serve as a useful prompt for the initiation of prophylaxis. However, procedures with requirements for extensive patient preparation may require antibiotic administration after induction of anaesthesia to fulfil the requirement of administration within 60 minutes before the first incision. Use of a surgical safety checklist may be helpful to veterinary staff to ensure appropriate timing of antibiotic administration (discussed further in section 19.4).

Concern regarding the potential impact of the pre-operative administration of antimicrobial prophylaxis on bacterial culture results has been raised as a potential justification for delaying the initiation of prophylaxis until after samples for culture have been collected at surgery. A study in dogs undergoing cystotomy for calculi removal compared culture results of urine and bladder mucosal biopsy samples collected when antibiotics were administered at induction of anaesthesia (as per guidelines for prophylaxis) with samples collected when antibiotic administration was withheld until after sample collection. No difference in positive culture results or bacterial isolates between the two groups was detected, although case numbers for statistical analysis were small (Buote et al., 2012). At the current time, there is insufficient evidence to support delaying the initiation of prophylaxis until after sample collection.

Redosing intervals

The β-lactam antibiotics frequently used for prophylaxis are bactericidal with time-dependent activity and a minimal post-antibiotic effect. This means that antibiotic concentrations should be kept above the minimum inhibitory concentration (MIC; the lowest concentration of antimicrobial that inhibits growth of the target pathogen) for a significant proportion of the dosing interval to ensure optimal efficacy, and that there is minimal persistent suppression of bacterial growth once the concentration of antibiotic falls below the MIC (McKellar et al., 2004; Papich, 2014). Convention states that intraoperative redosing of time-dependent antibiotic agents for prophylaxis is indicated if the duration of the surgical procedure exceeds two elimination half-lives of the antibiotic agent administered (Marcellin-Little et al., 1996; Bratzler et al., 2013). One elimination half-life is defined as the time taken for a drug concentration to reduce by half and has been reported as approximately 1 hour for cefazolin and cefuroxime with IV administration at standard recommended doses in dogs and for cefazolin in cats (Marcellin-Little et al., 1996; Albarellos et al., 2016, 2017; Gonzalez et al., 2017). Conversely, intraoperative redosing is not considered necessary if the surgical procedure is complete before two elimination half-lives of the antibiotic agent have passed.

Studies focusing on the pharmacokinetics of antibiotic agents commonly used for surgical prophylaxis are continuously advancing our understanding of the distribution, elimination and duration of action of antibiotics against specific pathogen targets that may be commonly encountered in small animal surgical patients (Albarellos et al., 2016, 2017; Gonzalez et al.,

Faye Swinbourne

2017). Application of the findings of these studies to clinical patients provides an opportunity to redefine historic recommendations relating to redosing intervals that have traditionally been based solely on elimination half-life. This carries the potential for extended redosing intervals, and possibly single-dose prophylaxis (Albarellos et al., 2016; Gonzalez et al., 2017). Most information to date has been gleaned from experimental work; however, the early application of these concepts to clinical patients has shown promise in attaining effective serum concentrations of antibiotic that exceed the MIC of commonly encountered pathogens during small animal surgical procedures (Cagnardi et al., 2018). Further clinical research is required to specifically determine the impact of extended redosing intervals on SSI risk in small animal patients. The ability to reduce the requirement for intraoperative redosing of antibiotics, or remove it completely for procedures of a defined duration, would serve to reduce antibiotic use in surgical patients.

Duration of antibiotic administration

For the purpose of prophylaxis, effective antibiotic concentrations should persist in the tissues of the surgical site for as long as bacterial contamination may occur, which equates to the duration of the surgical procedure and until the surgical site has been closed. Theoretically, the risk of surgical site contamination may persist until a fibrin seal has formed at the incision, which typically occurs by 3–5 hours post-operatively. Covering the surgical site with a dressing in the early post-operative period may help to reduce contamination before a fibrin seal is present, although a clinical benefit of this practice has not been identified (Dumville et al., 2016; Giannetto and Aktay, 2019).

Human guidelines for duration of antibiotic administration for the purpose of surgical prophylaxis state that antibiotics should generally be discontinued at the end of surgery (Bratzler et al., 2013). A systematic review and meta-analysis investigated the occurrence of SSIs in over 19,000 human surgical patients where surgical antimicrobial prophylaxis was either discontinued upon completion of surgery or continued into the post-operative period. The authors did not identify a benefit of post-operative continuation of prophylaxis in reducing the incidence of SSIs when best practice standards were followed in terms of the timing of initiation and redosing of

antibiotics (de Jonge et al., 2020). In addition to a lack of evidence to reliably support a clinical benefit of continued antimicrobial prophylaxis beyond the end of surgery in human patients, this practice is recognized as a risk factor for adverse post-operative events such as the development of Clostridioides difficile-associated colitis in surgical patients (Bratzler et al., 2013). It is reasonable to extrapolate these recommendations relating to the duration of antimicrobial prophylaxis to dogs and cats undergoing surgery, while acknowledging that additional consideration may need to be given to the potential for interference and contamination of the surgical site post-operatively in veterinary species. Some of the differences in post-operative management for veterinary patients may be negated by use of an Elizabethan collar to prevent the patient from traumatizing the surgical site and personal protective equipment for staff handling the surgical wound or dressings.

For clean-contaminated surgical procedures, human guidelines state that additional antimicrobial prophylaxis should not be administered after the surgical incision is closed (Berríos-Torres et al., 2017). In the absence of suitable veterinary studies, these recommendations are likely to be transferable to dogs and cats. When considering the potential for the development of infection following a contaminated surgical procedure, extension of antimicrobial prophylaxis into the post-operative period may be appropriate. However, the provision of prescriptive recommendations is not possible due to the wide variety of procedures within this wound classification category and potential for the nature of the contaminants to vary widely in terms of magnitude and virulence, depending on the source of the contamination. When continuation of post-operative antimicrobial prophylaxis is warranted, determining the appropriate duration of prophylaxis is highly subjective: an extension of 24–48 hours beyond the end of surgery is most frequently implemented following intraoperative events such as a break in aseptic technique or gross spillage of luminal content. Ultimately, the decision to extend antimicrobial prophylaxis beyond closure of the surgical incision should be made with consideration for the nature of the inoculum (e.g. urine versus faecal contamination) and any other factors that may influence susceptibility to infection such as the immune status of the host. Extended durations of antimicrobial prophylaxis will have implications for commensal microbial populations and selection for resistance, and therefore the decision to extend antibiotic use post-operatively must be weighed against the potential adverse effects of this practice.

USE OF ANTIBIOTICS IN THE POST-OPERATIVE PERIOD FOLLOWING ORTHOPAEDIC SURGERY.

The extension of antibiotic administration into the post-operative period for clean orthopaedic surgery has sparked considerable debate, particularly in relation to the proximal tibial osteotomy techniques performed for management of cranial cruciate ligament rupture in dogs. One of the most commonly performed osteotomy techniques, tibial plateau levelling osteotomy (TPLO), has been associated with a relatively high incidence of SSI when compared with other clean orthopaedic procedures involving use of an implant. Proposed reasons for this include the need for extensive soft-tissue dissection with resultant vascular disruption, limited soft-tissue coverage of the surgical site, prolonged surgical time, thermal bone necrosis and instability of the osteotomy site (Kim *et al.*, 2008; Solano *et al.*, 2015). The incidence of SSIs following TPLO varies widely, with reports in the literature ranging from 2% to 26%; the majority of studies report an SSI incidence within the lower half of this range and those reporting an incidence of over 15% mostly report outcomes in dogs with a body weight over 50 kg (Fitzpatrick and Solano, 2010; Frey *et al.*, 2010; Nazarali *et al.*, 2014, Nazarali *et al.*, 2015; Atwood *et al.*, 2015; Solano *et al.*, 2015; Aiken *et al.*, 2015; Brown *et al.*, 2016; Hans *et al.*, 2017; Spencer and Daye, 2018; Lopez *et al.*, 2018; Tuan *et al.*, 2019; Giannetto and Aktay, 2019; Hagen *et al.*, 2020). SSIs following TPLO may be associated with significant patient morbidity, a need for implant removal for resolution of the infection and increased costs (Fitzpatrick and Solano, 2010; Nazarali *et al.*, 2014; Nicoll *et al.*, 2014; Brown *et al.*, 2016). In an attempt to reduce SSI risk and associated morbidity, the continuation of oral antibiotics post-operatively has become commonplace following TPLO in some institutions. The choice of antibiotic agent and duration of therapy varies enormously both within and among institutions, with little standardization and decision making often left to the discretion of the individual surgeon (Weese and Halling, 2006). Given the fact that TPLO is commonly performed in dogs, the practice of extended antibiotic administration is likely to have significant implications for overall antibiotic consumption and associated adverse effects.

Studies attempting to determine the impact of extended antibiotic administration into the post-operative period on the incidence of SSIs following TPLO vary greatly in terms of design, peri-operative prophylaxis protocols and duration of post-operative antibiotic administration, which limits the ability to make meaningful comparisons. A systematic review investigating the efficacy of post-operative antibiotic use after TPLO in dogs concluded that the level of evidence provided by the included studies was low to moderate, the studies with the highest level of evidence did not provide evidence of the benefit of antibiotic use, and there was insufficient evidence to support the use of post-operative antibiotics to reduce the risk of SSIs in dogs after TPLO (Budsberg *et al.*, 2021). Studies reporting SSI incidence in relation to another commonly performed tibial osteotomy technique in dogs, tibial tuberosity advancement (TTA), are fewer in number and have the same limitations as those investigating TPLO. One retrospective study specifically investigated the impact of post-operative antibiotic use on rates of infection and implant removal after TTA in 1768 canine stifles and did not identify a benefit with the use of post-operative antibiotics (Ferrell *et al.*, 2019). The same study reported a significant risk of developing an oxacillin-resistant infection with the use of prophylactic post-operative antibiotics, and oxacillin-resistant infection was associated with a requirement for implant removal to obtain infection resolution. Other studies have reported a potential association with post-operative antibiotic use and the isolation of methicillin-resistant *Staphylococcus* spp. following TPLO, suggesting that any potential benefit of a reduction in SSI incidence associated with the extension of antibiotic administration could be countered by the isolation of drug-resistant pathogens (Atwood *et al.*, 2015; Giannetto and Aktay, 2019). Additionally, post-operative antibiotic administration following TPLO has been associated with delays in the clinical detection of SSI and a requirement for extended antibiotic courses to achieve resolution of infection (Fitzpatrick and Solano, 2010).

There is currently insufficient evidence to support the use of post-operative antibiotic administration in dogs and cats undergoing clean orthopaedic implant surgery. While implant-associated SSIs can present significant treatment challenges and there is an understandable drive to reduce SSI risk in such patients, the consequences of antibiotic overuse cannot be overstated. It is encouraging that reported SSI rates for clean orthopaedic (including TPLO) and neurosurgeries where post-operative antibiotic was not administered are comparable to those reported with the use of post-operative antibiotic (Välkki *et al.*, 2020). Ultimately, there is a need for further prospective, robustly designed and suitably powered studies with standardized antibiotic regimes to further our understanding of the role of antibiotics in reducing SSI risk for these types of surgery (Budsberg *et al.*, 2021). Active SSI surveillance should be utilized to reduce the potential for SSIs to go undetected after patient discharge (Turk *et al.*, 2015; Garcia Stickney and Thieman Mankin, 2018). The role of stricter measures relating to aseptic protocol for clean implant surgery warrants further consideration, with a focus on reducing contamination of the surgical site rather than relying on antibiotic prophylaxis to address contamination (Stine *et al.*, 2018).

19.3 Therapeutic Antibiotic Use in Surgical Patients

Bacterial disease requiring surgical intervention in small animal patients is often the result of translocation of opportunistic pathogens that are part of the individual's commensal microbial flora normally residing remote from the site of infection where they do not pose pathogenic potential. Oropharyngeal commensal organisms are commonly isolated from the pleural exudate of dogs and cats with pyothorax, with inhaled plant material believed to be the vehicle responsible for transfer of bacteria from the oropharynx to the pleural space in dogs (Walker *et al.*, 2000; Demetriou *et al.*, 2002; Lappin *et al.*, 2017). Ascending infection of opportunistic pathogens of the urogenital tract can result in conditions such as pyometra and bacterial prostatitis (Barsanti, 2012). Alternatively, bacterial disease may be the result of rupture of a viscus that contains commensal microbial flora, releasing bacteria into an otherwise sterile location where they are able to exert a pathogenic effect. A commonly encountered example in small animals is gastrointestinal perforation with resultant septic peritonitis. Finally, bacterial disease requiring surgical intervention may be the result of inoculation of bacteria from a traumatic incident, such as a dog

bite, or subsequent to a surgical intervention resulting in an SSI. Traumatic wounds that are heavily contaminated, or with established infection at the time of presentation, generally require a period of open wound management to reduce the bacterial burden and establish a healthy wound environment to allow healing to progress. A comprehensive review of the management of open wounds and SSIs is provided in Section 3 of this book and will not be discussed further here.

The formation of septic exudate and necrotic tissue is a common sequelae to bacterial infection. Both substances can accumulate in significant volumes at the site of infection, hampering the penetration and efficacy of systemically administered antibiotic agents and creating an environment that is not conducive to resolution of infection or tissue healing (Bergeron, 1986; Enoch and Harding, 2003). Consequently, a combination of surgical intervention and therapeutic antibiotic administration is usually required to effectively treat bacterial disease of this nature. When infection is in a location amenable to surgery, surgical debridement enables removal of devitalized, necrotic tissue, septic exudate and foreign material, which will reduce the bacterial burden, remove tissue barriers to antibiotic penetration, and improve perfusion, optimizing response to concurrent antibiotic administration. When the site of infection is not amenable to surgical debridement, usually due to the proximity of vital anatomic structures, drainage of exudate via single aspiration or by placement of an indwelling drain is commonly performed. Drainage is unlikely to be as effective as surgical debridement in removing non-viable tissue and reducing bacterial burden; however, it can provide significant benefit in terms of patient stabilization, particularly in the acute setting. In the presence of significant tissue necrosis and septic exudate, treatment of bacterial disease by administering systemic antibiotics alone (without surgical debridement or drainage of exudate) is highly likely to result in treatment failure. In addition to an unfavourable clinical outcome, the administered antibiotic will impact patient bacterial populations, both commensal and those implicated in the disease process, with potentially grave consequences for the development of bacterial resistance and future treatment outcomes. Likewise, in such situations, surgery alone without the concurrent administration of an appropriate antibiotic agent could result in treatment failure due to the inability of surgery to effectively clear the bacterial burden, particularly when infection occurs in locations not amenable to radical tissue resection. An exception to this is superficial abscessation of the dermis and subcutaneous tissues of an immunocompetent patient; in this instance, establishing drainage may well be effective and the only intervention necessary to successfully resolve infection, and is therefore an appropriate first-line treatment approach if the individual remains systemically well.

19.3.1 Diagnosis of bacterial disease

The definitive diagnosis of a bacterial disease process requires specific diagnostic testing; however, patient history, signalment and presenting clinical signs may raise suspicion of bacterial disease, prompting early investigation for infection. As an example, a springer spaniel presenting with pyrexia and tachypnoea warrants assessment for the presence of pleural fluid, and sampling and analysis of fluid if identified, because the breed is over-represented for pyothorax (Demetriou et al., 2002). A systemically unwell patient presenting after recent gastrointestinal surgery should be evaluated for the presence of free peritoneal fluid (with sampling and analysis) because this presentation is suggestive of gastrointestinal surgical site dehiscence and septic peritonitis. While the presence of clinical findings such as pyrexia and a purulent exudate can be suggestive of a bacterial aetiology, they should not be used in isolation to make diagnoses and treatment decisions. The presence of bacteria and their likely clinical significance should always be confirmed by laboratory testing. This approach will minimize the risk of antibiotic use for non-bacterial disease, provide information about causative agents (including identification and susceptibility) and facilitate surveillance of infectious disease, all of which will encourage the rational and prudent use of therapeutic antibiotic administration.

When a bacterial aetiology is suspected, sampling of the involved tissue or exudate is indicated to confirm or exclude the presence of bacteria. Sampling commonly takes the form of needle aspiration or tissue biopsy. Sampling may be performed purely with the intent of obtaining tissue or fluid for analysis, or can be performed with both diagnostic and therapeutic intent if the volume of exudate or diseased tissue removed improves clinical signs and reduces the bacterial burden. Examples of the latter scenario include the aspiration of pleural exudate

for the stabilization of individuals with pyothorax, and surgical debridement of necrotic tissue and foreign material associated with sublumbar abscessation. These interventions will reduce bacterial load and are likely to enhance the efficacy of concurrent therapeutic antibiotic administration.

In-house diagnostic testing for the confirmation of a bacterial component to a disease process typically takes the form of cytological analysis. This can be extremely useful in the emergency setting when a bacterial aetiology is suspected and early initiation of treatment (either surgery, antibiotic administration or a combination of the two) is indicated due to systemic involvement. When needle aspirates or fluid samples have been obtained, fresh smears can be made, air dried and stained with Romanowsky stains such as Diff-Quik. In-house microscopic examination of prepared slides will allow the detection of bacterial cocci and rods where present. The presence of inflammatory cells, predominantly neutrophils in the case of an acute infectious process, are likely to be observed when identified bacteria are clinically significant, and the presence of intracellular bacteria demonstrates a host response to bacterial infection by the action of phagocytosis. Importantly, detection of bacteria without a concurrent inflammatory response on cytological assessment is likely to represent the presence of bacterial contaminants rather than bacteria that are clinically significant. While in-house cytology can be extremely useful in rapidly supporting a clinical suspicion of bacterial disease, concurrent sample submission to an external laboratory is indicated in every instance to confirm a bacterial component to the disease process, isolate and identify pathogens likely to be of clinical significance, and perform antimicrobial susceptibility testing. This information will serve to ensure the use of antibiotics only when clinically indicated and guide decision making relating to agent selection, with the aim of optimizing treatment efficacy and minimizing the likelihood of inappropriate antibiotic use.

Culture of bacterial colonies on growth medium is the traditional method of isolating bacteria and is frequently used in surgical patients due to the ability to provide fresh tissue samples for culture from individuals undergoing surgical intervention. It is important to bear in mind that contaminants, rather than clinically significant pathogens, may be identified by culture and therefore any culture result must be interpreted within the context of the clinical setting (Guardabassi et al., 2018). Culture may be negative even in the presence of bacterial disease, particularly if the causative bacteria are challenging to culture due to their fastidious nature, as is often the case with anaerobes (Love and Jones, 2012). Use of molecular techniques such as polymerase chain reaction (PCR) assays and DNA sequencing to identify bacteria can prove beneficial when an elusive pathogen is encountered. These techniques are extremely sensitive and have the potential to detect contaminants and commensals that are not clinically significant, even when present in very low numbers, again highlighting the importance of interpreting any positive result with consideration for the individual patient and suspected disease process (Guardabassi et al., 2018).

Following the isolation and identification of a pathogen of likely clinical significance, antimicrobial susceptibility testing should be performed to aid the selection of an appropriate antibiotic agent for treatment. Susceptibility testing typically takes the form of serial dilutions of antibiotic to determine the MIC of a given antibiotic agent for the target pathogen, or agar diffusion testing, which identifies zones of inhibition of bacterial growth around antibiotic-impregnated discs on an agar plate, which can then be used to confer isolate susceptibility or resistance to the given antibiotic agent. It is important to remember that antimicrobial susceptibility is determined by in vitro testing, and a positive response to treatment in vivo is not guaranteed. Even when an isolated pathogen is classified as susceptible to a given antibiotic agent, the ability to achieve effective concentrations of antibiotic in the target tissue is critical if treatment is to be effective. In the event of a negative culture result due to an inability to successfully identify fastidious organisms, or if a pathogen is identified by molecular techniques precluding susceptibility testing, knowledge of antimicrobial susceptibility and resistance patterns for a given isolate can be used to guide the selection of antibiotic agent for isolates that are predictably susceptible (Love and Jones, 2012; Guardabassi et al., 2018).

19.3.2 Antibiotic regimens for therapeutic purposes

When using antibiotics therapeutically, there is a requirement to balance the need for effective treatment of the bacterial disease against the potential for adverse effects of antibiotic use (Weese et al., 2015). Selection of antibiotic

regimes with consideration for factors such as appropriate agent choice for the target pathogen, timely initiation of therapy, and optimal dosing and duration of therapy will serve to optimize treatment efficacy while minimizing the adverse consequences of antibiotic use for the individual patient and wider population.

Agent selection

The choice of therapeutic antibiotic should be based on the results of culture and susceptibility testing. This will allow targeted treatment of causative bacterial isolates, which will maximize treatment efficacy and minimize effects on wider, non-target bacterial populations and the selection for resistance. Such an approach may not be possible when delaying therapy until culture results are available risks adversely affecting patient outcome due to the presence, or imminent risk, of systemic progression of disease. Examples of this scenario in surgical patients include those presenting with conditions such as pyothorax and septic peritonitis. These conditions carry the risk of systemic involvement in the form of bacteraemia and sepsis, and the prompt administration of antibiotic therapy has been associated with improved patient outcomes (Summers et al., 2021). When treatment must be initiated before the results of culture and susceptibility testing are available, empirical therapy is necessary, with agent choice based on the likely pathogens present for the presenting condition and known susceptibility patterns. The temptation to prescribe agents with an overly broad spectrum of action, or use of multiple agents to increase the spectrum of coverage without a clear clinical indication to do so, should be avoided due to the increased potential to impact non-target bacterial species. A summary of bacterial surgical disorders of the dog and cat that may require empirical therapy pending culture results, the likely pathogens involved, and suggested empirical antibiotic protocols is provided in Table 19.3. Agents considered critically important for use in human medicine, such as the fluoroquinolones, should generally not be used without culture and susceptibility testing results to support their use. Administration of fluoroquinolones for the empirical treatment of dogs and cats presenting with life-threatening infections is considered an exception; however, their use should be reviewed on receipt of the culture and

Table 19.3. Bacterial surgical disorders in dogs and cats, the likely pathogens and suggested empirical antibiotic protocols pending culture and susceptibility testing results. Recommendations extrapolated from Allerton and Nuttall (2021).

Surgical disorder	Likely pathogen(s)	Suggested antibiotic protocol for empirical therapy pending culture result
Pyothorax	Anaerobes, e.g. *Bacteroides*, *Clostridium*, *Peptostreptococcus*, *Fusobacterium* and *Actinomyces* spp. Enterobacteriaceae, e.g. *Escherichia coli* (mainly in dogs) *Pasteurella* spp. (mainly in cats) *Nocardia* spp. (both cats and dogs)	Fluoroquinolone + amoxicillin (± clavulanate) *or* fluoroquinolone + clindamycin
Septic peritonitis secondary to intestinal dehiscence or perforation	Gram-negative bacilli, e.g. *E. coli* Gram-positive cocci, e.g. *Enterococcus* and *Streptococcus* spp. Anaerobes, e.g. *Clostridium* spp.	Fluoroquinolone + amoxicillin-clavulanate *or* fluoroquinolone + metronidazole (*or* cefuroxime + metronidazole; this combination is used commonly in human septic peritonitis and offers an alternative to use of a fluoroquinolone, but additional Gram-negative cover may be required in some cases)
Bacterial prostatitis with abscessation	Predominantly *E.coli* Gram-positive cocci, e.g. *Staphylococcus* spp., *Streptococcus* spp.	Trimethoprim sulfonamide *or* fluoroquinolone
Bite wound	Gram-negative, e.g. *Pasteurella* spp., *E. coli*, and Gram-positive, e.g. *Staphylococcus* spp., β-haemolytic *Streptococcus* spp., aerobes Anaerobes, e.g. *Fusobacterium*, *Bacteroides* and *Clostridium* spp. Where there are fistulas or draining nodules, consider *Actinomyces* or *Nocardia* spp. or mycobacteria	Amoxicillin-clavulanate *or* clindamycin
Open wound/fracture	Predominantly *Staphylococcus pseudintermedius* Other Gram-positive cocci, e.g. *Streptococcus* or *Enterococcus* spp. Gram-negative isolates, e.g. *E. coli*, *Pasteurella* spp. ± Anaerobes	First- or second-generation cephalosporin *or* amoxicillin-clavulanate

susceptibility testing results, with amendments to the empirical regime as necessary to ensure a targeted approach to treatment. The potential for a negative culture result due to the fastidious nature of causative pathogens should also be considered. For example, anaerobes implicated in pyothorax may not be successfully cultured, but administration of antibiotic with anaerobic coverage is recommended for the duration of treatment of pyothorax (Lappin *et al.*, 2017). Clinical progress should also be considered when making adjustments to therapeutic regimes, rather than focusing on laboratory results alone. Repeat culture and susceptibility testing is strongly advised when the response to treatment is not as expected or clinical deterioration is noted after an initial favourable response.

Faye Swinbourne

Route of antibiotic administration

For the majority of bacterial disease processes requiring surgical intervention, antibiotic therapy should be initiated at the time of diagnosis. IV administration is typically the most appropriate route to achieve peak serum and tissue antibiotic concentrations as rapidly as possible (Boothe and Boothe, 2015). Timely antibiotic administration is key to the management of severe, life-threatening infection. The early administration of antibiotics has been associated with improved outcome in dogs: individuals showing signs of septic shock are more likely to survive if antibiotics are administered within 3 hours of a diagnosis of sepsis (Summers *et al.*, 2021). Recommendations in human patients are to administer IV antibiotics as soon as possible after recognition of sepsis and septic shock (Rhodes *et al.*, 2017). IV administration is generally continued into the post-operative period until the patient is haemodynamically stable, eating well, and there are no gastrointestinal signs that may hamper the reliable intake and absorption of oral medication. At this stage, antibiotic administration can be changed from the IV to the oral route.

The local application of antibiotics directly to the site of infection has several potential advantages over systemic administration. Higher local antibiotic concentrations in the wound bed may enhance therapeutic efficacy in the presence of biofilm, reduced systemic antibiotic exposure may lessen patient toxicity risk and the impact on commensal microbial populations, and removal of a reliance on perfusion for antibiotic delivery could be advantageous when treating infection at avascular sites (McHugh *et al.*, 2011; Hayes *et al.*, 2013). Possible drawbacks to the local application of antibiotic include tissue toxicity at the site of implantation and systemic effects should significant absorption occur (Edmiston *et al.*, 2017). The delivery vehicle that holds and elutes the antibiotic may incite an inflammatory response locally (with consequences for wound healing) or may serve as a nidus for infection if made from non-absorbable materials (Hayes *et al.*, 2013). The potential for insufficient dwell times and sustained release of antibiotic at subtherapeutic concentrations from sites of local application raises concern regarding contribution to resistance (Webb and Spencer, 2007; Hayes *et al.*, 2013; Edmiston *et al.*, 2017). The concurrent use of systemic and local antibiotic therapy is not uncommon and this approach is likely to negate many of the proposed benefits of local antibiotic use. Traditionally, poly(methylmethacrylate) (PMMA) bone cement has been a commonly used carrier for the local application of antibiotic to a surgical site. PMMA bone cement is non-absorbable, and an exothermic reaction occurs during preparation meaning the impregnated antibiotic agent must be heat stable if efficacy is to be preserved (Webb and Spencer, 2007). Due to these limitations, biodegradable alternatives that incite less tissue reaction have gained favour as delivery vehicles for the local application of antibiotics. Biodegradable carrier options such as collagen sponge or calcium sulfate beads can negate the need for surgical removal of the carrier after treatment, although local inflammation at the site of implantation may still serve to negatively impact tissue healing, with implications for infection persistence in some instances (Hayes *et al.*, 2013). In small animal patients, the most frequently reported applications for the therapeutic use of local antibiotics include the management of intra-articular and implant-associated infection (Hayes *et al.*, 2013). The local application of an amikacin-infused collagen sponge at the site of implant removal has been successfully used to manage SSIs following TPLO in dogs without concurrent systemic antibiotic administration (Lee *et al.*, 2019). Calcium sulfate antibiotic-impregnated beads have been used to manage SSIs following orthopaedic surgery in dogs, although the importance of culture and susceptibility testing to guide antibiotic choice cannot be overemphasized: treatment failure is frequently encountered because causative bacteria isolated from intraoperative samples are commonly resistant to empirically selected local antibiotics (Peterson *et al.*, 2021). There is still a paucity of data regarding the elution, efficacy and potential systemic effects of local antibiotic use with therapeutic intent in small animal patients, and additional research is required to further our understanding of the appropriate applications for this form of antibiotic use.

There is no evidence to support the intracavitary application of antibiotics to sites such as the peritoneal cavity or pleural space in small animal patients. In addition to an absence of supporting evidence for the efficacy of such applications, these practices have the potential to negatively affect local tissues and can have systemic effects that may contribute to toxicity and the development of resistance (Rappaport *et al.*, 1989).

Dosing and duration of antibiotic administration

Antibiotic dosing regimens are designed to ensure sufficient drug exposure during treatment to effectively eliminate target bacteria while minimizing selection for resistant bacterial populations. There are numerous considerations for agent concentration, dosing frequency and duration of treatment when designing regimens that optimize treatment efficacy yet protect against potential adverse effects of antibiotic use. These concepts are discussed further in Chapter 16 (this volume).

There is a lack of objective evidence on optimal treatment durations for most bacterial surgical diseases in dogs and cats. General recommendations for treatment duration can be found in clinical guidelines; however, there is likely to be wide variation in terms of disease severity and response to treatment among individuals. Ultimately, decision making should be guided by clinical progress on a case-by-case basis (Martinez et al., 2012; Lappin et al., 2017; Weese et al., 2019). Recommendations for duration of therapy are often in the region of 4–6 weeks for bacterial disease with the potential for systemic involvement and that is managed with a combination of surgical intervention and systemic antibiotic administration (Lappin et al., 2017; Weese et al., 2019). For conditions where the inciting cause of the infection can be confidently identified and addressed, such as septic peritonitis secondary to intestinal dehiscence, shorter durations of therapy may be appropriate if the clinical response to treatment is favourable. Thorough clinical assessment and the use of follow-up diagnostic imaging to confirm resolution of clinical disease is advised before antibiotic therapy is discontinued, for example the resolution of pleural or peritoneal effusion in patients with pyothorax or septic peritonitis, respectively. The duration of antibiotic administration is an important consideration because extension of treatment beyond that which is clinically required unnecessarily increases patient drug exposure. Longer durations of therapy can increase the proportion of resistant bacteria within an exposed population, increase the drug exposure necessary to suppress amplification of resistant pathogens, and encourage bacterial phenotypic changes to form 'persister' cells, which have the ability to evade antibiotic action (Martinez et al., 2012). Conversely, discontinuation of therapy prematurely risks recrudescence of infection, with

selection for pathogens with reduced susceptibility (Guardabassi et al., 2018). There is a balance to be found, with the optimal time for discontinuation of therapy likely to be the point at which the bacterial burden has been reduced to a level that the host defences can address. Multiple factors may influence this time point for a given individual, including ability to significantly reduce the bacterial burden with surgical debridement, the patient's systemic health and the initial clinical response to therapy. As an example, extensive mediastinitis in canine pyothorax is a situation where the degree of surgical debridement that can be achieved will be restricted by the proximity of vital structures, and, despite surgical intervention, there is a heavy reliance on the post-operative administration of systemic antibiotics to address the significant, persistent bacterial load after surgery.

In an attempt to reduce the potential adverse effects of antibiotic use, there is a move towards the use of shorter durations of therapy in human medicine, and this approach has been supported by a small number of veterinary studies to date (Weese et al., 2019). There is a great need for prospective, randomized trials in veterinary patients to develop our understanding of appropriate durations of therapy. The results of such studies may well provide a body of evidence to support shorter-duration therapies over the arbitrary, often lengthy durations currently implemented for many bacterial surgical disorders in dogs and cats.

19.4 Inappropriate Antibiotic Use in Surgical Patients

The inappropriate use of antibiotics generally refers to overuse or misuse where the antibiotic is administered when not clinically indicated, or selected agents, dosages or treatment durations are not appropriate for the target pathogen. There are numerous examples of inappropriate antibiotic use for the indication of antimicrobial prophylaxis in surgical patients. Use of antibiotic prophylactically for a procedure where the perceived infection risk is low, for example clean procedures in healthy individuals lasting less than 90 minutes and without the use of an implant, would be deemed inappropriate. Agent selection without due consideration for likely contaminants given the procedure and location of surgery may result in the use of an unsuitable antibiotic agent with poor activity against the causative pathogens of a potential SSI.

Faye Swinbourne

In addition, the timing of antibiotic administration in terms of first dose, intraoperative redosing and cessation of therapy has implications for the goal of obtaining an effective antibiotic concentration at the surgical site before the first incision is made and until the end of surgery.

Reported use of antimicrobial prophylaxis for routine, clean surgical procedures in veterinary patients ranges from 14% to 35% for castration, and from 25% to 50% for simple cutaneous mass excision, confirming that indiscriminate use of prophylaxis for clean surgical procedures is common (Knights et al., 2012; Hardefeldt et al., 2017; Stetter et al., 2021). The choice of antibiotic agent for prophylaxis is generally appropriate, with studies reporting use of β-lactams in over 90% of included procedures and reasonably infrequent use of agents considered to be critically important for human health. However, route of administration of prophylaxis may be less appropriate, with only 25% of respondents reporting IV administration of antibiotic in one study (Knights et al., 2012; Hardefeldt et al., 2017; Stetter et al., 2021). In terms of adherence to guidelines relating to the timing of initiation of prophylaxis and intraoperative redosing intervals, studies including dogs undergoing clean surgical procedures have reported appropriate timings for initial dosing for 72–84% of cases, and for redosing in 51–81% of cases (Weese and Halling, 2006; Välkki et al., 2020; Stetter et al., 2021). More general reporting of appropriate use of peri-operative antimicrobial prophylaxis has been attempted by combining factors such as timing of initiation, redosing and dose administered: in dogs undergoing clean surgical procedures, antibiotic regimes were considered appropriate using these criteria in only 43–57% of cases (Nazarali et al., 2014; Hagen et al., 2020).

There is a clear need for improved compliance with antimicrobial prophylaxis guidelines if we are to limit unnecessary contributions to antibiotic consumption, optimize efficacy of surgical prophylaxis and limit the adverse effects of antibiotic use for the individual patient and beyond. Reasons for failure to comply with prophylaxis guidelines include a lack of understanding relating to the principles and indications for prophylaxis, and a belief that the routine use of antibiotics peri-operatively will make up for deficits in infection control measures within the practice. There may be a reluctance to change long-standing prescribing habits for fear of encountering adverse outcomes more commonly, even when there is no evidence to support these assumptions. Measures to educate the practice team about indications for prophylaxis and the application of practice-wide policies relating to agent selection and timing of administration can serve to create a more logical and uniform approach to the prophylactic use of antibiotics in surgical patients. Use of a surgical checklist has been shown to reduce the frequency of SSIs in dogs and cats undergoing surgery (Bergström et al., 2016; Launcelott et al., 2019). Inclusion of checks relating to antimicrobial prophylaxis requirements may serve to encourage the timely administration of antibiotics pre-operatively and protect against shortfalls in adherence to recommendations relating to redosing intervals (Fig. 19.1). The use of a checklist can also improve communication between members of the theatre team and prompt consideration for changes to the indication for antibiotic use, which may occur because of intraoperative events such as a break in aseptic technique. Additional measures have proved beneficial in maximizing prophylaxis compliance in human surgical patients and include the delegation of responsibility for antibiotic administration to a specific member of the theatre team, education of all staff members to elicit an understanding of the clinical implications for non-adherence and computerized reminders for redosing; such measures are likely to be transferable to veterinary practice (Haney et al., 2020; Hassan et al., 2021).

Creation and implementation of a robust practice infection control policy should provide confidence in infection control measures and protect against using antibiotics as a safety net for concerns relating to potential shortfalls in best practice standards. A comprehensive infection control policy will include protocols relating to preparation of the surgical team, patient preparation, aseptic technique, instrument sterilization, theatre cleaning, antibiotic stewardship and SSI surveillance (see Sections 2 and 3 of this volume for further details).

19.5 Conclusion

The use of antibiotics clearly has an important role in the prevention and treatment of infection in small animal surgical patients. At the same time, the rational use of antibiotic is essential if antibiotic efficacy is to be preserved for future use and contribution to the development of resistance is to be limited. For prophylactic indications, there is a great need for a better understanding of which

Surgical Safety Checklist

SIGN IN (to be read out loud)

Before induction of anaesthesia

Which ward was the patient in? _____
Which kennel? _____

Has the patient had their identity confirmed, procedure verified and consent checked?
☐ Yes

Is the surgical site marked?
☐ Yes/not applicable

Is the anaesthetic machine and medication check complete?
☐ Yes

Does the patient have a:
Known allergy?
☐ Yes ☐ No
Difficult airway/aspiration risk?
☐ Yes ☐ No
Risk of >15% blood loss?
☐ No
☐ Yes and adequate IV access/fluids planned
☐ Patient position in theatre known?
☐ Antibiotics at induction? Yes/NA
☐ Estimated surgery time is............
☐ Team discusses perioperative plan & designates roles
☐ Any concerns?
☐ Who is prepping patient_____

TIME OUT (To be read out loud)

Before start of surgical incision
☐ **Theatre team introductions**

Surgeon, Anaesthetist and nurse/assistant:
☐ What is the patient's name? _____
☐ Procedure, site and position are confirmed.
_____
☐ Monopolar plate checked. Re-checked after re-positioning? ☐

Surgeon:
☐ Anticipated blood loss?
☐ Are there any specific equipment requirements or special investigations?
☐ Are there any critical or unexpected steps you want the team to know about?

Anaesthetist:
☐ Are there any patient specific concerns?
☐ What is the patient's ASA grade?
☐ What monitoring equipment and other specific levels of support are required e.g. blood?

Nurse/Assistant:
☐ Is the sterility of instrumentation confirmed?
Initials on pack? _____ Date? _____
☐ Purse string / rectal swabs / oral swabs been placed (underline those that apply)?
☐ Are there any equipment issues or concerns?
☐ Number of swabs counted --------

Surgical site infection completed.
☐ Antibiotic prophylaxis within the last 60 minutes
☐ Patient warming. State temperature_____
☐ Hair removal and Antisepsis

SIGN OUT (to be read out loud)

Before any member of the team leaves the operating room

Theatre Nurse/Assistant verbally confirms with the team:
☐ Has the name of the procedure been recorded?
☐ Has it been confirmed that instruments, swabs and sharps counts are complete
☐ Have the specimens been labelled (including patient name)? By whom ....
☐ Have samples been collected for research (e.g. PBS, DNA)
☐ Have any equipment problems been identified that need to be addressed?
☐ Have the purse string / rectal swabs / oral swabs been removed (underline those that apply)?

Surgeon, Anaesthetist and Theatre Nurse/Assistant:
☐ What are the key concerns for recovery?

Patient Details	
Name:	
Client:	
Case number:	
Procedure:	
Theatre Staff (Initials)	
Surgeon(s):	
Anaesthetist:	
Theatre Nurse/Assistant:	
Theatre number:	

One ☐ Two ☐ Three ☐ Four ☐

Modified from WHO Surgical Safety Checklist 2009

Fig. 19.1. Example of a surgical safety checklist. Modified from WHO (2009).

surgical procedures warrant the administration of prophylactic antibiotics, with current practices almost certainly contributing to the overuse of antibiotics for this indication. While the criteria for use of antibiotics for therapeutic purposes in surgical patients is somewhat better defined, advances in our understanding of optimal dosing regimens will help protect against the administration of unnecessarily long courses of treatment. If future research efforts provide support for such changes to the way antibiotics are administered, the net effect will be to considerably reduce antibiotic consumption in small animal surgical patients.

The reporting of SSIs associated with various clean surgical procedures in dogs and cats with a focus on the use, or rather lack of, surgical antimicrobial prophylaxis is gaining momentum. Continued research in the form of well-designed, prospective studies will help to further our understanding of the indications for prophylaxis and will ultimately improve prescribing practices. Additional components of infection prevention and control strategies in surgical patients, including a stringent approach to aseptic technique, are fundamental to reducing infection risk. Attention to these areas will serve to reduce the requirement for antibiotic use in surgical patients both prophylactically and therapeutically by minimizing contamination of the surgical site and the subsequent risk of infection.

References

Aiken, M.J., Hughes, T.K., Abercromby, R.H., Holmes, M.A. and Anderson, A.A. (2015) Prospective, randomized comparison of the effect of two antimicrobial regimes on surgical site infection rate in dogs undergoing orthopedic implant surgery. *Veterinary Surgery* 44(5), 661–667. DOI: 10.1111/vsu.12327.

Albarellos, G.A., Montoya, L., Lorenzini, P.M., Passini, S.M., Lupi, M.P. *et al.* (2016) Pharmacokinetics of cefuroxime after intravenous, intramuscular, and subcutaneous administration to dogs. *Journal of Veterinary Pharmacology and Therapeutics* 39(1), 40–44. DOI: 10.1111/jvp.12239.

Albarellos, G.A., Montoya, L., Passini, S.M., Lupi, M.P., Lorenzini, P.M. *et al.* (2017) Cefazolin pharmacokinetics in cats under surgical conditions. *Journal of Feline Medicine and Surgery* 19(10), 992–997. DOI: 10.1177/1098612X16666594.

Allerton, F. and Nuttall, T. (2021) Antimicrobial use: importance of bacterial culture and susceptibility testing. *In Practice* 43(9), 500–510. DOI: 10.1002/inpr.139.

Atwood, C., Maxwell, M., Butler, R. and Wills, R. (2015) Effects of incision closure method on infection prevalence following tibial plateau leveling osteotomy in dogs. *Canadian Veterinary Journal* 56(4), 375–381.

Barsanti, J.A. (2012) Genitourinary Infections. In: Greene, C.E. (ed.) *Infectious Diseases of the Dog and Cat*, 4th edn. Elsevier, St Louis, Missouri, pp. 1013–1044.

Beal, M.W., Brown, D.C. and Shofer, F.S. (2000) The effects of perioperative hypothermia and the duration of anesthesia on postoperative wound infection rate in clean wounds: a retrospective study. *Veterinary Surgery* 29(2), 123–127. DOI: 10.1111/j.1532-950x.2000.00123.x.

Bellows, J., Berg, M.L., Dennis, S., Harvey, R., Lobprise, H.B. *et al.* (2019) 2019 AAHA Dental Care Guidelines for Dogs and Cats. *Journal of the American Animal Hospital Association* 55(2), 49–69. DOI: 10.5326/JAAHA-MS-6933.

Bergeron, M.G. (1986) Tissue penetration of antibiotics. *Clinical Biochemistry* 19(2), 90–100. DOI: 10.1016/s0009-9120(86)80054-6.

Bergström, A., Dimopoulou, M. and Eldh, M. (2016) Reduction of surgical complications in dogs and cats by the use of a surgical safety checklist. *Veterinary Surgery* 45(5), 571–576. DOI: 10.1111/vsu.12482.

Berríos-Torres, S.I., Umscheid, C.A., Bratzler, D.W., Leas, B., Stone, E.C. *et al.* (2017) Centers for disease control and prevention guideline for the prevention of surgical site infection, 2017. *JAMA Surgery* 152(8), 784–791. DOI: 10.1001/jamasurg.2017.0904.

Boothe, D.M. and Boothe, H.W. (2015) Antimicrobial considerations in the perioperative patient. *Veterinary Clinics of North America: Small Animal Practice* 45(3), 585–608. DOI: 10.1016/j.cvsm.2015.01.006.

Bratzler, D.W., Dellinger, E.P., Olsen, K.M., Perl, T.M., Auwaerter, P.G. *et al.* (2013) Clinical practice guidelines for antimicrobial prophylaxis in surgery. *American Journal of Health-System Pharmacy* 70(3), 195–283. DOI: 10.2146/ajhp120568.

Brown, D.C., Conzemius, M.G., Shofer, F. and Swann, H. (1997) Epidemiologic evaluation of postoperative wound infections in dogs and cats. *Journal of the American Veterinary Medical Association* 210(9), 1302–1306.

Brown, G., Maddox, T. and Baglietto Siles, M.M. (2016) Client-assessed long-term outcome in dogs with surgical site infection following tibial plateau levelling osteotomy. *Veterinary Record* 179(16), 409. DOI: 10.1136/vr.103688.

BSAVA/SAMSoc (2018) *BSAVA/SAMSoc Guide to Responsible Use of Antibacterials: PROTECT ME.* British Small Animal Veterinary Association/Small Animal Medicine Society, Quedgeley, UK. Available at: www.bsavalibrary.com/content/book/10.22233/9781910443644 (accessed 30 October 2022).

Budsberg, S.C., Torres, B.T. and Sandberg, G.S. (2021) Efficacy of postoperative antibiotic use after tibial plateau leveling osteotomy in dogs: a systematic review. *Veterinary Surgery* 50, 729–739.

Buote, N.J., Kovak-McClaran, J.R., Loar, A.S. and Cherrone, K.L. (2012) The effect of preoperative antimicrobial administration on culture results in dogs undergoing cystotomy. *Journal of the American Veterinary Medical Association* 241, 1185–1189.

Burke J.F. (1961) The effective period of preventive antibiotic action in experimental incisions and dermal lesions. *Surgery* 50, 161–168.

Cagnardi, P., Di Cesare, F., Toutain, P.L., Bousquet-Mélou, A., Ravasio, G. et al. (2018) Population pharmacokinetic study of cefazolin used prophylactically in canine surgery for susceptibility testing breakpoint determination. *Frontiers in Pharmacology* 9, 1137. DOI: 10.3389/fphar.2018.01137.

Classen, D.C., Evans, R.S., Pestotnik, S.L., Horn, S.D., Menlove, R.L. et al. (1992) The timing of prophylactic administration of antibiotics and the risk of surgical-wound infection. *New England Journal of Medicine* 326, 281–286. DOI: 10.1056/NEJM199201303260501.

Clutterbuck, A.L., Woods, E.J., Knottenbelt, D.C., Clegg, P.D., Cochrane, C.A. et al. (2007) Biofilms and their relevance to veterinary medicine. *Veterinary Microbiology* 121(1–2), 1–17. DOI: 10.1016/j.vetmic.2006.12.029.

Costerton, J.W., Lewandowski, Z., Caldwell, D.E., Korber, D.R. and Lappin-Scott, H.M. (1995) Microbial biofilms. *Annual Review of Microbiology* 49, 711–745.

Daude-Lagravei, A., Carozzo, C., Fayolle, P., Yiguier, E., Viateau, Y. et al. (2001) Infection rates in surgical procedures: a comparison of cefalexin vs. a placebo. *Veterinary and Comparative Orthopaedics and Traumatology* 14(03), 146–150. DOI: 10.1055/s-0038-1632689.

de Jonge, S.W., Gans, S.L., Atema, J.J., Solomkin, J.S., Dellinger, P.E. et al. (2017) Timing of preoperative antibiotic prophylaxis in 54,552 patients and the risk of surgical site infection: A systematic review and meta-analysis. *Medicine* 96(29), e6903. DOI: 10.1097/MD.0000000000006903.

de Jonge, S.W., Boldingh, Q.J.J., Solomkin, J.S., Dellinger, E.P., Egger, M. et al. (2020) Effect of postoperative continuation of antibiotic prophylaxis on the incidence of surgical site infection: a systematic review and meta-analysis. *Lancet Infectious Diseases* 20(10), 1182–1192. DOI: 10.1016/S1473-3099(20)30084-0.

Demetriou, J.L., Foale, R.D., Ladlow, J., McGrotty, Y., Faulkner, J. et al. (2002) Canine and feline pyothorax: a retrospective study of 50 cases in the UK and Ireland. *Journal of Small Animal Practice* 43(9), 388–394. DOI: 10.1111/j.1748-5827.2002.tb00089.x.

Dumville, J.C., Gray, T.A., Walter, C.J., Sharp, C.A., Page, T. et al. (2016) Dressings for the prevention of surgical site infection. *Cochrane Database of Systematic*

Reviews 12(12), CD003091. DOI: 10.1002/14651858.CD003091.pub4.

Dyall, B. and Schmökel, H. (2017) Tibial tuberosity advancement in small-breed dogs using TTA Rapid implants: complications and outcome. *Journal of Small Animal Practice* 58(6), 314–322. DOI: 10.1111/jsap.12654.

Dyall, B.A.R. and Schmökel, H.G. (2018) Surgical site infection rate after hemilaminectomy and laminectomy in dogs without perioperative antibiotic therapy. *Veterinary and Comparative Orthopaedics and Traumatology* 31(3), 202–213. DOI: 10.1055/s-0038-1639365.

Edmiston, C.E., Jr, Leaper, D., Spencer, M., Truitt, K., Litz Fauerbach, L. et al. (2017) Considering a new domain for antimicrobial stewardship: topical antibiotics in the open surgical wound. *American Journal of Infection Control* 45(11), 1259–1266. DOI: 10.1016/j.ajic.2017.04.012.

Enoch, S. and Harding, K. (2003) Wound bed preparation: the science behind the removal of barriers to healing. *Wounds* 15, 213–229.

Espinel-Rupérez, J., Martín-Ríos, M.D., Salazar, V., Baquero-Artigao, M.R. and Ortiz-Díez, G. (2019) Incidence of surgical site infection in dogs undergoing soft tissue surgery: risk factors and economic impact. *Veterinary Record* 6, e000233.

Eugster, S., Schawalder, P., Gaschen, F. and Boerlin, P. (2004) A prospective study of postoperative surgical site infections in dogs and cats. *Veterinary Surgery* 33(5), 542–550. DOI: 10.1111/j.1532-950X.2004.04076.x.

Felippe, W.A.B., Werneck, G.L. and Santoro-Lopes, G. (2007) Surgical site infection among women discharged with a drain *in situ* after breast cancer surgery. *World Journal of Surgery* 31(12), 2293–2299. DOI: 10.1007/s00268-007-9248-3.

Ferrell, C.L., Barnhart, M.D. and Herman, E. (2019) Impact of postoperative antibiotics on rates of infection and implant removal after tibial tuberosity advancement in 1,768 canine stifles. *Veterinary Surgery* 48(5), 694–699. DOI: 10.1111/vsu.13250.

Fitzpatrick, N. and Solano, M.A. (2010) Predictive variables for complications after TPLO with stifle inspection by arthrotomy in 1000 consecutive dogs. *Veterinary Surgery* 39(4), 460–474. DOI: 10.1111/j.1532-950X.2010.00663.x.

Frey, T.N., Hoelzler, M.G., Scavelli, T.D., Fulcher, R.P. and Bastian, R.P. (2010) Risk factors for surgical site infection-inflammation in dogs undergoing surgery for rupture of the cranial cruciate ligament: 902 cases (2005-2006). *Journal of the American Veterinary Medical Association* 236(1), 88–94. DOI: 10.2460/javma.236.1.88.

Garcia, C., Benitez, M.E., Grant, D.C. and Barry, S.L. (2020) Subclinical bacteriuria and surgical site infections in dogs with cranial cruciate ligament disease.

Veterinary Surgery 49(7), 1292–1300. DOI: 10.1111/vsu.13503.

Garcia Stickney, D.N. and Thieman Mankin, K.M. (2018) The impact of postdischarge surveillance on surgical site infection diagnosis. *Veterinary Surgery* 47(1), 66–73. DOI: 10.1111/vsu.12738.

Giannetto, J.J. and Aktay, S.A. (2019) Prospective evaluation of surgical wound dressings and the incidence of surgical site infections in dogs undergoing a tibial plateau levelling osteotomy. *Veterinary and Comparative Orthopaedics and Traumatology* 32(1), 18–25. DOI: 10.1055/s-0038-1676352.

Gonzalez, O.J., Renberg, W.C., Roush, J.K., KuKanich, B. and Warner, M. (2017) Pharmacokinetics of cefazolin for prophylactic administration to dogs. *American Journal of Veterinary Research* 78(6), 695–701. DOI: 10.2460/ajvr.78.6.695.

Gosling, M.J. and Martínez-Taboada, F. (2018) Adverse reactions to two intravenous antibiotics (Augmentin and Zinacef) used for surgical prophylaxis in dogs. *Veterinary Record* 182(3), 80. DOI: 10.1136/vr.104496.

Greene, C.E. and Marks, S.L. (2012) Gastrointestinal and intra-abdominal infections. In: Greene, C.E. (ed.) *Infectious Diseases of the Dog and Cat,* 4th edn. Elsevier, St Louis, Missouri, pp. 955–956.

Guardabassi, L., Apley, M., Olsen, J.E., Toutain, P.L. and Weese, S. (2018) Optimization of antimicrobial treatment to minimize resistance selection. *Microbiology Spectrum* 6, ARBA–0018. DOI: 10.1128/microbiolspec.ARBA-0018-2017.

Hagen, C., Singh, A., Weese, J.S., Marshall, Q., Linden, A.Z. *et al.* (2020) Contributing factors to surgical site infection after tibial plateau leveling osteotomy: A follow-up retrospective study. *Veterinary Surgery* 9(5), 930–939. DOI: 10.1111.vsu.13436.

Haney, V., Maman, S., Prozesky, J., Bezinover, D. and Karamchandani, K. (2020) Improving intraoperative administration of surgical antimicrobial prophylaxis: a quality improvement report. *British Medical Journal* 9(3), e001042. DOI: 10.1136/bmjoq-2020-001042.

Hans, E.C., Barnhart, M.D., Kennedy, S.C. and Naber, S.J. (2017) Comparison of complications following tibial tuberosity advancement and tibial plateau levelling osteotomy in very large and giant dogs 50 kg or more in body weight. *Veterinary and Comparative Orthopaedics and Traumatology* 30, 299–305.

Hardefeldt, L.Y., Browning, G.F., Thursky, K., Gilkerson, J.R., Billman-Jacobe, H. *et al.* (2017) Antimicrobials used for surgical prophylaxis by companion animal veterinarians in Australia. *Veterinary Microbiology* 203, 301–307. DOI: 10.1016/j.vetmic.2017.03.027.

Hassan, S., Chan, V., Stevens, J. and Stupans, I. (2021) Factors that influence adherence to surgical antimicrobial prophylaxis (SAP) guidelines: a systematic review. *Systematic Reviews* 10(1), 29. DOI: 10.1186/s13643-021-01577-w.

Hayes, G., Moens, N. and Gibson, T. (2013) A review of local antibiotic implants and applications to veterinary orthopaedic surgery. *Veterinary and Comparative Orthopaedics and Traumatology* 26(4), 251–259. DOI: 10.3415/VCOT-12-05-0065.

Holmberg, D.L. (1985) The use of Prophylactic Penicillin in orthopedic surgery: a clinical trial. *Veterinary Surgery* 14(2), 160–165. DOI: 10.1111/j.1532-950X.1985.tb00850.x.

Kim, S.E., Pozzi, A., Kowaleski, M.P. and Lewis, D.D. (2008) Tibial osteotomies for cranial cruciate ligament insufficiency in dogs. *Veterinary Surgery* 37(2), 111–125. DOI: 10.1111/j.1532-950X.2007.00361.x.

Knights, C.B., Mateus, A. and Baines, S.J. (2012) Current British veterinary attitudes to the use of perioperative antimicrobials in small animal surgery. *Veterinary Record* 170(25), 646. DOI: 10.1136/vr.100292.

Lappin, M.R., Blondeau, J., Boothe, D., Breitschwerdt, E.B., Guardabassi, L. *et al.* (2017) Antimicrobial use guidelines for treatment of respiratory tract disease in dogs and cats: antimicrobial guidelines working group of the international society for companion animal infectious diseases. *Journal of Veterinary Internal Medicine* 31(2), 279–294. DOI: 10.1111/jvim.14627.

Launcelott, Z.A., Lustgarten, J., Sung, J., Samuels, S., Davis, S. *et al.* (2019) Effects of a surgical checklist on decreasing incisional infections following foreign body removal from the gastrointestinal tract in dogs. *Canadian Veterinary Journal* 60(1), 67–72.

Lee, S.J., Frederick, S.W. and Cross, A.R. (2019) Use of an amikacin-infused collagen sponge concurrent with implant removal for treatment of tibial plateau leveling osteotomy surgical site infection in 31 cases. *Veterinary Surgery* 48(5), 700–706. DOI: 10.1111/vsu.13249.

Leigh, H., Harðardottir, H., Schöffmann, G. and Panti, A. (2019) Suspected anaphylaxis after intravenous administration of cefuroxime (Zinacef) in two dogs, with descriptions of arterial blood gas abnormalities over time. *Veterinary Record Case Reports* 7(4), e000922. DOI: 10.1136/vetreccr-2019-000922.

Leta, T.H., Gjertsen, J.-E., Dale, H., Hallan, G., Lygre, S.H.L *et al.* (2021) Antibiotic-loaded bone cement in prevention of periprosthetic joint infections in primary total knee arthroplasty: a register-based multicentre randomised controlled non-inferiority trial (ALBA trial). *British Medical Journal* 11(1), e041096. DOI: 10.1136/bmjopen-2020-041096.

Lopez, D.J., VanDeventer, G.M., Krotscheck, U., Aryazand, Y., McConkey, M.J. *et al.* (2018) Retrospective study of factors associated with surgical site infection in dogs following tibial plateau leveling osteotomy. *Journal of the American Veterinary Medical Association* 253(3), 315–321. DOI: 10.2460/javma.253.3.315.

Love, B.C. and Jones, R.L. (2012) Laboratory diagnosis of bacterial infections. In: Greene, C.E. (ed.) *Infectious*

Diseases of the Dog and Cat, 4th edn. Elsevier, St Louis, Missouri, pp. 277–283.

Marcellin-Little, D.J., Papich, M.G., Richardson, D.C. and DeYoung, D.J. (1996) Pharmacokinetic model for cefazolin distribution during total hip arthroplasty in dogs. *American Journal of Veterinary Research* 57, 720–723.

Martinez, M.N., Papich, M.G. and Drusano, G.L. (2012) Dosing regimen matters: the importance of early intervention and rapid attainment of the pharmacokinetic/pharmacodynamic target. *Antimicrobial Agents and Chemotherapy* 56(6), 2795–2805. DOI: 10.1128/AAC.05360-11.

McHugh, S.M., Collins, C.J., Corrigan, M.A., Hill, A.D.K. and Humphreys, H. (2011) The role of topical antibiotics used as prophylaxis in surgical site infection prevention. *Journal of Antimicrobial Chemotherapy* 66(4), 693–701. DOI: 10.1093/jac/dkr009.

McKellar, Q.A., Sanchez Bruni, S.F. and Jones, D.G. (2004) Pharmacokinetic/pharmacodynamic relationships of antimicrobial drugs used in veterinary medicine. *Journal of Veterinary Pharmacology and Therapeutics* 27(6), 503–514. DOI: 10.1111/j.1365-2885.2004.00603.x.

Miles, A.A. (1956) Nonspecific defense reactions in bacterial infections. *Annals of the New York Academy of Sciences* 66(2), 356–369. DOI: 10.1111/j.1749-6632.1956.tb40141.x.

Miles, A.A., Miles, E.M. and Burke, J. (1957) The value and duration of defence reactions of the skin to the primary lodgement of bacteria. *British Journal of Experimental Pathology* 38(1), 79–96.

National Research Council (1964) Report of an ad hoc committee of the committee on trauma. Postoperative wound infections: the influence of ultraviolet irradiation of the operating room and of various other factors. *Annals of Surgery* 160(Suppl. 2), 1–192.

Nazarali, A., Singh, A. and Weese, J.S. (2014) Perioperative administration of antimicrobials during tibial plateau leveling osteotomy. *Veterinary Surgery* 43(8), 966–971. DOI: 10.1111/j.1532-950X.2014.12269.x.

Nazarali, A., Singh, A., Moens, N.M.M., Gatineau, M., Sereda, C., et al. (2015) Association between methicillin-resistant *Staphylococcus pseudintermedius* carriage and the development of surgical site infections following tibial plateau leveling osteotomy in dogs. *Journal of the American Veterinary Medical Association* 247(8), 909–916. DOI: 10.2460/javma.247.8.909.

Nicholson, M., Beal, M., Shofer, F. and Brown, D.C. (2002) Epidemiologic evaluation of postoperative wound infection in clean-contaminated wounds: a retrospective study of 239 dogs and cats. *Veterinary Surgery* 31(6), 577–581. DOI: 10.1053/jvet.2002.34661.

Nicoll, C., Singh, A. and Weese, J.S. (2014) Economic impact of tibial plateau leveling osteotomy surgical site

infection in dogs. *Veterinary Surgery* 43(8), 899–902. DOI: 10.1111/j.1532-950X.2014.12175.x.

Norgate, D. and Bruniges, N. (2016) Suspected anaphylaxis following intravenous amoxicillin clavulanate administration under general anaesthesia in nine dogs. *Veterinary Record Case Reports* 4(1), e000295. DOI: 10.1136/vetreccr-2016-000295.

Papich, M.G. (2014) Pharmacokinetic-pharmacodynamic (PK-PD) modeling and the rational selection of dosage regimes for the prudent use of antimicrobial drugs. *Veterinary Microbiology* 171(3–4), 480–486. DOI: 10.1016/j.vetmic.2013.12.021.

Pennington, Z., Lubelski, D., Molina, C., Westbroek, E.M., Ahmed, A.K. et al. (2019) Prolonged postsurgical drain retention increases risk for deep wound infection after spine surgery. *World Neurosurgery* 130, e846–e853. DOI: 10.1016/j.wneu.2019.07.013.

Peterson, L.C., Kim, S.E., Lewis, D.D., Johnson, M.D. and Ferrigno, C.R.A. (2021) Calcium sulfate antibiotic-impregnated bead implantation for deep surgical site infection associated with orthopedic surgery in small animals. *Veterinary Surgery* 50(4), 748–757. DOI: 10.1111/vsu.13570.

Rappaport, W.D., Holcomb, M., Valente, J. and Chvapil, M. (1989) Antibiotic irrigation and the formation of intraabdominal adhesions. *American Journal of Surgery* 158(5), 435–437. DOI: 10.1016/0002-9610(89)90281-x.

Rhodes, A., Evans, L.E., Alhazzani, W., Levy, M.M., Antonelli, M. et al. (2017) Surviving sepsis campaign: international guidelines for management of sepsis and septic shock: 2016. *Intensive Care Medicine* 43(3), 304–377. DOI: 10.1007/s00134-017-4683-6.

Schmökel, H., Skytte, D. and Barsch, M. (2021) Infection rate treating radial and ulnar fractures using bone plate fixation without antibiotic prophylaxis. *Journal of Small Animal Practice* 62(12), 1079–1084. DOI: 10.1111/jsap.13407.

Sebastian, S., Liu, Y., Christensen, R., Raina, D.B., Tägil, M. et al. (2020) Antibiotic containing bone cement in prevention of hip and knee prosthetic joint infections: a systematic review and meta-analysis. *Journal of Orthopaedic Translation* 23, 53–60. DOI: 10.1016/j.jot.2020.04.005.

Shapiro, M. and Sacks, T. (1982) A decisive period in cefoxitin prophylaxis of experimental synergistic wound infection produced by *Bacteroides fragilis* and *Escherichia coli*. *Israel Journal of Medical Sciences* 18(8), 863–865.

Solano, M.A., Danielski, A., Kovach, K., Fitzpatrick, N. and Farrell, M. (2015) Locking plate and screw fixation after tibial plateau leveling osteotomy reduces postoperative infection rate in dogs over 50 kg. *Veterinary Surgery* 44(1), 59–64. DOI: 10.1111/j.1532-950X.2014.12212.x.

Spencer, D.D. and Daye, R.M. (2018) A prospective, randomized, double-blinded, placebo-controlled clinical study on postoperative antibiotherapy in 150 arthroscopy-assisted tibial plateau leveling osteotomies in dogs. *Veterinary Surgery* 47(8), E79–E87. DOI: 10.1111/vsu.12958.

Stetter, J., Boge, G.S., Grönlund, U. and Bergström, A. (2021) Risk factors for surgical site infection associated with clean surgical procedures in dogs. *Research in Veterinary Science* 136, 616–621. DOI: 10.1016/j.rvsc.2021.04.012.

Stine, S.L., Odum, S.M. and Mertens, W.D. (2018) Protocol changes to reduce implant-associated infection rate after tibial plateau leveling osteotomy: 703 dogs, 811 TPLO (2006-2014). *Veterinary Surgery* 47(4), 481–489. DOI: 10.1111/vsu.12796.

Stone, H.H., Hooper, C.A., Kolb, L.D., Geheber, C.E. and Dawkins, E.J. (1976) Antibiotic prophylaxis in gastric, biliary and colonic surgery. *Annals of Surgery* 184(4), 443–452. DOI: 10.1097/00000658-197610000-00007.

Summers, A.M., Vezzi, N., Gravelyn, T., Culler, C. and Guillaumin, J. (2021) Clinical features and outcome of septic shock in dogs: 37 Cases (2008-2015). *Journal of Veterinary Emergency and Critical Care* 31(3), 360–370. DOI: 10.1111/vec.13038.

Thieman Mankin, K.M. and Cohen, N.D. (2020) Randomized, controlled clinical trial to assess the effect of antimicrobial-impregnated suture on the incidence of surgical site infections in dogs and cats. *Journal of the American Veterinary Medical Association* 257(1), 62–69. DOI: 10.2460/javma.257.1.62.

Tuan, J., Solano, M.A. and Danielski, A. (2019) Risk of infection after double locking plate and screw fixation of tibial plateau leveling osteotomies in dogs weighing greater than 50 kilograms. *Veterinary Surgery* 48(7), 1211–1217. DOI: 10.1111/vsu.13308.

Turk, R., Singh, A. and Weese, J.S. (2015) Prospective surgical site infection surveillance in dogs. *Veterinary Surgery* 44(1), 2–8. DOI: 10.1111/j.1532-950X.2014.12267.x.

Välkki, K.J., Thomson, K.H., Grönthal, T.S.C., Junnila, J.J.T., Rantala, M.H.J. *et al.* (2020) Antimicrobial prophylaxis is considered sufficient to preserve an acceptable surgical site infection rate in clean orthopaedic and neurosurgeries in dogs. *Acta Veterinaria Scandinavica* 62(1), 53. DOI: 10.1186/s13028-020-00545-z.

van Kasteren, M.E.E., Manniën, J., Ott, A., Kullberg, B.-J., de Boer, A.S. *et al.* (2007) Antibiotic prophylaxis and the risk of surgical site infections following total hip arthroplasty: timely administration is the most important factor. *Clinical Infectious Diseases* 44(7), 921–927. DOI: 10.1086/512192.

Vasseur, P.B., Paul, H.A., Enos, L.R. and Hirsh, D.C. (1985) Infection rates in clean surgical procedures: a comparison of ampicillin prophylaxis vs a placebo. *Journal of the American Veterinary Medical Association* 187(8), 825–827.

Vasseur, P.B., Levy, J., Dowd, E. and Eliot, J. (1988) Surgical wound infection rates in dogs and cats. Data from a teaching hospital. *Veterinary Surgery* 17, 60–64.

VMD (2013) The veterinary medicines regulations 2013. Veterinary Medicines Directorate, Addlestone, UK. Available at: www.legislation.gov.uk/uksi/2013/2033/contents/made (accessed 21 November 2022).

Walker, A.L., Jang, S.S. and Hirsh, D.C. (2000) Bacteria associated with pyothorax of dogs and cats: 98 cases (1989-1998). *Journal of the American Veterinary Medical Association* 216(3), 359–363. DOI: 10.2460/javma.2000.216.359.

Webb, J.C.J. and Spencer, R.F. (2007) The role of polymethylmethacrylate bone cement in modern orthopaedic surgery. *Journal of Bone and Joint Surgery* 89-B(7), 851–857. DOI: 10.1302/0301-620X.89B7.19148.

Weese, J.S. and Halling, K.B. (2006) Perioperative administration of antimicrobials associated with elective surgery for cranial cruciate ligament rupture in dogs: 83 cases (2003-2005). *Journal of the American Veterinary Medical Association* 229(1), 92–95. DOI: 10.2460/javma.229.1.92.

Weese, J.S., Blondeau, J., Boothe, D., Guardabassi, L.G., Gumley, N. *et al.* (2019) International Society for Companion Animal Infectious Diseases (ISCAID) guidelines for the diagnosis and management of bacterial urinary tract infections in dogs and cats. *Veterinary Journal* 247, 8–25. DOI: 10.1016/j.tvjl.2019.02.008.

Weese, J.S., Faires, M.C., Frank, L.A., Reynolds, L.M. and Battisti, A. (2012) Factors associated with methicillin-resistant versus methicillin-susceptible *Staphylococcus pseudintermedius* infection in dogs. *Journal of the American Veterinary Medical Association* 240(12), 1450–1455. DOI: 10.2460/javma.240.12.1450.

Weese, J.S., Giguère, S., Guardabassi, L., Morley, P.S., Papich, M. *et al.* (2015) ACVIM consensus statement on therapeutic antimicrobial use in animals and antimicrobial resistance. *Journal of Veterinary Internal Medicine* 29(2), 487–498. DOI: 10.1111/jvim.12562.

Whittem, T.L., Johnson, A.L., Smith, C.W., Schaeffer, D.J., Coolman, B.R. *et al.* (1999) Effect of perioperative prophylactic antimicrobial treatment in dogs undergoing elective orthopedic surgery. *Journal of the American Veterinary Medical Association* 215(2), 212–216.

WHO (2009) WHO surgical safety checklist. World Health Organization, Geneva, Switzerland. Available at: www.who.int/teams/integrated-health-services/patient-safety/research/safe-surgery/tool-and-resources (accessed 2 November 2022).

Williams, R.W., Cole, S. and Holt, D.E. (2020) Microorganisms associated with incisional infections after gastrointestinal surgery in dogs and cats.

Veterinary Surgery 49(7), 1301–1306. DOI: 10.1111/vsu.13495.

Windahl, U., Bengtsson, B., Nyman, A.K. and Holst, B.S. (2015) The distribution of pathogens and their antimicrobial susceptibility patterns among canine surgical wound infections in Sweden in relation to different risk factors. *Acta Veterinaria Scandinavica* 57(1), 11. DOI: 10.1186/s13028-015-0102-6.

20 Antimicrobial Use in Medical (Including Chemotherapy) Patients

Fergus Allerton*

Willows Veterinary Centre & Referral Service, Shirley, Solihull, UK

20.1 Introduction

Across Europe, multiple, independent antimicrobial stewardship guidelines have been produced providing recommendations for rational antimicrobial use in cats and dogs (Allerton *et al.*, 2021b). Further system-specific guidance has been produced by the International Society for Companion Animal Infectious Diseases (ISCAID) for management of respiratory tract disease, urinary tract disease and superficial bacterial folliculitis (Hillier *et al.*, 2014; Lappin *et al.*, 2017; Weese *et al.*, 2019). Veterinarians can also seek information relating to antimicrobial selection and dosing from reference texts on infectious disease in small animals (Greene, 2012), internal medicine (Ettinger *et al.*, 2017; Nelson and Couto, 2019) and drug formularies (Plumb, 2018; Allerton, 2020).

Inevitably, guidelines cannot cover the entire spectrum of potential clinical presentations, and whenever a gap is present, users must either select the most appropriately matched recommendation given the observed clinical signs ('symptom mapping') or pursue additional investigations to reduce the diagnostic uncertainty. A common theme in antimicrobial use guidelines is the promotion of organism identification via cytology, bacterial culture and advanced microbiological techniques; a recommendation to this effect was identified in all evaluated European antimicrobial stewardship guidelines (Allerton *et al.*, 2021b). Demonstration of an infectious aetiology may confer greater confidence to prescribe antimicrobials, although there are important exceptions, such as subclinical bacteriuria in cats (Dorsch *et al.*, 2019), dogs (Weese *et al.*, 2019) and people (Zalmanovici Trestioreanu *et al.*, 2015) where antimicrobial therapy is not warranted despite the presence of bacterial organisms.

Given the financial limitations inherent to veterinary medicine, guidelines must account for syndromic-based diagnoses and, where appropriate, support empirical antibiotic therapy decisions. Furthermore, demonstration of a causative infectious agent is not always feasible, as collection of a representative sample may be technically challenging (e.g. cholecystocentesis) or potentially unsafe for the patient (e.g. tracheal wash or bronchoalveolar lavage in a respiratory-compromised animal). In such cases, the decision to prescribe may, reasonably, be reliant on a suspicion of infection. One of the important functions of antimicrobial use guidelines is to identify situations where a combination of clinical signs may have a sufficient positive predictive value to warrant instigation of antimicrobial therapy while avoiding use where an infectious aetiology is less likely. This dichotomy may best be illustrated by the differing significance of lower urinary tract signs in dogs and cats. In female dogs presenting with dysuria, haematuria and pollakiuria, the likelihood that a urinary tract infection (UTI) is present is high (Sørensen *et al.*, 2019). However, a similar clinical presentation in a cat would rarely be attributable to bacterial involvement; feline interstitial cystitis (a sterile condition) is a much more probable explanation (Dorsch *et al.*, 2019).

20.2 Treatment of Sepsis

Given the health risks from multidrug resistance, it is understandable that the underlying message of much antimicrobial use guidance, as here, espouses the reduction (or at least optimization) of

*fergus.allerton@willows.uk.net

antimicrobial use. Promotion of rational use and antimicrobial stewardship is essential to reduce the future development of untreatable infections. However, it is still important to recognize that there are situations where antibiotics can make a life-saving difference. Of an estimated 49 million sepsis cases worldwide in people in 2017, there were 11 million sepsis-related deaths, with nearly 3 million of these being children under the age of 5 years (Rudd *et al.*, 2020). Mortality rates for sepsis in people range from 15% to 56% (Bauer *et al.*, 2020), in part reflecting differing levels of access to effective antibiotics. It is estimated that sepsis accounted for nearly 20% of all global deaths (Rudd *et al.*, 2020), emphasizing the need for timely and efficacious therapeutic intervention. The incidence of sepsis among veterinary patients is unknown, but the mortality rate is of a similar magnitude at 20–65% (Abelson *et al.*, 2013; Dickinson *et al.*, 2015).

Given the time-critical implications to patient well-being, in the management of sepsis, treatment must sometimes be started before the presence of infection is proven. A delay in instigating antibiotics has been associated with poorer outcomes in people with sepsis (Kumar, 2016; Levy *et al.*, 2018), as well as in severe bacterial infections (Zasowski *et al.*, 2020) and acute bacterial meningitis (Køster-Rasmussen *et al.*, 2008). The concept of patient harm through delay could be seen as an argument to abandon stewardship principles in certain scenarios and use antibiotics 'just in case'. It is thus important to find ways to view sepsis and antimicrobial resistance (AMR) as two sides of the same coin, rather than as competitors (Fitzpatrick *et al.*, 2019).

Whenever clinicians act without diagnostic certainty, they must carefully balance the risks of failing to treat an active infection against overdiagnosis, overtreatment and potentiating AMR. In an ideal world, antibiotic prescription frequency would correlate directly with the likelihood of significant bacterial infection (Fig. 20.1). Unsurprisingly, actual prescribing habits will manifest with both overprescribers (situated above the line) and their parsimonious colleagues (the underprescribers) who (hypothetically at least) risk increased patient morbidity by withholding treatment. Treading the fine line in the middle remains the aim of the game.

The first critical step in the pathway of sepsis management is to accurately recognize a septic patient. Such a consideration should only be envisaged in a pet with a sepsis-compatible history,

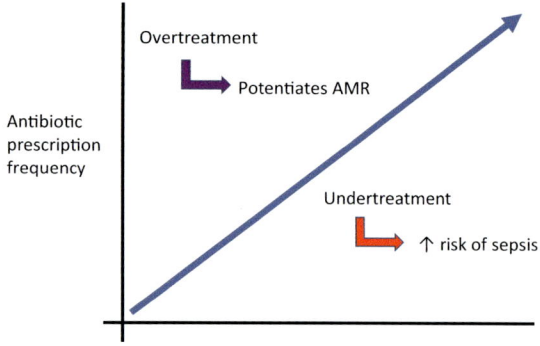

Fig. 20.1. Graphical representation of the dependence of antibiotic prescription on the likelihood of significant bacterial infection. AMR, antimicrobial resistance.

clinical signs and physical examination findings to avoid false positives. The currently accepted definition of sepsis in cats and dogs is based on the presence of sufficient criteria (minimum of two out of four) of the systemic inflammatory response syndrome (SIRS) *and* demonstration of an infectious cause (see Table 20.1) (Hauptman *et al.*, 1997; Brady *et al.*, 2000; Greiner *et al.*, 2008; Babyak and Sharp, 2016). The latter part of this equation is typically more challenging and more time consuming. It is important to remember that SIRS is a clinical state and not a disease itself; an underlying cause of the patient's malaise must still be sought. This investigation is particularly relevant when determining the need for antibiotic therapy, because SIRS can also be seen in association with non-infectious insults (e.g. pancreatitis).

The 2016 Sepsis-3 consensus (applicable to people) defines sepsis as life-threatening organ dysfunction caused by a dysregulated host response to infection (Singer *et al.*, 2016). Organ dysfunction is suspected based on the criteria described in the sequential organ failure assessment (SOFA) score (Vincent *et al.*, 1998). Recently, the prognostic value of a quick SOFA (qSOFA) score has been assessed in veterinary patients with sepsis (Stastny *et al.*, 2022). The qSOFA score is determined by assigning 1 point for each observable change in mentation (dullness, obtundation or stupor), respiration (respiratory rate greater than 22 breaths min^{-1}) or systolic blood pressure (hypotension less than 100 mmHg measured by Doppler). Dogs with qSOFA scores over 2 were found to be more likely to die or be euthanized (Stastny *et al.*, 2022);

Fergus Allerton

Table 20.1. Criteria for systemic inflammatory response syndrome.

Criterion	Cat	Dog
Temperature (°C)	<37.8 or ≥39.7	<38.1 or ≥39.2
Heart rate (beats min^{-1})	<140 or >225	>120
Respiratory rate (breaths min^{-1})	>40	>20
White blood cell count (× 10^9 l^{-1})	<5.0 or >19.5	<6.0 or >16
Band cells (%)	>5	>5

however, the potential of the score to differentiate SIRS from sepsis has not been investigated. Severely affected septic patients may manifest organ dysfunction, hypoperfusion and hypotension. Animals with septic shock may present with hypotension that is refractory to volume expansion consequent to the prolonged presence of bacteria within the bloodstream.

The suspicion of sepsis should be increased in any pet presenting with an acute (and marked) clinical deterioration or that has a known septic focus (e.g. pyothorax, septic peritonitis, mastitis, septic arthritis or pyometra (Goggs and Letendre, 2019)). Demonstration of a putative pathogen should be sufficient to settle the question regarding the need for antibiotic therapy. But what happens when the presence of bacteria (or their causative role) cannot readily be established? Are there any indicators (or combinations thereof) that automatically warrant antibiotic treatment? Frustratingly, septic animals often have a vague presentation. Clinical signs may include lethargy, weakness, gastrointestinal signs (vomiting, diarrhoea, loss of appetite, abdominal discomfort), altered respiration (tachypnoea, dyspnoea, polypnoea), pyrexia, focal swelling (e.g. periarticular) and malodorous wounds. Reliable, patient-side biomarkers are eagerly sought to differentiate infection from inflammation (and determine a need for antibiotics), but these are yet to be made commercially available in cats and dogs.

In patients with an abdominal effusion, confirmation of septic peritonitis can be achieved cytologically with a high (up to 100%) specificity if intracellular bacteria are seen (Bonczynski et al., 2003). However, failing to detect bacteria does not exclude the presence of infection because sensitivity reaches only 70%. Effusion and blood biomarkers have been evaluated as potential surrogate markers

of infection; effusion lactate greater than 4.2 mmol l^{-1} was considered the most discriminant biomarker with a sensitivity of 72% and specificity of 84% for septic peritonitis (Martiny and Goggs, 2019). The blood-effusion glucose gradient (with a cutoff of less than 2.06 mmol l^{-1}) was more sensitive (90%) but less specific (67%) in this population (Martiny and Goggs, 2019). Despite their limitations, at least these biomarkers are readily available in practice and can afford additional confidence to guide antibiotic use decisions. In people, levels of procalcitonin increased in parallel with the severity of the inflammatory insult and may be more specific indicators of infection than other acute-phase proteins (Schuetz et al., 2011). Efforts to validate a procalcitonin assay in dogs have been disappointing to date (Floras et al., 2014; Battaglia et al., 2020), but this remains a promising opportunity for the future in both dogs (Goggs et al., 2018) and cats (Cho et al., 2021).

In summary, in people, both the seriousness of sepsis and the need for rapid and effective antibiotic therapy are well established. By extrapolation and, supported by the limited data available for dogs and cats, similar conclusions may be assumed in these species. When sepsis is suspected, the decision to use antibiotics is a logical sequitur. The choice of this antibiotic may be guided by consideration of the most probable bacterial pathogen based on the apparent provenance of infection. The most common bacteria isolated from septic cats and dogs are Gram-negative (e.g. Escherichia coli), although mixed infections and pure Gram-positive infections (usually enterococci or streptococci) are also described. Table 20.2 lists some of the more commonly isolated bacteria from different infections that can provoke a septic state. More precise organism identification (or at least a more finely narrowed list of possibilities) may be achieved by recognizing bacterial morphology (rods or cocci) as well as staining patterns (e.g. Gram staining) while awaiting the culture and antibiotic susceptibility testing results (Allerton and Nuttall, 2021).

Where a particular bacterium is implicated or suspected, a knowledge of typical resistance patterns can help guide antibiotic selection (Allerton and Nuttall, 2021). In septic patients, sample collection should ideally be performed prior to starting antibiotic medication. Where a septic focus is not evident, submission of blood cultures is recommended. Empirical antibiotic selection should factor in the most likely causal organism, the origin

Table 20.2. Common bacterial pathogens that could be implicated as causes of bacteraemia/sepsis by site of infection.

Site of suspected infection	Potential bacterial pathogens	
	Dog	Cat
Soft tissue and skin (e.g. deep pyoderma and wounds)	***Staphylococcus spp.*** *Pseudomonas spp.* *Escherichia coli* *Enterococcus* spp.	***Pasteurella* spp.**
Urinary tract	***Escherichia coli*** *Staphylococcus* spp. *Proteus mirabilis*	***Escherichia coli*** *Enterococcus spp.* *Staphylococcus* spp.
Bone and joint	***Staphylococcus* spp.** *Streptococcus* spp. *Escherichia coli*	
Gastrointestinal tract (e.g. septic peritonitis)	***Escherichia coli*** *Enterococcus* spp. *Pasteurella* spp. *Staphylococcus* spp.	*Escherichia coli* *Enterococcus* spp. *Pasteurella* spp. *Staphylococcus* spp.
Hepatobiliary infections (e.g. hepatic abscess, biliary peritonitis)	***Escherichia coli*** *Enterococcus* spp. *Bacteroides* spp. *Clostridium* spp.	***Escherichia coli*** *Enterococcus* spp. *Bacteroides* spp. *Clostridium* spp.
Respiratory tract (e.g. bronchopneumonia and pneumonia)	*Escherichia coli* *Bordetella bronchiseptica* *Streptococcus* spp.	*Pasteurella* spp. *Bordetella bronchiseptica* *Mycoplasma* spp.
Pyothorax	*Pasteurella* spp. *Escherichia coli* *Staphylococcus* spp. *Corynebacterium* *Nocardia*	***Pasteurella* spp.** *Bacteroides* spp. *Fusobacterium* spp.
Reproductive tract (e.g. pyometra)	***Escherichia coli*** *Staphylococcus* spp. *Streptococcus* spp.	
Mastitis	***Escherichia coli*** *Staphylococcus* spp. *Streptococcus* spp.	
Central nervous system, ocular, prostate[a]	***Escherichia coli*** *Staphylococcus* spp. *Streptococcus* spp.	

The organisms encountered most frequently are shown in bold.

[a]These sites should be considered separately, and medications must be lipid soluble in order to cross the protective barriers.

of the infection and the capacity of the antibiotic to penetrate the relevant tissues, as well as consideration of any recent antibiotic use or hospital stay in the patient. Patient outcome was not affected in dogs with septic peritonitis whether or not empirical antibiotic selection was appropriate (based on antibiotic susceptibility testing) (Dickinson *et al.*, 2015; Kalafut *et al.*, 2018). However, for dogs that received antibiotic therapy in the 30 days prior to the diagnosis, there was an increased likelihood of being given inappropriate antibiotics at the time of surgery (Dickinson *et al.*, 2015).

If the septic focus is uncertain, initial treatment should cover Gram-positive, Gram-negative, aerobic and anaerobic bacteria. A broad-spectrum product such as amoxicillin-clavulanate supplemented with an aminoglycoside or a fluoroquinolone (to improve the Gram-negative coverage) is proposed in many antibiotic use guidelines (e.g. AFVAC, 2017; BSAVA/SAMSoc, 2018; Danish

Fergus Allerton

Veterinary Association, 2018). As soon as culture results become available, treatment should be de-escalated (i.e. the spectrum of cover narrowed) in accordance with the susceptibility profile. Should the culture prove to be negative but an underlying bacterial aetiology remains likely, de-escalation of treatment should be based on regular clinical re-evaluation of the patient.

Chemotherapy disrupts cell division and replication. As granulocytes have the shortest lifespan (4–8 h for neutrophils), impaired neutrophil production, especially around the nadir for that chemotherapeutic agent, can lead to significant neutropenia. Should the neutrophil count drop below 1×10^9 l^{-1}, there is an increased chance that the patient may develop infection and sepsis. Chemotherapy-induced neutropenia may be identified during routine haematological screening at or around the anticipated nadir. This induced absence of natural immunity increases the risk of sepsis. Therefore, it is critically important to protect vulnerable patients from this threat and to identify patients that may already be affected by bacterial infection. Clinical signs of chemotherapy-induced neutropenia, including lethargy, weakness and inappetance, are common but may also be attributable to the primary neoplastic process or to effects of the chemotherapy that are not mediated in the bone marrow. Documentation of pyrexia as well as other signs of sepsis (tachycardia, brick-red mucous membranes, hypotension and altered mentation) should alert the clinician to the possibility of an important infection and the need for prompt intervention.

Appropriate antimicrobial prophylaxis can be warranted in the context of the critical infection risk in chemotherapy patients. The recommendations to use antibiotics for chemotherapy-induced neutropenia are guided by the absolute neutrophil count. When the neutrophils are below 0.75×10^9 l^{-1}, the use of a broad-spectrum antibiotic is recommended for 3 days, or until the count increases above this threshold (Bisson *et al.*, 2018). For more details of the approach to immunosuppressed patients, see Chapter 15 (this volume).

The rationale for using antibiotic therapy in patients with sepsis is clear cut. However, as outlined above, the index of suspicion of a septic state is variable, and veterinarians must apply clinical reasoning to guide their prescribing habits. For pets presenting in more clinically stable situations, the critical need for antibiotic therapy is inherently less, and there is an opportunity to delay antibiotic treatment to observe the patient's clinical progression. Any decision to prescribe or not to prescribe is multifactorial. Weighing up these choices to maintain rational antibiotic use will be the focus of the next section.

20.3 To Use or Not To Use?

Antibiotic use guidelines detail multiple common presentations where the recommendation is that antibiotic administration is *unnecessary*. Animals in this category are more likely to be managed as outpatients, and the responsible veterinarian should reassure themselves that recovery is not dependent on antibiotic therapy. Herein lies the key dilemma based on an asymmetric calculation. In favour of antibiotic prescription, the clinician may cite the clinical benefit *should* there be an underlying infectious aetiology and the avoidance/limitation of clinical deterioration *should* sepsis develop. External factors including perceived client pressure and practice policy may also play a role. However, antibiotics (similar to all medications) can cause adverse effects that may be harmful to the patient, and there is a nebulous risk of promoting AMR, imposing a danger of the patient developing future infections that are more challenging to treat and, from a One Health perspective, increasing the number of multidrug-resistant bacteria in the environment.

In an era where clinicians increasingly endeavour to adhere to evidence-based veterinary medicine, it would be ideal if we could refer to the results of randomized controlled trials comparing meaningful outcomes for pets managed with and without antibiotics for each indication. Sadly, this information is rarely available, and recommendations are inescapably based on expert opinion, extrapolation from other species and anecdotal experience. Consultation data reviewed by the Small Animal Veterinary Surveillance Network (SAVSNET) and the Veterinary Companion Animal Surveillance System (VetCompass) offer an indication of the proportion of consultations in which antibiotic therapy is prescribed. This can be further broken down according to the principal motive for consultation.

20.3.1 Gastrointestinal disease

Accounting for 3% of all canine consultations and 2% of those in cats, gastrointestinal disease

(Singleton *et al.*, 2019a) is a frequent issue in small animal veterinary medicine. In a recent SAVSNET survey, half of all cases of canine acute diarrhoea (duration of less than 3 days) were prescribed an antibiotic (Singleton *et al.*, 2019b), matching previous surveillance data showing that 45–70% of dogs presenting with diarrhoea received antibiotics (Anholt *et al.*, 2014; Jones *et al.*, 2014; Singleton *et al.*, 2017). The likelihood of antibiotic prescription was higher if the diarrhoea contained blood or if the dog was pyrexic at presentation, although 36% of normothermic dogs with mild, acute, non-haemorrhagic diarrhoea were still prescribed antibiotics (Singleton *et al.*, 2019b). Although the rationale for individual clinical decisions cannot be reviewed retrospectively, this study alone described more than 1000 instances of systemic antibiotic prescription for a condition that is typically benign and likely to resolve without such treatment.

Indeed, all 15 of the antibiotic use guidelines identified in Europe (Allerton *et al.*, 2021b) recommend not using antibiotics to manage acute diarrhoea. A review of enteropathogenic bacteria also advised against the need for antibiotics stating: 'Most bacterial enteropathogens are associated with self-limiting diarrhoea, and injudicious administration of antimicrobials could be more harmful than beneficial' (Marks *et al.*, 2011). Even in the case of acute haemorrhagic diarrhoea syndrome (AHDS), previously termed haemorrhagic gastroenteritis, there is increasing evidence to suggest that antibiotics are not required (Unterer *et al.*, 2011, 2015; Mortier *et al.*, 2015). Encouragingly, this is one area where a randomized, placebo-controlled trial has been completed demonstrating the non-inferiority, in terms of morbidity and mortality, for dogs with AHDS of receiving a placebo compared with systemic amoxicillin-clavulanate (Unterer *et al.*, 2015). Another randomized trial performed in primary practice found no difference in outcome for dogs receiving amoxicillin-clavulanate versus those on amoxicillin-clavulanate and metronidazole (Ortiz *et al.*, 2018).

Another randomized, double-blinded, placebo-controlled clinical trial looked at the effect of metronidazole treatment on the duration of acute diarrhoea (Langlois *et al.*, 2020). A statistically significant reduction in the duration of diarrhoea was found in the metronidazole-treated group (mean time reduced from 3.6 to 2.1 days). While this study supports antibiotic use in this patient cohort, it is important to balance the clinical benefit against the wider impact of treatment. When evaluating the value of antibiotic treatments (or absence thereof), study investigators must select outcomes that are relevant to the principal stakeholders (in this case, the pet, the owner and wider society). While even a modest reduction in the duration of diarrhoea is likely to be appreciated by owners, the implications of increased use of metronidazole could include host-level effects, such as perturbation of the gastrointestinal microbiome (Pilla *et al.*, 2020), occasional risk of drug toxicity and long-term loss of efficacy (Gobeli *et al.*, 2012), as well as wider societal risks from potentiating AMR.

Avoidance (or at least judicial use) of antimicrobials is also recommended for the management of chronic diarrhoea (Cerquetella *et al.*, 2020); this group of veterinary gastroenterologists positioned antibiotic use *after* exhaustion of appropriate dietary trials and ideally with supportive histopathology from gastrointestinal biopsies. This advice represents a fundamental change in the classic approach to chronic enteropathy cases whereby a therapeutic trial with metronidazole, tylosin or oxytetracycline was frequently performed to address potential antibiotic-responsive diarrhoea. However, the proportion of cases that benefit from such treatment is likely to be small (Volkmann *et al.*, 2017), and non-antibiotic treatments (e.g. prebiotics, probiotics or faecal matter transplantation) hold promise to address intestinal dysbiosis and improve clinical signs without recourse to antibiotics.

The bottom line is that gastrointestinal disease offers very few indications for justified antibiotic use. For pets with acute or chronic diarrhoea (and/or vomiting), deferral of antibiotic therapy is recommended unless the patient has concurrent signs consistent with sepsis (see earlier). Given the frequency of consultation for gastrointestinal disease, adoption of non-antibiotic therapies could greatly reduce total antibiotic use with minimal to no detriment to our patients.

20.3.2 Respiratory tract disease

Respiratory disease accounts for approximately 1% of all consultations in both cats and dogs (Arsevska *et al.*, 2018; Singleton *et al.*, 2019c). Coughing was the most frequently reported clinical sign in dogs (68%), while sneezing (46%) and nasal discharge (30%) were more commonly seen in cats (Singleton *et al.*, 2019c). Data for 2019 found that systemic antibiotics were prescribed in 37% of consultations for canine respiratory disease compared with 49% for cats; these figures were nearly 25% lower than 5 years earlier, while other pharmaceutical classes remained unchanged (Singleton *et al.*, 2019c), which may be interpreted as improved antibiotic stewardship.

Feline upper respiratory tract disease (fURTD) describes a cluster of clinical signs (ocular and nasal discharge, sneezing and conjunctivitis). Viral pathogens (feline herpes virus 1 and feline calicivirus) are implicated in the majority of cases. However, bacteria including *Chlamydophila felis*, *Bordetella bronchiseptica* and *Mycoplasma* spp. may play a primary role in some cats. The aspect of the nasal discharge can offer some indication of secondary bacterial involvement (deemed more likely if there is a mucopurulent or purulent component). However, even if acute bacterial involvement is suspected, the ISCAID working group recommend a period of observation without immediate use of antibiotics (Lappin *et al.*, 2017). Intervention with antibiotics is only appropriate within this initial 10-day observation period if the cat presents with concurrent pyrexia, lethargy or anorexia alongside mucopurulent nasal discharge; additional supportive measures (appetite stimulation, assisted nutrition and analgesia) may be considered in the first instance. Most cats with fURTD will improve within 10 days with or without antibiotics. Data from Switzerland (Hubbuch *et al.*, 2020) suggest that these recommendations (despite being included in the national AntibioticScout stewardship tool) are infrequently followed, as 68% of cats with acute fURTD in 2018 were administered antibiotics for a median duration of 10 days. This was down from 77% of cases in 2016 (Hubbuch *et al.*, 2020).

There is no denying that fURTD can be a frustrating condition to manage, especially as the chronic form can be both persistent and recurrent, causing debilitation and impaired quality of life for some cats. In cats with signs lasting more than 10 days and where a bacterial component is identified (based on compatible clinical signs and exclusion of other explanations via appropriate diagnostic investigations), a therapeutic antibiotic trial may be warranted. The ISCAID working group advise selecting an antibiotic for this purpose on the basis of culture and susceptibility test results using samples from nasal lavage/brushings or nasal tissue biopsy, rather than culture of the nasal discharge (Lappin *et al.*, 2017). It should be remembered that a complete cure may not be achievable, and the cat may experience repeat opportunistic infections, potentially with antibiotic-resistant bacteria. For this reason, the use of antibiotics in fURTD should be restricted to cats with severe clinical signs.

Canine infectious respiratory disease complex (kennel cough or canine infectious tracheobronchitis) can be caused by several viruses (canine parainfluenza, canine adenovirus type 2, canine herpesvirus and others) with or without involvement of bacteria (*B. bronchiseptica* or *Mycoplasma canis*). Despite this acknowledged bacterial component, guidelines recommend delaying antibiotic therapy in the first 10 days of clinical signs to allow time for spontaneous recovery. The dog's immune system will be able to clear the infection effectively in the vast majority of cases, negating the need for antibiotics. A similar positive outcome may be anticipated in most people with a new cough without antibiotics; despite guidance to refrain from prescribing antibiotics in such cases, respiratory disease remains an important example of overprescription in people (Dekker *et al.*, 2015; Imanpour *et al.*, 2017).

Inflammation of the lungs (pneumonia or pneumonitis) can have a bacterial aetiology in dogs and cats, most commonly secondary to viral or parasitic infections, inhaled foreign bodies or aspiration events. Various bacteria have been isolated from small animal patients with pneumonia including *E. coli*, *Klebsiella pneumoniae*, *Pasteurella multocida*, *Streptococcus canis*, *B. bronchiseptica*, and *Enterococcus*, *Mycoplasma* and *Pseudomonas* spp. The presentation of respiratory signs (cough, tachypnoea/dyspnoea/polypnoea) with associated pyrexia is indicative of the presence of pneumonia. Clinicopathological findings (neutrophilic leucocytosis and increased C-reactive protein) and thoracic radiological findings (alveolar lung disease) may be seen with bacterial involvement, but collection of a transtracheal wash or bronchoalveolar lavage is necessary for pathogen demonstration and identification. Not all small animals are sufficiently stable for such procedures; a bronchoalveolar lavage fluid sample was collected in less than 6% of dogs with suspected aspiration pneumonia seen at two tertiary referral practices in the USA (Howard *et al.*, 2021).

Urgent empirical antibiotic therapy to treat suspected bacterial pneumonia has been recommended even in situations where samples are not or cannot be collected (Lappin *et al.*, 2017). However, there is an increasing recognition that antibiotics may not be required for all cases of aspiration, as clinical signs may be a consequence of chemical pneumonitis rather than bacterial infection. Indeed, antibiotic drug administration in people with aspiration pneumonia is considered controversial (Dragan et al., 2018); a distinct clinical benefit is rare, and treatment could generate selective pressures favouring antibiotic-resistant strains, posing an increased risk for patients that experience repeat aspiration events.

A recent study by Cook et al. (2021) reported the successful management of 14 cases of aspiration pneumopathy (compatible radiographic or endotracheal wash findings) without the use of antibiotics. Of note, some of the dogs included in this study presented with signs of respiratory distress, hypoxaemia, pyrexia and evidence of systemic inflammation (increased C-reactive protein, and neutrophilia or neutropenia), but still made a rapid (within 12–36 h) and complete recovery without antibiotic treatment. This is insufficient evidence to withhold antibiotics in all cases of suspected aspiration, and a thorough assessment of patient stability and the severity of respiratory distress is necessary to determine the decision. Close monitoring during the initial 24 h (with delayed antibiotic instigation) may be appropriate, provided the patient makes a clinical improvement. This is an area that would benefit from additional investigation to establish optimal antibiotic protocols across the spectrum of presentations where a dog has or is suspected to have aspirated.

As observed for gastrointestinal disease, dogs and cats presenting with signs of respiratory tract disease should be critically appraised prior to considering antibiotic use. The need for antibiotic therapy is likely to be appropriate in just a minority of presentations, and there would appear to be considerable further scope to reduce antibiotic prescription in this context. While the presence of bacteria in parts of the respiratory tract may be demonstrable, their causative role in disease pathogenicity is less convincingly established. Furthermore, the possibility of spontaneous patient recovery should not be overlooked, and an approach of patient observation, during which antibiotic therapy is delayed, may be applicable in most situations. Antibiotics can be introduced later in any patient that fails to improve or deteriorates clinically during monitoring.

20.3.3 Urinary tract disease

Bacterial UTIs, typically diagnosed presumptively based on clinical signs alone, account for 6–12% of antimicrobial prescriptions in dogs (Rantala et al., 2004; De Briyne et al., 2014; Lutz et al., 2020). Female dogs are markedly over-represented due to their shorter urethral length. The previous classification system of uncomplicated or complicated UTIs mirrored the terminology used in human medicine. However, there are important interspecies differences. A novel nomenclature has been introduced, defining all initial or infrequent (fewer than three episodes of cystitis in the preceding year) presentations in non-gravid females as 'canine sporadic cystitis', even if urinary tract abnormalities or comorbidities are present (Weese et al., 2019).

Sporadic cystitis may be suspected based on the presentation of compatible lower urinary tract signs (pollakiuria, dysuria/stranguria and haematuria). Retrospective analysis showed that 46–65% of dogs with one or more of this triad of clinical signs had bacterial infection confirmed by culture (Windahl et al., 2014; Sørensen et al., 2018, 2019). Bacterial culture and antimicrobial susceptibility testing are recommended to confirm bacterial involvement and optimize antimicrobial selection. It is recognized that samples for culture may not be collected routinely in veterinary practice and empirical therapy is routinely instigated presumptively. In human medicine, cultures were requested in only 10–40% of cases of suspected UTI, despite high levels (74–94%) of antibiotic use (Ironmonger et al., 2016; Spek et al., 2020). All guidelines must strike a balance between dogmatism and pragmatism, recognizing both the financial and practical implications of mandating additional diagnostics.

The guidance relating to antibiotic use for management of UTIs must take into account the location of infection. Involvement of the upper urinary tract (e.g. pyelonephritis) or prostate imposes different considerations in terms of diagnostic investigations and antibiotic selection. Table 20.3 offers a summary of guideline recommendations (informed largely by the updated ISCAID guidelines for the diagnosis and management of bacterial UTIs in dogs and cats; Weese et al., 2019) for different presentations of canine UTI.

The presence of bacteria in the urine may be demonstrated in patients absent lower urinary tracts signs (a state of subclinical bacteriuria). This finding may arise due to the inclusion of bacterial culture

Table 20.3. A summary of guidance for antibiotic decision making when managing urinary tract infections in dogs. Based on the recommendations of Weese et al. (2019).

	Sporadic cystitis	Recurrent cystitis	Prostatitis	Pyelonephritis	Subclinical bacteriuria
Population at risk	Healthy non-pregnant females or neutered males	Healthy non-pregnant females or neutered males	Intact male dogs	All dogs	All dogs *including* those with hyperadrenocorticism and diabetes mellitus
Compatible clinical signs	Pollakiuria Dysuria/stranguria Haematuria	Three or more episodes of sporadic cystitis in the preceding 12 months *or* a single recurrence in the preceding 3 months	Pollakiuria Dysuria/stranguria Haematuria	Pyrexia Lethargy Polyuria/polydipsia Renal pain Note that some dogs have vague signs only	None (by definition)
Diagnostics	Urine culture recommended[a]	Urine culture essential; identify risk factors and comorbidities via imaging ± cystoscopy + mucosal biopsies	Prostate palpation (per rectum) Blood work Urine ± prostatic fluid culture Ultrasound (size and structure)	Blood work: azotaemia, peripheral neutrophilia ± left shift Urinalysis: cylindruria. Urine culture essential (consider pyelocentesis)	Urine culture *not* indicated
Treatment	Consider analgesics only pending culture results	Initial approach as for sporadic cystitis	Prostatic abscesses require surgical or ultrasound-guided percutaneous drainage Consider castration	Start antibiotic therapy immediately	NA
Antibiotic	Follow AST *or* amoxicillin (if available) > amoxicillin-clavulanate Trimethoprim-sulfonamides	Guided by AST	Fluoroquinolone Trimethoprim-sulphonamides	Fluoroquinolone (enrofloxacin (not cats), marbofloxacin) IV or PO (if eating) Guided by AST once available	None
Duration	3–5 days	3–5 days for reinfection 7–14 days for persistent/relapsing infections	4–6 weeks for chronic prostatitis Consider a shorter course if acute	10–14 days	NA

Continued

Table 20.3. Continued

	Sporadic cystitis	Recurrent cystitis	Prostatitis	Pyelonephritis	Subclinical bacteriuria
Monitoring	Pursue further investigations (urinalysis and research of complicating factors) if no clinical response within 48 h of starting antibiotics	Consider urinalysis after 5–7 days of treatment	Monitor prostatic size via palpation/imaging	Repeat blood work and urinalysis 1–2 weeks after antibiotic cessation	NA
Additional points	Rely on clinical resolution. Post-treatment urinalysis *not* recommended unless LUT signs persist	Consider urinalysis 5–7 days after cessation of antibiotics			In dogs unable to display LUT signs (e.g. spinal cord injury), consider antibiotic treatment if systemic signs (e.g. pyrexia) develop

[a]Samples for culture should be collected by cystocentesis wherever possible and processed within 24 h. Voided (or catheter-collected) samples should be interpreted with caution due to risk of contamination.

AST, antimicrobial susceptibility testing; IV, intravenous; LUT; lower urinary tract; NA, not applicable; PO, per os.

Fergus Allerton

in many commercial laboratory urine profiles and should be managed appropriately to avoid unnecessary antibiotic use. There is no evidence that pets with subclinical bacteriuria are likely to progress to a clinically relevant infection. Subclinical bacteriuria is reported in 2–12% of healthy dogs (McGhie *et al.*, 2014; Wan *et al.*, 2014; Garcia *et al.*, 2020) and 1–13% of healthy cats (Eggertsdóttir *et al.*, 2011; White *et al.*, 2016). Importantly, in people there is a widely accepted consensus (backed by systematic reviews and meta-analyses) that antibiotic treatment is not indicated for management of subclinical bacteriuria (Zalmanovici Trestioreanu *et al.*, 2015; Köves *et al.*, 2017).

When cystitis becomes a recurrent issue (either due to relapse of persistence of a stubborn infection or repeated reinfection), further investigations should be pursued to look for a potential nidus of infection or underlying anatomic or immunological mechanisms that predispose the patient to recurrence. Certain comorbidities, including endocrine disease (diabetes mellitus and hyperadrenocorticism), immunosuppressive therapies or chronic kidney disease, can impair bacterial clearance. Abnormal urogenital conformation (e.g. vulval hooding or ectopic ureters) can impair innate defences against ascending bacteria. The presence of uroliths or bladder mucosal changes (e.g. polypoid cystitis) or concurrent prostatitis can harbour bacterial infections beyond standard antibiotic course lengths, prompting recurrence upon treatment withdrawal.

As mentioned in the introduction to this chapter, lower urinary tract disease in cats should be considered differently. Only a small minority of cats (1–8%) with lower urinary tract signs will have an underlying bacterial cause (Kruger *et al.*, 1991; Buffington *et al.*, 1997; Gerber *et al.*, 2005). Feline idiopathic (or interstitial) cystitis or urolithiasis accounts for the vast majority of such presentations. Consequently, feline lower urinary tract disease should not routinely be managed with antibiotics. This is one of the conditions included in the British Small Animal Veterinary Association (BSAVA)/Small Animal Medicine Society (SAMSoc) non-prescription form. If a UTI is confirmed in a cat, the recommendations outlined for dogs can be applied accordingly.

20.4 The Non-Prescription Form

Veterinarians can feel pressurized by clients to provide antibiotics (Smith *et al.*, 2018). Owner expectations may be derived from their pet's apparent prior favourable response to antibiotics or extrapolation of their own experience. Doctors reported similar constraints, prompting the creation of resources to support doctor–patient communication regarding the advantages and disadvantages of antibiotic prescription. Doctors can make use of a delayed prescription practice (whereby an antibiotic prescription is provided but postdated for several days in the future) or provide a non-prescription form that offers advice for management of a condition without recourse to antibiotics. A Cochrane collaboration analysis of three different prescribing strategies used in people (immediate antibiotic prescription, delayed prescription or no prescription) found no difference in patient outcome across the groups and a marked reduction in antibiotic use for the non-prescription cohort compared with both immediate and delayed approaches (Spurling *et al.*, 2017).

A non-prescription form (see Fig. 17.2, Chapter 17, this volume) has been produced by BSAVA and SAMSoc to support vets to share a message of rational antibiotic use with the pet owner. The objective of this form is to demonstrate that a clinical decision (in the best interests of their pet) has been made not to prescribe antibiotics. Alternative options for case management are incorporated (e.g. recommendation to feed a bland diet in the case of acute diarrhoea or to increase water turnover for cats with feline lower urinary tract disease) as well as safety netting advice to get back in contact with the vet should there be any clinical deterioration or failure to improve in a specified timeframe. The utility of this resource has not been investigated in a veterinary setting.

20.5 Conditions of Use

The sections above provide some suggestions as to when antibiotic prescription may be appropriate in cats and dogs with sepsis or gastrointestinal, respiratory or urinary tract disease. The remainder of this chapter will focus on the means of antibiotic administration and the important considerations when choosing the optimal antibiotic molecule.

The European Medicines Agency (EMA) Antimicrobial Advice Ad Hoc Expert Group (AMEG) has recently categorized antibiotics based on the need for their use in veterinary medicine alongside the potential consequences to public

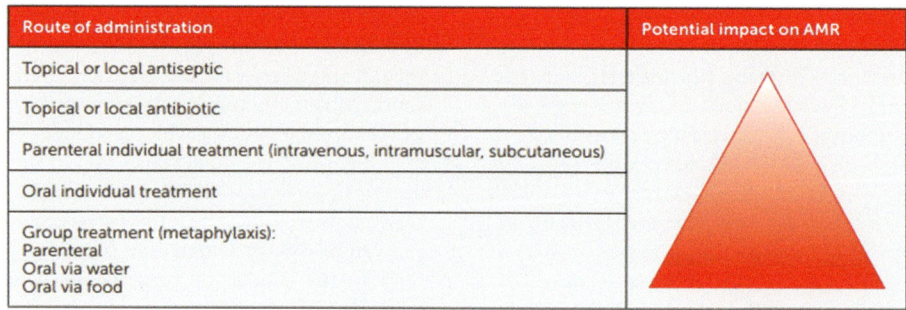

Route of administration	Potential impact on AMR
Topical or local antiseptic	
Topical or local antibiotic	
Parenteral individual treatment (intravenous, intramuscular, subcutaneous)	
Oral individual treatment	
Group treatment (metaphylaxis): Parenteral Oral via water Oral via food	

Fig. 20.2. A modified version of the European Medicines Agency pyramid of means of antibiotic administration. Reproduced from Nuttall (2021) courtesy of BSAVA/Companion.

health from increased AMR (EMA, 2020a) (see Chapter 17, this volume, for more details on antibiotic tiers). The AMEG document also takes into account the likely impact of the route of drug administration on AMR (Fig. 20.2) (Nuttall, 2021). Topical or local treatment can achieve high therapeutic concentrations at the site of infection while minimizing exposure of non-target bacteria at other sites (e.g. the gastrointestinal microbiome). Systemic administration inevitably treats the whole organism, including the bacteria that make up the microbiome. Parenteral therapy may result in a more modest impact on the gut microbiome compared with oral therapy (Rochegüe *et al.*, 2021). With the increasing availability of microbiome analysis, it is likely that awareness of the negative effects of antibiotics on the microbiome will improve in the coming years, opening the door to restorative treatments (Connelly *et al.*, 2019; Pilla *et al.*, 2020).

Intravenous antibiotic therapy is recommended initially for the management of severe life-threatening infections to ensure that adequate antibiotic concentrations are reached at the site of infection (McCarthy and Avent, 2020). Evidently, the intravenous route is also preferable in pets that are dehydrated, unable to take oral drugs or are vomiting. Parenteral treatment may be considered in pets that have a temperament that precludes oral drug administration. That said, this does not justify the selection of a long-acting injectable antibiotic purely for reasons of convenience. Transition from intravenous to oral medication is recommended to facilitate discharge from hospital and to reduce the risk of catheter-associated infections (phlebitis).

20.6 Will It Get to Where It Is Needed?

To be effective, antibiotic administered by any route needs to be able to access the target site of infection. For this reason, nitrofurantoin is only an appropriate option for the treatment of UTIs as it will fail to achieve therapeutic levels in any other tissues. Similarly, oral neomycin is not absorbed from the gastrointestinal tract meaning that it is only appropriate to treat enteric bacteria. Antibiotics used to treat prostatitis must adequately cross the blood–prostate barrier. Weakly alkaline, lipid soluble antibiotics with a high pKa are most suitable including trimethoprim (but not the sulphonamides) and the fluoroquinolones (Niżański *et al.*, 2014). These two antibiotic classes are therefore recommended options for the management of prostatitis.

20.7 Broad Versus Narrow Spectrum

Amoxicillin is a time-dependent, broad-spectrum antibiotic with efficacy against Gram-positive and -negative bacteria implicated as uropathogens in dogs and cats. Amoxicillin is also concentrated in urine, potentially overcoming β-lactamase resistance. Amoxicillin is considered equipotent with amoxicillin-clavulanate in the management of UTIs in small animals (Weese *et al.*, 2019) and is a narrower-spectrum agent. Selection of the minimum spectrum of activity necessary helps reduce bacterial exposure to antibiotics, reducing promotion of resistance. However, currently, amoxicillin-clavulanate remains the most commonly prescribed antimicrobial tablet in Europe (EMA, 2020b), accounting for 44% of antimicrobial prescriptions in first-opinion practices in the UK (Mateus *et al.*,

Fergus Allerton

2011). The EMA AMEG guidelines categorize amoxicillin-clavulanate in the higher ('caution') category compared with amoxicillin ('prudence'), emphasizing that from a stewardship perspective, the latter would be preferred (EMA, 2020a). Hopefully, with increased familiarity and altered practice stocking policies, a transition towards a lower-tier antibiotic approach will be possible without any negative impact on treatment efficacy.

20.8 Could Antibiotics Make Things Worse?

Avoidance of harm is a key principle of veterinary medicine. Any and all medications have the potential to elicit adverse effects in the recipient, some of which may be anticipated while others are idiosyncratic. Acute kidney injury and nosocomial *Clostridioides difficile* infections are well-documented, serious, adverse effects associated with antibiotic use in people (Patek *et al.*, 2020; Lee *et al.*, 2021) but a whole range of complications can arise from antibiotic use (Mohsen *et al.*, 2020), at significant cost to the health system (Beringer *et al.*, 1998). Figure 20.3 from the BSAVA/SAMSoc (2018) PROTECT ME poster lists some of the more commonly seen adverse effects associated with antibiotic use in cats and dogs. Interestingly, a study in the USA found that physician concern relating to joint damage in children caused by fluoroquinolones has driven avoidance of the antibiotic class in this patient cohort (Patel and Goldman, 2016). Inadvertently, the fear of a relatively uncommon adverse effect has contributed to improved antibiotic stewardship. Given that adverse effects are greatly underreported in veterinary medicine, wherever possible, steps should be taken to minimize negative patient impact during antibiotic treatment.

20.9 Shorter is Better

Until recently, a parting refrain from the doctor has been to 'always complete the course'. This advice was derived from the fear of bacterial resistance emerging in undertreated patients. However, antibiotic course length is inherently arbitrary at the best of times and based on multiples of five or seven for convenience purposes, rather than any experimentally measured properties of the target infection. In medicine, things are starting to change

as Constantine units are abandoned in favour of shorter (evidence-based) courses of antibiotic. The new idea is that shorter is better, and certainly non-inferiority of shorter-duration antibiotic courses has been demonstrated via randomized controlled trials for multiple infectious conditions (Spellberg, 2018; Spellberg and Rice, 2019). Administration of antibiotics beyond what is absolutely necessary imposes a selective pressure favouring resistance and increases the likelihood of drug-related adverse events.

Relatively few trials have been performed comparing different antibiotic treatment durations in cats and dogs. A 3-day course of enrofloxacin was not inferior to 14 days of amoxicillin-clavulanate for the treatment of bacterial UTIs in dogs (Westropp *et al.*, 2012). Similarly, a short (3-day) course of trimethoprim/sulfonamide was non-inferior to 10 days of cephalexin in sporadic cystitis in female dogs (Clare *et al.*, 2014). However, these studies are also comparing different antibiotics, limiting the conclusions that can be drawn. An ongoing study – the Stop on Sunday trial (Allerton *et al.*, 2021a) – is looking to establish the optimal duration of amoxicillin-clavulanate for treatment of presumptive UTIs in female dogs. This project (and others under way in Denmark and the USA) will hopefully generate robust data to inform the optimal duration of antibiotic treatment for this common presentation, minimizing unnecessary overtreatment.

Outdated recommendations for prolonged antibiotic courses (for example, 4–6 weeks of antibiotics for aspiration pneumonia or complicated cystitis) are being replaced by shorter and more dynamic approaches (Lappin *et al.*, 2017; Weese *et al.*, 2019). The use of surrogate markers of inflammation such as C-reactive protein to guide the decision to discontinue therapy in aspiration pneumonia (Viitanen *et al.*, 2017) has the potential to benefit the patient and simultaneously improve antibiotic stewardship.

20.10 Conclusion

All prescribers must critically evaluate their patients and decide first whether or not there is a requirement for an antibiotic and then select a preferred agent, dose and duration. Antibiotic use guidance, based predominantly on expert opinion and extrapolation from recommendations from human medicine,

ADVERSE REACTIONS TO ANTIBACTERIALS

This list is not comprehensive.

Antimicrobial	Adverse effect	At risk group	Recommendation
Aminoglycosides	Nephrotoxicity	Dogs/cats with pre-existing renal disease, volume or electrolyte depletion	Avoid in at risk animals or when close monitoring is not available Do not exceed 7 days treatment duration Monitor urine for casts
	Ototoxicity	Cats	
Amoxicillin/ clavulanate (intravenous use)	Urticaria, hypotension Anaphylactoid reactions	Dogs under general anaesthesia	Caution with intravenous use in anaesthetized patients
Doxycycline or clindamycin	Oesophageal irritation ± stricture	Cats (>dogs)	Ensure administration with food or water
Enrofloxacin	Retinal degeneration leading to partial, temporary or total blindness	Cats	Alternative fluoroquinolones preferred in cats
Fluoroquinolones	Defective cartilage development leading to severe lameness	Young dogs	Avoid in growing animals
Metronidazole	Dose-dependent neurotoxicity	Dogs	Caution with higher doses
Penicillins	Immediate and delayed hypersensitivity reactions	Dogs/cats	Avoid in penicillin-sensitive animals/ owners
Potentiated sulphonamides	Keratoconjunctivitis sicca Hepatic necrosis (rare) Immune complex reactions (polyarthritis, anaemia, thrombocytopenia)	Dogs esp. Dobermanns, Samoyeds and Miniature Schnauzers	Avoid in specified breeds Monitor Schirmer Tear Test before and during use

Fig. 20.3. Some of the adverse effects associated with certain commonly used antibiotics. Reproduced from the PROTECT ME poster courtesy of BSAVA/SAMSoc (BSAVA/BSAVA/SAMSoc, 2018).

Fergus Allerton

can support veterinary practitioners in reaching an optimal decision that will optimize the outcome for their patient while minimizing the promotion of AMR. Antibiotic stewardship is essential to help preserve antibiotic efficacy for future generations of people, cats and dogs, swinging the pendulum back towards effective management of infectious disease.

References

Abelson, A.L., Buckley, G.J. and Rozanski, E.A. (2013) Positive impact of an emergency department protocol on time to antimicrobial administration in dogs with septic peritonitis. *Journal of Veterinary Emergency and Critical Care (San Antonio, Tex* 23(5), 551–556. DOI: 10.1111/vec.12092.

AFVAC (2017) Guide de bonnes pratiques. Fiches de recommandations pour un bon usage des antibiotiques: filière animaux de compagnie. L'Association Française des Vétérinaires pour Animaux de Compagnie, Paris. Available at: www.veterinaire.fr/fileadmin/user_upload/images/CRO/Languedoc-Roussillon/actualites/AB_afvac-fiches-antibiotiques-nov16.pdf (accessed 2 November 2022).

Allerton, F. (ed.) (2020) *BSAVA Small Animal Formulary*, 10th edn. British Small Animal Veterinary Association, Quedgeley, UK.

Allerton, F. and Nuttall, T. (2021) Antimicrobial use: importance of bacterial culture and susceptibility testing. *In Practice* 43(9), 500–510. DOI: 10.1002/inpr.139.

Allerton, F., Pouwels, K.B., Bazelle, J., Caddy, S., Cauvin, A, et al. (2021b) Prospective trial of different antimicrobial treatment durations for presumptive canine urinary tract infections. *BMC Veterinary Research* 17(1), 299. DOI: 10.1186/s12917-021-02974-y.

Allerton, F., Prior, C., Bagcigil, A.F., Broens, E., Callens, B, et al. (2021a) Overview and evaluation of existing guidelines for rational antimicrobial use in small-animal veterinary practice in Europe. *Antibiotics* 10(4), 409. DOI: 10.3390/antibiotics10040409.

Anholt, R.M., Berezowski, J., Ribble, C.S., Russell, M.L. and Stephen, C. (2014) Using informatics and the electronic medical record to describe antimicrobial use in the clinical management of diarrhea cases at 12 companion animal practices. *PloS One* 9(7), e103190. DOI: 10.1371/journal.pone.0103190.

Arsevska, E., Priestnall, S.L., Singleton, D.A., Jones, P.H., Smyth, S. et al. (2018) Small animal disease surveillance: respiratory disease 2017. *Veterinary Record* 182(13), 369–373. DOI: 10.1136/vr.k1426.

Babyak, J.M. and Sharp, C.R. (2016) Epidemiology of systemic inflammatory response syndrome and sepsis in cats hospitalized in a veterinary teaching hospital. *Journal of the American Veterinary Medical Association* 249(1), 65–71. DOI: 10.2460/javma.249.1.65.

Battaglia, F., Meucci, V., Tognetti, R., Bonelli, F., Sgorbini, M. *et al.* (2020) Procalcitonin detection in veterinary species: investigation of commercial ELISA kits. *Animals* 10(9), E1511. DOI: 10.3390/ani10091511.

Bauer, M., Gerlach, H., Vogelmann, T., Preissing, F., Stiefel, J. *et al.* (2020) Mortality in sepsis and septic shock in Europe, North America and Australia between 2009 and 2019- results from a systematic review and meta-analysis. *Critical Care* 24(1), 239. DOI: 10.1186/s13054-020-02950-2.

Beringer, P.M., Wong-Beringer, A. and Rho, J.P. (1998) Economic aspects of antibacterial adverse effects. *PharmacoEconomics* 13, 35–49. DOI: 10.2165/00019053-199813010-00004.

Bisson, J.L., Argyle, D.J. and Argyle, S.A. (2018) Antibiotic prophylaxis in veterinary cancer chemotherapy: a review and recommendations. *Veterinary and Comparative Oncology* 16(3), 301–310. DOI: 10.1111/vco.12406.

Bonczynski, J.J., Ludwig, L.L., Barton, L.J., Loar, A. and Peterson, M.E. (2003) Comparison of peritoneal fluid and peripheral blood pH, bicarbonate, glucose, and lactate concentration as a diagnostic tool for septic peritonitis in dogs and cats. *Veterinary Surgery* 32(2), 161–166. DOI: 10.1053/jvet.2003.50005.

Brady, C.A., Otto, C.M., Van Winkle, T.J. and King, L.G. (2000) Severe sepsis in cats: 29 cases (1986-1998). *Journal of the American Veterinary Medical Association* 217(4), 531–535. DOI: 10.2460/javma.2000.217.531.

BSAVA/SAMSoc (2018) *BSAVA/SAMSoc Guide to Responsible Use of Antibacterials: PROTECT ME*. British Small Animal Veterinary Association/Small Animal Medicine Society, Quedgeley, UK. Available at: www.bsavalibrary.com/content/book/10.22233/9781910443644 (accessed 2 November 2022).

Buffington, C.A., Chew, D.J., Kendall, M.S., Scrivani, P.V., Thompson, S.B. *et al.* (1997) Clinical evaluation of cats with nonobstructive urinary tract diseases. *Journal of the American Veterinary Medical Association* 210(1), 46–50.

Cerquetella, M., Rossi, G., Suchodolski, J.S., Schmitz, S.S., Allenspach, K. *et al.* (2020) Proposal for rational antibacterial use in the diagnosis and treatment of dogs with chronic diarrhoea. *Journal of Small Animal Practice* 61(4), 211–215. DOI: 10.1111/jsap.13122.

Cho, J.-G., Oh, Y.-I., Song, K.-H. and Seo, K.-W. (2021) Evaluation and comparison of serum procalcitonin and heparin-binding protein levels as biomarkers of bacterial infection in cats. *Journal of Feline Medicine and Surgery* 23(4), 370–374. DOI: 10.1177/1098612X20959973.

Clare, S., Hartmann, F.A., Jooss, M., Bachar, E., Wong, Y.Y. *et al.* (2014) Short- and long-term cure rates of short-duration trimethoprim-sulfamethoxazole treatment in female dogs with uncomplicated bacterial cystitis. *Journal of Veterinary Internal Medicine* 28(3), 818–826. DOI: 10.1111/jvim.12324.

Connelly, S., Fanelli, B., Hasan, N.A., Colwell, R.R. and Kaleko, M. (2019) Low dose oral beta-lactamase protects the gut microbiome from oral beta-lactam-mediated damage in dogs. *AIMS Public Health* 6(4), 477–487. DOI: 10.3934/publichealth.2019.4.477.

Cook, S., Greensmith, T. and Humm, K. (2021) Successful management of aspiration pneumopathy without antimicrobial agents: 14 dogs (2014-2021). *Journal of Small Animal Practice* 62(12), 1108–1113. DOI: 10.1111/jsap.13409.

Danish Veterinary Association (2018) *Antibiotic Use Guidelines for Companion Animal Practice*. Available at: www.ddd.dk/media/2175/assembled_final.pdf (accessed 1 May 2022).

De Briyne, N., Atkinson, J., Pokludová, L. and Borriello, S.P. (2014) Antibiotics used most commonly to treat animals in Europe. *Veterinary Record* 175(13), 325. DOI: 10.1136/vr.102462.

Dekker, A.R.J., Verheij, T.J.M. and van der Velden, A.W. (2015) Inappropriate antibiotic prescription for respiratory tract indications: most prominent in adult patients. *Family Practice* 32(4), 401–407. DOI: 10.1093/fampra/cmv019.

Dickinson, A.E., Summers, J.F., Wignal, J., Boag, A.K. and Keir, I. (2015) Impact of appropriate empirical antimicrobial therapy on outcome of dogs with septic peritonitis. *Journal of Veterinary Emergency and Critical Care* 25(1), 152–159. DOI: 10.1111/vec.12273.

Dorsch, R., Teichmann-Knorrn, S. and Sjetne Lund, H. (2019) Urinary tract infection and subclinical bacteriuria in cats: a clinical update. *Journal of Feline Medicine and Surgery* 21(11), 1023–1038. DOI: 10.1177/1098612X19880435.

Dragan, V., Wei, Y., Elligsen, M., Kiss, A., Walker, S.A.N. *et al.* (2018) Prophylactic antimicrobial therapy for acute aspiration pneumonitis. *Clinical Infectious Diseases* 67(4), 513–518. DOI: 10.1093/cid/ciy120.

Eggertsdóttir, A.V., Sævik, B.K., Halvorsen, I. and Sørum, H. (2011) Occurrence of occult bacteriuria in healthy cats. *Journal of Feline Medicine and Surgery* 13(10), 800–803. DOI: 10.1016/j.jfms.2011.07.004.

EMA (2020a) *EMA Categorisation of Antibiotics for Use in Animals for Prudent and Responsible Use*. European Medicines Agency, Amsterdam, Netherlands. Available at: www.ema.europa.eu/en/documents/report/infographic-categorisation-antibiotics-use-animals-prudent-responsible-use_en.pdf (accessed 2 November 2022).

EMA (2020b) *Sales of Veterinary Antimicrobial Agents in 31 European Countries in 2018*. European Surveillance of Veterinary Antimicrobial Consumption (ESVAC), 10th Report. European Medicines Agency, Amsterdam, Netherlands. Available at: www.ema.europa.eu/en/documents/report/sales-veterinary-antimicrobial-agents-31-european-countries-2018-trends-2010-2018-tenth-esvac-report_en.pdf (accessed 2 November 2022).

Ettinger, S.J., Feldman, E.C. and Côté, E. (eds) (2017) *Textbook of Veterinary Internal Medicine: Diseases of the Dog and the Cat*, 8th edn. Elsevier, St Louis, Missouri.

Fitzpatrick, F., Tarrant, C., Hamilton, V., Kiernan, F.M., Jenkins, D. *et al.* (2019) Sepsis and antimicrobial stewardship: two sides of the same coin. *BMJ Quality & Safety* 28(9), 758–761. DOI: 10.1136/bmjqs-2019-009445.

Floras, A.N.K., Holowaychuk, M.K., Hodgins, D.C., Marr, H.S., Birkenheuer, A. *et al.* (2014) Investigation of a commercial ELISA for the detection of canine procalcitonin. *Journal of Veterinary Internal Medicine* 28(2), 599–602. DOI: 10.1111/jvim.12309.

Garcia, C., Benitez, M.E., Grant, D.C. and Barry, S.L. (2020) Subclinical bacteriuria and surgical site infections in dogs with cranial cruciate ligament disease. *Veterinary Surgery* 49(7), 1292–1300. DOI: 10.1111/vsu.13503.

Gerber, B., Boretti, F.S., Kley, S., Laluha, P., Müller, C. *et al.* (2005) Evaluation of clinical signs and causes of lower urinary tract disease in European cats. *Journal of Small Animal Practice* 46(12), 571–577. DOI: 10.1111/j.1748-5827.2005.tb00288.x.

Gobeli, S., Berset, C., Burgener, I. and Perreten, V. (2012) Antimicrobial susceptibility of canine *Clostridium perfringens* strains from Switzerland. *Schweizer Archiv Fur Tierheilkunde* 154(6), 247–250. DOI: 10.1024/0036-7281/a000340.

Goggs, R. and Letendre, J.A. (2019) Evaluation of the host cytokine response in dogs with sepsis and noninfectious systemic inflammatory response syndrome. *Journal of Veterinary Emergency and Critical Care* 29(6), 593–603. DOI: 10.1111/vec.12903.

Goggs, R., Milloway, M., Troia, R. and Giunti, M. (2018) Plasma procalcitonin concentrations are increased in dogs with sepsis. *Veterinary Record Open* 5(1), e000255. DOI: 10.1136/vetreco-2017-000255.

Greene, C.E. (ed) (2012) *Infectious Diseases of the Dog and Cat*, 4th edn. Elsevier, St Louis, Missouri.

Greiner, M., Wolf, G. and Hartmann, K. (2008) A retrospective study of the clinical presentation of 140 dogs and 39 cats with bacteraemia. *Journal of Small Animal Practice* 49(8), 378–383. DOI: 10.1111/j.1748-5827.2008.00546.x.

Hauptman, J.G., Walshaw, R. and Olivier, N.B. (1997) Evaluation of the sensitivity and specificity of diagnostic criteria for sepsis in dogs. *Veterinary Surgery* 26(5), 393–397. DOI: 10.1111/j.1532-950x.1997.tb01699.x.

Hillier, A., Lloyd, D.H., Weese, J.S., Blondeau, J.M., Boothe, D. *et al.* (2014) Guidelines for the diagnosis and antimicrobial therapy of canine superficial bacterial folliculitis (Antimicrobial Guidelines Working

Fergus Allerton

Group of the International Society for Companion Animal Infectious Diseases). *Veterinary Dermatology* 25(3), 163–e43. DOI: 10.1111/vde.12118.

Howard, J., Reinero, C.R., Almond, G., Vientos-Plotts, A., Cohn, L.A. *et al*. (2021) Bacterial infection in dogs with aspiration pneumonia at 2 tertiary referral practices. *Journal of Veterinary Internal Medicine* 35(6), 2763–2771. DOI: 10.1111/jvim.16310.

Hubbuch, A., Schmitt, K., Lehner, C., Hartnack, S., Schuller, S. *et al*. (2020) Antimicrobial prescriptions in cats in Switzerland before and after the introduction of an online antimicrobial stewardship tool. *BMC Veterinary Research* 16(1), 229. DOI: 10.1186/s12917-020-02447-8.

Imanpour, S., Nwaiwu, O., McMaughan, D.K., DeSalvo, B. and Bashir, A. (2017) Factors associated with antibiotic prescriptions for the viral origin diseases in office-based practices, 2006-2012. *JRSM Open* 8(8), 2054270417717668. DOI: 10.1177/2054270417717668.

Ironmonger, D., Edeghere, O., Gossain, S. and Hawkey, P.M. (2016) Use of antimicrobial resistance information and prescribing guidance for management of urinary tract infections: survey of general practitioners in the West Midlands. *BMC Infectious Diseases* 16, 226. DOI: 10.1186/s12879-016-1559-2.

Jones, P.H., Dawson, S., Gaskell, R.M., Coyne, K.P., Tierney, A. *et al*. (2014) Surveillance of diarrhoea in small animal practice through the Small Animal Veterinary Surveillance Network (SAVSNET). *Veterinary Journal* 201(3), 412–418. DOI: 10.1016/j.tvjl.2014.05.044.

Kalafut, S.R., Schwartz, P., Currao, R.L., Levien, A.S. and Moore, G.E. (2018) Comparison of initial and postlavage bacterial culture results of septic peritonitis in dogs and cats. *Journal of the American Animal Hospital Association* 54(5), 257–266. DOI: 10.5326/JAAHA-MS-6651.

Køster-Rasmussen, R., Korshin, A. and Meyer, C.N. (2008) Antibiotic treatment delay and outcome in acute bacterial meningitis. *Journal of Infection* 57(6), 449–454. DOI: 10.1016/j.jinf.2008.09.033.

Köves, B., Cai, T., Veeratterapillay, R., Pickard, R., Seisen, T. *et al*. (2017) Benefits and harms of treatment of asymptomatic bacteriuria: a systematic review and meta-analysis by the European Association of Urology Urological Infection Guidelines Panel. *European Urology* 72(6), 865–868. DOI: 10.1016/j.eururo.2017.07.014.

Kruger, J.M., Osborne, C.A., Goyal, S.M., Wickstrom, S.L., Johnston, G.R. *et al*. (1991) Clinical evaluation of cats with lower urinary tract disease. *Journal of the American Veterinary Medical Association* 199(2), 211–216.

Kumar, A. (2016) Systematic bias in meta-analyses of time to antimicrobial in sepsis studies. *Critical Care Medicine* 44(4), e234–5. DOI: 10.1097/CCM.0000000000001512.

Langlois, D.K., Koenigshof, A.M. and Mani, R. (2020) Metronidazole treatment of acute diarrhea in dogs: a randomized double blinded placebo-controlled clinical trial. *Journal of Veterinary Internal Medicine* 34(1), 98–104. DOI: 10.1111/jvim.15664.

Lappin, M.R., Blondeau, J., Boothe, D., Breitschwerdt, E.B., Guardabassi, L, *et al*. (2017) Antimicrobial use guidelines for treatment of respiratory tract disease in dogs and cats: antimicrobial guidelines working group of the International Society for Companion Animal Infectious Diseases. *Journal of Veterinary Internal Medicine* 31(2), 279–294. DOI: 10.1111/jvim.14627.

Lee, J.D., Heintz, B.H., Mosher, H.J., Livorsi, D.J., Egge, J.A, *et al*. (2021) Risk of acute kidney injury and *Clostridioides difficile* infection with piperacillin/tazobactam, cefepime, and meropenem with or without vancomycin. *Clinical Infectious Diseases* 73(7), e1579–e1586. DOI: 10.1093/cid/ciaa1902.

Levy, M.M., Evans, L.E. and Rhodes, A. (2018) The surviving sepsis campaign bundle: 2018 update. *Critical Care Medicine* 46(6), 997–1000. DOI: 10.1097/CCM.0000000000003119.

Lutz, B., Lehner, C., Schmitt, K., Willi, B., Schüpbach, G. *et al*. (2020) Antimicrobial prescriptions and adherence to prudent use guidelines for selected canine diseases in Switzerland in 2016. *Veterinary Record Open* 7(1), e000370. DOI: 10.1136/vetreco-2019-000370.

Marks, S.L., Rankin, S.C., Byrne, B.A. and Weese, J.S. (2011) Enteropathogenic bacteria in dogs and cats: diagnosis, epidemiology, treatment, and control. *Journal of Veterinary Internal Medicine* 25(6), 1195–1208. DOI: 10.1111/j.1939-1676.2011.00821.x.

Martiny, P. and Goggs, R. (2019) Biomarker guided diagnosis of septic peritonitis in dogs. *Frontiers in Veterinary Science* 6, 208. DOI: 10.3389/fvets.2019.00208.

Mateus, A., Brodbelt, D.C., Barber, N. and Stärk, K.D.C. (2011) Antimicrobial usage in dogs and cats in first opinion veterinary practices in the UK. *Journal of Small Animal Practice* 52(10), 515–521. DOI: 10.1111/j.1748-5827.2011.01098.x.

McCarthy, K. and Avent, M. (2020) Oral or intravenous antibiotics? *Australian Prescriber* 43(2), 45–48. DOI: 10.18773/austprescr.2020.008.

McGhie, J.A., Stayt, J. and Hosgood, G.L. (2014) Prevalence of bacteriuria in dogs without clinical signs of urinary tract infection presenting for elective surgical procedures. *Australian Veterinary Journal* 92(1–2), 33–37. DOI: 10.1111/avj.12140.

Mohsen, S., Dickinson, J.A. and Somayaji, R. (2020) Update on the adverse effects of antimicrobial therapies in community practice. *Canadian Family Physician* 66(9), 651–659.

Mortier, F., Strohmeyer, K., Hartmann, K. and Unterer, S. (2015) Acute haemorrhagic diarrhoea syndrome in dogs: 108 cases. *Veterinary Record* 176(24), 627. DOI: 10.1136/vr.103090.

Nelson, R.W. and Couto, C.G. (eds) (2019) *Small Animal Internal Medicine*, 6th edn. Elsevier, St Louis, Missouri.

Niżański, W., Levy, X., Ochota, M. and Pasikowska, J. (2014) Pharmacological treatment for common prostatic conditions in dogs - benign prostatic hyperplasia and prostatitis: an update. *Reproduction in Domestic Animals* 49 Suppl 2, 8–15. DOI: 10.1111/rda.12297.

Nuttall, T. (2021) Notes on…: antimicrobial resistance. *BSAVA Companion* 2021, 39–39.

Ortiz, V., Klein, L., Channell, S., Simpson, B., Wright, B. *et al.* (2018) Evaluating the effect of metronidazole plus amoxicillin-clavulanate versus amoxicillin-clavulanate alone in canine haemorrhagic diarrhoea: a randomised controlled trial in primary care practice. *Journal of Small Animal Practice* 59(7), 398–403. DOI: 10.1111/jsap.12862.

Patek, T.M., Teng, C., Kennedy, K.E., Alvarez, C.A. and Frei, C.R. (2020) Comparing acute kidney injury reports among antibiotics: a pharmacovigilance study of the FDA Adverse Event Reporting System (FAERS). *Drug Safety* 43(1), 17–22. DOI: 10.1007/s40264-019-00873-8.

Patel, K. and Goldman, J.L. (2016) Safety concerns surrounding quinolone use in children. *Journal of Clinical Pharmacology* 56(9), 1060–1075. DOI: 10.1002/jcph.715.

Pilla, R., Gaschen, F.P., Barr, J.W., Olson, E., Honneffer, J. *et al.* (2020) Effects of metronidazole on the fecal microbiome and metabolome in healthy dogs. *Journal of Veterinary Internal Medicine* 34(5), 1853–1866. DOI: 10.1111/jvim.15871.

Plumb, D.C. (2018) *Plumb's Veterinary Drug Handbook*, 9th edn. Wiley, Ames, Iowa.

Rantala, M., Hölsö, K., Lillas, A., Huovinen, P. and Kaartinen, L. (2004) Survey of condition-based prescribing of antimicrobial drugs for dogs at a veterinary teaching hospital. *Veterinary Record* 155(9), 259–262. DOI: 10.1136/vr.155.9.259.

Rochegüe, T., Haenni, M., Mondot, S., Astruc, C., Cazeau, G. *et al.* (2021) Impact of antibiotic therapies on resistance genes dynamic and composition of the animal gut microbiota. *Animals* 11(11), 3280. DOI: 10.3390/ani11113280.

Rudd, K.E., Johnson, S.C., Agesa, K.M., Shackelford, K.A., Tsoi, D. *et al.* (2020) Global, regional, and national sepsis incidence and mortality, 1990-2017: analysis for the global burden of disease study. *Lancet* 395(10219), 200–211. DOI: 10.1016/S0140-6736(19)32989-7.

Schuetz, P., Albrich, W. and Mueller, B. (2011) Procalcitonin for diagnosis of infection and guide to antibiotic decisions: past, present and future. *BMC Medicine* 9, 107. DOI: 10.1186/1741-7015-9-107.

Singer, M., Deutschman, C.S., Seymour, C.W., Shankar-Hari, M., Annane, D. *et al.* (2016) The third international consensus definitions for sepsis and septic shock (Sepsis-3). *Journal of the American Medical Association* 315(8), 801–810. DOI: 10.1001/jama.2016.0287.

Singleton, D.A., Sánchez-Vizcaíno, F., Dawson, S., Jones, P.H., Noble, P.J.M. *et al.* (2017) Patterns of antimicrobial agent prescription in a sentinel population of canine and feline veterinary practices in the United Kingdom. *Veterinary Journal* 224, 18–24. DOI: 10.1016/j.tvjl.2017.03.010.

Singleton, D.A., Noble, P.J.M., Sánchez-Vizcaíno, F., Dawson, S., Pinchbeck, G.L. *et al.* (2019a) Pharmaceutical prescription in canine acute diarrhoea: a longitudinal electronic health record analysis of first opinion veterinary practices. *Frontiers in Veterinary Science* 6, 218. DOI: 10.3389/fvets.2019.00218.

Singleton, D.A., Stavisky, J., Jewell, C., Smyth, S., Brant, B. *et al.* (2019b) Small animal disease surveillance 2019: respiratory disease, antibiotic prescription and canine infectious respiratory disease complex. *Veterinary Record* 184(21), 640–645. DOI: 10.1136/vr.l3128.

Singleton, D.A., Arsevska, E., Smyth, S., Barker, E.N., Jewell, C. *et al.* (2019c) Small animal disease surveillance: gastrointestinal disease, antibacterial prescription and *Tritrichomonas foetus*. *Veterinary Record* 184(7), 211–216. DOI: 10.1136/vr.l722.

Smith, M., King, C., Davis, M., Dickson, A., Park, J. *et al.* (2018) Pet owner and vet interactions: exploring the drivers of AMR. *Antimicrobial Resistance and Infection Control* 7, 46. DOI: 10.1186/s13756-018-0341-1.

Sørensen, T.M., Bjørnvad, C.R., Cordoba, G., Damborg, P., Guardabassi, L. *et al.* (2018) Effects of diagnostic work-up on medical decision-making for canine urinary tract infection: an observational study in Danish small animal practices. *Journal of Veterinary Internal Medicine* 32(2), 743–751. DOI: 10.1111/jvim.15048.

Sørensen, T.M., Holmslykke, M., Nordlund, M., Siersma, V. and Jessen, L.R. (2019) Pre-test probability of urinary tract infection in dogs with clinical signs of lower urinary tract disease. *Veterinary Journal* 247, 65–70. DOI: 10.1016/j.tvjl.2019.03.003.

Spek, M., Cals, J.W.L., Oudhuis, G.J., Savelkoul, P.H.M. and de Bont, E.G.P.M. (2020) Workload, diagnostic work-up and treatment of urinary tract infections in adults during out-of-hours primary care: a retrospective cohort study. *BMC Family Practice* 21(1), 231. DOI: 10.1186/s12875-020-01305-8.

Spellberg, B. (2018) The maturing antibiotic mantra: "shorter is still better." *Journal of Hospital Medicine* 13(5), 361.. DOI: 10.12788/jhm.2904.

Spellberg, B. and Rice, L.B. (2019) Duration of antibiotic therapy: shorter is better. *Annals of Internal Medicine* 171(3), 210–211. DOI: 10.7326/M19-1509.

Spurling, G.K., Del Mar, C.B., Dooley, L., Foxlee, R. and Farley, R. (2017) Delayed antibiotic prescriptions for respiratory infections. *The Cochrane Database of Systematic Reviews* 9(9), CD004417. DOI: 10.1002/14651858.CD004417.pub5.

Stastny, T., Koenigshof, A.M., Brado, G.E., Chan, E.K. and Levy, N.A. (2022) Retrospective evaluation of the prognostic utility of quick sequential organ failure assessment scores in dogs with surgically treated sepsis (2011-2018): 204 cases. *Journal of Veterinary Emergency and Critical Care* 32(1), 68–74. DOI: 10.1111/vec.13101.

Unterer, S., Strohmeyer, K., Kruse, B.D., Sauter-Louis, C. and Hartmann, K. (2011) Treatment of aseptic dogs with hemorrhagic gastroenteritis with amoxicillin/clavulanic acid: a prospective blinded study. *Journal of Veterinary Internal Medicine* 25(5), 973–979. DOI: 10.1111/j.1939-1676.2011.00765.x.

Unterer, S., Lechner, E., Mueller, R.S., Wolf, G., Straubinger, R.K. *et al.* (2015) Prospective study of bacteraemia in acute haemorrhagic diarrhoea syndrome in dogs. *Veterinary Record* 176(12), 309. DOI: 10.1136/vr.102521.

Viitanen, S.J., Lappalainen, A.K., Christensen, M.B., Sankari, S. and Rajamäki, M.M. (2017) The utility of acute-phase proteins in the assessment of treatment response in dogs with bacterial pneumonia. *Journal of Veterinary Internal Medicine* 31(1), 124–133. DOI: 10.1111/jvim.14631.

Vincent, J.L., de Mendonça, A., Cantraine, F., Moreno, R., Takala, J, *et al.* (1998) Use of the SOFA score to assess the incidence of organ dysfunction/failure in intensive care units: results of a multicenter, prospective study. Working group on "sepsis-related problems" of the European Society of Intensive Care Medicine. *Critical Care Medicine* 26(11), 1793–1800. DOI: 10.1097/00003246-199811000-00016.

Volkmann, M., Steiner, J.M., Fosgate, G.T., Zentek, J., Hartmann, S. *et al.* (2017) Chronic diarrhea in dogs - retrospective study in 136 cases. *Journal of Veterinary Internal Medicine* 31(4), 1043–1055. DOI: 10.1111/jvim.14739.

Wan, S.Y., Hartmann, F.A., Jooss, M.K. and Viviano, K.R. (2014) Prevalence and clinical outcome of subclinical bacteriuria in female dogs. *Journal of the American Veterinary Medical Association* 245(1), 106–112. DOI: 10.2460/javma.245.1.106.

Weese, J.S., Blondeau, J., Boothe, D., Guardabassi, L.G., Gumley, N. *et al.* (2019) International Society for Companion Animal Infectious Diseases (ISCAID) guidelines for the diagnosis and management of bacterial urinary tract infections in dogs and cats. *Veterinary Journal* 247, 8–25. DOI: 10.1016/j.tvjl.2019.02.008.

Westropp, J.L., Sykes, J.E., Irom, S., Daniels, J.B., Smith, A. *et al.* (2012) Evaluation of the efficacy and safety of high dose short duration enrofloxacin treatment regimen for uncomplicated urinary tract infections in dogs. *Journal of Veterinary Internal Medicine* 26(3), 506–512. DOI: 10.1111/j.1939-1676.2012.00914.x.

White, J.D., Cave, N.J., Grinberg, A., Thomas, D.G. and Heuer, C. (2016) Subclinical bacteriuria in older cats and its association with survival. *Journal of Veterinary Internal Medicine* 30(6), 1824–1829. DOI: 10.1111/jvim.14598.

Windahl, U., Holst, B.S., Nyman, A., Grönlund, U. and Bengtsson, B. (2014) Characterisation of bacterial growth and antimicrobial susceptibility patterns in canine urinary tract infections. *BMC Veterinary Research* 10, 217. DOI: 10.1186/s12917-014-0217-4.

Zalmanovici Trestioreanu, A., Lador, A., Sauerbrun-Cutler, M.T. and Leibovici, L. (2015) Antibiotics for asymptomatic bacteriuria. *Cochrane Database of Systematic Reviews* 4(4), CD009534. DOI: 10.1002/14651858.CD009534.pub2.

Zasowski, E.J., Bassetti, M., Blasi, F., Goossens, H., Rello, J. *et al.* (2020) A systematic review of the effect of delayed appropriate antibiotic treatment on the outcomes of patients with severe bacterial infections. *Chest* 158(3), 929–938. DOI: 10.1016/j.chest.2020.03.087.

Index